Handbook of
Obstetric Anesthesia

T0204605

Handbook of Obstetric Anesthesia

Mark C. Norris, M.D.
Department of Anesthesiology
Washington University
St. Louis, Missouri

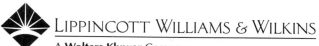

LIPPINCOTT WILLIAMS & WILKINS

A **Wolters Kluwer** Company

Philadelphia · Baltimore · New York · London
Buenos Aires · Hong Kong · Sydney · Tokyo

Acquisitions Editor: R. Craig Percy
Developmental Editor: Kristen Kirchner
Manufacturing Manager: Timothy Reynolds
Supervising Editor: Toni Ann Scaramuzzo
Production Editor: Colophon
Cover Designer: Jeane E. Norton
Compositor: Circle Graphics
Printer: R.R. Donnelley

© 2000 by LIPPINCOTT WILLIAMS & WILKINS.
227 East Washington Square
Philadelphia, PA 19106-3780 USA
LLW.com

Printed in the USA

Library of Congress Cataloging-in-Publication Data

Handbook of obstetric anesthesia / [edited by] Mark C. Norris.
    p. ; cm.
    Includes bibliographical references and index.
    ISBN 0-7817-1859-7 (alk. paper)
    1. Anesthesia in obstetrics—Handbooks, manuals, etc.
    I. Norris, Mark C.
    [DNLM: 1. Anesthesia, Obstetrical—
Handbooks. 2. Obstetric Surgical
Procedures—Handbooks. WO 231 H2365 2000]
    RG732.H335 2000
    617.9'682—dc21

                          99-044562

10 9 8 7 6 5 4 3 2 1

To Alice, Cynthia, Pam,
Rich, and Fazeela,
my steadfast friends

Contents

Part III: After Delivery

Preface

This handbook is more than just an abridged version of *Obstetric Anesthesia,* Second Edition. Here, I have provided focused information about anesthetic care for parturients. I have removed much of the background and historical information and emphasized current approaches to care. In addition, the management suggestions and anesthetic techniques are mine and often differ from the approaches suggested in *Obstetric Anesthesia.* I hope the reader will find the anesthetic techniques useful and will derive enough information from the remaining text to understand the reasoning behind them.

A word about references. Most of the information contained in this handbook has come from multiple sources, including other textbooks and journal articles. I have directly cited only a few of these many sources. The choice of citations was ultimately arbitrary. Most of what I included were either specific clinical trials that I thought were important to the topic at hand, or relatively recent articles that address clinically important new topics. I make no other claims about the relative merits of either included or nonincluded sources. Readers interested in specific sources should consult *Obstetric Anesthesia.*

In addition to the contributors to *Obstetric Anesthesia,* I would like to acknowledge the invaluable assistance of my secretary Ruthann Griffin and the contributions of my colleagues at Lippincott Williams & Wilkins. This book never would have happened without the dedication (and nagging) of Craig Percy. In addition, Kristen Kirchner provided essential assistance in reviewing, collating, and organizing the various parts of each chapter.

Acknowledgments

My thanks to the contributors to the second edition of *Obstetric Anesthesia*, without whom this handbook would not be possible. Your work looks as good the second time through as it did the first:

George Allen III, M.D.

Audrey S. Alleyne, M.D.

Valerie A. Arkoosh, M.D.

James A. Bartelsmeyer, M.D.

Richard B. Becker, M.D.

Yaakov Beilin, M.D.

Howard H. Bernstein, M.D.

David J. Birnbach, M.D.

Walter U. Brown, M.D.

Sherrie Buchmeier, R.D.M.S., R.T., L.P.N.

Linda Chan, M.D.

Steven L. Clark, M.D.

John G. D'Alessio, M.D.

M. Joanne Douglas, M.D.

John W. Downing, M.B.

Robert L. Eberle, M.D.

Fazeela Ferouz, M.D.

Steven T. Fogel, M.D.

Robert R. Gaiser, M.D.

Raphael Y. Gershon, M.D.

Beth Glosten, M.D.

Evan Goodman, M.D.

Holly C. Gunn, M.D.

Joy Hawkins, M.D.

Norman L. Herman, M.D., Ph.D.

Quinn Hogan, M.D.

William L. Holcomb, Jr., M.D.

H. Jane Huffnagle, D.O.

Suzanne Lynne Huffnagle, D.O.

BettyLou Koffel, M.D.

Jacob C. Langer, M.D.

Gabriela Rocha Lauretti, M.D., M.Sc., Ph.D.

Kathleen A. Leavitt, M.D.

Sung-Hee Rhim Lee, M.D.

Barbara L. Leighton, M.D.

Carol Ann Lennon, M.D.

Ji-Bin Liu, M.D.

Andrew M. Malinow, M.D.

Beth H. Minzter, M.D.

Holly A. Muir, M.D.

L Michael Newman, M.D., Ph.D.

C. E. P. Orlikowsky, M.D.

Craig M. Palmer, M.D.

Jaya Ramanathan, M.D.

Ramiah Ramasubramanian, M.D.

Edward T. Riley, M.D.

David Anthony Rocke, F.C.A.(SA.)

C. C. Rout, M.D.

Divina Juson Santos, M.D.

Jaye M. Shyken, M.D.

Baha M. Sibai, M.D.

Christopher M. Viscomi, M.D.

Richard N. Wissler, M.D., Ph.D.

Mark I. Zakowski, M.D.

Barbara Zucker-Pinchoff, M.D.

Handbook of
Obstetric Anesthesia

Physiologic Adaptation to Pregnancy: The Healthy Parturient

The pregnant woman experiences physiologic changes in every organ system. This transformation begins in the weeks after conception and continues postpartum. Understanding the progressive nature of these events helps the obstetric anesthesiologist confidently approach both the peripartum gravida and the pregnant surgical patient.

CARDIOVASCULAR SYSTEM

Physical Examination

1. S1
   a. Amplified by 12 weeks' gestation
   b. Exaggerated splitting
2. S2
   a. Less respiratory variation
   b. Exaggerated splitting
3. S3
   a. Audible in 84% by 20 weeks' gestation
   b. Volume peaks at 30 weeks.
   c. Usually disappears within 8 days of delivery
4. Murmurs
   a. Systolic ejection murmur in 96%
   b. Diastolic flow murmur in 18%
   c. Onset correlates most closely with rises in blood volume, not cardiac output.
5. Other findings
   a. Normal ECG
   b. Normal systolic function
   c. Pericardial effusion by echocardiography during third trimester in 9%
   d. All changes usually resolve within 4 weeks after delivery.

Hemodynamic Measurements

1. Increase
   a. Cardiac output (up to 50%)
   b. Heart rate (17% to 26%)
   c. Stroke volume (greater increase than heart rate)
   d. Changes begin during the first 8 weeks of gestation. These changes do not occur in pregnancies that are destined to fail.
2. Decrease
   a. Blood pressure (11%)
   b. Systemic vascular resistance
   c. Pulmonary vascular resistance
   d. Colloid oncotic pressure
3. Cardiac output
   a. Increases progressively throughout pregnancy

       i.   When measured in the supine position, cardiac output peaks between 24 and 32 weeks EGA and then falls to nonpregnant levels by term. Compression of the inferior vena cava (IVC) by the enlarging uterus decreases venous return and cardiac output (see below).

      ii.   When measured in the lateral position, cardiac output continues to increase throughout the third trimester.

4. Left ventricular function
   a. Shortening characteristics remain unchanged at term in spite of left ventricular enlargement.
   b. Contractility decreases postpartum, suggesting augmentation at term.
   c. Left ventricular mass increases due to increased wall thickness.
   d. Contractility is independent of the loading conditions.

Measurement Techniques

1. Pulsed-Doppler or suprasternal window continuous-wave ultrasound measurements correlate reasonably well with thermodilution cardiac output. However, during periods of hemorrhage, this consistency disappears.
   a. Accurate Doppler ultrasound cardiac output estimates require a constant aortic cross-sectional area.
   b. Variations in aortic area modify the estimated velocity of flow. Elevations in cardiac output detected by Doppler ultrasound could, then, be artifacts of an increasing aortic area.
   c. To mimic the changes in cardiac output reported during pregnancy, the aortic cross-sectional area would have to expand by 30% to 45%.
2. During the late third trimester, thoracic electrical bioimpedance correlates well with standard oxygen extraction (Fick) measurements of cardiac index only in the left and right lateral positions.

Pressures

1. Maternal systemic blood pressure
   a. Nadir is at 16 to 20 weeks' gestation.
   b. Then it increases toward term.
2. Diastolic pressure rises less than systolic pressure.
3. Central venous pressure (CVP) and pulmonary artery occlusion pressure (PAOP) remain stable.
4. Colloid oncotic pressure (COP) decreases 14%. Lower COP may predispose to pulmonary edema in the face of elevated PAOP.

Etiology

Cardiac Output

1. The heart must supply both the mother and fetus.
2. The metabolic needs of the pregnancy do not provide an adequate explanation for these cardiovascular changes.

3. Oxygen delivery usually exceeds fetal metabolic needs.
   a. First trimester
      i. Cardiac output increases 30% to 0%.
      ii. Oxygen consumption rises only 10%.
   b. Smaller a–v oxygen difference.

Blood Pressure
1. Systemic vascular resistance decreases before stroke volume and cardiac output increase.
   a. The fall in peripheral vascular resistance may incite the increase in plasma volume, which then increases cardiac output.
   b. Decreased resistance persists throughout the pregnancy.
2. The hormonal changes of early pregnancy may be the true triggers.
   a. Estrogen production rises rapidly after conception.
      i. In sheep, a 4-hour infusion of conjugated estrogens elevates cardiac output (+32%) and heart rate (+50%), and lowers MAP (–10%) and systemic vascular resistance (–19%).
      ii. Estrogen enhances myocardial contractility.
   b. Digitalis-like factor (DLIF) concentration increases during pregnancy.
   c. Relaxin, known to rise early in pregnancy, increases heart rate, left ventricular systolic pressure, and contractility in rats.

Effects of Positioning
1. During the third trimester, maternal cardiac output, stroke volume, and systolic and diastolic blood pressure decrease in
   a. Supine position
   b. Lithotomy position
   c. Right lateral decubitus position
2. Peripheral vascular resistance increases in these positions.
3. Incompletely answered questions about this phenomenon, called the supine hypotensive syndrome or aortocaval compression
   a. Why do some patients exhibit the syndrome more often or more severely than do others?
   b. What are the effects of labor on the syndrome?
   c. How can one prevent its occurrence?

Incidence and Etiology
1. Right atrial pressure declines in the supine position, limiting stroke volume and cardiac output.
   a. Most parturients, decreased cardiac output offset by
      i. Tachycardia.
      ii. Increased systemic vascular resistance.
      iii. Systolic blood pressure remains unchanged.
   b. Some patients become hypotensive with
      i. Bradycardia.
      ii. Decreased systemic vascular resistance.
   c. Fifteen percent to 20% of third-trimester patients exhibit hypotension or tachycardia when lying supine.

      d. Regional or general anesthesia compromises the gravida's ability to compensate for a fall in venous return.

      e. Labor, uteroplacental insufficiency, and fetal size also may affect the incidence and severity of supine hypotension.

2. Possible etiologies
    a. Compression of the inferior vena cava (IVC)
       i. The term uterus completely obstructs the IVC at its bifurcation when the parturient lies supine.
       ii. Blood returns to the heart through the azygous and vertebral veins.
       iii. Supine hypotension can occur without IVC obstruction.
       iv. IVC obstruction decreases right atrial pressure but does not invariably lower blood pressure and cardiac output.

    b. Simultaneous or isolated compression of the aorta
       i. Femoral artery hypotension occurs earlier and more often than brachial artery hypotension.
       ii. Usually, femoral artery systolic pressure decreases more than diastolic pressure.
       iii. Angiograms show the uterus displacing the subrenal aorta laterally, cranially, and dorsally.

Labor and Aortocaval Compression

1. Uterine contractions may be necessary to elicit the signs of aortic compression.
    a. The relaxed uterus produces less aortic compression than does the contracted uterus.
    b. During a contraction, compression, mostly limited to L4–L5, can completely occlude the aorta.
    c. Contractions occasionally eliminate foot pulse oximeter tracings.
    d. In actively laboring women
       i. Dorsalis pedis artery ultrasound flow velocities decrease by 80% in both the supine and the lateral positions during contractions.
       ii. Painful uterine contractions may cause aortic compression through vasoconstriction by endogenous catecholamines.
       iii. Dorsalis pedis artery flow velocity is often unchanged by contractions with epidural analgesia.
    e. Others report that uterine contractions relieve aortic compression.

2. Uterine contractions may relieve IVC obstruction.
    a. In the supine position, uterine contractions augment cardiac output (25%) and stroke volume (33%) while lowering heart rate (15%).
    b. In the lateral position, these values change very little with each contraction.

Prevention

1. The standard pelvic tilt position does not consistently relieve IVC compression.

2. Lateral position
    a. May not completely relieve IVC compression
    b. Does prevent aortic compression

Summary
1. The supine position may harm some gravidae.
   a. Up to 20% will experience hypotension or decreased uterine blood flow when supine.
   b. IVC compression impairs
      i. Venous return.
      ii. Cardiac output.
      iii. Uterine blood flow.
      iv. Fetal oxygen delivery.
   c. Uterine contractions may
      i. Alleviate IVC compression.
      ii. Exacerbate aortic compression.
   d. A 10-degree lateral tilt will ameliorate aortocaval compression in most gravidae.
   e. Depending in part on the position of the fetal body within the uterus, a given gravida may respond better in the left or right lateral position.

Anesthetic Implications
1. Normal cardiac output and uterine artery perfusion depend on adequate venous return.
   a. Neuraxial local anesthetics
      i. Loss of sympathetic tone
         (1) Peripheral vasodilation
         (2) Venous pooling
      ii. Vasodilation increases the likelihood of supine hypotension.
   b. Acute intravenous hydration before induction
      i. May increase blood volume.
      ii. May help maintain maternal cardiac output.
2. Aortocaval compression may complicate maternal and fetal resuscitation.
   a. Partial IVC occlusion hinders resuscitation of dogs given 20 mg per kilogram of intravenous bupivacaine.
   b. Adequate maternal resuscitation may require delivery of the fetus to completely eliminate the deleterious effects of aortocaval compression.

Receptors and Reflexes
1. Pregnancy blunts
   a. Vasoconstriction and vasodilation in response to α- and β-adrenergic stimulation.
   b. Catecholamine secretion in response to physiologic stress.
   c. Chronotropic response to isoproterenol.
      i. Blunted more than expected from increased plasma volume.
      ii. The chronotropic response to 15 μg of intravenous epinephrine also decreases.
      iii. A circulating pregnancy-related inhibitory factor may be responsible.
2. Anesthetic implications
   a. Decreased responsiveness to α- and β-adrenergic agonists limits the precision of a chronotropic intravenous test dose.

b. Beta-adrenergic agents are preferable for the treatment of maternal hypotension because α-adrenergic agents constrict the uterine arteries and impair uteroplacental blood flow.

Uterine Artery

1. Blood flow increases
   a. Three and a half percent of cardiac output in early pregnancy.
   b. Twelve percent at term.
   c. Fifty milliliters per minute at 10 weeks' gestation.
   d. Two hundred milliliters per minute at 28 weeks.
   e. Five hundred milliliters per minute at term.
2. The resistance of the uterine artery to blood flow steadily declines.
   a. Causes
      i. Arteriovenous anastomoses in the uterus
      ii. Uterine artery vasodilation secondary to estrogens and angiotensin II
3. The uterine artery dilates normally in response to sodium nitroprusside and hydralazine and constricts normally with norepinephrine.

Effects of Labor

1. Each contraction
   a. Squeezes about 300 mL of blood from the uterus into the central circulation.
   b. Relieves IVC compression.
   c. Increases (first stage of labor)
      i. Cardiac output (22%).
         (1) Apex 18 seconds before the uterus attains maximum amniotic fluid pressure
      ii. Stroke volume (27%).
      iii. Systolic and diastolic blood pressure (10 to 20 mm Hg).
   d. Causes
      i. Autotransfused blood.
      ii. Augmented venous return.
      iii. Pain-induced catecholamine release.
2. Both the process of labor and individual contractions affect cardiac output.
   a. Caudal analgesia
      i. Prevents the progressive rise in cardiac output during labor.
      ii. But, has no effect on the increases that coincide with each contraction.
   b. Basal cardiac output increases progressively throughout labor, reaching 13% above baseline by 8-cm cervical dilation.
   c. Second stage
      i. Expulsive efforts impair cardiac output and stroke volume due to decreased venous return.
3. Gravidae with limited cardiac reserve frequently benefit from early labor analgesia and limited expulsive efforts.

Effects of Delivery
1. Cardiac output, stroke volume, and heart rate
   a. Increase immediately after delivery.
   b. Decline to their prelabor values within 24 hours.
   c. Causes of cardiac output increase
      i. Central shift of blood from the now-empty uterus
      ii. Marked decrease in IVC compression
   d. Cardiac output returns to prelabor values within the first hour.
2. Abdominal delivery
   a. Cardiac output, stroke volume, and heart rate change less than with vaginal delivery.
   b. Greater blood loss explains these differences.
   c. Type of anesthesia does not influence these changes.
3. Postpartum hemodynamics rapidly return to prelabor, term values.
4. Transition to nonpregnant values takes longer.
   a. Cardiac output
      i. Increased for the first 24 hours postpartum
      ii. Progressively falls, decreasing 25% from term values by the tenth postnatal day
   b. Heart rate (20%), stroke volume (18%), cardiac output (28%), and contractility decrease by 2 weeks after delivery.
   c. Maternal systolic and diastolic pressure
      i. May decrease for the first 2 postpartum days.
      ii. Significantly increase by the fourth to sixth postpartum day.
   d. Central venous pressures rise in the first 24 hours if oxytocic drugs are given.
   e. If blood loss is excessive (greater than 500 mL):
      i. Heart rate increases.
      ii. Stroke volume falls for 48 hours.
5. Type of anesthesia does not alter the effects of delivery on maternal hemodynamics.

Plasma Volume
1. Increases during the first 24 weeks of gestation to 1,500 mL (50% larger than before conception).
   a. Some increment takes place by the end of the first trimester.
   b. Most occurs during the second trimester.
   c. There is only a slight increase in the third trimester.
   d. Plasma volume plateaus between 24 and 40 weeks' gestation at 70 mL per kilogram.
2. The expanded plasma volume
   a. Enhances circulation to the uterus.
   b. Meets excretory needs of the kidneys.
   c. Helps radiate body heat produced by the elevated metabolic rate.
   d. Protects the fetus from the impaired venous return and decreased cardiac output of aortocaval compression.
   e. Safeguards against blood loss at delivery.
3. Possible etiologies
   a. The fall in systemic vascular resistance and blood pressure produce a reflex rise in blood volume.

   b. Estrogens also stimulate the renin-angiotensin system, resulting in sodium and water retention.
4. Red Cells
   a. Red cell mass increases by 18%.
   b. Red blood cell volume rises more slowly and to a lesser extent than does plasma volume.
      i. Mean red cell volume remains constant at 27 mL per kilogram.
      ii. Plasma volume changes from 50 to 70 mL per kilogram.
      iii. This discrepancy causes decrease in hematocrit with pregnancy.
      iv. A normal or elevated hematocrit during pregnancy may signify intravascular volume depletion.
   c. Erythropoietin
      i. Is synthesized by the kidneys.
      ii. Stimulates red cell production.
      iii. Urinary excretion peaks between 20 and 28 weeks' gestation.
      iv. Action is augmented by human placental lactogen.
   d. Chorionic somatotropin, prolactin, and progesterone also stimulate erythropoiesis.
5. White cells
   a. Increase during pregnancy
      i. Mostly neutrophils are responsible for this elevation.
      ii. Monocytes may contribute.
      iii. Lymphocytes, eosinophils, and basophils generally decline.
6. Delivery
   a. Normal blood loss
      i. Five hundred milliliters at vaginal delivery
      ii. One thousand milliliters at abdominal delivery
   b. Response
      i. Blood volume rapidly decreases (to nonpregnant normal).
      ii. Hematocrit changes very little.
      iii. Total red blood cell volume falls rapidly.
      iv. Red cell volume per kilogram of body weight remains stable.
   c. Plasma volume
      i. Declines over 3 to 5 days.
      ii. Reaches preconception levels by 8 weeks' postpartum.
   d. Blood loss at delivery rarely necessitates transfusion, as the rapid decrement in plasma volume helps maintain hematocrit.
   e. Postpartum, a drop in hematocrit suggests continuing blood loss.

RESPIRATORY SYSTEM
Physical Examination
1. Increased intraabdominal contents at term
   a. Elevate the diaphragm.
   b. Widen the transverse diameter of the chest by 2 cm.
2. Gestation does not impair diaphragmatic motion.

3. Roentgenograms reveal
    a. Increased lung markings.
    b. A widened subcostal angle.
4. Upper airway
    a. Hyperemia of the nasal turbinates
    b. Facial edema
    c. Severe laryngeal edema may occur without stridor.

Lung Volumes

1. Etiology
    a. Physical changes
        i.   Elevation of the diaphragm
        ii. Increase in the chest diameter
    b. Hormonal and metabolic factors also play a major role.
2. Tidal volume increases, beginning in the first trimester, to 28% above nonpregnant values at term.
3. Functional residual capacity (FRC) is progressively compressed.
4. Residual volume and expiratory reserve volume (ERV) also fall.
5. Total lung capacity and vital capacity change little.
6. Inspiratory capacity rises 10% at term.
7. Expiratory capacity decreases 20%.
8. Inconsistent changes in closing volume
9. Airway closure occurs during normal tidal breathing if closing volume exceeds ERV.
    a. Can adversely affect gas exchange
    b. May explain the mild supine hypoxemia often seen in term parturients
    c. Late in gestation, airway closure occurs above or closer to FRC than it does in the nonpregnant state.
        i.   Airway closure may be due to decreased FRC, not increased closing volume.
        ii. Most often, position does not alter closing volume, but FRC falls further in the supine position.
        iii. Hypoxemia often follows.
             (1) Nocturnal hypoxemia (SpO_2 less than 95) occurs more often during pregnancy.
             (2) Mean SpO_2 decreases compared with nonpregnant values (95.2% versus 98.5%).
10. Dead space
    a. No change in anatomic dead space
    b. Decreased physiologic dead space (VD/VT).
        i.   Pregnancy must considerably reduce alveolar dead space.
        ii. A smaller alveolar dead space improves the efficiency of ventilation and lowers the gradient between alveolar and end-tidal carbon dioxide.
11. Intrapulmonary increases
    a. Two percent to 5% in nonpregnant subjects
    b. Thirteen percent to 15% in term gravidae
    c. May explain some of the dyspnea on exertion reported during pregnancy

Flow

1. No change
    a. FEV_1

      b. Flow–volume loops
      c. Lung compliance
2. Total pulmonary resistance (made up of airways resistance and tissue resistance) falls significantly.
      a. Decreased airway resistance predominates.
3. Specific airway conductance rises during pregnancy, suggesting increased cross-sectional area of the airway.
      a. For a given alveolar pressure, there is a significantly higher flow of air during pregnancy due to smooth muscle relaxation.
      b. Normally, bronchial muscle constricts in response to hypocapnia.
      c. Bronchodilation in the face of hyperventilation requires a bronchodilating mechanism.
      d. Progesterone
         i. Increases β-adrenergic activity.
         ii. Promotes smooth muscle relaxation.

Minute Ventilation

1. Rises 19% to 50% by term
      a. Increase begins very soon after conception.
      b. Respiratory rate increases 9%.
      c. Tidal volume increases 28%.
2. Increase in minute ventilation is more than required changes in oxygen consumption and carbon dioxide production.
3. Exercise
      a. Further increases minute ventilation and oxygen consumption.
      b. A decrease in pulmonary reserve becomes apparent.
4. The alveolar hyperventilation of pregnancy reflects hypersensitivity of the respiratory centers.
      a. Progesterone stimulates respiration without changing the basal metabolic rate.
      b. Carbon dioxide sensitivity curves shift to the left during pregnancy.
         i. A parturient can hold her breath until she attains a p_aCO_2 of 39.2 mm Hg.
         ii. Nonpregnant subjects can reach 48.2 mm Hg.
         iii. Progesterone administration to males and postmenopausal women duplicates these changes.
         iv. Sensitivity to carbon dioxide is the same in the first and third trimesters but falls dramatically after delivery.
5. Nitrogen washout also reflects alveolar hyperventilation.
      a. The time needed to reach an end-tidal nitrogen of 2% when breathing 100% oxygen:
         i. Before conception: 130 seconds
         ii. At 13 to 26 weeks' EGA: 108 seconds
         iii. At 26 to 42 weeks: 80 seconds[1]
      b. Clinically, rapid nitrogen washout allows adequate maternal denitrogenation with four vital capacity breaths of 100% oxygen.
      c. Four vital capacity breaths and 3 minutes of breathing 100% oxygen yield similar p_aO_2 values.

Oxygen Consumption

1. At term, the parturient consumes 20% to 30% more oxygen than at 12 to 14 weeks postpartum.
2. Most of this oxygen supplies the fetus.
3. Demands by the placenta, uterus, and breasts account for most of the remainder.

Pulmonary Gas Exchange

1. Diffusion capacity
   a. Does not change or increases early in gestation.
   b. Later decreases return diffusion capacity at term to nonpregnant values.
2. The alveolar–arterial gradient (p_AO_2–p_aO_2)
   a. Does not differ between the first trimester and term.
   b. Increases in the supine position compared with the sitting position (twenty millimeters of mercury vs. fourteen point three millimeters of mercury, respectively).
   c. Most likely represents the relationship between a diminished FRC and a slightly elevated closing volume.
   d. At term, under general anesthesia for abdominal delivery, mean p_aO_2–p_aO_2 gradient is 138 mm Hg at an inspired oxygen concentration of 67.5%.
3. The hyperventilation of pregnancy lowers end-tidal carbon dioxide.
4. Gestation also affects the arterial to end-tidal carbon dioxide difference.
   a. In anesthetized, nonpregnant women, arterial carbon dioxide (p_aCO_2) is 3.5 to 5.3 mm Hg higher than the end-tidal carbon dioxide.
   b. After conception, this gradient narrows.[2]
      i. In early gestation p_aCO_2 is only 0.5 mm Hg higher than end-tidal carbon dioxide.
      ii. By the end of the first trimester, the end-tidal carbon dioxide approximates p_aCO_2.
      iii. At term, under general anesthesia, the gradient can reverse, and 50% of parturients have a higher end-tidal carbon dioxide than arterial carbon dioxide.
      iv. The capnogram shows a steep phase III slope.
      v. This trend reverses with delivery.
         (1) Mean p_aCO_2 is 0.03 to 0.78 mm Hg above end-tidal carbon dioxide by 25 minutes postpartum.
         (2) Still, up to 31% of postpartum patients have higher end-tidal than arterial carbon dioxide.
         (3) During general anesthesia for postpartum tubal ligation, the mean p_aCO_2–$P_{ET}CO_2$ gradient remains low at 0.6 mm Hg.
         (4) Regression analysis suggests that the relationship between arterial and end-tidal carbon dioxide returns to normal by 8 days after delivery.
   c. Etiology
      i. Increased
         (1) Minute ventilation
         (2) Cardiac output
         (3) Blood volume

ii. Decreased alveolar dead space

d. End-tidal carbon dioxide values can accurately predict the degree of maternal hyperventilation and prevent uterine vasoconstriction-induced hypocarbia.

Maternal–Fetal Gas Exchange

1. The placenta consumes oxygen and produces carbon dioxide.
2. Placental metabolism contributes to a considerable maternal–fetal carbon dioxide gradient.
    a. Fetal pCO_2 averages 11.3 mm Hg higher than maternal p_aCO_2.
    b. Fetal pCO_2, but not pO_2, correlates with maternal p_aCO_2.
    c. The carbon dioxide gradient does not correlate with maternal p_aO_2.
3. Maternal–fetal oxygen gradient varies with maternal p_aO_2.
    a. Umbilical vein pO_2 rises moderately in response to maternal hyperoxia.
    b. Fetal oxygen uptake and uterine blood flow do not correlate with maternal p_aO_2.
    c. These relationships allow administration of high oxygen concentrations to the mother without exposing the fetus to the hazards of hyperoxia.
4. The oxygen hemoglobin dissociation curves
    a. Overlap the normal range.
    b. Most lie to the right of their nonpregnant position.
    c. p50 increases significantly during gestation.
        i. Nonpregnant: 26.7 mm Hg
        ii. First trimester: 27.8 mm Hg
        iii. Second trimester: 28.8 mm Hg
        iv. Third trimester: 30.4 mm Hg
    d. The elevated p50 aids oxygen delivery to the uteroplacental unit.
    e. The respiratory alkalosis of pregnancy pushes the oxygen hemoglobin dissociation curve to the left and increases 2,3-diphosphoglycerate (DPG) production.
        i. Maternal 2,3-DPG levels rise by 30% above nonpregnant values.
        ii. The higher concentration of 2,3-DPG pushes the dissociation curve back to the right.
    f. Preeclampsia shifts the oxygen hemoglobin dissociation curve to the left with a p50 of 25.1 mm Hg.

Blood Gas Analysis

1. p_aCO_2 decreases to 26 to 32 mm Hg.
    a. The supine position does not change p_aCO_2.
2. p_aO_2 rises slightly to 92 to 106 mm Hg (mean oxygen saturation, 97.2%).
    a. The supine position impairs oxygen exchange
        i. Average p_aO_2 falls from 101.2 to 94.6 mm Hg.
        ii. Capillary pO_2 also is higher (13 mm Hg) in the sitting versus the supine position.
        iii. Increased volume of abdominal contents and elevated closing volume may cause this mild supine hypoxemia.

       iv. Aortocaval compression also could contribute:
         (1) Hindering venous return.
         (2) Widening the arteriovenous oxygen difference.

3. The metabolic compensation to this respiratory alkalosis induces:
   a. A fall in plasma bicarbonate concentration (16 to 21 mEq/L).
   b. A near-normal or slightly elevated pH (7.405 to 7.42).
   c. This adjustment begins early in pregnancy.
   d. Persistently low intracellular pH values provide a continual stimulus to hyperventilation.

4. Etiology
   a. Acid-base changes begin immediately after conception.
   b. They resemble acclimatization to high altitude.
   c. A hormonal basis seems likely.
      i. Both progesterone and estrogens may be involved.
      ii. Other important mediators may include prostaglandins, cyclic guanine monophosphate, and cyclic adenosine phosphate.
   d. Progesterone augments the respiratory response to hypercarbia. It may:
      i. Modify the permeability of chemoreceptor cells.
      ii. Directly stimulate the central respiratory or hypothalamic neurons in contact with the blood.

Effects of Labor

1. Forced vital capacity, FEV_1, and maximum voluntary ventilation do not change.
2. Pain induces maternal hyperventilation.
   a. During the first stage of labor, uterine contractions increase oxygen consumption (63%) and minute ventilation (74%).
   b. Hyperventilation during early labor is out of proportion to metabolic demand.
   c. p_aCO_2 falls 6 to 7 mm Hg.
   d. Second stage
      i. Mean p_aCO_2 is 22.3 mm Hg between contractions.
      ii. Mean p_aCo_2 is 16.2 mm Hg during contractions.
      iii. pH and p_aO_2 increase.
   e. Maternal hyperventilation can modify fetal acid-base status.
      i. The most alkalotic mothers (p_aCO_2 less than 17 mm Hg) deliver acidotic infants.
      ii. Uterine blood flow decreases if p_aCO_2 reaches a critical level.
   f. Adequate analgesia eliminates these changes.
      i. Contractions do not significantly modify respiratory measurements in women receiving lumbar epidural analgesia.
      ii. Therefore, epidural block effectively decreases the work of breathing during labor.
      iii. Even during expulsive efforts of the second stage, analgesia minimizes oxygen consumption and minute ventilation.

3. Hypoxemia also may arise during labor.
    a. Oxygen saturation falls below 90% in 49% of laboring women.
    b. Risk is increased with systemic narcotics and inhalation analgesia.

Effects of Delivery
1. Early
    a. Alveolar hyperventilation and sensitivity of respiratory centers to carbon dioxide suddenly decrease.
    b. Vital capacity, total lung capacity, and maximum breathing capacity fall markedly.
2. FRC and residual volume return to normal within 48 hours.
3. Tidal volume begins to decline within 5 days.
4. Within 2 weeks
    a. CO_2 production and O_2 consumption approach normal.
    b. Minute ventilation and oxygen uptake remain elevated for up to 2 weeks.

Anesthetic Implications
1. Decreased FRC and increased oxygen consumption
    a. Limit oxygen reserve.
    b. p_aO_2 falls rapidly with apnea.
        i.   Critical hypoxemia can occur with alarming speed.
        ii. Rapid intubation or oxygenation (by mask with cricoid pressure) by experienced personnel prevents disaster.
2. Mechanical hyperventilation may lower fetal p_aO_2.
    a. Uterine artery constriction may produce fetal asphyxia with severe hypoxia and metabolic acidosis
    b. May limit maternal cardiac output and, therefore, placental blood flow.
    c. Maintain maternal arterial and end-tidal CO_2 near 30 mm Hg.
3. Although maternal hypercapnia may increase oxygen supply to the fetus, it is not clinically indicated.
4. Due to the differences between fetal and maternal hemoglobin, increasing maternal F_IO_2 from 50% to 100% raises maternal p_aO_2 but has little effect on fetal pO_2.
5. High F_IO_2 can maximize maternal oxygenation without compromising the fetus.
6. Sitting minimizes the negative respiratory effects of pregnancy.
    a. Gravidae with significant respiratory disease can best be evaluated and cared for when upright.

RENAL SYSTEM
Physical Changes
1. Ureteral dilatation
    a. The gravid uterus
    b. Progesterone
    c. Occurs above the pelvic brim
    d. Manifests early in pregnancy
    e. May persist up to 12 weeks postpartum

2. Postpartum intravenous pyelograms reveal a mean kidney length 1.5 cm greater than that measured in nonpregnant women.

Glomerular Filtration
1. First two trimesters
   a. Glomerular filtration rate (GFR) increases 50%.
      i. Blood urea nitrogen (BUN): 6 to 8 mg per 100 mL
      ii. Creatinine: 0.4 to 0.6 mg per 100 mL
   b. Effective renal plasma flow (ERPF) increases.
2. Third trimester
   a. ERPF decreases.
   b. GFR is unchanged.
   c. Creatinine production must increase.
      i. Serum creatinine concentration rises.
      ii. Clearance does not change.
3. Serial measurements of creatinine clearance reveal the early and progressive nature of the changes in GFR.
   a. Creatinine clearance approximates GFR and increases 25% by the fourth week of gestation.
   b. By the ninth week, clearance rises 45%.
   c. Despite these increases, the kidney retains the capacity to vasodilate and increase GFR in response to an acute protein load.
   d. Thus, GFR can increase by more than one mechanism.
4. Etiology
   a. Elevated blood volume contributes to augmented glomerular filtration but fails to explain early changes.
   b. A hormonal mechanism seems likely
      i. Changes in creatinine clearance also occur during the normal menstrual cycle.
      ii. Women destined to have spontaneous abortions do not show sustained changes in creatinine clearance.

Tubular Function
1. Glucose
   a. The ability to reabsorb glucose universally declines.
   b. With minor degrees of glycosuria, tubular function returns to normal after delivery.
   c. Parturients who exhibit more glycosuria have post-partum evidence of tubular damage.
   d. The mechanism of glucosuria is unclear.
      i. Persistent tubular damage suggests involvement of more than just a larger filtered glucose load.
      ii. Glycosuria normally resolves within 1 week of delivery, faster than carbohydrate metabolism normalizes, suggesting an alteration of tubular function.
2. Sodium
   a. Retention is essential to increased plasma volume.
   b. Five hundred to 850 mEq of sodium are retained during pregnancy.
   c. Increased renin and aldosterone contribute to sodium retention.

    i. The uteroplacental unit contributes to elevated prorenin production.
  d. Aldosterone secretion compensates for natriuretic effects of pregnancy.
    i. Sodium loss promoted by:
     (1) Increased GFR.
     (2) Progesterone's competitive inhibition of aldosterone's action at distal tubular sites.
3. Potassium
  a. Three hundred milliequivalents are retained.
  b. Progesterone inhibits excretion by antagonizing aldosterone.
  c. Plasma potassium concentration decreases by 10%.
4. Bicarbonate
  a. Reclamation remains normal.
  b. Renal acidifying mechanisms are unchanged.
5. Plasma osmolality
  a. Decreases 8 to 10 mOsmol/kg by the tenth week of gestation.
  b. The osmotic threshold for thirst declines.
  c. The threshold for arginine vasopressin (AVP) secretion declines.
  d. The parturient drinks more to maintain the lower osmolality.
  e. Renin activity remains elevated for 2 to 7 days after delivery.

Implications
1. Pregnancy modifies the interpretation of diagnostic studies that detect dilated ureters or increased kidney size.
2. Ureteral dilatation contributes to frequent urinary tract infection.
  a. The risk of preterm labor increases with infection.
3. A gravida with significant renal disease may maintain a normal BUN and creatinine.
  a. Slight elevation of these values suggests a need for diagnostic evaluation.
4. Glycosuria may be normal during pregnancy.
5. Pregnancy modifies renal handling of drugs and may have significant effects on pharmacokinetics.

GASTROINTESTINAL SYSTEM
1. Progesterone decreases gastric motility during pregnancy.
2. Progesterone-treated male rats have impaired esophageal, antral, and colonic contractile activity.
3. Progesterone and estradiol treatment inhibit the gastrointestinal contractile response elicited by acetylcholine and gastrin.

Esophagus
1. Lower esophageal sphincter (LES) tone
  a. Unchanged at 16 weeks
  b. Response to agents that normally increase tone is attenuated.

   c. Becomes progressively weaker during pregnancy.
   d. Reaches a nadir at 36 weeks.
2. Intragastric pressure rises during gestation.
3. Lower intraesophageal pressure falls.
4. Pressure difference between the stomach and esophagus
   a. Nonpregnant: 7 mm Hg
   b. Pregnant: 3.4 mm Hg
5. Peristaltic speed and amplitude decline.
6. Elevated abdominal pressure and altered stomach position
   a. Higher incidence of hiatal hernia
   b. Up to 70% complain of heartburn and associated esophagitis.
   c. Esophagitis correlates with the lowest gradients across the LES and pyloric sphincter relaxation.

Stomach

Gastric Emptying

1. Conflicting data
   a. Barium meals and induced vomiting
      i.   No delay in gastric emptying during labor without sedation
   b. Double-sampling technique
      i.   Longer mean emptying time in term pregnant women than in nonpregnant subjects
      ii. However, gastric volume 30 minutes after a meal is not significantly different between the two groups.
      iii. Labor (without analgesics or sedatives)
         (1) Further slows emptying of the final 100 to 200 mL of test solution.
         (2) Gastric volume at 30 minutes is greater than in nonpregnant women.
2. Paracetamol (acetaminophen) absorption also measures gastric emptying.
   a. Absorbed only in the small bowel
   b. Blood concentration of correlates with gastric emptying
   c. Delayed gastric emptying is first seen between 8 and 14 weeks.
   d. No delay noted
      i.   Third trimester
      ii. First 24 to 48 hours postpartum
   e. Systemic opioids significantly slow paracetamol absorption in laboring patients.
   f. Metoclopramide accelerates gastric emptying in pregnant patients given systemic narcotics.
   g. Ranitidine may decrease gastric volume, whether or not opioids have been given.
3. Noninvasive gastric impedance can measure gastric emptying.
   a. Pregnancy alone, even in the third trimester, does not slow gastric emptying.
   b. Postpartum patients who had received opiate analgesia had significantly prolonged 70%, 50%, and 30% emptying times.
   c. However, the impedance technique does not always permit measurement of the final 20% to 30% of gastric fluid.

      d. That volume approximates the final 100 to 200 mL portion of the 750-mL test volume used in the double-sampling technique.

      e. Therefore, rapid initial emptying followed by delayed complete emptying is possible.

      f. Opiates significantly prolong both emptying phases in pregnant patients.

4. Motilin
   a. Stimulates gastrointestinal smooth muscle contraction.
   b. Pregnancy markedly decreases both fasting and glucose-induced motilin secretion.
   c. Motilin may partially mediate the smooth muscle relaxation attributed to progesterone.

Gastric Secretions

1. Gastrin
   a. Partially controls gastric acid secretion.
   b. Increases LES tone.
   c. Inhibits the pyloric sphincter.
2. Gastrin and pregnancy
   a. The fetus, the placenta, or both, produce gastrin.
   b. There is no change in serum concentration during the first trimester.
   c. Production rises progressively throughout the second and third trimesters, as well as during labor.
   d. The volume of acid secreted by the stomach, pancreas, and small intestine increases.

Postpartum

1. Opioids during labor delay gastric emptying after delivery.
2. Normal emptying times are reached by 4 to 5 days postpartum.
3. Postpartum studies of volume and pH suggest that 33% to 73% of patients undergoing postpartum tubal sterilization still meet at-risk criteria for aspiration pneumonitis.

Gallbladder

1. Progesterone inhibits cholecystokinin release from the intestinal mucosa.
2. The contractile response to cholecystokinin diminishes during pregnancy.
   a. The gallbladder incompletely empties, particularly in the second and third trimesters.
   b. May contribute to cholesterol gallstones during pregnancy.

Liver

1. Signs of pregnancy can mimic liver disease.
   a. Spider angiomata
   b. Palmar erythema
   c. Eighty percent of normal parturients have prolonged retention of Bromsulphalein.
   d. Plasma protein concentration decreases.
      i. Albumin concentration falls 20% to 30%.

   ii. Albumin concentration remains low for 6 to 7 weeks postpartum.

  e. Some proteins increase during pregnancy.

2. Smooth endoplasmic reticulum proliferates, indicating a rise in hepatic microsomal activity.
3. Steroid hormones competitively inhibit oxidative enzymes but do not impair conjugation.
4. Certain liver enzymes show higher activities, particularly after the fifth month of gestation.
   a. Glucose-6-phosphate dehydrogenase
   b. Aminolevulinic acid synthetase
   c. Gammaglutamyl transpeptidase
   d. Transferase (AST and ALT)
   e. Lactic dehydrogenase
   f. Placental production raises the serum concentration of alkaline phosphatase by 200% to 400%.
5. Liver ribonucleic acid content markedly increases.

Implications

1. Pay careful attention to acid aspiration prophylaxis.
   a. Risk of regurgitation is increased.
      i. Increased gastric volume
         (1) Delayed emptying
         (2) Larger volume of secretions
      ii. Decreased LES tone
      iii. Elevated intragastric pressure
   b. Alternatives
      i. Avoidance of general anesthesia
      ii. Early regional anesthesia
      iii. When general anesthesia is required, consider:
         (1) Nonparticulate antacids.
         (2) H2-receptor antagonists.
         (3) Metoclopramide.
         (4) Rapid sequence induction with cricoid pressure.
2. Liver disease
   a. Pregnancy complicates the diagnosis of hepatic disease.
   b. While mild-to-moderate elevation of liver enzymes may be normal in pregnancy, they should not be overlooked.
   c. Protein drug binding may increase or decrease, depending on the specific drugs involved.

COAGULATION

1. Pregnancy activates the clotting system.
2. All factors except XI and XIII increase.
   a. The most significant elevations:
      i. Factors VII, VIII, X
      ii. Fibrinogen
3. Platelets
   a. Mean volume rises.
   b. Platelet count remains unchanged or falls.
   c. Platelet intracellular free calcium increases in the third trimester.

4. Fibrinolysis
    a. Plasma fibrinolytic activity decreases.
    b. Plasminogen concentration increases as early as 4 months' gestation.
    c. A compensated, accelerated state of fibrinolysis may occur during late pregnancy.
        i. May originate at the placental–uterine interface
            (1) Localized fibrin formation from platelet activation and coagulation
            (2) Active fibrinolysis follows.
        ii. Measuring indices of fibrinolysis in the peripheral blood may not detect uterine fibrinolysis.
5. Delivery
    a. Placental separation activates the clotting mechanism.
    b. Factor VIII activity transiently increases in uterine vein blood after delivery, shortening measured coagulation times.
    c. Fibrinolysis
        i. Twenty-one percent exhibit significant increases in fibrin degradation products during labor.
        ii. Thirty-two percent show the same immediately postpartum.
        iii. Fibrin degradation remains elevated in 10% of women 24 to 72 hours after delivery.
    d. Platelet count returns to normal 24 to 72 hours postpartum.

ENDOCRINE
Glucose/Insulin
1. Pregnancy lowers fasting glucose concentration.
2. Insulin
    a. Secretion rises throughout gestation.
    b. Tissue sensitivity to insulin diminishes.
    c. Degradation remains unchanged.
    d. Insulin resistance
        i. Caused by pregnancy-specific hormonal factors
        ii. Human placental lactogen (HPL) has antiinsulin activity.
        iii. Progesterone alone does not cause the changes in glucose and insulin metabolism.
    e. Insulin secretion declines precipitously after delivery, suggesting that the placenta holds the stimulus for insulin release.
3. Decreased buffering capacity predisposes the gravida to ketoacidosis.

Thyroid
1. Total serum thyroxine concentrations rise.
2. Thyroid-binding globulin concentration peaks in the third trimester.
3. Pituitary sensitivity to thyroid-stimulating hormone remains constant.
4. The percentage of free thyroxine in the serum falls.
5. Most parturients remain euthyroid.

6. Causes
   a. Progesterone
   b. Serum chorionic gonadotropin has intrinsic thyroid-stimulating activity and activates the thyroid gland.
      i. Concentration peaks between 9 and 18 weeks of gestation.
      ii. Suppression of thyroid-stimulating hormone production
7. The thyroid gland grows larger. Increased size may hinder rapid sequence induction.

Progesterone
1. May stimulate many physiologic changes of pregnancy
2. Plasma concentration
   a. Rises progressively throughout pregnancy.
   b. Abruptly declines after delivery of the placenta.

Prostaglandins
1. Peripheral concentrations increase during pregnancy.
2. Prostaglandin A compounds multiply most dramatically.
   a. Early in gestation, prostaglandin A–like material rises by 300%.
   b. Typical effects of prostaglandin A compounds
      i. Decreased systemic vascular resistance
      ii. Increased cardiac output
      iii. Both occur early in pregnancy and correlate with the elevation in prostaglandin A activity.
3. Prostaglandin E
   a. Increases in the third trimester.
   b. Peripheral production may be stimulated by angiotensin II.
      i. Prostaglandin E–induced vasodilation prevents angiotensin II–mediated hypertension.
      ii. Prostacyclin also may cause vasodilatation.

MUSCULOSKELETAL
1. Relaxin
   a. Initially secreted by the corpus luteum
   b. Concentration rises dramatically during the first trimester.
   c. Then, concentration declines to a stable level throughout the third trimester.
   d. Actions
      i. Softens the cervix
      ii. Inhibits uterine contractions
      iii. Relaxes the pubic symphysis
      iv. Peripheral joints become lax during the last trimester.
      v. Ligamentous laxity
         (1) May contribute to the high incidence of lower back pain with pregnancy.
         (2) May risk injury during the mechanical stress of labor.

CENTRAL NERVOUS SYSTEM

1. Pregnancy-mediated analgesia
   a. Pregnant animals are more tolerant to aversive stimuli.
   b. The antinociceptive threshold rises abruptly 1 to 2 days before parturition.
   c. This effect is reversed by intrathecal or systemic opioid antagonists.
   d. Etiology
      i. The placenta produces endorphins and enkephalins.
      ii. β-endorphin
         (1) Systemic secretion increases during labor.
         (2) Systemic secretion correlates with patient perceived pain intensity.
         (3) This large molecule does not cross the blood–brain barrier.
            (a) If this compound is important in mediating the changes in pain sensitivity in pregnancy or labor, its cerebrospinal fluid (CSF) concentrations also should rise.
            (b) They do not.
      iii. CSF 5-HIAA, a major metabolite of serotonin, increases with gestational age.
      iv. Progesterone
         (1) Plasma and CSF concentrations rise significantly with pregnancy.
         (2) CSF progesterone concentration falls rapidly postpartum.
2. Pregnant women require less spinal or epidural local anesthetic per spinal segment blocked than do nonpregnant controls.
   a. This change arises early in gestation and persists into the postpartum period.
   b. Although higher dermatomal levels develop as soon as 5 minutes after injection, pregnancy prolongs the time to complete epidural spread.
   c. Both mechanical and biochemical factors may have a role.
      i. Mechanical factors
         (1) May explain some, but not all, of the altered sensitivity to local anesthetics seen in pregnancy.
         (2) Abdominal compression, which mimics the effects of the gravid uterus, increases the spread of intrathecal tetracaine 4 mg.
         (3) The same dose of tetracaine spreads further still in parturients.
         (4) The gravid uterus elevates epidural but not CSF pressure.
      ii. α1-Acid glycoprotein (AAG)
         (1) CSF concentrations decrease during pregnancy.

(2) This decrease is unlikely to produce a clinically relevant increase in free bupivacaine concentrations.

iii. Increased sensitivity to local anesthetics

(1) Likely plays the largest role.

(2) Peripheral nerves are more vulnerable to local anesthetics during pregnancy.

(a) Faster onset of 50% block with bupivacaine in A, B, and C vagal fibers

(b) The dose–response curve to conduction blockade in isolated A and C nerve fibers shifts to the left.

(3) Prolonged (4 days), but not acute, exposure to progesterone makes nerve fibers more susceptible to local anesthetics.

3. General anesthetics
   a. Isoflurane minimum alveolar consentration (MAC) for transcutaneous tetanic electrical stimulus
      i. In nonpregnant women: 1.075%
      ii. At 8 to 12 weeks' gestation: 0.775%
      iii. Remains decreased 24 to 36 hours after delivery.
      iv. Equals nonpregnant values when measured more than 72 hours after delivery.[3]
   b. Pregnancy also decreases halothane and enflurane MAC by 27% and 30%, respectively.
   c. By 7 to 13 weeks' gestation, the dose of thiopental required to produce hypnosis and anesthesia is 17% to 18% lower in pregnant women compared with nonpregnant women.[4]

4. Implications
   a. Use lower doses of drug.
   b. Carefully assess individual patient responses.

PHARMACOKINETICS

1. Pregnancy alters drug binding and drug elimination.
   a. Albumin concentration falls.
   b. Hepatic microsomal activity rises.
2. The larger plasma volume increases renal blood flow and glomerular filtration.
3. Pharmacokinetic parameters do not show any consistent trend.
   a. Enhanced effects
      i. Prolonged elimination of bupivacaine, diazepam, thiopental, and theophylline
      ii. Increase in unbound fraction of diazepam, phenytoin, phenobarbital, and lidocaine
   b. Increased volume of distribution may decrease the response to thiopental and theophylline.
4. Plasma pseudocholinesterase
   a. Activity rapidly declines:
      i. Twenty percent during pregnancy.
      ii. Up to 60% after delivery.

     b. No structural abnormality
     c. Succinylcholine
        i. Increased volume of distribution during pregnancy counterbalances the decrease in pseudocholinesterase activity.
       ii. Postpartum, when plasma volume decreases before pseudocholinesterase activity recovers, succinylcholine paralysis persists about 3 minutes longer than in nonpregnant patients.

CONCLUSION

1. Adaptations to pregnancy affect every organ system, usually within several weeks of conception.
2. Change continues during and after parturition.
3. Cardiovascular system
   a. Increasing demands of the growing uterus and fetus
   b. Increases in plasma volume and cardiac output alter the hemodynamic responses to anesthetic interventions.
   c. Beginning in the second trimester, aortocaval compression can hinder uterine blood flow and maternal cardiac output.
   d. The larger plasma volume helps protect the parturient against blood loss at delivery.
4. Respiratory system
   a. A smaller FRC and a higher oxygen consumption render the parturient more susceptible to hypoxemia during apnea.
   b. Mechanical hyperventilation can lower uterine blood flow and incite fetal acidosis.
5. Gastrointestinal system
   a. Gastric emptying slows.
   b. Acid secretion increases.
   c. Intraabdominal pressure rises.
   d. The parturient is at greater risk of regurgitation and aspiration should her airway reflexes become impaired.
6. Pregnancy-related nervous system changes increase sensitivity to all anesthetics.

REFERENCES

1. Byrne F, Oduro-Dominah A, Kipling R. The effect of pregnancy on pulmonary nitrogen washout: A study of pre-oxygenation. *Anaesthesia* 1987;42:148.
2. Shakar KB, Moseley H, Ramasamy M. Arterial to end-tidal carbon dioxide tension difference during anaesthesia in early pregnancy. *Can J Anaesth* 1989;36:124.
3. Gin T, Chan MTV. Decreased minimum alveolar concentration of isoflurane in pregnant humans. *Anesthesiology* 1994;81:829.
4. Gin T, Mainland P, Chan MTV, Short TG. Decreased thiopental requirements in early pregnancy. *Anesthesiology* 1997;86:73.

Preoperative Evaluation of the Parturient with Coexisting Disease: Cardiac, Renal, and Hematologic Disease

Ultimately, preoperative evaluation of pregnant patients with coexisting disease requires answers to these questions:

How does the disease affect the pregnancy?
How does the pregnancy affect the disease?

Only then can a safe anesthetic be planned and administered.

CARDIAC DISEASE

1. Currently, many women with cardiac abnormalities successfully complete pregnancy. Although there are certain recognized risks (Table 2.1), the majority of women with mild disease or well-repaired cardiac defects tolerate pregnancy.
2. Heart disease complicates 0.5% to 4.0% of pregnancies worldwide.
   a. The incidence of rheumatic heart disease has declined.
   b. Increasing numbers of parturients present with corrected congenital heart disease.
3. Despite improved prognosis, hemodynamic changes associated with pregnancy may greatly increase the risk of maternal morbidity and mortality.
4. Maternal mortality is less than 1% in women with uncomplicated atrial septal defect, ventricular septal defect, patent ductus arteriosus, corrected tetralogy of Fallot, porcine valve replacement, and mitral valve stenosis (New York Heart Association [NYHA] class I or II).
5. The maternal mortality associated with pregnancy approaches 50% in women with pulmonary hypertension, complicated coarctation of the aorta, and Marfan syndrome with aortic involvement.

Normal Physiologic Changes of Pregnancy

1. The normal changes in the cardiovascular system during pregnancy (see Chapter 1) can simulate organic heart disease.
2. Healthy parturients often complain of fatigability, dyspnea, orthopnea, chest discomfort, or palpitations.
3. Symptoms that warrant investigation include paroxysmal nocturnal dyspnea, syncope with exertion, activity-related chest pain, and anasarca (Table 2.2).

Cardiac Disease and Pregnancy

Classification

1. A valuable way to assess severity of underlying heart disease is the NYHA classification of functional impairment (Table 2.3).

Table 2.1.   Recognized risks of heart disease during pregnancy

An inability of the mother to meet the physiologic demands of pregnancy

An inadequate supply of well-oxygenated blood for fetal nourishment

A worsening of maternal disease

Hereditary transmission with congenital heart disease

Infection, hemorrhage, or thromboembolism

2. Five percent to 10% of pregnant cardiac patients fall into NYHA class III or IV.
   a. Some of these women have a 75% to 90% risk of maternal mortality.
   b. Absent pulmonary hypertension, complicated congenital heart disease, and Marfan syndrome with aortic involvement, patients who are in classes III and IV have a 5% to 15% mortality and a 20% to 30% risk of fetal loss.

Diagnosis and Management during Pregnancy
1. Sole reliance on subjective signs and symptoms may lead to erroneous diagnosis of cardiac disease in the parturient.
2. Serial measurement of a host of noninvasive, objective parameters can provide important information.
   a. Intermittent measurements of peripheral oxygen saturation with a pulse oximeter may provide an early indication of cardiac failure.
   b. Vital capacity measurement may detect increases in blood volume that produce pulmonary vascular engorgement.

Table 2.2.   Signs and symptoms of maternal heart disease

Signs	Symptoms
Cyanosis	Severe dyspnea
Clubbing	Paroxysmal nocturnal dyspnea
Persistent neck vein distention	Hemoptysis
Systolic murmur > grade II/VI	Syncope with exertion
Diastolic murmur	Stress-related chest pain
Cardiomegaly	
Arrhythmia	
Loud P2	

Table 2.3.   New York Heart Association functional classification

Class I	Asymptomatic
Class II	Slight limitation of physical activities; comfortable at rest
Class III	Marked limitation with less than ordinary activity causing fatigue, palpitation, dyspnea, or angina; remains comfortable at rest
Class IV	Symptomatic at rest

    c. Electrocardiograms (ECGs) and Holter monitors can detect ischemia, arrhythmias, conduction defects, and axis deviations.

    d. Chest films, repeated as necessary, can diagnose or confirm progressive congestive heart failure, cardiomegaly, and pleural or pericardial effusions.

       i. A chest radiograph exposes the mother to a maximum of 80 mrad of radiation, approximately 50 mrad to the chest and 5 mrad to the gonads.

       ii. A dose of 0.5 rad is the recommended maximal radiation exposure to the pregnant woman, although some authors have suggested that even 10-rad exposure is safe.

       iii. Less than one case of malformation or cancer is expected per 1,000 patients irradiated by 1 rad in utero during the first 4 months of pregnancy.

       iv. No measurable risk is associated with a chest radiograph during pregnancy.

       v. Radionuclide techniques expose the mother to 500 to 800 mrad, and cardiac catheterization exposes the patient to as much as 28,000 mrad of radiation.

    e. Flow-directed right heart and pulmonary artery catheterization without fluoroscopy can assess valvular function and chamber pressures.

    f. Two-dimensional contrast echocardiography can evaluate valve and ventricular function.

Management at Term

    Good communication between the obstetric anesthesiologist and the obstetrician facilitates the care of these high-risk parturients. Invasive monitoring, antibiotic regimens, anticoagulation, termination of pregnancy, route of delivery, anesthetic management, maternal-fetal priorities, and the effects of various cardiac and uterine therapeutic modalities should be discussed before parturition.

MONITORING

    1. Pulmonary artery catheter

       a. Contraindicated in some patients with Eisenmenger syndrome, because in these patients, the risks (arrhythmias, passing a catheter through an atrial or septal

defect in the cardiac circulation, trauma, infection, and embolism) far outweigh the benefits.
    b. Isolated aortic stenosis may be managed without a pulmonary artery catheter because volume status can be easily assessed with a central venous pressure catheter.
    c. In general, reserve pulmonary artery catheterization is for pregnant women with NYHA class III and IV cardiac disease and patients with severe preeclampsia/eclampsia with end-organ disease, septic shock, hypovolemic shock, or thyroid storm.

ENDOCARDITIS PROPHYLAXIS

1. The genitourinary tract is second only to the oral cavity as a portal of entry for organisms that cause endocarditis.
2. American Heart Association guidelines
    a. High-risk patients
        i. Prosthetic valves
        ii. History of bacterial endocarditis
        iii. Complex cyanotic congenital heart lesions (tetralogy of Fallot)
        iv. Surgically constructed shunts
    b. Prophylaxis is *optional* for high-risk patients undergoing vaginal delivery or vaginal hysterectomy.
    c. Prophylaxis is *not* recommended for cesarean delivery.
    d. In the absence of localized infection, prophylaxis also is *not* recommended for:
        i. Urethral catheterization.
        ii. Uterine dilatation and curettage.
        iii. Therapeutic abortion.
        iv. Sterilization procedures.
        v. Insertion or removal of intrauterine devices.
3. Endocarditis prophylaxis for high-risk adults:
    a. Ampicillin 2 g intramuscularly (IM) or intravenously (IV)
    b. Plus gentamicin 1.5 mg per kilogram IM or IV (not to exceed 120 mg) 30 minutes before start of the procedure
    c. Plus ampicillin 1 g IM or IV or amoxicillin 1 g orally 6 hours after the procedure.
    d. For patients allergic to ampicillin or amoxicillin:
        i. Vancomycin 1 g IV over 1 to 2 hours
        ii. Plus gentamicin 1.5 mg per kilogram IV or IM 30 minutes before the start of the procedure.[1]

ANTICOAGULANTS

1. Certain patients must receive anticoagulants.
    a. Patients with mechanical valve prostheses
    b. Those with
        i. Cardiac valve disease
        ii. Chronic atrial fibrillation
        iii. A history of systemic emboli
2. Warfarin (Coumadin)
    a. Crosses the placenta and increases the danger of abnormal fetal development and congenital malformations, as well as abortion, stillbirth, and hemorrhage.

        i. These complications may be due to high-dose warfarin.

        ii. Risks may be minimal with low doses (5 mg or less daily).

    b. In the United States, heparin is the preferred anticoagulant used during gestation because it does not cross the placenta.

3. Risks of heparin
   a. Maternal thrombocytopenia
   b. Thromboembolism
   c. Osteoporosis
   d. Rare hypersensitivity reactions
   e. Retroplacental hemorrhage
   f. Abruptio-placentae, which can result in prematurity, stillbirth, and spontaneous abortion
   g. Otherwise, heparin is safe for the fetus.

4. Low-molecular-weight heparin (LMWH)
   a. Safety in pregnancy has not been clearly elucidated.
   b. Less platelet aggregation
   c. Does not cross the placenta
   d. Reduced association with osteoporosis
   e. Does not prolong activated thromboplastin time (aPTT)
   f. Increases the risk of epidural hematoma after neuraxial block

5. Some physicians use heparin from conception through the first trimester (to avoid embryopathy) and resume warfarin in midpregnancy. Others fear fetal bleeding at all stages of development and avoid warfarin throughout.

6. At term, discontinue heparin therapy 24 hours before elective induction of labor or cesarean section.
   a. Should spontaneous labor occur in a heparinized parturient, carefully monitor the aPTT (unless patient is receiving LMWH).
   b. If aPTT is prolonged near delivery, consider protamine sulfate unless the patient is receiving LMWH.

CHRONIC MEDICATIONS

1. Digoxin appears safe during pregnancy. Therapeutic serum concentrations lack apparent toxic fetal effects.

2. Lidocaine appears safe in the therapeutic range.

3. Quinidine and procainamide may induce premature labor. Chronic procainamide use may result in a lupus-like syndrome due to the development of maternal antinuclear antibodies.

4. Diuretics may reduce uteroplacental blood flow and yield fetal electrolyte imbalance, neonatal jaundice, thrombocytopenia, liver damage, and fetal death.

5. The β-adrenegetic blocking drugs (propranolol, labetalol, and esmolol)
   a. Cross the placenta.
   b. May cause
      i. Fetal bradycardia (esmolol).
      ii. Neonatal hypoglycemia.
      iii. Intrauterine growth retardation (IUGR) and low birth weight.

6. Calcium channel blockers
   a. Short-term use lacks adverse effects in the fetus or new-born infant.
   b. Can exert a tocolytic effect.
   c. In combination with magnesium sulfate, calcium channel blockers, particularly nifedipine, have been associated with hypotension and pronounced muscle weakness.
7. Amiodarone has been associated with preterm delivery, IUGR, and neonatal hypothyroidism.
8. Angiotensin-converting enzyme (ACE) inhibitors (captopril and enalapril)
   a. Use during the second or third trimester has been associated with
      i. Fetopathy
      ii. Renal tubular dysplasia
      iii. Hypocalvaria
      iv. IUGR
      v. Patent ductus arteriosus
   b. There is increased risk of preterm labor, oligohydramnios, and neonatal renal failure.

Specific Lesions
1. The parturient tolerates regurgitation better than stenosis.
2. Multivalvular regurgitation is not uncommon in normal pregnancy and occasionally persists into the early postpartum period.
   a. Regurgitation mainly right-sided:
      i. Tricuspid: 94.4%.
      ii. Pulmonary: 94.4%.
      iii. Mitral: 27.8%.
      iv. Aortic: 0%.
3. Chamber enlargement and valve annular dilation also are common.

MITRAL STENOSIS
1. Mitral stenosis is the most common acquired valvular disease in pregnancy (rheumatic origin).
   a. An obstructing lesion usually develops 10 to 20 years after the initial infection.
2. It may not tolerate the normal cardiovascular changes of pregnancy.
   a. Sudden life-threatening pulmonary edema may occur in previously asymptomatic patients.
   b. Symptoms occur in as many as 25% of affected gravidae (Table 2.4).
3. Progressive mitral stenosis
   a. Left ventricular volume decreases.
   b. The left atrium, pulmonic system, and right heart face an increase in both pressure and volume.
      i. The normal adult mitral valve area varies from 4 to 6 cm^2.
      ii. Stenotic lesions are graded as follows:
         (1) Mild: 1.5 to 2.5 cm^2.
         (2) Moderate: 1.0 to 1.5 cm^2.
         (3) Severe: less than 1 cm^2.

Table 2.4. Mitral valve disease: severe mitral stenosis

Symptoms

  Shortness of breath, dyspnea on exertion, orthopnea

  Recurrent bronchitis

  Hemoptysis

  Systemic embolism

  Acute pulmonary edema may occur with the onset of atrial fibrillation or acute pulmonary infection.

Physical findings

  First heart sound and mitral opening snap are loud with pliable valve, and faint with calcific valve.

  Diastolic murmur: low-frequency apical murmur is longer with more severe stenosis.

  ECG: left atrial enlargement or atrial fibrillation; right-axis deviation; rarely, right ventricular hypertrophy

  Chest radiograph: increased cardiac size, especially left atrium, calcification in mitral valve, pulmonary congestion

  Echocardiogram: left atrial dilation, decreased left ventricular performance, characteristic valve changes.

Hemodynamic findings

  Diastolic gradient between the pulmonary artery occlusion pressure and left ventricular diastolic pressure

Source: After Basta LL. *Cardiovascular disease.* New York: Medical Examination Publishing Co, 1983, with permission.

    c. Distal to the valve, the left ventricle is small to normal in size.

    d. Left ventricular end-diastolic pressure is in the normal range.

    e. Approximately one-third of patients have a depressed ejection fraction from either a chronic decrease in left ventricular volume or residual scarring from rheumatic myocarditis.

    f. Dilated left atrium
      i. May predispose to left lower lobe infections.
      ii. Severe dilation can cause left recurrent laryngeal nerve paralysis and dysphagia.

    g. Tachycardia, atrial fibrillation, or junctional rhythm may decrease stroke volume.

  4. Auscultation
    a. Accentuated first heart sound
    b. "Opening snap"
    c. Early diastolic sound heard best over the lower left sternal border
    d. A low-pitched apical diastolic "rumble"
    e. Evidence of mitral regurgitation, as well as involvement of other valves, is not uncommon.

  5. The ECG and chest radiograph will detect signs of advanced disease, such as atrial fibrillation or right ventricular hypertrophy.

6. Cardiac decompensation
   a. Most likely to occur at times of maximal increase in heart rate, systemic blood volume, cardiac output, and pulmonary blood volume
   b. Occurs with a transvalvular pressure gradient greater than 25 mm Hg
   c. Accompanying events
      i.   Atrial fibrillation
      ii. Paroxysmal tachycardia
      iii. Pulmonary vascular congestion
      iv. Infarction
7. Late-stage mitral stenosis
   a. Elevated pulmonary pressures produce persistent pulmonary hypertension and irreversible pulmonary arterial hyperplasia.
   b. Right heart failure
   c. Peripheral edema
   d. Hepatomegaly
   e. Ascites
   f. Distended neck veins
   g. Ventilation-perfusion mismatching, which worsens in the Trendelenburg position, is not uncommon.

MITRAL INSUFFICIENCY
1. Mitral insufficiency is often due to rheumatic fever.
2. It is usually associated with mitral stenosis, but there are other causes of regurgitant flow (Table 2.5).
3. It is generally better tolerated during pregnancy than is mitral stenosis.
4. Pathophysiology
   a. Failure of valve closure
      i. Left ventricular blood flows into the left atrium during ventricular systole.
      ii. Regurgitant flow depends on
          (1) The ventriculoatrial pressure gradient.
          (2) Regurgitant orifice size.
          (3) Heart rate affects.
              (a) Time for ventricular filling.
              (b) Duration of ventricular ejection.

Table 2.5. Etiology of mitral valve insufficiency

Rheumatic fever
Mitral valve prolapse
Chordae tendineae dysfunction and/or rupture
    Cardiac trauma
    Endocarditis
Papillary muscle dysfunction and/or rupture
    Cardiac trauma
    Endocarditis
Spatial disorientation
    Cardiomyopathy with left ventricular enlargement
    Idiopathic hypertrophic subaortic stenosis

    b. Regurgitant blood
       i. Raises left atrial pressure.
      ii. May produce pulmonary vascular congestion and pulmonary edema.
5. The increased left ventricular diastolic volume is generally tolerated.
    a. Ventricular compliance increases.
    b. Increased left ventricular end-diastolic volume does not raise left ventricular end-diastolic pressure, and oxygen consumption is not initially prohibitive.
    c. When regurgitant fraction is greater than 60% of left ventricular volume:
       i. Congestive heart failure.
      ii. Decreased left ventricular output.
     iii. Pulmonary hypertension.
     iv. Ultimately, right ventricular failure (Table 2.6).
6. Mitral insufficiency plus mitral stenosis
    a. Pressure and volume work increase.
    b. Symptoms are more severe.
    c. Symptoms occur earlier than in pure insufficiency.
    d. Fatigue is the most typical early symptom.

Table 2.6. Mitral valve insufficiency

	Chronic	Acute
Symptoms	Long-standing exertional dyspnea	Acute pulmonary edema, cardiogenic shock with papillary muscle rupture
Rhythm	Usually atrial fibrillation	Usually sinus rhythm
First heart sound	Faint	Faint
Third heart sound (S3)	May be audible	May be audible
S4 gallop	No	Very common
Heart size	Large	Normal or slightly enlarged
Left atrial size	Markedly increased	Slightly increased
Left ventricular hypertrophy on ECG	Common	Uncommon
Echocardiogram	Chamber size, valve characteristics depend on etiology	Chamber size, typical changes of flail valve leaflet
Left atrial pressure	Not considerably increased	Very prominent V wave may approach aortic diastolic pressure

Source: After Basta LL. *Cardiovascular disease.* New York: Medical Examination Publishing Co, 1983, with permission.

7. Findings
   a. Apical holosystolic murmur radiating to the left axilla
   b. ECG may show left atrial enlargement or fibrillation, and left ventricular hypertrophy.
   c. With significant insufficiency, chest radiograph may show cardiomegaly and pulmonary vascular congestion.
8. Tachycardia of pregnancy may improve mitral regurgitation.
   a. The area of the regurgitant orifice may decrease in the faster heart.
      i. Mitral valve prolapse with regurgitation is the exception to this principle.
      ii. Prolapse of redundant mitral leaflets worsens with a smaller ventricular valve orifice as caused by tachycardia.
   b. Lower systemic vascular resistance improves forward flow.
   c. Any increase in systemic vascular resistance may worsen regurgitation.

MITRAL VALVE PROLAPSE

1. Affects 5% to 10% of young adults, mainly women of child-bearing age
2. Complicates 1.2% of pregnancies
3. Findings
   a. Physical examination
      i. Mid to late systolic click followed by a systolic murmur
      ii. Heard best at the lower left sternal border or cardiac apex
   b. ECG and chest radiograph are nonspecific.
   c. Echocardiography reveals pathologic protrusion of the mitral leaflet into the left atrium during systole.
4. Symptoms include atypical chest pain, dyspnea, fatigue, dizziness, palpitations, anxiety, syncope, and sudden death.
5. Structural abnormalities
   a. Elongated chordae tendineae
   b. Large redundant mitral leaflets
   c. The familial form of mitral valve prolapse shows myxomatous degenerative changes.
6. Pathophysiology
   a. The mitral valve is too large for the ventricle.
   b. Redundant leaflets prolapse into the left atrium as ventricular volume decreases in mid and late systole.
   c. Prolapse worsens with decreases in ventricular volume.
      i. Increased myocardial contractility
      ii. Decreased preload
      iii. Tachycardia
      iv. Straining
      v. Excessive airway pressure
7. Depending on changes in vascular resistance and blood volume, pregnancy may enhance or diminish the signs of mitral valve prolapse. Cardiac compromise is common during pregnancy.

AORTIC STENOSIS

1. Pathophysiology
   a. Left ventricular outflow obstruction
      i. Normal aortic valve area: 2.5 to 3.5 cm^2
      ii. Advanced aortic stenosis: valve area less than 0.75 cm^2
      iii. Stroke volume is decreased and fixed.
   b. Concentric left ventricular hypertrophy and elevated left ventricular chamber pressure
      i. Reduced subendocardial blood flow
      ii. Ischemia and ventricular failure follow.
   c. Atrial contraction maintains cardiac output.
      i. Normally, atrial contraction augments stroke volume by 20%.
      ii. With aortic stenosis, atrial contraction may contribute as much as 40%.
      iii. Loss of atrial function (atrial fibrillation or junctional rhythms) may be lethal.
2. Findings
   a. Harsh systolic ejection murmur, heard at the base of the heart, that radiates to the carotid arteries
   b. Slowly rising and prolonged arterial pulse
   c. Fourth heart sound
   d. Paradoxically split second heart sound
3. History may reveal syncope, angina, or dyspnea on exertion (Table 2.7).
4. Effects of pregnancy
   a. Increased oxygen requirements risk ischemic injury.
   b. Increased plasma volume may raise pressure in the noncompliant left ventricle, increasing myocardial oxygen demand and encouraging pulmonary transudation of fluid.
5. Pregnancy outcome
   a. Generally satisfactory
   b. Severe aortic stenosis
      i. Risks maternal mortality (up to 17%)
         (1) Cardiac output depends on adequate blood volume.
         (2) Sudden maternal blood volume loss (i.e., delivery) can be catastrophic.
      ii. Valvular surgery during pregnancy is advised when the aortic valve gradient exceeds 70 mm Hg.
      iii. If hemodynamically severe aortic stenosis is diagnosed before pregnancy, advance surgical correction is advisable.
6. Fetal effects
   a. Decreased cardiac output may hinder uteroplacental blood flow; IUGR and congenital anomalies may follow.
   b. Fetal mortality is 32% in women with uncorrected aortic stenosis.
   c. Correction before conception reduces the fetal mortality rate to about 12%.

Table 2.7.   Severe aortic stenosis

Symptoms	Angina; syncope; paroxysmal nocturnal dyspnea; congestive heart failure (rare)
Physical findings	Slow carotid upstroke; left ventricular enlargement, if marked, signifies poor left ventricular performance; faint or absent aortic closure sound in calcific aortic stenosis; long ejection murmur that peaks in mid-systole heard maximally over the second space to the right of the sternum
Chest radiograph	Left ventricular enlargement; pulmonary congestion possible; aortic valve calcification
Electrocardiogram	Left ventricular hypertrophy and "strain"
Echocardiogram	Thickened valve with limited mobility; increased left ventricular wall thickness and decreased left ventricular performance
Cardiac catheterization	Large systolic gradient across aortic valve (>50 mm Hg)

Source: After Basta LL. *Cardiovascular disease.* New York: Medical Examination Publishing Co, 1983, with permission.

AORTIC INSUFFICIENCY
1. Unusual in pregnant women
   a. Etiology
      i. Most often rheumatic disease
      ii. Congenital or in relationship with either rheumatoid arthritis or systemic lupus erythematous
      iii. Marfan syndrome (aortic root dilatation and subsequent regurgitation)
      iv. Trauma and dissection (acute regurgitation)
2. Preconception dilation of the ascending aorta is an important predictor of aortic dissection.
   a. Risk increases steadily when the aortic diameter is greater than or equal to 4 cm.
      i. These parturients should have monthly transthoracic echocardiographic assessment.
      ii. Some suggest surgical correction during gestation when or before the aortic root reaches 5.5 cm, or elective cesarean delivery.
3. Symptoms/findings (chronic insufficiency)
   a. Twenty-year latency
   b. Fatigue and dyspnea (may be worse at rest than during exercise)

    c. Pulse pressure increased

    d. Pulse

       i. Rapid upstroke

       ii. Rapid decline

       iii. Bisferious pulse (a double impulse during systole) possible

    e. A high-pitched, blowing, diastolic decrescendo murmur along the sternal border is heard best with the patient sitting upright during end-expiration.

    f. The ECG, chest radiograph, and echocardiogram may help make the diagnosis (Table 2.8).

4. Pathophysiology

    a. An incompetent valve allows regurgitation of blood into the left ventricle.

       i. Ventricular strain

       ii. Dilation

       iii. Ultimately, cardiac failure

    b. The regurgitant blood adds to normal ventricular filling.

       i. The left ventricle sees a chronically elevated volume.

       ii. Chamber size increases.

       iii. Walls thicken eccentrically.

    c. In the most advanced state, pulmonary hypertension and right ventricular failure arise.

    d. Bradycardia

       i. Ventricular distention

       ii. Increased left atrial pressure

       iii. Pulmonary congestion

5. Effects of pregnancy

    a. Usually well tolerated

    b. Increased plasma volume may help maintain cardiac output.

    c. Decreased systemic vascular resistance and a faster pulse encourage forward flow.

IDIOPATHIC HYPERTROPHIC SUBAORTIC STENOSIS

1. Uncommon autosomal dominant inherited disorder

2. Disproportionate hypertrophy of the intraventricular septum

    a. An abnormally large septum bulges into the left ventricular chamber.

    b. It obstructs the ventricular outflow tract in mid to late systole.

3. Outflow obstruction worsens with

    a. Tachycardia.

    b. Increased myocardial contractility.

    c. Hypovolemia.

4. Findings

    a. Systolic ejection murmur at the base of the heart

       i. Murmur increases with maneuvers that lower left ventricular volume.

    b. ECG

       i. Left ventricular hypertrophy

       ii. Large septal Q waves

Table 2.8.   Aortic insufficiency

Severe	
Symptoms	Left ventricular failure; uncommonly angina or syncope
Physical findings	Wide pulse pressure; aortic diastolic pressure <40 mm Hg; enlarged left ventricle; typical auscultatory findings
Chest radiograph	Left ventricular enlargement; pulmonary congestion possible
Electrocardiogram	Left ventricular hypertrophy with T-wave inversion in severe cases
Echocardiogram	Shows left ventricular dimensions, wall thickness, and performance
Acute	
Symptoms	Recent history of pulmonary edema, features of low cardiac output
Physical findings	Frequently not prominent; aortic diastolic pressure is not considerably reduced, and the pulse pressure is not distinctly wide; left ventricular enlargement may not be impressive; aortic diastolic murmur may be short and faint; loud S3 common
Chest radiograph	Pulmonary edema with only slightly enlarged heart
Electrocardiogram	May be normal
Echocardiogram	May provide important clues to the diagnosis; diastolic mitral valve closure; high-frequency diastolic vibrations of the mitral leaflet and hyperkinetic left ventricle

Source: After Basta LL. *Cardiovascular disease.* New York: Medical Examination Publishing Co, 1983, with permission.

      c.   Echocardiogram
         i.   Thickened ventricular septum
        ii.   Abnormal anterior movement of the mitral valve during systole
  5.   Symptoms include dyspnea, chest pain, and palpitations.
      a.   Increased catecholamine secretion worsens symptoms.
      b.   There is a 1% to 3% chance of sudden death per year.
  6.   Effects of pregnancy
      a.   Usually positive
         i.   Elevated plasma volume
        ii.   Autotransfusion of blood from the contracting uterus at placental delivery
      b.   Worsening of symptoms has been reported.
  7.   Despite potential fetal hazards of IUGR and newborn bradycardia, β-blockade usually is continued throughout gestation.

CONGENITAL HEART DISEASE

1. Occurs with 1% of live births in the United States
2. Increasing numbers of women with congenital heart lesions are reaching childbearing age.
   a. Many have partially or fully corrected lesions.
   b. Functional deterioration risk is greatest with
      i. Cyanotic heart defects.
      ii. Lesions that lead to pulmonary hypertension.
   c. Corrected lesions that result in residual hypoxemia have been associated with a high rate of spontaneous abortion, poor fetal growth, and premature delivery.
   d. Corrective maternal surgery is most often done before conception to optimize maternal and fetal condition.
3. The obstetric anesthesiologist needs to know
   a. The medical and surgical history of the mother.
   b. The pathophysiology of a parturient's particular lesion.
4. The obstetric anesthesiologist may need to review
   a. ECG.
   b. Chest radiograph.
   c. Echocardiogram.
   d. Cardiac catheterization.

LEFT-TO-RIGHT SHUNTS

Atrial Septal Defect

1. Defects include
   a. Ostium primum.
   b. Ostium secundum.
   c. Sinus venosus.
2. The majority discovered and repaired in childhood.
3. Long-term prognosis after repair is good.
4. Ostium secundum
   a. Located near foramen ovale and adjacent tissue
   b. More common in women
   c. Supraventricular arrhythmias are common, especially if repair occurred after the onset of atrial fibrillation or flutter.
5. Findings
   a. A persistently split second heart sound is best heard at the base of the heart.
   b. Systolic ejection murmur
   c. ECG: right-axis deviation
   d. Chest radiograph may show prominent pulmonary vasculature.
6. Shunting
   a. Left-to-right
      i. Worsens with
         (1) Increased systemic vascular resistance.
         (2) Decreased pulmonary vascular resistance.
   b. Right-to-left
      i. Can follow acute increases in pulmonary vascular resistance
7. In the absence of large left-to-right shunting or secondary pulmonary hypertension, parturients with atrial septal defects tolerate pregnancy well.

Ventricular Septal Defect

1. More common than atrial septal defects
2. Membranous or muscular
3. Appear during embryogenesis
4. Different sizes
5. Multiple locations
6. Most close spontaneously in childhood.
7. Remaining lesions are usually surgically corrected before conception.
   a. Repair can damage the bundle of His, which lies at the posterior margin of the ventricular septum, producing arrhythmias.
8. On physical examination, a loud holosystolic murmur is heard best along the left sternal border.
9. Effects of pregnancy
   a. No pulmonary congestion
      i. Fatigue and malaise are common.
      ii. Otherwise, the patient tolerates pregnancy well.
      iii. The predominant risk is endocarditis.
   b. Increased systemic vascular resistance is poorly tolerated.
      i. Increases left-to-right shunting
      ii. Pulmonary hypertension
      iii. Increased right ventricular work
   c. Decreased systemic vascular resistance also causes problems.
      i. Right-to-left shunting (worse with pulmonary hypertension)
         (1) Maternal hypoxemia
         (2) Fetal hypoxemia

RIGHT-TO-LEFT SHUNTS

Tetralogy of Fallot

1. Most common cause of right-to-left shunt
2. Anatomically characterized by
   a. Ventricular septal defect
   b. Aorta overrides the pulmonary outflow tract
   c. Infundibular pulmonary artery stenosis with obstruction of outflow from the right ventricle
   d. Right ventricular hypertrophy (Fig. 2.1)
3. Seventy percent of patients have a bicuspid aortic valve, and the distal pulmonary artery may be hypoplastic or absent.
4. Physiologic state is determined by the degree of right ventricular and pulmonary artery hypertrophy.
   a. Right-to-left shunting occurs after pulmonary vascular resistance exceeds systemic vascular resistance.
      i. Blood following the path of least resistance is shunted through an atrial or septal defect before oxygenation in the lung.
      ii. Cyanosis due to arterial hypoxemia is apparent by 6 months of age.
      iii. Hypercyanotic attacks, or "tet spells":
         (1) Classically treated with β-adrenergic blockade to decrease spasm of the pathologic infundibular cardiac muscle.

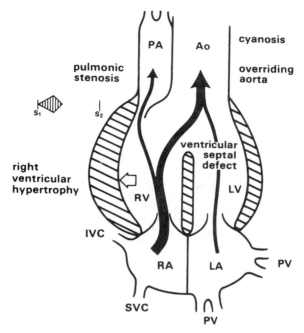

Fig. 2.1. Hemodynamic characteristics of tetralogy of Fallot. Note that the four defects in this disease result from abnormal development of the pulmonary infundibulum. Right ventricular (*RV*) hypertrophy is due to the fact that pressures are equal in both ventricles. Ao, aorta; IVC, inferior vena cava; LA, left atrium; LV, left ventricle; PA, pulmonary artery; PV, pulmonary vein; RA, right atrium; RV, right ventricle; SVC, superior vena cava. (Source: From Basta LL. *Cardiovascular disease.* New York: Medical Examination Publishing Co, 1983, with permission.)

    (2) Recurrence of attacks is an indication for surgical correction.
 5. Survival to childbearing age requires corrective surgery.
  a. Closure of the ventricular septal defect
  b. Resection of the infundibular stenosis, or pulmonary valvulotomy
 6. Findings in uncorrected tetralogy of Fallot:
  a. Ejection murmur heard over the left sternal border, resulting from blood flow across the infundibular pulmonary stenosis
  b. Right ventricular heave
  c. Chest radiograph shows diminished pulmonary vasculature.
  d. ECG shows right-axis deviation and right ventricular hypertrophy.

e. Arterial blood gas
   i. Normal pH and p_aCO_2.
   ii. Regardless of inspired oxygen tension, these women have a markedly reduced p_aO_2.
f. A hematocrit greater than 60% combined with an arterial oxygen saturation less than 80%, syncopal episodes, and right ventricular hypertension are all poor prognostic indicators.
g. The echocardiogram reveals an aorta overriding the ventricular septum.

7. Fetal morbidity and mortality
   a. The perinatal mortality rate approaches 20%.
   b. Risk increases with the severity of maternal cyanosis.
   c. Spontaneous abortions, prematurity, and IUGR are common.
   d. Congenital heart defects approach 15% to 20% in the offspring of mothers with tetralogy of Fallot.
   e. Palliation or surgical correction improves outcome for both mother and fetus.

8. Dynamic right ventricular outflow obstruction
   a. The muscular infundibular area dilates or constricts, depending on the inotropic state of the myocardium and the volume of the central circulation.
   b. Decreased peripheral vascular resistance increases outflow obstruction and right-to-left intracardiac shunt.
   c. Compression of the vena cava decreases venous return and right heart volume, which also may increase outflow obstruction and worsen the right-to-left intracardiac shunt.
   d. Autotransfusion associated with uterine contraction during labor and after delivery will improve venous blood return and may diminish the magnitude of right-to-left intracardiac shunt.

Eisenmenger Syndrome

1. Pulmonary vascular resistance exceeds systemic vascular resistance, reversing intracardiac shunt and producing cyanosis.
2. Eisenmenger syndrome may occur in up to 50% of untreated patients with a large ventricular septal defect and in 10% of patients with an atrial septal defect.
3. Pathophysiology
   a. Left-to-right intracardiac shunt progressively increases right heart volume and pulmonary vascular resistance.
   b. As the pulmonary vascular resistance and right-sided pressures increase, bidirectional or right-to-left shunting begins.
4. This syndrome contraindicates surgical correction of the underlying congenital heart defect because pulmonary vascular resistance is irreversibly elevated.
5. Prognosis
   a. Maternal mortality may exceed 50%, and fetal mortality may approach 30%.
   b. Prognosis is worse in the face of advanced medial and intimal pulmonary vascular thickening.

    c. Although pregnancy is discouraged in these women, prolonged bed rest, anticoagulation, and oxygen therapy improve maternal and fetal outcomes.

6. Pregnancy aggravates Eisenmenger syndrome.
   a. Systemic vascular resistance decreases, but pulmonary vascular resistance remains fixed.
   b. Right-to-left shunting, hypoxemia, and cyanosis progressively increase.
   c. Labor and delivery
      i. The pain and stress of labor, acute blood loss at delivery, and autotransfusion of uterine blood in the third stage of labor put these patients at very high risk.
      ii. Expulsive efforts may overload the right heart and increase the right-to-left shunt, or cause complete right heart failure.

7. These women have little cardiac reserve.
   a. Risk is greatest
      i. Late in pregnancy.
      ii. When supine without uterine displacement.
      iii. During labor and delivery or surgery.
      iv. Early postpartum.
   b. Sudden death may occur.
      i. Causes include embolism, arrhythmia, myocardial infarction, right heart overload, and sudden decreases in systemic vascular resistance.
      ii. Emboli may affect the coronary or cerebral circulation.

8. Management
   a. Finger pulse oximetry may be an ideal noninvasive indicator of shunt fraction and direction.
   b. The pulmonary vasculature may respond to oxygen or be irreversibly fixed.

PERIPARTUM CARDIOMYOPATHY

1. Reported incidence ranges from 1 in 1,300 to 15,000 pregnancies.
2. Mortality rate is between 30% and 60%.
3. Diagnostic criteria
   a. Development of cardiac failure in the last month of pregnancy or within 5 months after delivery
   b. Absence of a defined etiology for the cardiac failure
   c. Absence of demonstrable heart disease before the last month of gestation
4. Outcome
   a. Correlates with recovery of left ventricular function
   b. Patients whose ventricular failure does not resolve within 6 months have an especially poor prognosis.
   c. Heart transplantation is an option for patients with severe disease unresponsive to conventional treatment. Patients who have undergone heart transplantation after an episode of severe peripartum cardiomyopathy have later became pregnant, delivered, and survived.
   d. The recurrence risk in subsequent pregnancies is at least 50%, with a 60% mortality.

5. Diagnosis
    a. The final diagnosis is one of exclusion.
    b. Signs and symptoms are of left ventricular failure. Central and systemic emboli occur in up to 25% of cases.
    c. Early diagnosis is difficult: Many parturients complain of fatigue, dyspnea on exertion, and edema.
    d. The increased blood volume and cardiac output at term and peripartum may raise pulmonary capillary pressure and incite congestive heart failure in women with impaired ventricular function.
    e. The differential diagnosis includes amniotic fluid or pulmonary embolism, β-mimetic tocolytic therapy, or preeclampsia.
    f. Echocardiography may show a dilated hypokinetic left ventricle.
    g. Endomyocardial biopsy reveals fibrous deposition, mural thrombi, and generalized degenerative changes.
6. Postulated etiologies of peripartum cardiomyopathy include inadequate nutrition, viral myocarditis, preeclampsia, immunologic disorders, advanced maternal age, multiple gestation, obesity, and breastfeeding.

MYOCARDIAL INFARCTION

1. Incidence during pregnancy: 1 in 10,000.
    a. Increasing incidence may be related to advanced maternal age, hypertension, and smoking.
    b. Risk factors
        i. Use of bromocriptine, collagen vascular disease, Kawasaki disease, cocaine abuse, aortic valve disease, sickle cell chronic lung disease, hyperlipidemia, diabetes mellitus, and pheochromocytoma.
2. Etiology
    a. Coronary artery disease is involved in the vast majority of cases.
    b. Thrombosis, aneurysm, spasm, obstruction, or dissection of the coronary vasculature may occur as well.
    c. Coronary vasospasm
        i. Cocaine
        ii. Increased serum renin–angiotensin concentrations due to diminished venous return at the end of pregnancy.
    d. Thromboembolic phenomena from the hypercoagulable state of pregnancy
3. The mortality rate of acute myocardial infarction during pregnancy ranges from 21% to 50%. Poor prognostic factors are
    a. Occurrence of the infarct in the third trimester.
    b. Age of the patient less than 35 years.
    c. Delivery within 2 weeks of infarct.
    d. Delivery by cesarean section.
    e. Cardiac risk to the patient in subsequent pregnancies is associated with residual left ventricular dysfunction, underlying coronary anatomy, and the presence of ongoing ischemia.

4. Evaluation
    a. History: Elicit information about obesity, smoking, hyperlipidemia, hypertension, arrhythmias, angina, heart disease, obstetric history, and drug usage.
    b. Physical examination: Look for carotid bruit, arrhythmia, extra heart sounds, or pulmonary congestion.
    c. Serial 12-lead ECG and cardiac isoenzymes are standard.
    d. Laboratory: hematocrit, serum electrolytes, blood urea nitrogen and creatinine, coagulation profile, and baseline arterial blood gas
    e. Echocardiography to examine left ventricular function
5. Pathophysiology
    a. Adequate coronary artery blood flow and oxygen content are required to avert myocardial injury.
    b. Mean aortic root diastolic pressure minus the left ventricular end-diastolic pressure determines coronary blood flow or perfusion pressure to the left ventricle.
    c. Many factors affect the oxygen content of blood perfusing the coronary arteries. Among them are hemoglobin, arterial oxygen saturation, pH, temperature, and 2,3-diphosphoglyceric acid (2,3-DPG).
    d. The major determinant of myocardial oxygen demand is heart rate. Other factors include preload, afterload, and contractility.
6. The increased heart rate, stroke volume, plasma volume, metabolic rate, V/Q mismatching, and oxygen consumption of the term parturient allow her myocardium little reserve.

PRIMARY PULMONARY HYPERTENSION

1. A very lethal, uncommon disorder that occurs most often in young women
    a. Death often takes place within 2 years of onset of symptoms.
    b. Pregnancy and primary pulmonary hypertension combined produce a maternal mortality rate of 50%.
2. Pathophysiology
    a. Fixed, nonreactive pulmonary vasculature increases right ventricular work, leading to muscular hypertrophy.
    b. A noncompliant right ventricle eventually impairs the left heart output.
    c. The end result is cardiac failure.
3. Signs and symptoms include syncope, hemoptysis, and chest pain. A right ventricular heave and a loud second heart sound are present. Peripheral cyanosis and clubbing are not uncommon.
4. Effects of pregnancy
    a. Increased plasma volume, cardiac output, and oxygen consumption augment the workload of the already strained right heart.
    b. Uterine compression of the vena cava and acute blood loss at delivery decrease venous return, left ventricular filling, and cardiac output.
    c. Despite these physiologic changes, which often result in maternal death, cases with positive outcome have been reported.

RENAL DISEASE
Renal Function and Pregnancy

1. Renal calyces, pelvis, and ureters dilate as ureteral smooth muscle hypertrophies, creating a physiologic hydroureter.
   a. Dextrorotation of the gravid uterus can worsen the dilation on the right side of the urinary collecting system.
   b. The mechanism of ureteral smooth muscle hypertrophy is unknown. Increased progesterone, gonadotropins, and prostaglandin E1 have been suggested. Compression of the ureters by the iliac artery and enlarged uterine veins also play a role.
   c. These changes may allow stasis, leading to bacteriuria, and can make renal obstruction difficult to diagnose.
2. Glomerular filtration rate increases 30% to 50%, and renal plasma flow rises 60% to 80%.
   a. Postulated mechanisms
      i. Vasodilation of preglomerular and postglomerular resistance vessels
      ii. Progesterone-mediated changes in pressor receptors
      iii. Altered responses to renin–angiotensin control
      iv. Reduction in vascular tone may reset volume and osmoreceptors that help maintain volume homeostasis during pregnancy.
   b. Creatinine and urea nitrogen production remain unchanged, so their serum concentrations fall. Values considered normal in the nonpregnant state may suggest renal dysfunction in the parturient.
3. Osmoregulation
   a. There is an average 8- to 10-mOsmol per kilogram decrease in plasma osmolality.
   b. This decrement in the nonparturient would produce a significant diuresis, yet the gravida appears to adjust both vasopressin secretion and thirst to maintain this lower osmolality.
4. Water regulation
   a. The parturient retains 7 to 8 L of total body water.
      i. Two liters of intravascular water, which contain 290 mEq of sodium, and 155 mEq of potassium
      ii. At term, there are 1.2 L of amniotic fluid, 700 mL of water in the uterus, 300 mL in the placenta, and 400 mL in the breasts.
   b. Water excretion is reduced in late gestation.
      i. This may relate to the hemodynamic effects of maternal posture.
      ii. The clinical usefulness of random specific gravity measurements in the supine third-trimester gravida is questionable.

Glucose

1. Glucosuria occurs frequently.
   a. The parturient cannot increase glucose reabsorption in parallel with the larger amount of filtered glucose.
   b. Urinary glucose sampling may be unreliable in evaluating pregnant diabetic patients.

2. Changes in renal handling of glucose may not indicate renal pathology.

Sodium
1. Sodium is the principal regulator of volume homeostasis.
2. Reabsorption accounts for the largest renal adjustment in pregnancy.
   a. Total body sodium increases by 1,000 mEq.
   b. Sixty percent remains maternal.

Acid-Base Balance
1. Plasma bicarbonate concentration decreases 4 mEq per liter in response to maternal respiratory alkalosis.
2. The average p_aCO2 is 31 mm Hg; pH, 7.44; and serum bicarbonate, 20 mEq per liter.
3. The reduced total buffering capacity raises the risk of severe acidosis during pregnancy.

Evaluation of Renal Dysfunction
1. A reliable diagnosis of underlying renal disease can be accomplished easily during pregnancy.
2. The initial workup: history, physical examination, and laboratory data
   a. Clues in the history may include hematuria, polyuria, nocturia, and enuresis.
   b. Symptoms of urinary tract infection include dysuria, urgency, and foul-smelling urine.
   c. Look for a history of hypertension, diabetes, gout, or renal disease in both the patient and her family.
   d. Electrolyte disturbances may present as weakness, paresthesia, and areflexia, or as cardiac problems.
   e. The first voided urine in the morning is usually concentrated and requires careful examination.
      i. Proteinuria generally indicates a derangement in glomerular permeability.
         (1) With pregnancy, daily protein excretion may reach 250 mg.
         (2) Proteinuria between 150 mg and 2 g daily may signal chronic interstitial nephritis or nephrosclerosis.
         (3) Heavy proteinuria, more than 2 g daily, may occur in chronic glomerulonephritis, diabetic nephropathy, systemic lupus erythematosus, membranous glomerulonephritis, lipoid nephrosis, and focal glomerulosclerosis.
      ii. Tubular epithelial cells can be seen in tubular necrosis and nephrotoxic nephritis.
      iii. The Maltese cross of epithelial cells filled with lipid is typical of the nephrotic syndrome.
      iv. Hematuria
         (1) Microscopic hematuria may be induced by exercise, acute febrile illness, or kidney trauma.
         (2) Significant hematuria may suggest glomerulonephritis, systemic lupus erythematosus, or periarteritis.

(3) Red and white blood cell casts indicate primary renal pathology.
f. Laboratory data
   i. Hematocrit, serum blood urea nitrogen and creatinine, electrolytes, uric acid, and creatinine clearance.
      (1) In pregnancy, both the serum blood urea nitrogen and creatinine concentration decrease.
      (2) Normal concentrations found in the parturient are suspicious.
g. Abdominal radiographs are usually avoided, and an intravenous pyelogram is seldom needed.
h. Renal biopsy is technically difficult in the parturient. The increase in renal blood flow presents a further risk.
3. Uremia affects multiple organ systems.
   a. The immune system is compromised.
   b. Platelet function may be depressed.
   c. Autonomic neuropathies and central nervous system irritability are not uncommon.
   d. Gastric emptying is prolonged.
   e. Erythropoietin deficiency produces anemia. Both anemia and decreased concentrations of 2,3-DPG may compromise of fetal oxygen delivery.

Prognosis
1. Severe renal insufficiency (serum creatinine greater than 2.5 mg per deciliter or creatinine clearance less than 50 mL per minute)
   a. These women usually do not become pregnant.
   b. If they do conceive, 50% have poor fetal outcomes and will exhibit end-stage renal disease within 1 year.
2. Moderate renal insufficiency: increased spontaneous abortion, hypertension, worsening renal function, and obstetric complications
3. Mildly depressed renal function: better fetal outcomes; fewer advance to end-stage renal disease
4. Other important outcome determinants
   a. Chronic hypertension
      i. Uncontrolled hypertension and concurrent renal insufficiency can cause progression to end-stage renal disease.
      ii. Hypertension before conception increases the risk of IUGR fivefold and doubles the premature delivery rate.
   b. Onset of hypertension during pregnancy
   c. Patients with glomerular disease may experience worsening renal status with the increased glomerular filtration of pregnancy.
5. Hematocrit affects oxygen delivery to the fetus.
   a. The anemia of renal disease, secondary to depressed erythropoietin production, will decrease oxygen-carrying capacity.
   b. The incidence of IUGR may increase.

Pyelonephritis

1. Frequent during pregnancy
2. Dilatation of the collecting system, *Escherichia coli* virulence factor, and host ligands may contribute to gestational pyelonephritis.
3. If improperly managed, pyelonephritis can produce considerable morbidity.
   a. Low birth weight, increased perinatal mortality, anemia, preeclampsia, and premature rupture of membranes
   b. Untreated, pyelonephritis may lead to adult respiratory distress syndrome and death.
4. Common symptoms include fever, chills, nausea, vomiting, costovertebral angle tenderness, and urinary complaints.

Glomerulonephritis

1. Gram-positive or gram-negative bacterial pathogens trigger immune glomerulonephritis.
   a. May present as focal, diffuse, proliferative, or lupus type
   b. May lead to the nephrotic syndrome in the presence of sufficient proteinuria
   c. Edema and hypertension are not uncommon.
   d. Microscopic hematuria with red blood cell casts, low serum complement, and a rising antistreptolysin titer suggest the diagnosis of acute poststreptococcal glomerulonephritis.
   e. Significant proteinuria is a risk factor for impaired renal function in the postpartum period.
2. Berger disease or IgA nephropathy
   a. May present with hematuria but minimal proteinuria
   b. Prognosis is generally good in the absence of hypertension.
   c. Pregnancy does not adversely influence the natural course of IgA nephropathy.
3. The fetus seems protected from the maternal glomerulonephritides. Possible explanations:
   a. The antigen–antibody complexes are too large to cross the placental circulation.
   b. The fetal glomeruli do not react in the same manner to the complexes.
   c. The glomerular pressure (a possible factor in the development of this disease) is too low in the fetus.
   d. Perinatal mortality may reach 18%, however.

Systemic Lupus Erythematosus

1. Complicates 1 in 1,600 to 5,000 pregnancies
2. An autoimmune disorder with antigen–antibody complexes forming and depositing in tissues
3. Etiology unknown
4. Lupus and pregnancy
   a. Most common clinical manifestations include arthralgias, fever, skin lesions, and renal disease.
   b. Serum complement concentration falls, antibodies against DNA arise, and the lupus anticoagulant appears.

    c. The impact of pregnancy on systemic lupus erythematosus is controversial.

    d. Significant maternal and fetal morbidity and mortality (increased risk of obstetric complications, fetal loss, prematurity, and IUGR) have been reported.

5. Lupus anticoagulant

    a. Might bind with platelet membranes, inciting aggregation and an increased incidence of thrombosis in the deep veins, peripheral arteries, retinal vessels, placenta, pulmonary vessels, and brain

    b. The partial thromboplastin time, and rarely the prothrombin time, may be prolonged. Changes in these tests do not correlate with clinical hemorrhage.

6. Anticardiolipin antibodies

    a. Associated with thrombocytopenia and thrombocytopathy

    b. Can make blood cross-matching difficult

7. A transient or permanent deterioration in renal function may occur. Proteinuria, hypertension, and reduced creatinine clearance correlate with a poor prognosis.

8. Fetal effects

    a. Immunoglobulin–complement complexes can deposit in trophoblastic tissue.

    b. Fetal heart block and endocardial fibroelastosis are not infrequent.

    c. The risks of abortion, perinatal mortality, and premature delivery increase.

Diabetic Nephropathy

1. Primary finding: localized nodular or diffuse glomerulosclerosis, or thickening of the glomerular basement membrane. Vascular disease of both large and small renal vessels can cause severe scarring of the renal interstitium.

2. In the presence of proteinuria and diminished renal function, most parturients are hypertensive.

    a. Probably secondary to renal vascular disease

3. The prognosis relates to the degree of proteinuria.

    a. More than 3 g in 24 hours correlates with a rapid progression to renal insufficiency.

4. Effect of pregnancy

    a. No increased risk or acceleration of renal failure in patients with mild-to-moderate disease

    b. Parturients with moderate-to-severe disease have a greater than 40% chance of disease acceleration.

5. Preeclampsia occurs more often in these women, and, when severe, perinatal mortality may approach 25%.

Calculi

1. Incidence

    a. Does not rise during pregnancy.

    b. Remains between 0.1% and 1.0%.

2. Risk factors

    a. Calcium

        i. Intestinal absorption of calcium increases during pregnancy, and urinary calcium excretion usually exceeds 250 mg in a 24-hour period.

      ii. Hypercalciuria accounts for more than 40% of calculi in the parturient.
  b. Urinary tract infections predispose to recurrent stone formation.
      i. Urease-containing organisms alkalinize the urine, allowing precipitation of calcium.
3. Although incidence remains the same, dilation of the gravid renal pelvis and ureter may ease passage of any calculi.

Nephrotic Syndrome

1. Proteinuria, hypoalbuminemia, hyperlipidemia, and edema characterize this syndrome.
2. Diagnosis may be confused with normal physiologic changes of pregnancy.
  a. Increases in urinary protein may simply be a consequence of the increments in renal hemodynamics, changes in the glomerular barrier, or rise in renal vein pressure.
      i. Serum albumin decreases 0.5 to 1.0 g per deciliter in normal gestation.
      ii. Edema may follow (reduced plasma oncotic pressure).
  b. More cholesterol and other circulating lipids are found in both normal pregnancy and in nephrotic syndrome.
3. Etiology
  a. Most common: preeclampsia
  b. Others: diabetic glomerulosclerosis, lupus nephritis, lipoid nephrosis, renal vein thrombosis, amyloidosis, and drug reaction
4. Consequences of protein loss
  a. The patient may be effectively hypothyroid or immunodeficient.
  b. Intravascular volume depletion. With uteroplacental blood flow at risk, patient positioning is crucial.

Hemodialysis

1. There are a few reports of conception and parturition with chronic maternal hemodialysis.
2. These women are at greater risk of spontaneous abortion, delivery of a low-birth-weight infant, and premature labor and delivery.
3. Risk of premature labor, vaginal bleeding, and systemic hypotension is greatest immediately at the cessation of dialysis.
4. Dialysates containing both glucose and bicarbonate have been recommended for the gravida in renal failure.
5. Risks during dialysis
  a. Hypoxemia and hypercarbia secondary to hypoventilation after excessive HCO_3 removal
  b. Hypotension from intravascular volume depletion and acetate in the dialysate
  c. Bleeding from heparinization
  d. Thrombocytopenia and bleeding from platelet retention on the dialysis membrane
  e. Altered pseudocholinesterase concentrations and platelet function

f. Premature contractions secondary to the depletion of progesterone by hemodialysis

6. In early gestation, or in the presence of IUGR or oligohydramnios, limit the volume of maternal fluid removed, as hemodialysis results in amniotic fluid shifts.

Peritoneal Dialysis (CAPD)

1. The conception rate of reproductive-age women receiving peritoneal dialysis is reported to be 0.2% per year.
   a. Pregnancy in CAPD patients is associated with hypertension, bleeding, anemia, peritonitis, and premature delivery.
   b. Only 40% of these pregnancies result in surviving infants.
   c. Interestingly, hemodialysis patients become pregnant about twice as often as CAPD women.
2. Management of CAPD during pregnancy
   a. Volume and frequency of exchanges are adjusted to achieve a total creatinine clearance of greater than 15 mL per minute.
   b. CAPD may offer a more constant biochemical and extracellular environment for the fetus, with fewer episodes of hypotension.

Acute Renal Failure

1. Many complications may cause acute renal failure in the gravida (Table 2.9).
2. Most common etiology: hypovolemia, renal hypoperfusion, and subsequent ischemia. Persistent hypovolemia may reduce cortical blood flow and lead to acute tubular necrosis.
3. Other causes
   a. Disseminated intravascular coagulation from amniotic fluid embolism, intrauterine fetal death, placental abruption, or major transfusion reaction
   b. A fall in urinary prostaglandin E2 is associated with the increased renal vascular resistance and decreased renal blood flow in preeclampsia.

Table 2.9.   Causes of acute renal failure in obstetrics

Antepartum	Postpartum
Abortion	Uterine atony
Placenta previa	Retained placenta
Placenta abruption	Amniotic fluid embolism
Hyperemesis gravidarum	Uterine rupture
Pregnancy-induced hypertension	Vaginal/cervical tear
Preeclampsia	Hemolytic uremic syndrome
Chorioamnionitis	Septic abortion
Acute fatty liver	
Pyelonephritis	

4. The cortical necrosis that can follow acute renal failure in the gravida usually results from fibrin deposits in the renal vasculature.
5. Prognosis
   a. Renal vascular injury, especially from cortical necrosis and hemolytic uremia syndrome, has been associated with poor prognosis.
   b. Recently, preeclampsia/eclampsia complicated by abruptio placentae has carried a worse maternal and renal prognosis.
   c. The outcome of acute tubular necrosis ranges from mild and short-lasting tubular damage to chronic renal failure from sclerosis of any remaining nephrons.
6. Nephrotoxic renal failure
   a. Exogenous toxins
      i. Radiographic contrast media
      ii. Antibiotics
      iii. Nonsteroidal antiinflammatory drugs
   b. Endogenous toxins include hemoglobin, myoglobin, uric acid, oxalic acid, and myelomatous proteins from multiple myeloma.
7. Urinary tract obstruction secondary to the gravid uterus, polyhydramnios, nephrolithiasis, pelvic and broad ligament hematoma, or surgical damage also can cause acute renal failure.
8. Diagnosis
   a. Separate prerenal, intrinsic renal, or postrenal causes
   b. History may reveal use of nephrotoxic agents.
   c. Look for history of cardiac disease, hepatic disease, or recent muscle damage.
   d. Physical examination should concentrate on signs and symptoms of dehydration and hypovolemia.
   e. Laboratory evaluation: urinalysis, hematocrit, and serum blood urea nitrogen/creatinine ratio (Table 2.10)

Table 2.10. Urinary findings: prerenal and intrinsic renal disease

	Prerenal	Intrinsic Renal
Urine sediment	Not remarkable	Renal epithelial cells and casts; granular, muddy, pigmented cells
Urine osmolality (mOsmol/kg)	>500	<350
Urine sodium (mEq/L)	<20	>40
Urine specific gravity	>1.020	<1.015
Urine:plasma creatinine concentration ratio	>40	<20

HEMATOLOGIC DISEASE
Anemia
1. Most common hematologic complication of pregnancy
2. Incidence ranges from 20% to 80%.
    a. Data from the Center for Disease Control's Pregnancy Nutritional Surveillance System suggests a prevalence of 20% to 40% in low-income women in the United States.
    b. The incidence is highest in the 15- to 19-year age group and in Black women of all ages.
3. Symptoms include fatigue, dyspnea, palpitations with mild physical activity, intolerance to exertion, dizziness, headache, irritability, difficulty sleeping, anorexia, and bowel irregularities. Many patients are asymptomatic.
4. Anemia is most commonly found on routine laboratory testing.
5. The average red blood cell size (mean corpuscular volume [MCV]) provides useful information regarding the mechanism of anemia.
    a. Macrocytosis coincides with both folate and vitamin B12-deficiency anemia.
    b. Microcytosis occurs with iron deficiency, thalassemia, and lead poisoning.
    c. Hemoglobin content, red cell size distribution, reticulocyte count, and iron stores also may provide useful diagnostic information.
6. Fetal effects
    a. The degree of maternal anemia that results in risk to the fetus or neonate remains unclear.
    b. Although reports of decreased birth weight, prematurity, and perinatal death exist, it is difficult to control for poor nutrition and low socioeconomic status.
    c. Fetal risk may increase progressively as hemoglobin falls below 10 g per deciliter.
7. High-output congestive heart failure with intravascular volume overload is common in severe anemia. The gravida is therefore at an even greater risk of this complication.

Iron-deficiency Anemia
1. The majority of the body's iron is stored in hemoglobin.
2. During pregnancy, the demands on iron stores are increased, and iron deficiency anemia results when these stores become depleted.
    a. Approximately 1,000 mg of additional iron is needed during pregnancy.
    b. Most adult women maintain a 500-mg iron storage pool.
    c. Iron is preferentially delivered to the fetus secondary to the heavy concentration of transferrin receptors on the placental trophoblastic membranes.
    d. Lack of bleeding due to amenorrhea during pregnancy saves approximately 200 mg of iron.
    e. Bleeding, multiple gestation, chronic illness, poor appetite, poor nutrition, and nausea and vomiting can cause further iron depletion.
3. Maternal and fetal effects of iron-deficiency anemia, particularly when developing early in pregnancy, may include

preeclampsia, low birth weight, premature labor, and still-birth.

4. Iron-deficiency anemia may be difficult to diagnose during pregnancy.
    a. A microcytic, hypochromic red blood cell smear is a late finding.
    b. MCV typically increases during the first 2 months of gestation.
    c. Transferrin and total iron-binding capacity rise during pregnancy, making the iron-to-transferrin ratio low, even in gravid women without iron deficiency.
    d. The most sensitive test in the parturient for iron-deficiency anemia is measurement of serum ferritin.

5. Treatment
    a. Oral iron (30 to 120 mg of elemental iron daily)
    b. Absorption varies and is reduced by 40% to 50% when iron is taken with meals.
    c. The most common untoward effect from oral iron preparations is gastrointestinal irritation.
    d. The reticulocyte count increases by the second week of treatment with iron supplementation.
    e. Iron has been given parenterally; however, possible untoward reactions include anaphylaxis, headache, malaise, fever, arthralgias, lymphadenopathy, phlebitis, dizziness, and nausea and vomiting. Still, intravenous iron therapy during pregnancy may be an effective method of regenerating iron stores in severely iron-deficient patients who cannot use oral preparations.

Megaloblastic Anemia

1. Commonly acquired nutritional anemia
2. Most common in countries or socioeconomic groups with poor nutrition
3. Folic acid and vitamin B12 deficiencies are the usual causes.
    a. The pregnant patient is unlikely to develop a vitamin B12 deficiency.
        i. Vitamin B12 has an integral role in all DNA replication, and a significant deficiency should result in sterility.
        ii. Normally, there are large stores of vitamin B12, making this an unlikely source of anemia.
    b. Folic acid
        i. Essential cofactor in nucleic acid synthesis
        ii. Most likely source of megaloblastic anemia in the gravida
        iii. Pure folate deficiency results in a macrocytic anemia or may even cause pancytopenia.
        iv. During pregnancy, the growing fetus induces a 50% rise in folate requirements.
        v. The total body stores of this vitamin are small and short-lived.
        vi. Sources of folate
            (1) The main dietary source is green leafy vegetables. Excessive cooking decreases available folate.

(2) Some drugs, such as oral contraceptives and phenytoin, hinder the absorption of folic acid.

(3) Nausea and vomiting may significantly impair intake.

(4) Unless the diet is supplemented, negative folate balance usually arises in the third trimester.

4. Signs and symptoms

   a. Significant anemia (Hb = 6 to 9 g per deciliter)

   b. Symptoms consistent with both a decreased intravascular volume and a diminished oxygen-carrying capacity. These may include weakness, dizziness, light-headedness, and palpitations.

   c. Common physical findings are pale skin, tachycardia, and a systolic flow murmur.

   d. Not uncommonly, patients with long-standing disease complain of diarrhea, as well as sore tongue and mouth.

   e. Because of associated peripheral nerve demyelination, patients with vitamin B12 deficiency, may manifest numbness and paresthesia of the extremities, ataxia, poor coordination, and eventually, mental status changes, which range from minimal forgetfulness to dementia and psychosis.

5. Diagnosis

   a. Low erythrocyte count

   b. Significant macrocytosis (MCV greater than 100)

   c. Low reticulocyte count

   d. Peripheral blood smear usually reveals anisocytosis, poikilocytosis, and macroovalocytis.

   e. Iron-deficiency anemia frequently complicates folate deficiency, making interpretation of a peripheral smear difficult.

   f. A definitive diagnosis frequently requires a bone marrow aspirate, which characteristically appears cellular with a decreased myeloid-to-erythroid ratio.

   g. Other findings may include purpura, hemolytic jaundice, thrombocytopenia, and bleeding diathesis.

6. When the diagnosis is confirmed, rapid reversal can occur with appropriate therapy.

7. Megaloblastic anemia has been linked to prematurity, low birth weights, preeclampsia, and abruptio placenta.

Thalassemias

1. Normal adult hemoglobin is 95% hemoglobin A and consists of two α and two β chains that form a tetramine protein.

2. Of the six different, possible globin chains in the human genome, the α and β chains are affected most in the thalassemias (Table 2.11).

   a. All forms of thalassemia are autosomal recessive traits.

   b. With suppression or absence of α- or β-chain synthesis, hemoglobin precipitation and shortened red blood cell lifespan occur.

3. The α-hemoglobin monomer is encoded on four genes.

   a. The absence of all four α-globin chains is incompatible with life and results in hydrops fetalis. The γ tetramers

Table 2.11. Composition of hemoglobins found in normal human development and abnormal hemoglobins found in thalassemia

Globin Chains	Hemoglobin	State
$\alpha_2\beta_2$	A	Adult
$\alpha_2\delta_2$	A_2	Adult
$\alpha_2{}^A\gamma_2$	F	Fetus
$\alpha_2{}^G\gamma_2$	F	Fetus
$\alpha_2\varepsilon_2$	Gower 2	Embryo
$\xi_2\varepsilon_2$	Gower 1	Embryo
$\xi_2\gamma_2$	Portland	Embryo
β_2	H	α-thalassemia
γ_4	Bart's	α-thalassemia
α_2 precipitate	—	β-thalassemia

      that form have such high oxygen affinity that release to tissues does not occur. High-output congestive heart failure and end-organ ischemia cause fetal death.

    b. In the absence of three α chains, hemoglobin H is formed.

    c. The presence of two normal α chains results in α-thalassemia minor, and these patients usually have a mild anemia.

    d. The presence of three normal α chains generally does not cause anemia.

    e. Patients with α-thalassemia trait and hemoglobin H disease have no increased incidence of fetal wastage with normal hemoglobin. However, maternal splenomegaly and bone marrow hyperplasia are not uncommon.

4. The β chain is encoded by only two genes.

    a. β-Thalassemia major is homozygous,

    b. β-Thalassemia minor is heterozygous.

    c. β-Thalassemia major is detected several months after birth as a severe anemia.

        i. Infants will require frequent transfusions.

        ii. Complications of excessive iron may result in death by the second or third decade.

        iii. Few women with β-thalassemia major reach reproductive age.

            (1) At puberty, these women are frequently amenorrheic due to hypogonadotropic hypogonadism.

            (2) Pregnancy, when it does occur, does not have a deleterious effect on the course of thalassemia.

            (3) Even β-thalassemia major patients who are transfusion dependent can have a successful pregnancy outcome.

        (4)   Anemia, hepatosplenomegaly, bone deformities, and cardiomyopathy, however, may complicate pregnancy.

        (5)   A higher rate for cesarean birth is common due to cephalopelvic disproportion from characteristic short stature and small pelvis of many thalassemia patients.

    d.   β-Thalassemia minor produces either a mild anemia or a completely normal hemoglobin.

Sickle Cell Anemia

1.   Error in the sixth position on the β-globin chain
    a.   Valine substituted for glutamic acid
    b.   This change produces instability of the β chain and decreased solubility of the hemoglobin molecule.
    c.   When oxygen tension falls, the hemoglobin molecule will precipitate and produce the characteristic sickle-shaped red blood cells.
    d.   Heterozygous sickle cell patients
        i.   Twenty-five percent to 40% hemoglobin S.
        ii.   Hemoglobin unlikely to polymerize and precipitate unless hypoxia is severe (p_aO_2 less than 20 mm Hg).
    e.   Homozygous patients
        i.   May have 75% to 100% hemoglobin S
        ii.   Sickling develops at a p_aO_2 of 60 mm Hg.
        iii.   Acidosis worsens sickling by shifting the oxyhemoglobin dissociation curve to the right.
        iv.   The p50 of the parturient is shifted to the right at term secondary to 2,3-DPG and also may potentiate maternal sickling.

2.   The combination of hemoglobin S with other abnormal hemoglobins produces sickle cell disease. In the United States, the most frequent types are hemoglobin SS, hemoglobin SC, and hemoglobin S/β-thalassemia.

3.   Pregnancy and abnormal hemoglobin
    a.   Increased oxygen consumption may be associated with significant morbidity.
    b.   Pregnant women with sickle cell disease increase cardiac output by changing left ventricular end-diastolic volume rather than increasing heart rate or fractional shortening. In the face of additional physiologic stress, these patients could be at risk for cardiovascular compromise if significant diastolic dysfunction occurs.
    c.   Parturients with sickle cell trait tend to have a benign course, and the disease poses little risk to mother or fetus.
    d.   A woman with homozygous sickle cell anemia (hemoglobin SS) is likely to have impaired fertility and limited survival.
        i.   The mortality rate of the homozygous gravida has decreased in recent years with comprehensive and aggressive prenatal care.
        ii.   Nonsickle-related antepartum and intrapartum complication rates are comparable to those of other African-American women.

     iii.   These patients are at high risk for vaso-occlusive and aplastic crises.

     iv.   Thrombotic events in the placenta may lead to fetal loss and IUGR.

Dysplasias

Leukemia

1. Rare during pregnancy
   a. Malignancy complicates an estimated 1 in 1,000 pregnancies.
   b. The incidence of leukemia is less than 1 in 75,000 pregnancies. This low rate may reflect the relative infertility of women with leukemia.
2. The diagnosis of acute leukemia during pregnancy usually requires immediate and aggressive treatment, as mean survival without treatment is approximately 2 months.
   a. Many agents used to treat leukemia are relatively safe during the second and third trimesters of pregnancy.
   b. Some antileukemic cytotoxic drugs can produce teratogenicity, IUGR, and premature birth.
   c. Not infrequently, fetal death, prematurity, and teratogenesis occur.
   d. Aggressive and appropriate management of some patients with acute leukemia (promyelocytic disease) can result in live births with complete remission of disease.
   e. Cardiac or pulmonary complications, as well as thrombocytopenia, disseminated intravascular coagulation, and opportunistic infection, often produce significant mortality.
3. Chronic myeloid leukemia
   a. Indolent course
   b. Aggressive treatment may be delayed.
   c. Pregnancy lacks effect on the course of chronic leukemia, with more than 90% of women and 80% of fetuses surviving to delivery.
4. Symptoms
   a. The main defect in the leukemias is deregulation of precursor cell differentiation. Subsequently, one cell line proliferates in the bone marrow at the expense of other cell lines.
   b. Hemolysis, diminished red blood cell replacement, thrombocytopenia, and granulocytopenia cause maternal anemia, hemorrhage, and an increased susceptibility to infection.
   c. The gravida's liver, spleen, kidney, lymph node, skin, brain, and meninges may be affected.

Lymphoma

1. The incidence of lymphoma in pregnancy is unknown.
2. From case reports, pregnancy does not adversely affect the course of disease.
3. Prognosis of non-Hodgkin lymphoma in pregnancy is poor due to the insidious nature of the tumor, and treatment during pregnancy has a tendency toward adverse outcomes.

Thrombocytopenia

IDIOPATHIC THROMBOCYTOPENIA PURPURA (ITP)

1. Autoimmune disease caused by an immunoglobulin G (IgG) antibody
   a. Low platelet count
   b. Otherwise normal peripheral blood smear and normal complete blood count
2. Most common in young women and not uncommon in the parturient
3. Maternal mortality may be as high as 5%, and perinatal mortality ranges from 6% to 17%.
4. IgG antibody can cross the placenta and produce thrombocytopenia in the fetus.
   a. No strong correlation exists between maternal and infant platelet counts.
   b. The severity of infant thrombocytopenia may be proportional to the amount of antiplatelet antibody that is transferred across the placenta.
   c. Mothers with a previous splenectomy are at a reduced risk of having thrombocytopenic infants.
   d. A relationship between IgG antibody protein binding in the maternal serum and infant thrombocytopenia also may exist.
5. Intracranial hemorrhage is a major risk for both mother and fetus.
6. Chronic ITP may present with easy bruising and petechiae, menorrhagia, or epistaxis.
7. Treatment
   a. According to the clinical guidelines proposed by the American Society of Hematology,[1] pregnant women with ITP and platelet counts greater than 50,000 per liter do not routinely require treatment.[3]
   b. Treatment is reserved for women with platelet counts less than 10,000 per liter and women with platelet counts of 10,000 to 30,000 per liter who are bleeding or are in the second or third trimester of pregnancy.
   c. Intravenous IgG is the recommended initial treatment.
      i. Intravenous IgG raises the patient's serum IgG concentration and impairs reticuloendothelial cell function, sparing the sensitized platelets from clearance.
      ii. The platelet-elevating effect generally lasts less than 3 weeks, and treatment is repeated several times throughout pregnancy.
   d. Glucocorticoid therapy, usually 1 to 2 mg per kilograms per day of oral prednisone or pulsed high-dose oral dexamethasone also may be started and then tapered when the platelet count begins to rise.
      i. To elevate both the maternal and fetal platelet counts, parturients with low platelet counts have their steroid regimens increased in the final weeks of gestation.
      ii. Because placental enzymes inactivate most of the administered prednisone, some substitute dexamethasone or betamethasone.

e. Splenectomy has been advocated for the parturient resistant to steroids and intravenous IgG.
    i. Attempt to schedule surgery during the second trimester.
        (1) The risk of preterm labor is reduced.
        (2) The gravid uterus does not interfere with surgical exposure.
    ii. Splenectomy is usually avoided in asymptomatic parturients with platelet counts greater than 10,000 per liter.
f. Immunosuppressive therapy
    i. Reserved for the most refractory cases
    ii. Administration is limited to after fetal organogenesis.
g. Platelet transfusions
    i. Only effective for several hours
    ii. Usage is reserved for severe bleeding or when surgery is planned.
h. Treatment risks
    i. Steroid related: maternal hyperglycemia, hypertension, and postpartum psychosis, fetal adrenal suppression
    ii. Platelet transfusion may place the parturient at risk for a transfusion-related complication.
    iii. Splenectomy during pregnancy has high risk of fetal loss.
8. Although platelet count falls in the face of autoimmune hyperdestruction, the platelets present are usually younger, larger, and superfunctional.

GESTATIONAL THROMBOCYTOPENIA

1. Occurs in approximately 5% of parturients
2. Often an incidental finding during the late third trimester
    a. Other screening coagulation tests and bone marrow examination usually prove normal.
    b. Platelet count returns to normal in the postpartum period.
3. Not normally associated with increased bleeding or adverse maternal or fetal outcomes
4. No specific therapy is recommended, as there is no increased risk of bleeding.
5. Differential diagnosis
    a. Platelet count may drop to as low as 80,000 per milliliter during normal pregnancy.
    b. Patients with idiopathic immune thrombocytopenia cannot be distinguished from those with gestational thrombocytopenia by the platelet antiglobulin test currently used. Glycogen-specific assays may be more useful.

HUMAN IMMUNODEFICIENCY VIRUS

1. Human immunodeficiency virus (HIV)-positive parturients may manifest thrombocytopenia in the early asymptomatic stage, as well as in the advanced acquired immunodeficiency syndrome (AIDS)-related complex stage.

2. Several theories have been suggested to explain this association.
    a. Accelerated platelet destruction by autoantibodies
    b. Platelet sequestration in the spleen
    c. A production defect from bone marrow suppression
    d. Infection of megakaryocytes
3. Maternal hemorrhage and fetal thrombocytopenia are possible.
4. As early HIV infection develops into clinical AIDS, the platelet count and function may normalize.

PREECLAMPSIA AND ECLAMPSIA

1. Most common cause of thrombocytopenia in pregnancy
2. Approximately 15% of parturients with preeclampsia will have some form of consumptive thrombocytopenia.
3. The incidence is even greater in the patient with eclampsia.
4. Patients with preeclampsia who have a platelet count less than 100,000 per milliliter also may have other abnormal coagulation tests.
5. Platelet dysfunction may occur despite a normal platelet count. Platelet aggregation studies find both activated, hyperaggregable platelets and exhausted, hypoaggregable platelets in the circulation of patients with preeclampsia.

DRUG-INDUCED THROMBOCYTOPENIA

1. An extensive list of drugs can act as antigenic stimuli, resulting in an autoimmune thrombocytopenia, which is an indistinguishable idiopathic thrombocytopenia except that resolution occurs with cessation of the offending agent.
2. The typical drugs include aspirin, penicillin, streptomycin, sulfa drugs, phenobarbital, heparin, and isoniazid. Aspirin irreversibly acetylates cyclooxygenase, a thromboxane precursor, and impairs platelet function. Nonsteroidal antiinflammatory agents competitively inhibit cyclooxygenase reversibly.
3. Heparin-induced thrombocytopenia may have both immunologic and nonimmunologic mechanisms.
    a. Life-threatening arterial and venous thrombosis may occur in patients taking heparin.
    b. Platelet transfusions can worsen the clinical picture.
    c. The fetus is not directly affected, as heparin does not cross the placenta.
    d. Platelet function usually recovers within 5 days after termination of heparin therapy.

Hemophilias

VON WILLEBRAND DISEASE

1. Most common congenital hemorrhagic disorder
2. Results from a qualitative or quantitative defect of von Willebrand factor (vWF).
    a. vWF serves as a molecular bridge between platelets and damaged subendothelium on the vessel wall (Fig. 2.2).
    b. In addition, it modulates circulation of factor VIII.

Blood Flow

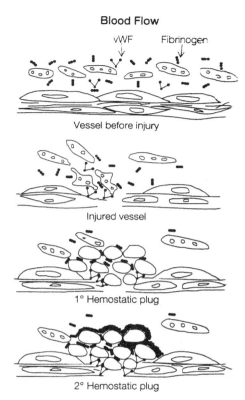

Fig. 2.2. Primary and secondary hemostasis in flowing blood after vessel injury. (Source: From Hawiger J. Formation and regulation of platelet and fibrin hemostatic plug. *Hum Pathol* 1987;18:111, with permission.)

    c. Defects in vWF are characterized by abnormal platelet function and a decrease in factor VIII.

    d. Classic, type 1 vWD
        i. Autosomal dominant with variable penetrance
        ii. Manifestations from no evidence of disease to a moderate reduction in hemostatic function range

    e. Type 2 vWD is usually associated with a qualitative defect in vWF.

    f. The recessively inherited type 3 vWD is characterized by a quantitative defect in vWF and results in severely decreased levels of factor VIII.

3. Factor VIII
    a. A protein complex consisting of
        i. von Willebrand factor (VIII:vWF).
           (1) A large glycoprotein
           (2) Allows aggregation of platelets to proceed

(3) Essential for the formation of a primary hemostatic plug after injury

(4) Also regulates the production and release of factor VIII:C

ii. Factor procoagulant activity (VIII:C).

(1) Factor VIII:C measures the biologic activity of factor VIII.

(2) This factor is part of the intrinsic coagulation cascade. It is needed for the formation of a definitive hemostatic plug.

b. Factor VIII-related antigen (VIIIR:Ag) represents the antigenic determinants of vWF.

4. Symptoms

a. Although not a primary platelet disorder, because vWF is essential for platelet aggregation, the pattern of bleeding is similar to that found in patients with dysfunctional platelets.

b. Patients may present with menorrhagia, epistaxis, and bleeding from mucous membranes or intravenous sites.

c. Mildly afflicted patients may have no symptoms.

5. Diagnosis

a. Often made following excessive surgical bleeding after dental extractions or minor surgery

b. Partial thromboplastin time is abnormal because of the decreased coagulant activity of factor VIII.

c. Bleeding time is prolonged secondary to the decrease in factor VIII:vWF.

6. Effects of pregnancy

a. In normal pregnancy, factor VIII:C and factor VIIIR:Ag increase 200% and 375%, respectively.

b. Parturients with vWD also show an increase in factor concentration, but, by term, they have only half the amounts that a normal parturient will have.

c. The increase in factor concentrations with gestation may improve coagulation.

d. There is no increase in maternal mortality or fetal loss.

e. These women are at high risk for postpartum hemorrhage, as factor VIII:C and factor VIIIR:Ag concentrations fall precipitously (within a few hours) to nonpregnant levels.

f. Bleeding problems tend to recur about 1 week postpartum, or at the time of abortion.

HEMOPHILIA A

1. A sex-linked recessive disorder characterized by a lack of procoagulant activity of factor VIII.

2. Female carriers have a genetic defect on one X chromosome and a second normal gene.

3. Pathophysiology

a. Clotting factor level is approximately 50% of normal.

b. Patients with factor VIII levels of at least 25% of normal clot without difficulty.

c. Patients with hemophilia A become symptomatic when factor VIII activity falls below 5%.

    d. Patients with less than 1% factor VIII activity have severe disease.

4. Symptoms
   a. Hemophiliac bleeding may occur up to days after injury, involve any organ, and, left untreated, may continue for days or weeks.
   b. Compartment syndromes, pseudophlebitis, or ischemic damage to compressed nerves may follow.
   c. Most often, these patients bleed into soft tissues, muscles, and weight-bearing joints.
5. Phenotypic hemophilia in women is extremely rare, and acquired hemophilia is an unusual cause of postpartum hemorrhage.
6. Pregnancy increases the concentration of factor VIII:C.
   a. Carriers may reach normal levels by term.
   b. With the rapid fall of factor VIII activity postpartum, abnormal bleeding following delivery may resume.
7. Affected male fetuses are at risk for scalp and intracranial hemorrhage during labor and delivery from the use of invasive monitoring techniques, prolonged labor, and instrumental deliveries.

Autologous Blood Donation

1. In recent years, concerns about the risk of blood transfusion have led to a significantly increased use of autologous blood donation in the nonobstetric population.
2. In the obstetric population, premature delivery and pre-existing anemia may limit autologous blood donation.
3. For patients undergoing elective cesarean sections, the donation procedure has been well tolerated. With a predonation level higher than 11 g per deciliter, there have been no adverse effects reported to either mother or fetus.
4. Most data suggest that autologous blood donation is not a cost-effective way to prevent transfusion related complications.

NOTE

1. See ref. 222 in Chapter 2, *Obstetric Anesthesia,* Second Edition.

REFERENCES

1. Dajani AS, Taubert KA, Wilson W, et al. Prevention of bacterial endocarditis recommendation by the American Heart Association. *JAMA* 1997;277:1794.
2. Horlocker TT, Wedel DJ. Neuraxial block and low-molecular-weight heparin: Balancing perioperative analgesia and thromboprophylaxis. *Reg Anesth Pain Med* 1998;23:S164.
3. The American Society of Hematology ITP Practice Guideline Panel. Diagnosis and treatment of idiopathic thrombocytopenic purpura: Recommendations of the American Society of Hematology. *Ann Intern Med* 1997;126:319.

Preoperative Evaluation of the Parturient with Coexisting Disease: Pulmonary and Neuromuscular Disease, Acquired Immunodeficiency Syndrome, and Substance Abuse

RESPIRATORY DISEASE

Asthma

1. Most common pulmonary disease in women of childbearing age
2. Complicates approximately 1% of pregnancies.

Pathophysiology

1. The tracheobronchial tree is more sensitive to a variety of stimuli.
2. Bronchospasm and the major symptoms of asthma (dyspnea, wheezing, and cough) occur in response to provocation.
3. Symptoms vary.
   a. Mild and almost undetectable
   b. Severe and unremitting syndrome of status asthmaticus
4. Physiologic effects
   a. Intermittent small-airway obstruction
      i. Is most marked on expiration (wheezing).
      ii. Leads to air trapping and hyperinflation.
   b. Hypersecretion of mucus
   c. Mucosal edema
   d. Smooth muscle hypercontractility
5. Factors that can precipitate bronchospasm include
   a. IgE-mediated hypersensitivity to inhaled irritants.
   b. Acute inflammatory disease.
   c. Cold.
   d. Exercise.
   e. Aspirin.
   f. Non–immune-mediated (direct) bronchoconstriction to inhaled substances (e.g., animal dander, dust, and smoke).
   g. Emotional stress.
   h. Mechanical stimulation (e.g., intubation of the trachea).
6. Several theories attempt to explain the pathophysiology of asthma.
   a. Asthma may represent an imbalance between the sympathetic and parasympathetic nervous systems.
      i. Vagal and α-adrenergic effects predominate over β-adrenergic action.

ii. Stimulation of parasympathetic airway fibers increases intracellular cyclic guanosine monophosphate (cGMP), which promotes bronchoconstriction and airflow obstruction.
b. Asthma patients may produce autoantibodies to β-adrenergic receptors.
c. Asthma may arise from inflammatory pulmonary changes that various stimuli produce in susceptible individuals.
   i. On reexposure of an individual to a particular allergen, an antigen–antibody complex forms and binds to specific mast cell receptors.
   ii. Mast cells degranulate and release vasoactive and cell-mediator biochemicals (histamine, leukotrienes, prostaglandins, platelet-activating factor, and cell chemotactic factors).
      (1) Mediators produce vascular and airway changes, which lead to symptoms.
      (2) Mediators also attract inflammatory cells (macrophages and eosinophils) that cause further capillary endothelial and airway epithelial cell damage. This damage increases vascular permeability and incites airway hyperreactivity, inciting additional bronchoconstriction and mucosal edema.

7. Clinical evidence of obstruction includes wheezing, hyperinflated lung volumes, and decreased forced expiratory volume. The ultimate effects of obstruction are ventilation—perfusion abnormalities with resultant hypoxemia and hypercarbia. Bronchoconstriction reverses when sympathetic stimulation of β_2 receptors increases intracellular cyclic adenosine monophosphate (cAMP). By interfering with bronchial smooth muscle actinomycin activity, cAMP produces muscle relaxation and bronchodilation.

Interaction with Pregnancy

EFFECT OF PREGNANCY ON ASTHMA

1. Few studies show a consistent effect of pregnancy on pre-existing asthma. Two things seem clear:
   a. Patients with severe asthma before pregnancy will have the most severe exacerbations during pregnancy.
   b. The course of asthma in previous pregnancies is the best predictor of the course in future pregnancies.
2. The most common causes for exacerbation are respiratory tract infection (59%) and noncompliance with therapeutic regimens (27%).
3. Pregnancy-related changes that may worsen asthma:
   a. Prostaglandin F2α (a known bronchoconstrictor) increases
   b. Changes in cell-mediated immunity may increase susceptibility to infection.
4. Pregnancy-related changes that may improve asthma:
   a. Plasma concentrations of cortisol and progesterone (which induce smooth muscle relaxation) rise.

b.   The correlation between serum progesterone concentration and airway response is weak. Therefore, if progesterone does improve asthma, it does not work alone.

EFFECT OF ASTHMA ON PREGNANCY

1.   Maternal asthma may increase the frequency of hemorrhage, hyperemesis, toxemia, neonatal deaths, preterm deliveries, and low-birth-weight infants.
2.   Maternal hypoxemia and respiratory alkalosis may severely compromise the fetus.
    a.   Maternal–fetal oxygen exchange depends on, among other things, maternal arterial oxygen tension and the oxygen affinity of maternal blood.
        i.   Maternal hypoxemia lessens the maternal–fetal oxygen diffusion gradient, hindering oxygen delivery to the fetus.
        ii. Maternal alkalosis causes a leftward shift of the oxyhemoglobin dissociation curve, resulting in a greater affinity of maternal hemoglobin for oxygen and less exchange to the fetus.
    b.   The fetus rapidly develops hypoxemia and risks vital organ damage when its oxygen supply is compromised.
3.   Status asthmaticus during pregnancy can harm both mother and fetus.
4.   Aggressive management of asthma to prevent episodes of status asthmaticus may improve pregnancy outcome.

Pharmacotherapy

1.   Management goals in treating asthma include:
    a.   Identification and removal of precipitating factors.
    b.   Proper rest, nutrition, and hydration.
    c.   Aggressive antibiotic treatment of infection.
    d.   Pharmacotherapy where indicated.
2.   Pharmacotherapy for pregnant asthmatics differs very little from that used in the nonpregnant patient. The available evidence suggest that commonly employed drugs are safe for use in the pregnant patient.

BRONCHODILATOR AGENTS

1.   β-Agonists
    a.   β-Adrenergic stimulation relaxes bronchial smooth muscle by increasing intracellular concentrations of cAMP.
    b.   β-Agonist bronchodilators are safe for use throughout pregnancy.
    c.   β-Agonists may interfere with normal labor due to uterine relaxation and may contribute to postpartum uterine atony and hemorrhage.
    d.   Terbutaline, metaproterenol, salmeterol, and albuterol are the most β_2-selective agents.
    e.   Aerosol administration speeds onset and reduces the side effects from systemic absorption.
    f.   Epinephrine
        i.   Has α-adrenergic (possible uteroplacental vasoconstriction) effects along with nonspecific β-adrenergic activity

ii. While not a first line treatment for acute asthma, do not hesitate to use epinephrine in cases of life-threatening bronchospasm refractory to other therapies.

2. Parasympatholytics
    a. Ipratropium bromide relaxes bronchial smooth muscles by competitive inhibition of vagus-mediated broncho-constriction.
    b. Aerosol administration minimizes systemic anticholinergic effects (e.g., tachycardia, dry mouth).

3. Methylxanthines
    a. Theophylline and its water-soluble salt aminophylline are methylxanthines.
    b. The exact mechanism of action of these agents is unknown. Methylxanthines may
        i. Inhibit phosphodiesterase, the enzyme responsible for the breakdown of cAMP.
        ii. Modulate the interaction of actinomycin and calcium.
        iii. Antagonize prostaglandins.
        iv. Inhibit adenosine
            (1) Releases endogenous catecholamines
            (2) Attenuates the release of mast cell mediators.
    c. Methylxanthines have a long record of safe use in pregnancy and have traditionally been used as adjuvants to β-agonist therapy. However, aminophylline does not significantly enhance the bronchodilation provided by standard β-agonist—steroid therapy in adult asthma exacerbations.

ANTIINFLAMMATORY AGENTS

1. Steroids
    a. Steroids function by altering protein production, inhibiting mediator release, and suppressing inflammatory mediator action.
    b. Steroids regulate protein synthesis through gene induction. Glucocorticoids activate cell receptors. The activated receptor complex binds to the nucleus and then to gene regulators. The regulator then activates or inhibits gene transcription and ultimately increases or decreases protein production by that gene.
    c. During an acute asthma exacerbation, steroids increase the synthesis of proteins that inhibit the production of prostaglandins and platelet-activating factor. They also increase the synthesis of new β_2 receptors.
    d. Steroids increase the responsiveness of β receptors to catecholamines, potentiate β-agonist bronchodilation, and reverse β-receptor fatigue from prolonged stimulation.
    e. Steroids reduce airway edema by inhibiting the release of chemical mediators and suppressing their adverse effect on microvascular permeability.
    f. Finally, steroids inhibit the formation of inflammatory cell chemotactic mediators and inactivate inflammatory cells already involved in the asthma process.
    g. Steroid use in pregnancy

   i.   Similar to use in treating nonpregnant asthmatics
  ii.   Although high-dose systemic steroids may be life-saving in treating acute asthma, some therapeutic actions have a lengthy onset. Use alternative therapies to medicate the attack until steroid onset.
 iii.   Steroid use in the chronic asthmatic
      (1) Use the lowest effective dose.
      (2) Aerosol administration may help eliminate or reduce systemic steroid use. It also localizes the action of steroids and reduces systemic side effects, thereby minimizing the risk of adrenal suppression.
      (3) If patients have used high-dose systemic steroids for 1 month or longer, adrenal suppression is possible. Taper doses when discontinuing the drug.
      (4) During periods of increased physiologic stress, these patients may require steroid supplementation.
  2. Cromolyn sodium
     a. Is an aerosol agent.
     b. Prevents degranulation of mast cells by membrane stabilization.
     c. It is safe in pregnancy, but only as a prophylactic agent.
     d. Do not use it to treat acute bronchospasm because it cannot counter effects of previously released substances.

Evaluation
  1. History is the most valuable tool in evaluating a stable asthmatic (Table 3.1). Asking the patient how she rates her current ability to breathe provides a rough idea of the degree of bronchospasm.

Table 3.1.   Pertinent history in parturients with acute exacerbation of asthma

Previous attacks
   Number
   Severity
   Duration
Previous emergency room visits
   Number
   Most recent
Previous need for intubation and mechanical ventilation
Course of asthma in previous pregnancies
Current therapy
   Medications
   Compliance
Known precipitating factors
Environmental exposures
Recent or current upper respiratory infection
Coexisting pulmonary or cardiac problems

2. In an acute crisis, however, management of hypoxia and respiratory compromise take precedence over gathering history.
3. Physical examination
   a. General appearance: Marked tachypnea, cyanosis, and fatigue signal impending respiratory failure.
   b. Wheezing is evidence of diffuse bronchoconstriction and is a sign of air exchange; lack of wheezing is more serious and denotes inability to ventilate.
   c. Increasing use of accessory muscles and nostril flaring point to worsening distress.
   d. Note the patient's ability to converse. A patient who can speak in sentences is less ill than one working so hard to breathe that she cannot speak at all.
   e. Tachycardia is a compensatory response to stress and hypoxia; bradycardia may precede hypoxic cardiac arrest. A decrease in heart rate of 15 beats per minute or greater with inspiration (pulsus paradoxus) is a nonspecific indication of a severe attack.
   f. An elevated temperature may signal acute infection.
4. Other data
   a. A complete blood count may suggest acute infection.
   b. Gram stain any sputum.
   c. Evaluate a chest radiograph for any acute underlying infectious process, hyperinflation, pneumothorax, or pneumomediastinum.
   d. An arterial blood gas can be critical in evaluating severity.
      i. Remember that blood gas values normally change in pregnancy.
      ii. The blood gas will uniformly show hypoxemia; therefore, this parameter is not as useful as a pH and p_aCO_2.
      iii. If the patient has alkalosis and lower-than-normal pregnancy p_aCO_2 (32 mm Hg), the attack is mild.
      iv. If the observed pH and p_aCO_2 are normal for pregnancy, the attack is more severe.
      v. Acidosis and hypercapnia (pH = 7.35, p_aCO_2 = 35 to 38 mm Hg) signal impending respiratory failure, especially combined with a p_aO_2 less than 60 mm Hg.
5. Serial spirometry can determine the efficacy of therapy.
6. For a summary of the treatment of acute asthma, refer to Table 3.2.

Differential Diagnosis

1. The initial reaction to acute respiratory distress may be to assume that its etiology is asthma. However, the following causes of respiratory distress should be eliminated:
   a. Acute upper airway obstruction
   b. Pulmonary embolism
   c. Anaphylaxis
   d. Congestive heart failure
   e. Acute infection
   f. Chronic obstructive pulmonary disease
   g. Aspiration pneumonitis

Table 3.2.   Treatment of acute asthma

Unstable Asthma	Stable Asthma
Correct hypoxemia and acidosis	Obtain history
Support ventilation, if necessary	Remove precipitating factors
Give supplemental oxygen	Hydrate
Give bronchodilators and steroids	Obtain clinical studies (labs, arterial blood gas, chest radiograph, spirometry, sputum stain)
Treat underlying cause	Initiate pharmacotherapy
Proceed to *stable asthma*	Bronchodilators
treatment when stable	Steroids
	Consider aminophylline
	Antibiotics for infection
	Repeat clinical studies to assess efficacy of therapy

Cystic Fibrosis (CF)

1. This multisystem, autosomal recessive disorder occurs in approximately 1 in 1,000 births. It is the most common lethal genetic disorder in Whites.
2. The disease is one of chronic exocrine gland dysfunction, but the underlying defect is unknown.
   a. These patients produce thick, tenacious mucus.
   b. They suffer pancreatic insufficiency with accompanying protein and fat malabsorption.
   c. Hepatobiliary disease with chronic cholestasis, fibrosis, and cirrhosis occurs.
   d. Abnormally high sweat duct excretion of sodium chloride is seen.
3. Patients typically are diagnosed early in childhood, but milder forms of the disease may not be recognized until much later.
4. The average survival of patients with CF is 20 to 30 years, with death usually from respiratory failure. Patients have persistent bronchial infections, usually with *Pseudomonas aeruginosa*. Chronic infection generates airway fibrosis and, later, parenchymal fibrosis, ventilation–perfusion mismatching, and hypoxemia.
5. Improved survival of CF patients has allowed women to reach childbearing age.
   a. The maternal outcome of pregnancy correlates with maternal condition before conception.
   b. Pregnancy does not influence the course of the disease.
   c. Maternal condition during gestation predicts perinatal outcome. Chronically, hypoxemic and malnourished

mothers have increased perinatal morbidity and mortality, whereas well-managed mothers with mild disease have improved outcomes.

6. Treatment of CF aims at the reparatory system
   a. Aggressive antibiotic therapy for infection, along with avid pharmacologic and physiotherapeutic measures to facilitate removal of secretions, are the mainstays of management.
   b. Additionally, pancreatic enzyme replacement will decrease gastrointestinal malabsorption, and vitamin K supplementations can correct bleeding problems that arise from poor hepatic function or malabsorption of fat-soluble vitamins.

7. The preanesthetic evaluation of the pregnant patient with CF focuses on the degree of respiratory compromise.
   a. Ensure that the patient is in the best possible pulmonary condition.
   b. Hydrate her well to help with secretions.
   c. If there is any suspicion of a pulmonary infection, obtain a sputum gram stain and initiate appropriate antibiotic therapy.
   d. Laboratory evaluation can detect electrolyte imbalance, acute infection, or coagulation defect.
   e. Arterial blood gas tensions or pulse oximetry will detect hypoxemia. Changes with time may help in assessing the degree of respiratory deterioration.

Cigarette Smoking

1. Smoking during pregnancy has adverse maternal and fetal consequences.
   a. For the mother, smoking increases airway irritability and mucus production, and impairs respiratory tract mucociliary function.
   b. The inhalation of carbon monoxide from smoke produces carboxyhemoglobin, shifting both maternal and fetal oxyhemoglobin dissociation curves leftward. This shift limits oxygen exchange between the mother and fetus and between the fetus and its vital organs.

2. Smoking is the leading risk factor for the development of pulmonary malignancies and chronic obstructive pulmonary disease (COPD).
   a. Because older women, who may have longer smoking histories, are having babies, anesthesiologists are likely to encounter COPD in the parturient.
   b. Superimposing the normal respiratory changes of pregnancy on the changes induced by COPD could produce so great an increase in the work of breathing that decompensation occurs.
   c. Fortunately, however, patients with COPD usually tolerate pregnancy.
   d. Monitor such women closely. It may be difficult to distinguish between the pregnancy-related dyspnea and that caused by worsening pulmonary function.

3. Smoking can complicate pregnancy in several ways.

a. Smokers have a higher incidence of ectopic pregnancy and placental complications, including abruption, previa, and premature calcification.

b. Fetal hazards include growth retardation, which is directly proportional to the number of cigarettes smoked, prematurity, and spontaneous abortion. These effects relate chiefly to chronic fetal hypoxemia (secondary to increased fetal carboxyhemoglobin) and uteroplacental hypoperfusion (from nicotine-induced vasospasm).

4. Treatment of pregnant smokers
    a. Urge cessation of smoking.
        i. In as little as 48 hours, the oxyhemoglobin dissociation curve resumes its normal configuration, increasing oxygen availability.
        ii. In 2 to 3 months, sputum production decreases and ciliary function improves.
    b. Treat any infection with antibiotics.
    c. Use bronchodilators for any bronchospastic component of airway disease.

5. The preanesthetic evaluation
    a. Determine the presence and severity of pulmonary disease.
    b. A history of decreased exercise tolerance and increased cough, sputum production, and dyspnea requires further evaluation.
    c. Laboratory evidence may be helpful.
        i. An elevated leukocyte count may indicate respiratory infection.
        ii. Arterial blood gas analysis may show hypoxemia or hypercarbia.

Sarcoidosis

1. Generalized granulomatous disease with a pulmonary predilection
2. Resulting fibrosis and a restrictive pattern of pulmonary disease can lead to hypoxemia, pulmonary hypertension, and cor pulmonale.
3. Steroids are often useful in the treatment of severe disease.
4. Pregnant patients generally tolerate existing sarcoidosis well.
    a. Monitor oxygenation closely.
    b. A small percentage of these patients have laryngeal involvement, so anticipate airway interference.

Pulmonary Infection

1. Pulmonary infections occur as commonly in pregnant women as in the general population.
2. Like the general population, pregnant women tolerate these illnesses well unless immunocompromised or otherwise afflicted with chronic disease.
    a. Treatment in these special cases must be aggressive.
    b. Prophylaxis with immunizations or pharmacologic agents may be beneficial.
3. The etiology of acute, community-acquired respiratory infection is most often viral (influenza). Such infections are rarely

from varicella. Bacterial infections are uncommon unless the patient is debilitated.
4. Isolate the infecting organism from blood or sputum, and tailor antibiotic therapy accordingly.
5. Fungal pulmonary infections are rare in healthy patients. With the rising number of immunocompromised patients with AIDS, the incidence of fungal infections will likely increase.

NERVOUS SYSTEM DISEASE

1. Pregnant women are susceptible to the same neurologic illnesses as are nonpregnant women.
2. Because improved diagnosis and therapy allow women with neurologic disease to survive to reproductive age, and because older women are becoming pregnant, anesthesiologists will encounter more pregnant patients with these problems.
3. The gross neurologic examination of the healthy gravida is not greatly altered from that of the nonpregnant patient.
   a. Motor function, sensation, and reflexes are the same.
   b. Edema or a changed center of gravity from pregnancy may alter gait.
   c. Cranial nerves are grossly intact, although normal pregnancy-induced hypertrophy of the pituitary gland occasionally alters a visual-field examination.

Seizure Disorders

1. Seizure disorders complicate approximately 0.5% of pregnancies.
2. Seizures are not themselves a disease but are the expression of an underlying neurologic problem.
3. Epilepsy is the ongoing tendency to have seizures.
   a. Seizures can be focal or general, or may begin in a localized fashion and spread to become generalized.
   b. The cerebral cortex, thalamus, and brainstem can be involved.
4. The most common etiology is idiopathic, but intracranial lesions, head trauma, metabolic derangement, hypoxia, cerebral inflammatory disease, and drug toxicity can cause seizures. In pregnancy, eclampsia also may account for seizures.
5. Epilepsy appears to increase the risk of maternal and fetal complications, particularly congenital malformations, prematurity, low birth weight, preeclampsia, stillbirth, hemorrhage, and obstetric intervention. Hypoxia and acidosis incurred during a prolonged seizure or status epilepticus can precipitate fetal distress and, if uncorrected, lead to maternal and fetal demise.
6. Pregnancy has a variable effect on seizure frequency.
   a. About one-fourth of women with seizure disorders experience an increased frequency of seizures, one-fourth have fewer seizures, and in half, the frequency of seizures does not change.
   b. Patients with secondary generalized and complex partial seizures are more likely to experience increased seizure frequency.
   c. Seizure control before pregnancy seems to be the best predictor of control during pregnancy.

d. Although the most common reason for an increase in seizure frequency during pregnancy is poor compliance with anticonvulsant therapy, pregnancy-induced changes in drug metabolism may account for some seizures.

Treatment

1. Anticonvulsants appear to act by reducing the spread of activity from hyperexcitable neurons to normal neurons.
2. They may be used singly or in combination.
   a. The simpler the regimen, the better the compliance and the less likely are side effects and adverse drug interactions.
3. Because all anticonvulsants commonly used in pregnancy have been variably charged with being teratogens, it is vitally important to weigh the risks and benefits of pharmacologic therapy. The American Academy of Pediatrics Select Committee on Anticonvulsants in Pregnancy has made the recommendations shown in Table 3.3.[1]
4. Phenytoin (Dilantin)
   a. The most commonly administered antiepileptic drug
   b. Effective for most types of seizures
   c. Site of action is the motor cortex, where it may promote sodium efflux from neurons, thus stabilizing the membrane hyperexcitability threshold.
   d. Clearance is via the liver.
   e. Maternal side effects include gastrointestinal distress, skin rash, pancytopenia, megaloblastic anemia, systemic lupus erythematous, gingival hyperplasia, and peripheral polyneuropathy.
   f. Toxic manifestations include ataxia, nystagmus, and dysarthria progressing to respiratory and circulatory depression.
   g. Phenytoin has been implicated as a causative factor in the increased incidence of congenital malformations in the offspring of epileptic women.

Table 3.3. Recommendations for use of anticonvulsants in pregnancy

1. Before conception, withdraw anticonvulsant medication from women who have been seizure-free for many years.
2. A woman taking anticonvulsants should be told that if she becomes pregnant, she will have approximately a 90% chance of having a normal baby. However, the risk of having a baby with mental retardation or congenital malformations is two to three times greater than average.
3. There is no reason to switch a woman from well-known anticonvulsants, such as phenytoin or phenobarbital, to less well known drugs.
4. Do not discontinue medication in women whose seizures are controlled by that medication because seizures may be deleterious to them and their fetuses.

        i.   It is difficult to separate the teratogenic role of the drug from the effects of the underlying disease.

       ii.   Genetic factors in epileptic women may contribute more strongly to birth defects than may any drug.

      iii.   Fetal malformations associated with phenytoin include craniofacial and limb malformations and fetal hydantoin syndrome: growth retardation, mental deficiency, and dysmorphic facial and limb features.

  h. Phenytoin also may cause deficiencies in folic acid and vitamin K-dependent clotting factors. Women should receive folic acid and vitamin K supplements during pregnancy to prevent megaloblastic anemia and hemorrhage.

5. Phenobarbital

  a. Major side effects are sedation, skin rash, and megaloblastic anemia.

  b. Toxic manifestations include nystagmus and ataxia.

  c. Phenobarbital is a potent inducer of hepatic microsomal enzymes and can enhance metabolism of other substances.

  d. Excretion is by the kidneys.

  e. Phenobarbital use correlates with a defects similar to fetal hydantoin syndrome.

  f. Like phenytoin, phenobarbital may cause folate deficiency and coagulopathy.

  g. Phenobarbital may cause neonatal depression and neonatal drug withdrawal.

6. Primidone (Mysoline) is partly metabolized to phenobarbital. Its uses, side effects, and cautions are similar to those for phenobarbital.

7. Carbamazepine (Tegretol)

  a. May be the safest and least teratogenic of the anticonvulsants.

  b. However, little is known about carbamazepine in pregnancy; use caution when considering prescribing it for a well-controlled pregnant epileptic who has been receiving phenytoin or phenobarbital.

  c. Side effects include dizziness, drowsiness, skin rash, and bone marrow depression with aplastic anemia and congestive heart failure.

  d. Neuromuscular symptoms are prominent at toxic drug concentrations.

  e. Elimination is mainly by the renal route.

8. Ethosuximide, clonazepam, trimethadione, and valproic acid

  a. Used to treat petit mal seizures

  b. The few data that exist for ethosuximide and clonazepam suggest that their use in pregnancy is relatively safe.

  c. Trimethadione is the most potent known teratogen among the anticonvulsants, and its use is contraindicated in women of reproductive age.

  d. Valproic acid is associated with craniofacial, limb, and heart malfunctions as well as neural tube defects.

ANTICONVULSANT PHARMACOKINETICS IN PREGNANCY

1. Pregnancy induces several maternal pharmacokinetic changes that may significantly alter serum concentrations of anticonvulsants.
   a. Total protein and albumin content falls and there is less drug–protein binding.
   b. Free fatty acid concentrations rise, displacing drugs from proteins.
   c. This combination allows a higher concentration of pharmacologically active free drug.
   d. Because protein binding is highly variable among individuals, the amount of free drug increase is unpredictable.
   e. Other pharmacologic changes combine to reduce the serum concentration of anticonvulsant drugs.
      i. Bowel absorption of phenytoin falls, probably as a result of decreased gastrointestinal motility and a change in gastric pH. Uptake of other anticonvulsants also may be impaired.
      ii. Volume of distribution increases, diluting serum drug concentrations.
         (1) Increased total body water
         (2) Accumulation of fat
         (3) The addition of fetal, placental, and uterine tissues
      iii. Drug clearance is more rapid.
         (1) Elevated estrogen and progesterone increase hepatic metabolism.
         (2) The drugs themselves may induce liver enzymes to speed metabolism.
      iv. These changes generally require increases in drug doses.
2. Monitor pregnant women taking anticonvulsants closely to ensure therapeutic drug concentrations.
   a. Estimate drug amounts from either plasma or saliva.
   b. Saliva drug concentration correlates well with plasma concentration of pharmacologically active drugs.
3. After delivery, because maternal physiology rapidly reverts to its prepregnancy state, decrease anticonvulsant doses to avoid toxicity.

STATUS EPILEPTICUS AND PREGNANCY

1. Status epilepticus is the repetitive occurrence of grand mal seizures, during which the patient does not regain consciousness. It is a medical emergency.
2. Without treatment, hypoxia, acidosis, and death ensue.
3. The prognosis depends on the promptness of therapy and the etiology of the seizure.
4. Abruptly halting anticonvulsant medication is the most common reason for seizures.
5. Treatment
   a. Maintain a patent airway.
   b. Give intravenous anticonvulsants.
      i. Because of the fatal nature of this condition if left untreated, do not consider the teratogenicity of agents employed.

      ii. Initial therapy
          a. Intravenous benzodiazepine
          b. Followed by phenytoin or phenobarbital
     iii. If these agents fail, induction of general anesthesia with an potent inhalation agent and the use of neuromuscular blocking agent may be needed.

Preoperative Evaluation

1. To avoid the surprise, confusion, and misdiagnosis arising from unexpected convulsions, identify epileptic patients immediately on arrival.
2. Determine
   a. Seizure type.
   b. Frequency of seizures during this and previous pregnancies.
   c. Anticonvulsant regimen.
   d. Compliance.
3. Measure serum or saliva concentrations of drugs and adjust to therapeutic ranges, if necessary.
4. Finally, do a brief baseline neurologic examination to help assess subsequent changes.

Myasthenia Gravis (MG)

1. Chronic autoimmune neuromuscular disorder caused by a loss of functional acetylcholine receptors at the postsynaptic membrane of the neuromuscular junction
   a. About 85% of patients have autoantibodies against acetylcholine receptors.
   b. In the remaining patients, autoantibodies binding to nonacetylcholine receptor neuromuscular junction determinants induce the receptor loss.
2. Incidence is approximately 1 in 15,000 to 20,000 adults.
   a. Usually manifests in the third decade
   b. Affects women twice as often as men
3. Characteristically, the disease produces exacerbations and remissions of muscle weakness and fatigue, especially of oculomotor, facial, laryngeal, and reparatory muscles.
   a. May be associated with cardiomegaly or other autoimmune diseases
   b. Emotional or physiologic stress, infection, electrolyte imbalance, aminoglycoside antibiotics, magnesium sulfate, and neuromuscular blocking agents can precipitate or aggravate muscle weakness.

Interaction with Pregnancy

1. Pregnancy affects MG in unpredictable ways.
   a. In approximately equal numbers of patients, the disease stays the same, gets worse, or gets better.
   b. The course of MG in previous pregnancies does not predict the course in subsequent pregnancies.
   c. Respiratory difficulty and inadequate expulsive efforts from muscle fatigue during the second stage are the only effects on labor and delivery.

      d. Stress or infection during labor may precipitate a myasthenic crisis with severe weakness with respiratory insufficiency.

      e. Cholinergic crisis also presents with severe weakness; however, these women have evidence of muscarinic receptor stimulation with nausea, vomiting, lacrimation, and diarrhea.

2. Because of transplacental transfer of antibodies, the newborn may show signs of MG.

    a. Symptoms may not appear for days.

    b. Some infants require treatment, but the condition usually is transient.

Treatment

1. The goal of treating MG is to increase the function of the acetylcholine receptors.

    a. Increase the amount of endogenous acetylcholine.

    b. Decrease the amount or function of acetylcholine receptor autoantibodies.

2. There are four current approaches to therapy:

    a. Administration of anticholinesterase drugs.

    b. Immunosuppression.

    c. Plasmapheresis.

    d. Surgical thymectomy.

3. Anticholinesterase drugs

    a. Edrophonium, neostigmine, and pyridostigmine

        i. Quaternary ammonium structures that reversibly inhibit of acetylcholinesterase.

           (1) Acetylcholinesterase is found anywhere in the body there is acetylcholine.

           (2) By converting acetylcholine to acetic acid and choline, acetylcholinesterase terminates the action of acetylcholine.

           (3) Inhibition of acetylcholinesterase increases the amount of acetylcholine available for neurotransmission and thereby augments the ability of skeletal muscle to respond to repetitive stimuli.

        ii. Edrophonium

           (1) Forms an electrostatic attachment to acetylcholinesterase.

           (2) Prevents the proper alignment of acetylcholine.

           (3) Because the electrostatically bound complex is weak, acetylcholine can easily compete for binding sites, and the therapeutic effect of edrophonium is short-lived.

           (4) The main use of edrophonium is in diagnosing MG and assessing the adequacy of anticholinesterase therapy.

               (a) Give intravenous edrophonium in small (1-mg) doses every minute or two until weakness improves.

> > (i) In new-onset MG, this test is diagnostic.
> > (ii) In treated patients, improvement shows that current therapy is inadequate.
> (b) Administering edrophonium to patients with weakness from cholinergic crisis (anticholinesterase overdose) will not improve symptoms.

iii. Neostigmine and pyridostigmine
  (1) Produce reversible carbamyl–ester complexes with acetylcholinesterase.
  (2) Competitively inhibit the enzyme interaction with acetylcholine and act longer than edrophonium.

iv. The pharmacologic effect of anticholinesterase agents is present at both muscarinic and nicotinic receptors.
  (1) Nicotinic receptors are responsible for effects at the neuromuscular junction.
  (2) Muscarinic receptors effect such responses as bradycardia, salivation, and emesis.
  (3) If necessary, control muscarinic side effects with anticholinergic agents.

v. Anticholinesterase agents impair the function of plasma cholinesterase and may prolong the actions of succinylcholine and ester local anesthetics.

vi. Continue anticholinesterase therapy throughout labor and delivery.
  (1) Because gastric absorption of drugs during labor may be erratic, administer by intravenous or intramuscular routes.
  (2) To prevent further muscle weakness, avoid agents with muscle-relaxing properties, such as neuromuscular blockers, magnesium sulfate, and certain antibiotics (e.g., gentamicin and erythromycin).

4. When anticholinesterase drugs are inadequate, immunosuppression may prove beneficial.
  a. The common immunosuppressants (prednisone, azathioprine, and cyclophosphamide) prevent the production of, or reduce the circulating concentration of, acetylcholine receptor antibodies.
  b. No controlled data prove the efficacy of these agents in pregnancy.
  c. Some immunosuppressants are potentially teratogenic (i.e., azathioprine and cyclophosphamide) and should be avoided during gestation.

5. Plasmapheresis
  a. Uncommon therapy for MG
  b. Aimed at reducing circulating autoantibodies
  c. Consider its use when conventional therapeutic measures have failed.
  d. Plasmapheresis may benefit the acetylcholine receptor antibody–negative subset of MG patients.

6. Surgical thymectomy
   a. Aims to remove the source of antibody production.
   b. Yields favorable remission rates.
   c. It is unclear which patients benefit most from thymectomy:
      i. Patients with moderate or advanced disease may benefit more than those with mild symptoms.
      ii. The presence of acetylcholine receptor antibodies and thymic hyperplasia may be the best predictors of a favorable response to thymectomy.
7. Table 3.4 provides a quick reference for MG.

Preoperative Evaluation
1. Assess the degree of neuromuscular weakness.
2. Look closely for evidence of respiratory compromise.
   a. Determine the ability to maintain a patent airway (e.g., can she cough and clear secretions?).
3. Catalogue the current drug regimen and previous therapies and their efficacies.
   a. If a patient who is treated with an anticholinesterase agent exhibits weakness, a trial of edrophonium may help determine the adequacy of her current regimen.

Table 3.4.   Summary of myasthenia gravis in pregnancy

Autoimmune	85% acetylcholine receptor
	15% nonacetylcholine-receptor autoantibodies
Onset	Third decade
Epidemiology	Women two times the frequency of men
Characteristics	Exacerbations and remissions of muscle fatigue
Associated diseases	Cardiomegaly
	Other autoimmune diseases
Precipitators	Stress
	Infection
	Electrolyte imbalance
	Neuromuscular blocking agents
Interaction with pregnancy	Unpredictable
	Early second-stage fatigue
Interaction with neonate	Transient MG syndrome
Diagnosis	Administer edrophonium until weakness improves
Treatment	Anticholinesterase
	Thymectomy
	Plasmapheresis
Cholinergic crisis	
Symptoms	Weakness
	Diarrhea
	Excessive salivation
Treatment	Anticholinergics (atropine)

    b. Consider anticholinergic crisis if edrophonium fails to alleviate symptoms.

4. Ask about coexisting major diseases.
5. A brief baseline neurologic examination may prove helpful in determining subsequent changes.

Multiple Sclerosis (MS)

1. A chronic, acquired disorder of the central nervous system (CNS)
2. Multiple, random areas of axonal demyelination (plaques) in the brain and spinal cord
3. Occurs most frequently during the peak reproductive years (20 to 40 years)
4. Affects women twice as often as it does men
5. Has a striking geographic distribution
    a. Higher prevalence in temperate zones than in tropical or subtropical zones
    b. Most likely to affect affluent urban dwellers
6. First-degree relatives of those affected have a 12- to 15-fold increase in incidence, pointing to a genetic predisposition. Sixty percent of patients have a common histocompatibility antigen (HLA-DW2).
7. Disease progression
    a. Some patients suffer a chronic, progressive course.
    b. Most experience periods of exacerbation and remission throughout their disease.
        i. These episodes occur at unpredictable intervals over many years.
        ii. Eventually, residual symptoms persist and the patient experiences disability
8. Typical symptoms include visual disturbances, spastic weakness, fatigue, bowel and bladder dysfunction, sexual dysfunction, gait disturbance, and incoordination. Less common symptoms include alterations in cognitive function and affective disorders.
    a. The symptomatology is a manifestation of the area of demyelination.
    b. For example, if demyelination occurs in the motor pathways, spastic weakness can result, whereas demyelination of frontal and periventricular areas correlates with psychological disturbances.
9. Theories of pathogenesis
    a. Infectious etiology
        i. Most widely held theory
        ii. A virus seems the most likely infectious agent.
            (1) Some viruses cause human and animal demyelinating diseases.
            (2) Presumably, the virus initiates an altered immune response in genetically susceptible individuals, and autoimmune destruction of myelin follows.
            (3) The viruses most often implicated are the measles virus and canine distemper virus.

10. A high-fat diet may be a risk factor for the development of MS.
    a. The pathogenetic mechanism may relate in some way to the predominantly lipid composition of the myelin sheath.
    b. Geographic areas such as Norway and Switzerland and affluent urban areas with diets especially high in animal fat have higher rates of MS.
    c. However, certain populations with a low incidence of MS and high-fat diets contradict this theory.
11. Trauma, especially of the head or spinal column, also may relate to the development of MS.
    a. Trauma alters the blood–brain barrier and may lead to plaque formation in vulnerable individuals.
    b. Others find no evidence that trauma is a causative factor in MS.
12. Industrial workers exposed to zinc have an elevated incidence of MS.
    a. Possibly, a zinc imbalance causes an immunoregulatory defect.
    b. If this were the case, these same workers also should exhibit greater numbers of other immunologically related diseases, but they do not.
13. Environmental exposure to an unknown agent in genetically predisposed individuals may damage oligodendrocyte precursor cells. This damage prevents production of sufficient numbers of oligodendrocytes to maintain myelin.

Diagnosis

1. Exclude other neurologic diseases.
2. Laboratory evidence of demyelination
    a. Slowed nerve conduction on evoked potential testing
    b. Computed tomography (CT) may reveal plaques that are areas of demyelination.
    c. Most patients have elevated CSF immunoglobulin G (IgG) with mononuclear pleocytosis.
    d. Elevated CSF myelin basic protein concentrations signify myelin destruction.

Treatment

1. There is no known cure for MS.
2. Treatment is supportive and aims to decrease the number and duration of exacerbations, decrease disability, and limit the progression of chronic disease.
3. Medical management of acute exacerbations centers around immunosuppressive therapy.
    a. Adrenocorticotropic hormone (ACTH)
        i. Stimulates the adrenal cortex to secrete cortisol, corticosteroid, and aldosterone.
        ii. Decreases the duration of acute exacerbations.
        iii. Lacks any long-term benefit.
    b. Corticosteroids
        i. Produce similar results more rapidly than ACTH.
        ii. Both drugs decrease synthesis of CSF IgG.

4. Treatment of chronic progressive MS is controversial. Possible therapies include azathioprine, cyclophosphamide, plasmapheresis, intrathecal interferon-β, total lymphoid irradiation, cyclosporin A, and monoclonal antibodies.

Interaction with Pregnancy

1. MS does not seem to adversely affect the course of pregnancy or the outcome of the fetus.
2. MS-related symptoms such as fatigue, weakness, and incoordination may influence pregnancy. These women may tire more readily during labor and have weaker, less effective expulsive efforts.
3. Drugs used to treat MS also may affect pregnancy.
   a. Corticosteroids are safe for treating MS in pregnancy.
   b. Chronic steroid administration may cause hypertension, fluid and electrolyte imbalance, catabolism and muscle wasting, anemia from gastrointestinal bleeding, poor wound healing, and susceptibility to infection.
   c. ACTH has not undergone controlled testing in pregnancy and is embryocidal.
4. Do not use azathioprine, cyclophosphamide, and the agents under investigation because of the known or potential risk of teratogenesis.
5. Neonatal effects
   a. There is no neonatal MS syndrome.
   b. These infants have an increased incidence of MS.
6. Progression of disease
   a. Neurologic deterioration is common during pregnancy. The normal, pregnancy-related hormonal changes, such as elevated plasma cortisol, may explain this phenomenon.
   b. The rate of exacerbation during the first postpartum months, is up to ten times the relapse rate during pregnancy.
7. Table 3.5 provides a quick reference for MS.

Preoperative Evaluation

1. Assess the degree of neuromuscular weakness and respiratory compromise.
2. Obtain a history of concurrent major illness and current drug therapy.
3. In those patients treated with chronic steroids, blood chemistries may be abnormal.
4. Perform a neurologic examination to aid in assessing any later exacerbation.

Neurofibromatosis

1. Chronically progressive, autosomal dominant disorder of the supportive tissues of the nervous system
2. It occurs in approximately 1 in 3,000 births.
3. It has a diverse clinical expression.
   a. Classically, patients have diagnostic cutaneous pigmentary changes (e.g., café au lait spots or axillary freckling).

Table 3.5.   Summary of multiple sclerosis and pregnancy

Pathology	Central nervous system demyelination
	Genetic predisposition (HLA-DW2)
Onset	20–40 yr
	Women affected two times more than men
Geographic distribution	Temperate zones
Pathogenic theories	Infectious agent (measles, canine distemper virus)
	High-fat diet
	Trauma
	Heavy-metal exposure
	Oligodendrocyte precursor damage
Interaction with pregnancy	Nonspecific, related to MS symptoms
	Higher risk of relapse postpartum
Interaction with neonate	No immediate interaction
Diagnosis	Evoked potentials: slow nerve conduction
	Computed tomography evidence of plaques
	Increased CSF IgG
	Increased CSF myelin basic protein

  b. Neurofibromas are tumors that arise from the Schwann cell sheaths and fibroblasts of peripheral, cranial, or autonomic nerves.
     i. Can be small and discrete or extensive masses
    ii. Usually involve the skin
   iii. Can occur in deeper nerves, blood vessels, and organs
    iv. Although usually a benign, cosmetic concern, neurofibromas can cause major neurologic or obstructive symptoms or undergo sarcomatous degeneration.
        (1) Airway compromise can occur with neurofibromas of the oropharynx, larynx, or mediastinum.
        (2) Neurofibromas are often very vascular and can cause severe hemorrhage.
        (3) Some patients have intracranial or spinal cord tumors and may develop intracranial hypertension, neurologic compromise, or seizures.
        (4) Cranial nerve involvement may lead to altered gag or swallowing reflexes.
     v. Disorders of bone growth are common.
        (1) Cervical spine involvement is a major concern during positioning for laryngoscopy or surgery.
        (2) Lumbar or thoracic spine involvement may make regional anesthesia impossible.

vi. Other organ involvement and associated diseases can include pulmonary parenchymal fibrosis leading to pulmonary hypertension, pheochromocytoma, hyperthyroidism, Wilms' tumor, neuroblastoma, and congenital heart lesions, especially pulmonary stenosis.

Treatment

1. Treatment of neurofibromatosis involves symptomatic drug therapy (e.g., anticonvulsants for seizures) and surgical removal of selected lesions.
2. Reserve surgery for those tumors that are particularly disfiguring or associated with obstructive symptoms or neurologic compromise.
3. Associated symptoms such as orthopedic deformity, endocrine dysfunction, or cancer also may require surgery.

Interaction with Pregnancy

1. During pregnancy, neurofibromas often enlarge, creating the potential for hemorrhage, increased obstruction, and neurologic compromise. Pelvic neurofibromas may preclude vaginal delivery or create pressure symptoms.
2. Pregnant women with neurofibromatosis also can be hypertensive, probably due to renal artery stenosis from vascular changes associated with the disease.
3. Patients may exhibit prolonged paralysis after nondepolarizing neuromuscular blocking agents. The response to succinylcholine may be either exaggerated or diminished.
4. Neurofibromatosis is an autosomal dominant disorder.
   a. Infants born of affected mothers have a 50% chance of developing the disease.
   b. Many of the signs and symptoms of this progressive disorder are absent at birth. Axillary freckling or the presence of five or more café au lait spots larger than 0.5 cm in diameter are diagnostic.

Preoperative Evaluation

1. Carefully search for problematic manifestations of the disease.
   a. A history of voice changes, symptoms of increased intracranial pressure, or neurologic changes should cause concern.
   b. A history of significant cardiopulmonary disease, endocrine dysfunction, and orthopedic malformation is important.
   c. Assess the airway carefully for possible obstruction and cervical spine involvement.
2. As with all patients with neurologic disease, perform a baseline examination.

Paraplegia and Quadriplegia

1. Improved treatment of spinal cord injury victims has allowed more women with these injuries to survive and bear children.

2.   Trauma, infection, tumors, and vascular lesions are the most common causes of spinal cord injury or transection.
   a.   The initial phase of an acute spinal cord transection is known as spinal shock.
      i.   Characteristics include flaccid paralysis and loss of sensation, temperature regulation, and spinal reflexes below the level of the lesion.
      ii. Characteristically, patients experience hypotension, bradycardia, cardiac dysrhythmias (especially premature ventricular contractions), and electrocardiographic changes consistent with ischemia.
      iii. Women are amenorrheic for 2 to 3 months following injury.
   b.   A lesion between C2 and C4, causing diaphragmatic denervation, may require immediate and permanent ventilatory support.
   c.   With lower lesions and intact diaphragmatic innervation, the patient can probably generate adequate tidal volumes but may not be able to cough and clear her airway.
      i.   Paralysis of the abdominal musculature does not allow the patient to generate the force required to cough.
      ii. Intraabdominal contents to shift and displace the diaphragm. The result is altered lung volumes, particularly a decreased functional residual capacity and decreased expiratory reserve volume.
      iii. Pulmonary aspiration and pneumonia are common.
   d.   Following the initial phase of injury, patients enter the chronic stage.
      i.   Spinal cord reflexes generally return.
      ii. Patients experience muscle spasm and sympathetic nervous system hyperactivity.
      iii. Other associated findings include chronic pulmonary and urinary tract infections, anemia, thermoregulatory dysfunction, and cardiovascular instability.
   e.   Renal failure resulting from chronic urinary tract infection or renal calculi is a major cause of morbidity and mortality.
      i.   Spinal cord transection often disrupts the motor innervation of the bladder and ureters, causing urinary stasis, chronic bladder infection, and pyelonephritis.
      ii. Chronic instrumentation for bladder elimination increases the risk of infection.
      iii. Good perineal hygiene, routine bladder emptying, and chronic suppression therapy can lessen the risk of infection.
   f.   Spinal cord injury patients often have anemia. Some of the most commonly proposed causes for this anemia are iron deficiency, renal failure from chronic infection, obstruction, or renal calculi, and anemia of chronic disease.

Autonomic Hyperreflexia

1. Can produce cardiovascular instability following the return of spinal cord reflexes after spinal shock
2. Results from the dissociation of sympathetic spinal reflexes (below the level of the transection) from controlling mechanisms in the CNS
3. Visceral or cutaneous stimulation, most commonly by distention of a hollow viscus, such as the bowel, bladder, or uterus, initiates the reflex.
   a. In neurologically intact individuals, visceral stimulation sends afferent signs that enter the spinal cord and elicit a sympathetic nervous system response. Descending impulses from the CNS normally regulate this response.
   b. Spinal cord injury disrupts the transmission of this regulatory information, resulting in sympathetic hyperactivity.
4. The level of the spinal cord lesion determines the incidence of autonomic hyperreflexia.
   a. Occurs in nearly all patients (85% with transections above T6)
   b. Unlikely to occur in those with lesions below T10
5. The most common manifestations are severe paroxysmal hypertension, tachycardia, bradycardia, headache, facial flushing, diaphoresis, piloerection, pupillary dilation, and nasal congestion.
6. Treatment
   a. Requires immediate attention: Severely elevated blood pressure can incite seizures and unconsciousness as well as retinal, cerebral, and subarachnoid hemorrhages.
   b. Rapidly control the blood pressure.
      i. Remove the initiating stimulus (e.g., empty a full bladder).
      ii. Initiate pharmacologic therapy with peripheral vasodilators such as ganglionic blocking drugs, α-adrenergic antagonists, direct vasodilators, or general or regional anesthesia.
      iii. Because of the disruption of regulatory pathways, centrally acting agents are ineffective.
7. Table 3.6 summarizes the consequences of spinal cord injury.

Interaction with Pregnancy

1. Women who suffer spinal cord injuries during pregnancy have a greater risk of stillbirth.
2. The level of injury will determine the patient's response to labor pain.
   a. Women with lesions below T11 to L1 will feel labor pain.
   b. Those with lesions from T10 to T5 to T6 will not have pain but can palpate contractions.
   c. Those with lesions above T5 to T6 are at high risk for autonomic hyperreflexia.
   d. Because women in these last two groups may find labor painless, premature, unsupervised delivery may occur.
   e. Labor also tends to progress rapidly.

Table 3.6.   Consequences of spinal cord injury

Acute	Chronic
Neural	**Neural**
Flaccid paralysis	Muscle spasm
Loss of sensation, temperature regulation, and spinal reflexes	Altered thermoregulation
Return of spinal reflexes	
Cardiovascular	**Cardiovascular**
Hypotension	Autonomic hyperreflexia
Bradycardia	with lesions above T6
Dysrhythmia	
ECG changes	
Respiratory	**Respiratory**
C2–C4 lesions require ventilatory support	C2–C4 lesions require ventilatory support
Lower lesions alter lung volumes and may impair the ability to protect the airway	Lower lesions alter lung volumes and may impair the ability to protect the airway
	Renal
	Failure from infection or calculi
Other	**Other**
Amenorrhea for 3 mo	Anemia

3. Additional problems include possible respiratory embarrassment from the distended uterus, profound anemia, and urinary obstruction with increased incidence of distention, infection, and autonomic hyperreflexia.

Preanesthetic Evaluation
1. Focuses on respiratory status
   a. The level of the lesion will gauge the need for ventilatory support.
   b. Assess the patient's ability to clear her airway.
   c. Consider the degree of respiratory compromise due to the gravid uterus.
   d. Be prepared to lend ventilatory assistance.
2. Knowing the level of transection also will determine the risk of autonomic hyperreflexia.
3. Laboratory data can help detect severe anemia and pulmonary or urinary tract infection.

Central Nervous System Neoplasms
1. CNS neoplasms are uncommon in women of reproductive age.
2. Pregnancy can precipitate or aggravate the symptoms of these lesions. The mechanism is unclear, but it is probably

related to tumor enlargement due to water retention or increased vascularity.

3. Tumors may be either metastatic or primary.
   a. Metastatic tumors of particular importance to women in this age group are those from breast and lung cancer and from choriocarcinoma.
   b. Except for metastatic choriocarcinoma, there is no difference in the distribution of brain tumors, the symptoms of which first occur in pregnant women and in nonpregnant women in the same age group.
4. Spinal hemangiomas seem to occur more frequently in the pregnant population.
5. Certain tumors seem to manifest symptoms at different times during gestation.
   a. Spinal hemangiomas generally present in the third trimester.
   b. Gliomas generally present in the first trimester.
   c. Meningiomas generally present progressively throughout pregnancy.
   d. Progesterone seems to positively correlate with tumor symptoms.
6. The diagnosis of CNS tumors in pregnant patients does not differ from their diagnosis in nonpregnant patients.
   a. Signs and symptoms suggestive of a CNS space-occupying lesion form the basis for diagnosis.
   b. Use CT and magnetic resonance imaging without hesitation.
7. Tumor-related symptoms may be difficult to distinguish from some pregnancy-related complaints.
   a. Typical symptoms of CNS tumors include nausea and vomiting, headache, visual changes, altered mental status, and convulsions.
   b. Other findings may include sensory or motor deficits.
8. Pregnancy should not alter or delay treatment of these tumors.
   a. Radiation treatment and chemotherapy (except for possible teratogens and surgery) should be used as indicated.
   b. If the mother's neurologic examination is stable and she shows no evidence of increased intracranial pressure, delay treatment until after delivery.
   c. A deteriorating status due to severe, uncontrolled intracranial hypertension requires immediate therapy, with pregnancy termination and surgery as necessary. Some measures that may be needed include:
      i. Intubation and hyperventilation.
      ii. Corticosteroids to reduce cerebral edema.
      iii. Drainage of CSF via ventricular shunting or ventriculostomy.
      iv. Administration of barbiturates.
   d. If possible, avoid hyperosmotic drugs such as mannitol, which may shift water from the fetus to the mother.
9. The preanesthetic evaluation of the parturient with known or suspected CNS lesions should focus on determining the

patient's level of consciousness and assessing her ability to maintain and protect her airway. Also look for intracranial hypertension and initiate therapy as appropriate. To immediately appreciate changes in neurologic status, frequent examinations are essential.

Cerebrovascular Disease

1. Uncommon in women of reproductive age
2. Events during pregnancy are a leading cause of maternal mortality.
3. Because these disorders are unusual in this age group, it is easy to attribute their symptoms to more common diseases, such as eclampsia or seizure disorders. As a consequence, crucial delays in therapy may result.
4. The cerebrovascular diseases most commonly seen in pregnancy include intracerebral hemorrhage and subarachnoid hemorrhage.
   a. Intracerebral hemorrhage
      i. Etiologies include hypertension, eclampsia, and metastatic choriocarcinoma.
      ii. Unless associated with a complication of gestation, pregnancy does not alter its incidence.
      iii. Hemorrhage is rare except when due to eclampsia or preeclampsia.
         (1) The presumed causes of bleeding in these instances are hypertension and vascular changes associated with preeclampsia.
         (2) Hemorrhage causes one-third of deaths due to eclampsia and preeclampsia.
         (3) Symptoms include headache, convulsions, mental status changes, and focal neurologic findings.
   b. Subarachnoid hemorrhage
      i. Complicates fewer than 1 in 10,000 pregnancies
      ii. Etiologies include cerebral aneurysm, arteriovenous malformation, metastatic choriocarcinoma, eclampsia, and disseminated intravascular coagulation. Aneurysm and arteriovenous malformation are the first and second most common causes.
         (1) Gravidas with aneurysms tend to be older (30 to 35 years) than those with arteriovenous malformations (20 to 25 years).
         (2) Aneurysms have a progressively increasing risk of rupture during the pregnancy, being highest between 30 and 40 weeks' gestation. They rarely rupture during labor.
         (3) Arteriovenous malformations may rupture at any time during pregnancy or labor or after delivery.
         (4) Ruptured aneurysms are generally more fatal than are ruptured arteriovenous malformations.

iii. Symptoms of subarachnoid hemorrhage include severe headaches, nausea, vomiting, altered mental status, nuchal rigidity, and focal neurologic deficit. Distinguishing a ruptured aneurysm from a ruptured arteriovenous malformation by neurologic examination is difficult and may require specific testing, such as CT and cerebral angiography.

5. The preanesthetic evaluation of the pregnant patient with cerebrovascular disorders is similar to that for a patient with CNS neoplasms.

HUMAN IMMUNODEFICIENCY VIRUS INFECTION
Epidemiology

1. Acquired immunodeficiency syndrome (AIDS) is a currently incurable disease complex that results from infection with the human immunodeficiency virus (HIV).
2. By the end of 1993, more than 300,000 cases of AIDS in the United States were reported to the Centers for Disease Control, and at least 1 million individuals in the United States were thought to be infected with HIV.
   a. Approximately 6,530 HIV-infected women gave birth in the United States in 1993, and, based on a 25% vertical transmission rate, an estimated 1,630 of their infants were infected with HIV.[2]
   b. In the United States, in areas with high prevalence, male-to-female HIV-seropositive ratios approach 1 : 1.
3. Eighty percent of reported cases of AIDS in adult women occur among those of reproductive age.
   a. A majority of these cases occur in intravenous drug abusers.
   b. About one-third result from heterosexual transmission.
   c. HIV seroprevalence in pregnant women is as high as 8 to 20 per 1,000.
   d. In areas if higher prevalence, routine HIV screening may be cost effective.
4. The interaction of pregnancy and HIV remains unclear.

Pathophysiology

1. AIDS results from immunosuppression by HIV-1, a large family of retroviruses that use host reverse transcriptase to produce, ultimately, core viral ribonucleic acid (RNA).
   a. The virus replicates by binding to the CD4 receptor on the membranes of T-cell lymphocytes, monocytes, macrophages, a small number of B-cell lymphocytes, glial cells, gut chromaffin cells, lymph nodes, skin, and rectal mucosal cells.
   b. Once inside the cell, the viral RNA is converted to DNA, which either integrates into the DNA of the host cell (proviral DNA) or remains unintegrated. Proviral DNA may lie dormant indefinitely, but the cell is permanently infected and will reduplicate the viral DNA with each cell division.
   c. Cell-free virus is found in various body fluids—synovial, cerebrospinal, pleural, peritoneal.

  d. After infection with HIV, many of the CD4 lymphocytes die or become dysfunctional. The mechanism of death for these cells is unknown, but the destruction of the helper T4 cell ultimately leads to significant defects in cell-mediated immunity.

2. The primary mode of transmission is via cells containing virus.

3. Infection with HIV is detected either by culture or serology.

  a. Culturing the virus yields unreliable results.

  b. Serologic tests for HIV antibodies are reproducible, sensitive, and specific.

    i. The enzyme-linked immunosorbent assay (ELISA) and rapid latex agglutination tests are sensitive but nonspecific.

    ii. Western blot immunophoresis and cytoplasmic membrane immunofluorescence tests are very specific but more often require repeating.

  c. Recently, rapid diagnostic assays have been developed that directly detect HIV antigens instead of HIV antibody.

  d. Identification of the pregnant woman with HIV infection requires a high degree of clinical suspicion.

    i. Look for risk factors.

      (1) A history of intravenous drug abuse

      (2) A sexual partner who is either HIV-positive or an intravenous drug user

      (3) Blood transfusion since 1978

    ii. Prevalence is highest in lower socioeconomic groups.

4. Initially, AIDS was recognized only in its end stages, when multiple opportunistic infections and unusual cancers occurred.

  a. Now, the disease is seen as a progression that depends on a multitude of factors, including extent of initial exposure.

  b. The progression of HIV-associated illness varies among individuals.

    i. The patient's immune response to the virus may slow viral replication.

    ii. Ultimately, the virus multiplies and overpowers the host immune system.

    iii. Then T4 count becomes extremely low, and the patient develops frequent infections by opportunistic bacteria, fungi, viruses, and progression of various cancers.

    iv. AIDS-associated cardiomyopathy, nephropathy, and dementia may complicate the course of this disease.

Treatment

1. Although HIV infection remains incurable, new drug therapies can slow the progression of AIDS and reduce the total viral load in HIV-infected patients.

2. Azidothymidine (AZT), now called zidovudine (ZDV)
   a. A thymidine analog
   b. Blocks the replication of HIV by inhibiting reverse tran-
      scriptase activity
   c. The first agent shown to improve the clinical and labo-
      ratory status of patients infected with HIV
   d. It penetrates the blood–brain barrier; concentrations in
      the CNS are approximately 30% to 50% of serum con-
      centrations.
3. Didanosine (ddI)
   a. Another nucleoside analog
   b. Interferes with reverse transcriptase
   c. Patients treated with ddI have a significant delay in
      progression to AIDS compared with those who had
      received prior ZDV therapy.
4. Zalcitabine (ddC) is another reverse transcriptase inhibitor
   that is approved for use in combination with ZDV in patients
   with CD4 counts less than 300 and evidence of clinical progression on ZDV alone.
5. Combination therapy with ZDV and ddI or ddC is under
   intense study and may make an attractive approach to com-
   bating AIDS and HIV infection.
6. Multiple other antiviral agents that act at different sites in
   the life cycle of HIV also are being evaluated.

Interaction with Pregnancy
1. There is no evidence that HIV infection or AIDS affects
   fertility.
2. Pregnancy may accelerate the course of disease in HIV-
   infected women.
   a. Cell-mediated immunity is depressed during preg-
      nancy, especially in the second and third trimesters.
   b. While some authors report an increased risk of progres-
      sion to AIDS within 28 to 60 months of delivery, others
      suggest that pregnancy does not accelerate the occur-
      rence of AIDS among HIV-positive women.
3. Similarly, pregnancy may increase the death rate in women
   with AIDS.
4. Confusion also exists about the effect of HIV infection on
   pregnancy.
   a. Despite a much higher incidence of complications (pre-
      mature rupture of membranes, low birth weight, and
      preterm birth), patient populations with risk factors
      such as low socioeconomic status, drug abuse, poor
      nutritional status, and poor prenatal care show little
      difference in maternal risk and outcome between HIV-
      seropositive and HIV-seronegative mothers.
   b. Women who abuse drugs have an increased risk of preg-
      nancy complications (spontaneous abortion, preterm
      deliveries, and low-birth-weight infants).
   c. Although the true effect of HIV infection on the course of
      pregnancy remains unclear, these patients are at high
      risk.

5. With the obstetric implications of HIV seropositivity and even AIDS still unclear, the issue of screening for HIV in pregnant women remains debatable.
    a. Testing and ZDV treatment of infected women and their infants can decrease the vertical transmission rate by half.
    b. Nevertheless, the debate over screening continues. The arguments for screening include the following:
        i.   Voluntary testing may miss a large percentage of positive individuals.
        ii. Perinatal transmission of the virus may be reduced.
        iii. Health care workers may be better protected.
    c. Those against screening point out:
        i.   The high cost of an effective screening program.
        ii. The high false-positive rates in low-prevalence populations.
        iii. The likelihood of discouraging prenatal care with mandatory HIV screening.
    d. Health care workers must rely on universal precautions for personal protection.
        i.   When handling blood or other body fluids, assume that all patients are infected.
        ii. Currently, testing for HIV is limited to those patients at high risk for the disease.
6. Perinatal transmission of HIV is a worsening problem.
    a. In most of these cases, infants will acquire the infection through vertical transmission from their mothers.
    b. Currently, about 30% of HIV-positive mothers in the United States transmit HIV to their newborn infants.
    c. Transmission may occur *in utero,* as virus has been isolated from an infant born by cesarean section.
    d. Exposure to maternal blood and body fluids at the time of birth is another possible route of HIV transmission. Avoid scalp electrodes and fetal blood sampling in the HIV-positive patient.
    e. Both elective cesarean section and maternal antiviral therapy (ZDV) appear to decrease the rate of vertical transmission. Combining these interventions is more effective than either one alone.[3]
    f. HIV is present in breast milk, and there are several cases in which transmission is thought to have occurred during breastfeeding.
    g. Risk factors
        i.   There is no association between risk of transmission and trimester during which exposure occurred.
        ii. Absence of maternal symptoms does not appear protective.
        iii. The efficiency of sexual transmission varies in different risk groups. Similar stratification may exist with transmission of the virus to offspring.

SUBSTANCE ABUSE

1. Drug use is a major public health problem in the United States.

2. Nicotine, alcohol, marijuana, and cocaine remain the most commonly abused substances.
   a. As many as 20% of parturients in the United States smoke cigarettes.
   b. Twelve percent abuse alcohol.
   c. Eleven percent to 20% report regular use of cocaine or crack.
3. Drug use in various settings reflects factors varying from availability to social acceptance.
4. The physiologic changes of pregnancy alter pharmacokinetic and pharmacodynamic behavior and then amplify cardiovascular and respiratory depressant effects of many addictive drugs.
5. Placental transfer and fetal effects
   a. The placenta, like the liver, can metabolize drugs, but environmental factors determine the quality and quantity of enzymes present.
   b. Drug abuse may decrease the number of placental neurotransmitter receptors, altering fetal and neonatal behavioral development.
   c. Any substance that affects the vascular tone of the placenta may alter placental blood flow and ultimately result in placental infarction and fetal compromise.
   d. Substances ingested, inhaled, or injected by the mother may cross the placenta and directly affect the fetus by one of several mechanisms:
      i. The drug or a metabolite may have direct fetal effects.
      ii. Drugs can induce hepatic enzymes and affect development via altered synthetic and degradation pathways.
      iii. The risk of disease transmission is greatest for the fetus of a substance abuser.
      iv. Maternal malnutrition, which so often accompanies substance abuse, increases the risk of neural tube defects and peripartum complications.
6. The course of gestation for substance abusers often depends on their ability and willingness to participate in counseling and detoxification programs. Up to 25% of substance abusers who seek prenatal care deny drug use. Even so, a widely focused approach seems the best way to address the multiple problems of these women. Such a program might include:
   a. Counseling.
   b. Detoxification and substitution therapy.
   c. Education about nutrition, drug effects, maternal care, and HIV prophylaxis.
   d. Screening for hepatitis, HIV, tuberculosis, and vaginal/cervical infections.
   e. Repeated evaluation of fetal condition.

Ethanol

1. Ethanol is a CNS depressant.
   a. It may induce behavioral stimulation by depressing inhibitory control mechanisms.

b. As intoxication advances, this initial excitatory phase is succeeded by a general impairment of nervous function.

c. A condition of general anesthesia ultimately prevails.

d. The CNS effects of alcohol are proportional to the blood alcohol concentration. They are most marked in the face of a rising alcohol concentration.

2. The rate-limiting step in alcohol metabolism is the conversion of ethanol to acetaldehyde by alcohol dehydrogenase.

   a. This enzyme has variable activity.

   b. Isoenzymes are coded by five genes. Variable expression of these genes occurs between races and individuals.

3. Alcohol exhibits cross-tolerance with most CNS depressant drugs.

   a. Acute intoxication increases the effects of cross-tolerant drugs.

   b. Chronic ingestion of alcohol decreases other drug effects.

   c. Tolerance does not alter the lethal blood concentration of alcohol.

4. Abrupt cessation of alcohol ingestion incites hyperactivity of all senses, hyperreflexia, muscle tension and tremor, over-alertness, anxiety, insomnia, and reduction of seizure threshold, commonly known as the alcohol withdrawal syndrome.

   a. Symptoms range from mild to severe and can appear as early as several hours after the last drink, but they more typically occur after 48 hours of abstinence.

   b. Delirium tremens

      i. A medical emergency characterized by extreme autonomic hyperactivity and global confusion

      ii. If left untreated, the mortality rate exceeds 40%.

      iii. Once established, delirium tremens cannot be rapidly reversed with alcohol.

      iv. Sedative therapy in withdrawal syndrome and delirium tremens involves replacement of alcohol with a cross-tolerant drug and calming the anxious, hallucinating, or delirious patient.

         (1) It is unknown which sedative best achieves these goals.

         (2) In the parturient, phenobarbital and clonidine are often recommended.

5. Chronic alcohol abuse affects multiple organ systems.

   a. In addition to CNS symptoms, chronic myelopathy, polyneuropathy, and myopathy may be present.

   b. These problems can complicate anesthetic management by altering recovery from muscle relaxants and regional or general anesthesia.

6. Acute cardiovascular effects of ethanol

   a. Myocardial depression

   b. Altered electrophysiology

   c. Atrial and ventricular dysrhythmias

   d. Chronic consumption results in cardiomyopathy and progressive myocardial dysfunction.

      i. The increased cardiac demand of pregnancy may result in cardiac failure in the pregnant alcohol abuser with significant myocardial disease.

     ii. Anesthetics that depress cardiac function may accelerate this process.

7. Respiratory complications are common among chronic alcohol abusers.

   a. Mild ventilation—perfusion mismatch and intrapulmonary shunting

   b. Chronic infection and aspiration pneumonia

   c. Alcohol further compounds the already higher risk of aspiration in the term parturient because it, too, decreases gastric motility and lowers esophageal sphincter tone.

8. Liver disease is common after ethanol abuse.

   a. Fatty infiltration, cirrhosis, portal hypertension, and hepatic encephalopathy can occur.

   b. Hepatocellular damage can yield hypoglycemia from impaired gluconeogenesis and induced glycogenolysis.

   c. Decreased drug metabolism and protein and coagulation factor synthesis may alter the anesthetic approach to the pregnant patient with alcoholic liver disease.

9. Gastrointestinal complications

   a. Gastritis, esophagitis, bleeding varices, and pancreatitis

   b. These contribute to an increased risk of aspiration pneumonia.

10. The stress response is altered. Cortisol, prolactin, epinephrine, norepinephrine, renin, angiotensin, and aldosterone rise, while growth hormone decreases.

11. Electrolyte abnormalities such as hyponatremia, hypokalemia, and hypomagnesemia may require correction. Correct hyponatremia slowly to avoid overcorrection and central pontine myelinolysis.

12. Fetal effects

   a. Ethanol does not affect umbilical arterial tone or placental blood flow.

   b. Ethanol blocks the placental transport of α-aminobutyric acid, implying inhibition of placental transfer of other nutrients.

   c. Alcohol increases fetal and subsequent neonatal morbidity in several ways.

      i. Maternal consumption has a dose-dependent effect on fetal and neonatal morbidity.

        (1) First-trimester exposure to more than 90 g per day produces developmental defects.

        (2) Exposure during the third trimester can cause growth retardation and a delayed rise in the lecithin–sphingomyelin ratio.

     ii. Ethanol decreases the conversion of dihomogammalinolenic acid (DGLA) to prostaglandin E1 (PGE1).

        (1) It inhibits delta-6-desaturase, an enzyme essential for a continued supply of DGLA.

        (2) As a result, these fetuses have low concentrations of PGE1.

(3) This deficiency may account for many of the changes noted with the fetal alcohol syndrome.
  (a) Growth deficiency
  (b) Major and minor birth defects
  (c) Abnormal mental and motor performance
  (d) Fetal or neonatal wastage
iii. Paternal exposure to ethanol also breeds fetal growth retardation and decreased DNA, RNA, and leucine synthesis.

Barbiturates
1. Have both presynaptic and postsynaptic effects on the neurotransmitter γ-amino-butyric acid (GABA) and its receptors
2. Reversibly depress the activity of all excitable tissues
   a. The CNS is most sensitive.
   b. All degrees of depression of the CNS, from mild sedation to general anesthesia, are achievable.
   c. Only very large doses or doses of extended duration have clinically detectable, direct effects on peripheral tissues.
3. Pharmacodynamic and pharmacokinetic tolerance can occur.
   a. Despite tolerance to mood-altering and other systemic effects, the lethal dose remains the same.
   b. With continued use, the therapeutic index falls and the risk of lethal overdose rises.
   c. Barbiturates exhibit cross-tolerance with ethanol.
   d. An abstinence syndrome similar to that occurring with ethanol can develop.
      i. The severity of withdrawal relates to the degree of tolerance and, therefore, the extent, duration, and continuity of abuse.
      ii. Symptomatology is very similar to the alcohol withdrawal syndrome.
         (1) Symptoms range from tremors, insomnia, and irritability to seizures, delirium, and hallucinations.
         (2) Convulsions are ominous.
      iii. Administration of barbiturates does not acutely reverse this syndrome.
4. Fetal effects
   a. Compromise of uteroplacental blood flow may occur.
   b. Behavioral and morphologic features of the fetal alcohol syndrome also appear, but there is no specific fetal defect.
   c. Induction of fetal hepatic enzymes tends to decrease neonatal bilirubin.
   d. Newborns of abusers or even therapeutic users (i.e., epileptics) may be dependent. Depending on the half-life of the barbiturate and the length of maternal use, withdrawal symptoms may arise up to 1 week after birth.

Benzodiazepines
1. Also exert their CNS effects via the GABA receptor

2. Not general neuronal depressants like barbiturates and ethanol
    a. There are wide differences in receptor selectivity.
    b. They are cross-tolerant with ethanol or barbiturates.
3. Withdrawal syndromes are best managed with additional benzodiazepines.
4. Although physostigmine or naloxone partially antagonize the CNS effects, flumazenil is a specific antagonist.
5. In the neonate, benzodiazepines impair thermoregulation, resulting in hypothermia.

Cocaine

1. Pharmacology
    a. Cocaine alkaloid, an ester of benzoic acid, undergoes hydrolysis to become ecgonine, which in turn is benzoylated and methylated to the base cocaine.
        i.   The hydrochloride salt of this base produces cocaine freebase, or "crack," when mixed with an alkali. This preparation is more stable on heating, vaporizes easily, and has a high bioavailability when smoked.
        ii. The bioavailability of topical intranasal cocaine is four to six times less than an equivalent intravenous dose, with peak plasma concentration proportional to the total dose.
        iii. Time to peak concentration, however, lengthens with increasing doses, as cocaine may limit its own absorption via vasoconstriction.
    b. The biologic half-life of cocaine is 0.5 to 1.5 hours.
        i.   Metabolism occurs via plasma and liver esterases, with liver hydrolysis producing the only active metabolite, norcocaine. Norcocaine has been detected in primate brain, where it inhibits the reuptake of norepinephrine more than cocaine.
        ii. Plasma from homozygotes for atypical cholinesterase has impaired *in vitro* decay of cocaine.
        iii. Acquired deficiencies of the enzyme (liver disease, malnutrition, plasmapheresis, anticholinesterase medications, and pregnancy) also impair hydrolysis.
    c. Sensitivity to cocaine may increase with pregnancy.
        i.   Changes in cocaine metabolism, alternations in central or peripheral adrenergic receptor sensitivity to norepinephrine, or differences in cocaine-induced cardiac responsiveness may be the reason.
        ii. In pregnant animals, liver cytochrome P_{450} concentrations fall by as much as 25%, and activity of glucuronyl transferase and monooxygenase declines.
        iii. Effects of progesterone
             (1) High concentrations of progesterone in pregnant ewes can delay cocaine metabolism or increase its bioactivity.

(2) Progesterone may either increase N-deme-thylation to norcocaine or enhance α-adrenergic receptor sensitivity.

d. In the neonate, esterase metabolites persist as long as 4 to 5 days after maternal cocaine use.

e. Mechanism of action
   i. Complex and incompletely understood
   ii. Additive effects on many neurotransmitter systems, including nerve conduction, autonomic sympathetic, and CNS functions
   iii. Several binding sites exist in both central and peripheral nervous systems.
   iv. The acute actions are brief and intense, resembling the neuropharmacologic and cardiovascular effects of amphetamines.
      (1) Tachycardia, increased myocardial contractility, vasoconstriction, bronchodilation, pupillary dilation, muscle tremors, and elevated temperature are predictable, even with low doses of intranasal or intravenous cocaine.
      (2) Arousal and euphoria proceed dysphoria, anxiety, somnolence, and drug craving.
      (3) During gestation, cocaine may stimulate cardiac output to a greater degree than in the nonpregnant state.
      (4) Uterine blood flow decreases, even with so-called recreational doses.
   v. Fetal effects include hypoxemia, hypertension, and tachycardia secondary to reduced uterine blood flow, direct drug effects, and increased fetal catecholamine concentrations.

f. Toxicity
   i. All users are at risk.
   ii. Toxicity may lead to sudden death.
   iii. It is characterized by unpredictable and rapid onset.
   iv. Manifestations include overstimulation of the respiratory, cardiovascular, and central nervous systems.
   v. Ultimately, seizures, profound depression, and cardiovascular collapse arise.
   vi. The syndrome of hypertension, altered mental status, and seizures may mimic preeclampsia or eclampsia. History of cocaine use or urine and blood drug screening may be an important determinant of ensuing therapy and management.

2. Perinatal risks
   a. Cocaine alkaloid, or "crack," is a highly potent, addictive, and relatively inexpensive form of cocaine that has more adverse perinatal effects than do other forms of cocaine.
   b. Epidemic rates of maternal crack use bring national estimates of fetal cocaine exposure into the range of 91,500 to 240,000 children per year.

   c. Maternal cocaine use increases the risk of a multitude of perinatal problems:

     i. Congenital urogenital abnormalities.

     ii. Lower mean birth weight.

     iii. Lower mean gestational age at delivery.

     iv. Preterm labor and delivery.

     v. Abruptio placentae.

     vi. Premature rupture of membranes.

     vii. Increased neonatal morbidity and mortality.

   d. Fetal cocaine exposure increases both the neonatal hospital costs and length of stay. At a national level, these costs add to almost $500 million per year.

Opioids

1. The physiologic effects of opioids in humans are well known. Except for a steeper dose–response curve, they are the same in the pregnant population.

2. Most maternal effects occur secondary to respiratory depression.

   a. Maternal hypercarbia and hypoxemia impair uterine blood flow.

   b. During withdrawal, heightened sympathetic tone further lowers uterine blood flow.

   c. These physiologic changes result in a placental abruption rate of 25%.

3. Neonatal effects

   a. Increased incidence of respiratory distress syndrome

   b. Increased risk of meconium aspiration

   c. Symptoms of withdrawal occur in up to 80% of (chronically) exposed infants.

   d. Maternal treatment, including prenatal care through methadone clinics, markedly lowers neonatal morbidity and mortality. However, treatment does not preclude an extremely high incidence of neonatal withdrawal syndrome among infants of methadone-dependent mothers.

   e. Long-term effects

     i. For their first 2 years of life, exposed infants are 250 to 500 g lighter and have a 1-cm smaller head circumference than do controls.

     ii. After 2 years of age, there are no growth or developmental differences, although an elevated incidence of central motor dysfunction persists until 5 years of age.

REFERENCES

1. American Academy of Pediatrics Committee on Drugs. Anticonvulsants and pregnancy. *Pediatrics* 1979;63:331.

2. Dais SF, Byers RH Jr, Lindegren ML, Caldwell MB, Karon JM, Gwinn M. Prevalence and incidence of vertically acquired HIV infection in the United States. *JAMA* 1995;274:952.

3. The International Perinatal HIV Group. The mode of delivery and the risk of vertical transmission of human immunodeficiency virus type 1: A meta-analysis of 15 prospective cohort studies. *N Engl J Med* 1999;340:977.

Pathophysiology and Obstetric Management of Preeclampsia

Hypertension complicates 7% to 10% of pregnancies and is a major cause of maternal morbidity and mortality. Clinically, hypertension manifests as a wide spectrum of disorders, ranging from mildly elevated blood pressure to severe disease involving all of the major organ systems. The revised Technical Bulletin from the American College of Obstetricians and Gynecologists, published in 1996, defined *hypertension during pregnancy* as a sustained blood pressure of 140 mm Hg systolic or 90 mm Hg diastolic.[1]

HYPERTENSIVE DISORDERS OF PREGNANCY

1. Hypertensive disorders of pregnancy can be broadly classified as chronic hypertension and pregnancy-induced hypertension (PIH).
2. PIH encompasses several clinical subsets, depending on end-organ effects.
   a. Preeclampsia: the development of hypertension with proteinuria after the twentieth week of gestation in a previously normotensive woman. Preeclampsia can be mild or severe (Table 4.1).
   b. Eclampsia: the development of convulsions or coma in women with preeclampsia without other precipitating causes of seizures
   c. HELLP syndrome: hemolysis, elevated liver enzymes, and low platelet count
   d. Chronic hypertension of pregnancy: elevated blood pressure of any etiology with no proteinuria, usually occurring before the twentieth week of gestation and persisting more than 6 weeks postpartum. The development of preeclampsia in pregnant women with chronic hypertension is classified as superimposed preeclampsia.
   e. Gestational hypertension: increased blood pressure arising in the second half of pregnancy or in the first 24 hours postpartum without evidence of edema or proteinuria. Blood pressure returns to normal within 10 days of delivery.
3. Although the terminology and the definitions are well described, the accurate diagnosis of various subsets of hypertension during pregnancy is often difficult.
   a. Poor documentation of blood pressures and inadequate assessment of renal function early in pregnancy can make differentiating preeclampsia from preexisting chronic hypertension and renal dysfunction an arduous task.
   b. The nonspecific signs of preeclampsia (proteinuria and generalized edema) are often present in normal pregnancy.
   c. There are no specific clinical or biochemical markers of preeclampsia.

Table 4.1. Clinical manifestations of severe disease in patients with pregnancy-induced hypertension

1. Systolic pressure of 160 mm Hg, or diastolic pressure 110 mm Hg on two occasions at least 6 h apart
2. Proteinuria of at least 5 g in 24-h urine collection (3+ or 4+ on semiquantitative assay)
3. Oliguria of <400 mL in 24 h
4. Cerebral or visual disturbances such as altered consciousness, headache, scotomas, or blurred vision
5. Pulmonary edema or cyanosis
6. Epigastric or right upper quadrant pain
7. Impaired liver function of unclear etiology
8. Thrombocytopenia

Source: American College of Obstetricians and Gynecologists. *Preeclampsia.* Technical Bulletin 219, 1996.

INCIDENCE AND PREDISPOSING FACTORS

1. Preeclampsia is primarily a disease of the young primigravida.
2. It also occurs in women older than 40 years, presumably due to the higher incidence of chronic hypertension in these women.
3. Preeclampsia complicates 6% to 7% of pregnancies in the United States. The incidence among young, Black primigravidae in inner-city hospitals is 20%.
4. Risk factors include:
   a. Preeclampsia during previous pregnancy.
   b. Molar pregnancy.
   c. Twin gestation.
   d. Hydrops fetalis.
   e. Diabetes mellitus.
   f. Chronic hypertension.
   g. Chronic renal disease.
   h. Antiphospholipid syndrome.
   i. African-American race, inadequate prenatal care, poor socioeconomic background, nutritional deficiencies, and a family history of PIH.

ETIOLOGY

1. Preeclampsia is a disease of unknown etiology.
2. It occurs only in human pregnancy.

Abnormal Response to Placentation

1. In preeclampsia, the maternal vasculature does not respond appropriately to the implantation and growth of placenta.
2. In the early stages of normal pregnancy, endovascular trophoblasts invade the decidual segments of the spiral arteries.
   a. A second wave of trophoblast migration follows at the sixteenth week of gestation.
   b. The second wave of migration invades the myometrial segments of the spiral arteries.

3. In preeclampsia, vascular changes involve only the decidual segments of the spiral arteries.
   a. The musculoelastic portions of the myometrial segments of the spiral arteries remain intact.
   b. The myometrial portion of the spiral artery is small and narrow and responds readily to vasomotor stimuli with vasoconstriction.
      i. Decreases placental perfusion
      ii. Produces areas of placental infarction
      iii. Predisposes to intrauterine growth retardation
4. This abnormal maternal response to placentation is the earliest pathognomonic feature of preeclampsia.

Thromboxane–Prostacyclin Imbalance

1. Thromboxane A_2 produced by the platelets, is a potent vasoconstrictor and induces platelet aggregation.
2. Prostacyclin, produced by the vascular endothelium and the renal cortex, is a potent vasodilator and an inhibitor of platelet aggregation.
3. The ratio of thromboxane A_2 to prostacyclin is consistently elevated in maternal serum, umbilical serum, amniotic fluid, and urine in women with preeclampsia compared with normotensive parturients.
4. Many authors consider the imbalance in the production of thromboxane A_2 and prostacyclin as an important etiologic factor of PIH.

Altered Platelet Calcium Metabolism

1. Intracellular free calcium is a major determinant of vascular smooth muscle tone.
2. Increased intracellular calcium and altered calcium metabolism are frequently present in preeclampsia and other hypertensive states.
3. An exaggerated response of platelet intracellular calcium to arginine vasopressin can be measured early in pregnancy and predicts subsequent preeclampsia.

Renin–Angiotensin–Aldosterone System

1. Plasma concentrations of renin, angiotensin II, and aldosterone
   a. Elevated in normal parturients versus nonpregnant controls
   b. In women with preeclampsia, however, the blood contains lower amounts of these compounds.
2. Vascular response to pressors (i.e., angiotensin II).
   a. Decreases in normal pregnancy.
   b. In preeclampsia, the pressor response to angiotensin II increases significantly, which may be a marker for early diagnosis of preeclampsia.

Sympathoadrenal Activity

1. Recent direct measurements, using microelectrodes, of postganglionic sympathetic nerve activity in skeletal muscle vasculature found that sympathetic nerve activity (expressed as bursts per minute) in women with preeclampsia was more

than three times higher than in normotensive pregnant women and twice as high as in hypertensive nonpregnant women.
2. Baroreflex-mediated control of heart rate (Valsalva maneuver) and non–baroreflex-mediated sympathoexcitatory stimulus (cold pressor test) were not significantly different between preeclamptic and normotensive women.
3. These results suggest that, in preeclampsia, the increases in the peripheral vascular resistance and blood pressure are partly mediated by a substantial enhancement of central sympathetic vasoconstrictor activity.

Digoxin-like Immunoreactive Substance (DLIS)
1. A natriuretic that produces vasoconstriction
2. Plasma concentration rises in preeclampsia.

Atrial Natriuretic Peptide (ANP)
1. A potent natriuretic, diuretic, and a vascular smooth muscle relaxant
2. ANP affects plasma volume and vascular tone.
3. The primary stimulus for ANP release is distention of atrial stretch receptors by expanded blood volume.
4. A potent stimulus for ANP release may be the increased plasma concentration of endothelin associated with severe preeclampsia.
5. The significance of elevated ANP in women with preeclampsia is unknown.

Endothelin and Nitric Oxide
1. Endothelin
   a. A vasoconstrictor ten times more potent than angiotensin II
   b. Endothelin is secreted in response to endothelial injury.
   c. Concentrations rise in patients with acute myocardial infarction, severe hypertension, acute and chronic renal failure, preeclampsia, and the hemolysis, elevated liver enzymes, and low platelet count (HELLP) syndrome.
2 . Nitric oxide (NO)
   a. Synthesized in the vascular endothelium
   b. A potent relaxant of vascular, gastrointestinal, and bronchial smooth muscles
   c. Studies of NO in women with PIH have yielded conflicting results.

PATHOPHYSIOLOGY
Intense vasospasm is the single most important pathophysiologic change in women with PIH. This process involves all major organs, including the uterus and placenta. Generalized vasospasm in turn decreases perfusion throughout the body, causing widespread organ dysfunction.

Cardiovascular System
Blood Volume
1. In mild preeclampsia, plasma volume is approximately 9% lower than in normotensive pregnant women.

2. Plasma volume is 30% to 40% lower in women with severe preeclampsia than in normal parturients of similar gestational age.
    a. Despite decreased plasma volume, extravascular and interstitial volume markedly increase.
    b. Hemoconcentration increases blood viscosity. Maternal hematocrit and hemoglobin concentrations correlate directly with the frequency of placental infarction and inversely with newborn weight.

Hemodynamic Profile

1. The hemodynamic changes that accompany severe preeclampsia are complex, difficult to study, and highly variable. Reasons for these problems include:
    a. Previous administration of antihypertensive medications or fluids.
    b. Concurrent medical problems, such as chronic hypertension.
    c. Duration and severity of preeclampsia.
    d. Labor.
    e. Mode of delivery.
    f. Small number of patients studied.
2. Untreated preeclamptic women have
    a. Lower cardiac output, stroke volume, and pulmonary artery occlusion pressure (PAOP) and higher systemic vascular resistance (SVR) compared with normotensive parturients.
    b. Despite the low cardiac output, left ventricular function is hyperdynamic.
3. Women with severe preeclampsia who have received various forms of treatment show a wide range of hemodynamic values.
    a. In general, these women have an elevated cardiac output, normal-to-high PAOP, and a normal-to-elevated SVR.
    b. Most also have hyperdynamic left ventricular function (Fig. 4.1).

CVP versus PAOP

1. In women with preeclampsia, changes in central venous pressure (CVP) often do not parallel changes in PAOP.
2. The reasons for the disparity are unclear.
    a. A placid right atrium may accommodate increased filling volume without simultaneous increases in pressure. This change would limit the sensitivity of CVP as a measure of intravascular volume.
    b. In severe preeclampsia, cardiac output may remain high despite the increased left ventricular afterload. This effort leads to higher left-sided intracavitary pressures compared with normal or low pressures in the right heart.
    c. Central redistribution of intravascular volume due to generalized vasospasm involving the capacitance vessels may produce the observed changes.

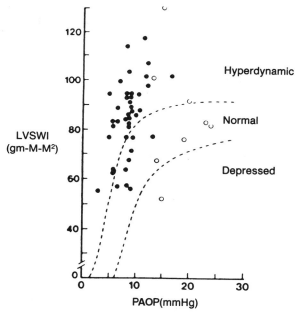

Fig. 4.1. Left ventricular stroke work index (*LVSWI*) versus pulmonary artery occlusion pressure (*PAOP*). Left ventricular function is hyperdynamic in most women with severe preeclampsia. (Source: From Mabie W, Ratts T, Sibai B. The central hemodynamics of severe preeclampsia. *Am J Obstet Gynecol* 1989;161:1443, with permission.)

Pulmonary Edema
1. Causes of cardiogenic pulmonary edema:
    a. Left ventricular dysfunction in the face of severe increases in SVR.
    b. Chronic hypertension.
    c. Peripartum cardiomyopathy and other conditions.
2. Causes of noncariogenic pulmonary edema:
    a. Increased pulmonary capillary permeability.
    b. Iatrogenic fluid overload.
    c. A reduction in plasma oncotic pressure (POP)–PAOP gradient.
        i. Hydrostatic pressure in the capillaries (PAOP) facilitates outward movement of fluids from capillaries. POP (πc) helps retain fluid and maintain intravascular volume. Approximately 70% of POP is exerted by plasma albumin, and the remaining 30% by globulins.

      ii.   In nonpregnant patients
         (1) POP averages 25.4 ± 2.3 mm Hg.
         (2) PAOP varies from 8 to 12 mm Hg.
         (3) POP–PAOP gradient is about 12 mm Hg.
      iii. In pregnancy
         (1) POP values range from 18 to 21 mm Hg.
         (2) PAOP averages 7.5 ± 1.8 mm Hg.
         (3) POP–PAOP gradient remains similar to nonpregnant values.
         (4) POP falls significantly after delivery, reaching its nadir 6 hours postpartum.
      iv. Women with severe PIH
         (1) Lower than normal values for POP both before and after delivery. Either renal loss or impaired synthesis of albumin (hepatic dysfunction) may produce the lower POP.
         (2) After delivery
            (a) POP falls from 17.9 ± 0.3 mm Hg to 13.7 ± 0.5 mm Hg.
           (b) PAOP increases significantly owing to the mobilization of extravascular edema fluid, iatrogenic fluid overload, and diminished renal output.
           (c) The lowering of POP with the simultaneous elevation of PAOP narrows the POP–PAOP gradient and may risk noncariogenic pulmonary edema.
3. Cardiac pulmonary edema and diastolic dysfunction
   a. One subset of women
      i. Markedly obese, with chronic hypertension and superimposed preeclampsia
      ii. All had severe hypertension, elevated cardiac output, elevated PAOP, normal SVR, normal POP, and pulmonary edema.
      iii. Echocardiography showed large chambers with thick walls, normal systolic function, and abnormal diastolic function.
      iv. In these women, pulmonary edema resulted from intrinsic volume overload in the presence of impaired left ventricular relaxation (diastolic dysfunction).
      v. Vasodilator therapy worsened the high-output state and pulmonary edema by further increasing cardiac output without lowering mean arterial pressure (MAP).
      vi. All patients responded well to diuretic therapy.[2]
   b. Hypertensive crisis and pulmonary edema
      i. Echocardiography usually shows impaired left ventricular diastolic filling with normal systolic function.
      ii. Less often, pulmonary edema is associated with impaired left ventricular systolic function.
4. While pulmonary edema associated with preeclampsia is most likely related to cardiac causes, further studies are needed to define the role of abnormally low POP-PAOP gradients.

Respiratory System
1. Upper airway edema associated with normal pregnancy worsens in preeclampsia. Occasionally, the edema can be severe enough to cause total airway obstruction.
2. The maternal oxyhemoglobin dissociation curve is shifted to the left due to decreased 2,3-diphosphoglycerate concentration or increased carboxyhemoglobin concentration. Such changes, in association with the preexisting marked decrease in uteroplacental blood flow, can significantly interfere with maternal-fetal oxygen transfer.

Coagulation Abnormalities
1. Preeclampsia is associated with microvascular endothelial damage and enhanced clotting.
    a. Plasma concentration of fibronectin, a marker of vascular endothelial damage, increases.
    b. Significant reductions in antithrombin III and α_2-antiplasmin signal enhanced clotting.
2. Platelet activation and platelet consumption with shortened platelet lifespan are characteristic.
    a. Increased concentration of platelet-specific proteins, such as β-thromboglobulin and platelet factor 4, suggest ongoing platelet aggregation and degranulation.
    b. Thrombocytopenia occurs in 15% to 20% of women with preeclampsia.
        i. The incidence is as high as 50% in those with severe disease.
        ii. The exact mechanism of thrombocytopenia is uncertain.
            (1) Women with preeclampsia and thrombocytopenia usually have increased mean platelet (larger than normal platelets), signifying increased platelet destruction.
            (2) Platelet destruction is not related to increased thrombin activity (disseminated intravascular coagulation [DIC]), as prothrombin time (PT), partial thromboplastin time (PPT), and the protamine sulfate paracoagulation assay are usually normal.
            (3) The presence of platelet-associated IgG suggests autoimmune-mediated platelet destruction.
    c. Besides affecting the number of platelets, preeclampsia also alters their function. Synthesis of platelet thromboxane A_2, an *in vitro* platelet function test, falls.
3. Although thrombocytopenia is a common finding in women with severe preeclampsia, clinically evident DIC is rare.
4. Monitoring
    a. Admission platelet count is an excellent predictor of subsequent platelet counts.
        i. The lower the admission platelet count, the higher the incidence of subsequent severe thrombocytopenia.
        ii. Signs of DIC, such as low fibrinogen or prolonged PT and PTT, do not occur in the absence of thrombocytopenia.

    b. Serial platelet counts alone are adequate in most women with severe preeclampsia.

    c. Estimation of PT, PTT, and fibrinogen concentration should be reserved for those cases complicated by a platelet count less than 100,000 per milliliter.

5. Resolution of thrombocytopenia

    a. In one study, mean time until platelet count exceeded 100,000 per milliliter was 67 ± 25 hours after delivery and 44 ± 17 hours from the platelet nadir.

    b. All women in this study had counts above 100,000 per milliliter by 111 hours after delivery and by 88 hours after the platelet nadir.[3]

Renal Function

1. Both glomerular filtration rate and renal plasma flow are significantly lower in women with preeclampsia than in normal parturients.

2. In addition, intrinsic renal structural abnormalities arise:

    a. Swelling of glomerular endothelial cells.

    b. Deposition of fibrin along the basement membrane.

    c. Narrowing or complete obliteration of the capillary lumen.

3. Renal glomerular endotheliosis is one of the important histopathologic markers of preeclampsia.

    a. The extent and severity of glomerular endotheliosis correlates with protein loss.

    b. Significant urinary protein loss lowers POP, leading to generalized edema.

4. In addition, PIH impairs renal excretion of sodium, increasing total body sodium.

5. Clearance of urea, uric acid, and creatinine decline, significantly increasing their serum concentrations.

Hepatic Function

1. Intense vasospasm of the hepatic arteriolar bed can cause mid-zonal necrosis and multiple areas of hepatic infarction.

2. Epigastric or right upper quadrant pain is symptomatic of small subcapsular hepatic hemorrhage. Rarely, severe spontaneous hepatic hemorrhage and rupture with sudden cardiovascular collapse can occur.

3. Hyperbilirubinemia and elevated liver enzymes, although frequent, seldom persist after delivery.

4. Pseudocholinesterase concentrations are significantly lower compared with healthy parturients; the duration of succinylcholine and ester type of local anesthetics may be prolonged.

Central Nervous System

1. Neurologic manifestations of preeclampsia include:

    a. Diffuse symptoms: severe headache, confusion, excitability, nausea, and vomiting.

    b. Focal signs: blurred vision, blindness, hyperreflexia, and hemiparesis.

    c. Seizures herald the onset of eclampsia.

        i. Eclamptic seizures may occur at any time and can lead to severe maternal morbidity and mortality.

     ii. Abnormal electroencephalographic findings are seen in 75% of eclamptic women and 50% of preeclamptic women.

     iii. Computed tomographic (CT) and magnetic resonance imaging (MRI) studies show ischemic lesions in the parietal and occipital lobes in patients with eclampsia.

     iv. Postmortem examinations of eclamptic women reveal cerebral edema and widespread hemorrhagic intracerebral lesions.

2. The etiology of eclamptic seizures is uncertain.
   a. Seizures may occur due to focal ischemia from widespread vasospasm of intracranial arteries.
   b. Seizures may be a form of hypertensive encephalopathy.
      i. Cerebral edema, due to loss of autoregulation, can occur during sudden and severe increases in MAP.
      ii. Cerebral blood flow velocities are markedly elevated in women with preeclampsia, and correlate with systemic arterial pressures.
   c. Cerebral edema, presumably vasogenic in origin, is a common finding on MRI scan in women with severe preeclampsia and eclampsia.

3. These studies have important anesthetic implications.
   a. Rapid sequence induction of general anesthesia and tracheal intubation can cause acute and severe elevations in maternal MAP in women with severe preeclampsia.
   b. The resultant rapid increase in the blood flow velocity or overdistension of intracerebral arteries can cause cerebral edema or hemorrhage.
   c. This risk underscores the importance of pretreatment with antihypertensive agents or β-adrenergic blocking drugs before tracheal intubation in women with severe preeclampsia.

The Uterus and Placenta

1. Uteroplacental blood flow is markedly decreased due to intense vasospasm.
2. The uterus is hypertonic and the placenta is often small, with areas of infarction, calcification, and fibrin deposition. The incidence of placental abruption is significantly higher.

OBSTETRIC MANAGEMENT OF PREECLAMPSIA
Mild Preeclampsia

1. All women with mild preeclampsia at or near term require immediate hospitalization for further evaluation and treatment.
2. Women with a favorable cervix should undergo induction and delivery without delay.
3. Management of mild preeclampsia detected early in pregnancy is controversial (Fig. 4.2).

Severe Preeclampsia

1. Management of women with severe preeclampsia is more aggressive.

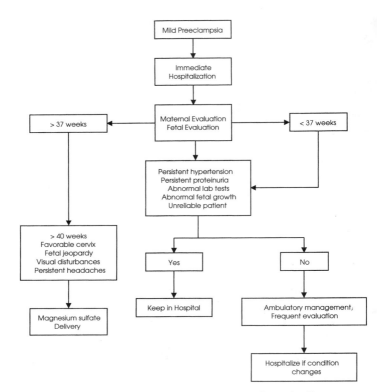

Fig. 4.2. Management of women with mild preeclampsia. (Source: From Sibai B. Preeclampsia-eclampsia. In: Beribri R, Berek S, Creasy R, Decherney A, Ryan KJ, eds. *Current problems in obstetrics, gynecology and fertility.* Chicago: Year Book Medical Publishers, 1990:9, with permission.)

2. All women with this diagnosis are admitted to the labor and delivery floor for observation, regardless of gestational age.
   a. Those women with gestational age beyond 35 weeks are delivered within 24 hours.
   b. Patients at 33 to 35 weeks' gestation receive steroids to accelerate fetal lung maturity and are then delivered.
   c. Women with resistant hypertension or maternal and fetal deterioration also are delivered within 24 hours, regardless of gestational age and fetal lung maturity.
3. Seizure prophylaxis with magnesium sulfate and blood pressure control also are common.
4. If patients presenting at less than 33 weeks' gestation respond well to therapy (as evidenced by diuresis and diastolic pressures below 110 mm Hg), close observation until the fetal lungs mature may be appropriate.

TREATMENT
1. The major goals of therapy are:
   a. Prevention of convulsions.
   b. Control and stabilization of blood pressure.
   c. Optimization of intravascular volume status.
2. Attaining these goals will contribute to safe delivery of a viable baby.

Seizure Prophylaxis
1. Prevention of eclampsia is an important goal of the care of women with preeclampsia.
2. In the United States, magnesium sulfate is the drug of choice for this purpose.
   a. Objective data to support this practice are limited and weak.[4]
      i. The frequency of seizures in untreated women with severe preeclampsia is low (3.2%).
      ii. The frequency of seizures in untreated women with mild preeclampsia is unknown.
   b. Despite its tocolytic effect, magnesium neither prolongs labor nor increases the risk of cesarean section.
   c. Maternal magnesium therapy may reduce the risk of cerebral palsy in very-low-birth-weight infants.[5]

Magnesium Sulfate
1. The mechanism by which magnesium prevents eclamptic seizures is unknown.
   a. In animals, magnesium ions specifically suppress experimentally induced electroencephalographic spike activity and neuronal burst response.
   b. Magnesium is a cerebral vasodilator and may prevent seizures by preventing cerebral ischemia.
   c. Magnesium may prevent seizures by an action at N-methyl-D-aspartate (NMDA) receptors.
2. Magnesium impairs neuromuscular function.
   a. It potentiates the action of nondepolarizing muscle relaxants.
   b. The severity of this effect correlates with the serum magnesium concentration.
3. Infusion of magnesium sulfate increases cardiac index by 12.5% and transiently lowers MAP without significantly changing other hemodynamic variables.
4. Magnesium rapidly crosses the placental barrier. With prolonged administration, fetal and maternal serum concentrations equilibrate. Neonatal hypotonia and respiratory depression may follow.
5. Therapeutic magnesium concentrations range from 5.0 to 7.0 mg per deciliter.
   a. Toxicity arises as the serum concentration approaches 9 mg per deciliter.
   b. Overdose, severely compromised renal function, or both, can produce toxic serum concentrations of magnesium.
      i. Respiratory arrest from impaired muscle strength and cardiac arrest (usually due to hypoxemia, but

potentially due to the negative inotropic effects of
magnesium) may follow.

    ii.   Treatment usually involves cardiorespiratory sup-
port and administration of calcium chloride.

6.   Some patients can have eclamptic seizures while receiving
magnesium infusion.

    a.   Give more intravenous magnesium or small doses of a
shortacting barbiturate or midazolam.

    b.   If convulsions persist, resort to tracheal intubation and
artificial ventilation to prevent pulmonary aspiration of
gastric contents.

Other Drugs for Prevention of Eclampsia

1.   European obstetricians opt for conventional anticonvulsants
such as diazepam, barbiturates, and chlormethiazol.

    a.   These drugs produce significant maternal and neonatal
sedation and respiratory depression.

    b.   Large doses of diazepam can cause neonatal hypother-
mia, jaundice, and respiratory depression.

2.   Phenytoin, a traditional anticonvulsant agent, has been
used to prevent and treat convulsions in preeclampsia
without adverse maternal or neonatal effects. Currently
available data suggest that magnesium is a more effective
anticonvulsant in women with preeclampsia.[6]

Treatment of Hypertension

Although magnesium sulfate transiently lowers maternal
blood pressure, other drugs are often needed to control hypertension in women with preeclampsia.

Hydralazine

1.   Commonly used antihypertensive agent in women with PIH
2.   Effects

    a.   In pregnant ewes, hydralazine reduces maternal blood
pressure and uterine vascular resistance while increasing uterine blood flow.

    b.   Doppler ultrasonographic studies have shown that
hydralazine does not alter placental or maternal renal
artery flow velocity waveforms, suggesting that placental and renal vascular resistance remains unaffected.

3.   Limitations

    a.   Slow and unpredictable onset, usually peaking 20 min-
utes after intravenous administration

    b.   Maternal tachycardia in response to decreased MAP
and SVR

Labetalol

1.   A combined α- and β-adrenergic blocking agent

    a. β-to-α blockade ratio of $3:1$ after oral administration
and $7:1$ after intravenous use

    b.   Labetalol produces less adrenergic blockade in the fetus
than in the mother.

2. In women with preeclampsia, labetalol decreases SVR without altering cardiac output.
3. Compared with hydralazine, labetalol has a more rapid onset and provides a smoother reduction of blood pressure.
4. Labetalol, in doses of 1 mg per kilogram, safely blunts the hypertensive response to endotracheal intubation during induction of general anesthesia in women with severe preeclampsia.
5. The major disadvantage of this drug is the widely varying dose requirement, which cannot be predicted by any clinical criteria.

Nifedipine
1. Most widely use calcium channel blocking agent in the treatment of PIH
2. Nifedipine lowers the blood pressure in a predictable manner when given orally in doses of 10 mg.
   a. Onset is within 10 to 30 minutes.
   b. Peak effect occurs in 40 to 75 minutes.
   c. The degree of blood pressure reduction is related to the pretreatment pressures; the higher the MAP, the greater the effect of the drug.
3. Nifedipine crosses the placental barrier, but does not alter the fetal hemodynamics.
4. Treatment of acute hypertension with immediate-release nifedipine is not recommended by the Cardiorenal Advisory Committee of the Food and Drug Administration due to the unpredictable nature of the resultant blood pressure decrease.

Potent Antihypertensive Drugs
1. Reserve more potent antihypertensive agents, such as nitroglycerin, nitroprusside, and trimethaphan, for specific indications:
   a. Acute hypertensive crisis
   b. Intractable hypertension unresponsive to conventional therapy.
   c. Prevention of severe hypertensive response to tracheal intubation under general anesthesia.
2. Administration of such potent antihypertensive agents requires continuous monitoring of maternal arterial pressure (via an indwelling radial artery catheter) and maternal electrocardiogram.

SODIUM NITROPRUSSIDE (SNP)
1. A potent arteriolar dilator
2. Rapid onset and short duration
3. Although fetal cyanide toxicity is a cause for concern, the use of low doses of SNP for short periods is safe. No adverse maternal or fetal effects have been reported in humans.
4. In women with PIH complicated by pulmonary congestion and heart failure, SNP dramatically decreases PAOP and produces significant hemodynamic improvement.

NITROGLYCERIN (NTG)

1. A venodilator
2. NTG reduces cardiac filling pressures by acting mainly on capacitance vessels.
3. In women with severe preeclampsia, NTG reduces MAP, PAOP, and cardiac index. Heart rate, stroke volume, and CVP do not change.
4. Volume expansion markedly impedes the hypotensive effects of the drug.
5. NTG blunts the hypertensive response to tracheal intubation in women with severe preeclampsia undergoing cesarean delivery under general anesthesia.
6. Both SNP and NTG cross the blood–brain barrier and increase cerebral blood flow and intracranial pressure.

TRIMETHAPHAN

1. Ganglionic blocking agent
2. Trimethaphan has limited placental transfer due to its high molecular weight.
3. Compensatory tachycardia, tachyphylaxis, histamine release, and possible prolongation of the action of succinylcholine can complicate its use.

HELLP SYNDROME

1. The syndrome of hemolysis, elevated liver enzymes, and low platelet count (HELLP) is a recognized complication of severe preeclampsia.
   a. The incidence varies from 2% to 12%.
   b. Seventy percent of cases occur antepartum and 30% postpartum.
   c. The risk is highest among older (age more than 25 years), White, multiparous women with a poor obstetric history.
2. Diagnosis
   a. Usually easy near term
   b. Early in pregnancy, women may present with nonspecific symptoms such as malaise, nausea and vomiting, and right upper quadrant pain.
      i. Adding to difficulty of diagnosis, hypertension and proteinuria may not be present.
      ii. HELLP may be misdiagnosed as viral hepatitis, gastroenteritis, peptic ulcer, cholecystitis, fatty liver of pregnancy, idiopathic thrombocytopenia, or hemolytic uremic syndrome.
   c. Appropriate diagnostic criteria include:
      i. Hemolysis:
         (1) Abnormal peripheral smear
         (2) Increased serum bilirubin (greater than 1.2 mg per deciliter)
         (3) Increased lactic dehydrogenase levels (greater than 600 IU per liter).
      ii. Elevated liver enzymes:
         (1) Serum glutamic oxaloacetic transaminase (SGOT) greater than 70 IU per liter

(2)   Increased   lactic   dehydrogenase   levels (greater than 600 IU/L)
iii.   Low platelet count: less than 100,000 per cubic millimeter.
3.   Patients with a diagnosis of HELLP syndrome should be immediately transferred to a tertiary care center for further evaluation and treatment.
4.   Initial management resembles that for women with severe preeclampsia.
   a.   First, stabilize the maternal condition, especially coagulation function.
   b.   Diagnosis of HELLP syndrome is not indication for immediate cesarean delivery.
   c.   Mode of delivery should be determined by coexisting obstetric factors.
   d.   Those developing laboratory evidence of DIC require immediate delivery, regardless of fetal gestational age.

PREVENTION OF PREECLAMPSIA
1.   Prevention of preeclampsia is difficult, as its etiology is unknown.
2.   Earlier recommendations of dietary salt restriction and diuretics simply reduced the blood volume with little or no beneficial effect on hypertension.
3.   Aspirin
   a.   Low-dose aspirin therapy may reduce the incidence of preeclampsia in specific subgroups of women but, this effect is of minimal clinical significance.
   b.   Aspirin therapy is associated with an increased risk of placental abruption.
   c.   Based on the available information, the American College of Obstetricians and Gynecologists does not recommend routine use of aspirin for prevention of preeclampsia.[6]

REFERENCES
1.   American College of Obstetricians and Gynecologists. Preeclampsia. Technical Bulletin 219, 1996.
2.   Mabie WC, Ratts TE, Ramanathan KB, Sibai BM. Circulatory congestion in obese hypertensive women: A subset of pulmonary edema in pregnancy. *Obstet Gynecol* 1988;72:553.
3.   Chandran R, Serra-Serra V, Redman CW. Spontaneous resolution of pre-eclampsia-related thrombocytopenia. *Br J Obstet Gynaecol* 1992;99:887.
4.   Duley L, Gulmezoglu AM, Henderson-Smart DJ. Anticonvulsants for women with pre-eclampsia. The Cochrane Database of Systematic Reviews 1998:4.
5.   Nelson KB, Grether JK. Can magnesium sulfate reduce the risk of cerebral palsy in very low birthweight infants? *Pediatrics* 1995;95:263.
6.   Lucas MJ, Leveno KJ, Cunningham FG. A comparison of magnesium sulfate with phenytoin for the prevention of eclampsia. *N Engl J Med* 1995;333:201.

Diabetes Mellitus in Pregnancy

1. Diabetes mellitus is a common cause of maternal and perinatal morbidity and mortality.
   a. In the United States, approximately 1.5 million women of childbearing age have diabetes.
   b. In addition, transient disturbances in glucose tolerance occur in 1% to 3% of pregnancies.
2. Diabetes mellitus is a chronic metabolic disorder caused by an absolute or relative lack of insulin.
3. There are two main types of disease in pregnancy:
   a. Preexisting, usually insulin dependent (IDDM).
   b. Gestational diabetes (GDM), which is carbohydrate intolerance of variable severity first recognized during pregnancy.
   c. Insulin deficiency causes:
      i. Hyperglycemia.
      ii. Abnormal protein and lipid metabolism.
      iii. Microangiopathy involving the retinal and renal vessels.
      iv. Peripheral neuropathy.
      v. Severe, uncontrolled diabetes culminates in catastrophic ketoacidosis, with a perinatal mortality rate of 50% to 90%.
4. Table 5.1 shows a widely used classification of diabetes.

EFFECTS OF DIABETES ON THE MOTHER

1. Major changes in glucose metabolism occur with pregnancy.
   a. Nonpregnant women, when fasted, maintain a basal plasma concentration of glucose by both the continuous release of glucose from hepatic glycogen stores and gluconeogenesis from amino acids and other glucose precursors. Insulin and glucagon control plasma glucose concentrations.
   b. In healthy, pregnant women, fasting for 12 hours (overnight) can produce a plasma glucose concentration of as low as 40 to 45 mg per deciliter.
      i. This rapid fall in plasma glucose reduces insulin secretion, leading in turn to ketosis.
      ii. Such exaggerated response to fasting is termed *accelerated starvation of pregnancy.*
         (1) Increases in maternal and fetal glucose utilization and in the volume of distribution for glucose are apparently responsible for this effect.
         (2) Accelerated starvation and maternal hypoglycemia increase production of ketoacids, which readily cross the placenta and accumulate in the fetus, causing acidosis.
   c. When healthy parturients eat, their plasma glucose concentration rises.

**Table 5.1.   Classification of glucose intolerance
in pregnant women**

Type I or insulin-dependent diabetes mellitus

Juvenile diabetes, juvenile-onset diabetes, ketosis-prone
diabetes

> Ketosis-prone; insulin-deficient due to islet cell loss; often asso-
> ciated with specific HLA types with predisposition to viral
> insulitis or autoimmune (islet cell antibody phenomena);
> occurs at any age: common in youth; these women are usually
> of normal weight but may be obese

Type II or non–insulin-dependent diabetes mellitus, nonobese, obese

Adult-onset diabetes, maturity-onset diabetes, ketosis-resistant
diabetes, stable diabetes

> Ketosis-resistant; more frequent in adults but occurs at any
> age; majority are overweight; may be seen in family aggre-
> gates as an autosomal dominant genetic trait; always require
> insulin for hyperglycemia during pregnancy but not "insulin-
> dependent"; previous history of "borderline diabetes,"
> impaired glucose tolerance, or treatment with oral hypo-
> glycemic agents;
> HbA1c >8% during first 20 weeks of gestation

Type III or gestational carbohydrate intolerance, nonobese, obese

Gestational diabetes

> Screening tests: all pregnant women; 50 g of oral glucose given
> randomly (need not be fasting) at 24 and 28 weeks of gesta-
> tion; a plasma glucose 1 h later >140 g/100 mL (7.8 mmol) is
> an indication for oral glucose tolerance test

Type IV or secondary diabetes

*Conditions and syndromes associated with impaired glucose
tolerance*

> Cystic fibrosis; endocrine disorders such as acromegaly, hyper-
> prolactinemia, Cushing's syndrome, insulin receptor abnor-
> malities, or aberrant forms of insulin, drugs, or chemical
> agents, renal dialysis, organ transplantation, certain genetic
> syndromes

    i.   This exaggerated hyperglycemic response to a car-
bohydrate load markedly increases insulin production.

      (1) Hypertrophy of the β cells of the islets of
Langerhans yields this hyperinsulinemic
response.

      (2) Most evident during the third trimester.

   ii. Persistent hyperglycemia signals hepatic resistance to insulin. The synergistic effects of placental hormones, human placental lactogen,
estrogen, and progesterone produce the insulin-
resistant characteristic during pregnancy.

2. Diabetes during pregnancy exaggerates all of these effects.
   a. In early pregnancy, maternal hypoglycemia frequently occurs and necessitates drastic reductions in insulin dose.
   b. During the latter half of pregnancy, insulin resistance develops, with a progressive increase in insulin requirements.
   c. Without tight metabolic control, these women are extremely prone to ketoacidosis.
3. The incidence of obstetric complications such as preeclampsia, hydramnios, and preterm labor is significantly higher in pregnant women with diabetes. Other serious complications of severe diabetes mellitus during pregnancy include diabetic retinopathy, nephropathy, hypertension, and coronary insufficiency.

EFFECTS OF DIABETES ON THE FETUS
Congenital Anomalies
1. The advent of insulin therapy in pregnancy reduced perinatal mortality to less than 5%.
2. Despite the general decline in perinatal morbidity and mortality, major congenital anomalies continue to occur at a rate of 6% to 12%, approximately two to four times that in the general population, and account for 40% of neonatal deaths among children of diabetic parturients.
3. The exact mechanism of these anomalies remains a mystery.
   a. Inadequate control of diabetes during the early stages of pregnancy, particularly organogenesis, may at least partly explain the high incidence of anomalies.
   b. Strict control of diabetes and maintenance of euglycemia beginning before conception or at very early gestation can significantly lower the incidence of congenital defects.

Macrosomia
1. Maternal hyperglycemia provides excessive quantities of glucose to the fetus.
   a. Glucose crosses the placenta by facilitated diffusion, a carrier-mediated and non-energy-dependent process.
   b. Hyperglycemia in the fetus increases insulin production and fuel utilization.
      i. Insulin is an anabolic hormone.
      ii. Increased fat deposition, hypertrophy of visceral organs, and increased skeletal growth occur.
2. Diabetes-induced macrosomia manifests as fetal fat deposition in the shoulders and trunk.
   a. The head is no longer the largest part of the delivering fetus.
   b. During vaginal delivery, macrosomia (fetal weight greater than 4,000 g) contributes to a high incidence of birth injuries, such as shoulder dystocia, facial nerve or brachial plexus injury, and asphyxia.
3. Despite good metabolic control, the incidence of macrosomia may be as high as 20% to 30%.

Neonatal Hypoglycemia

1. In infants of healthy, nondiabetic mothers, insulin concentration falls rapidly with the separation of placenta at delivery, compensating for the sudden cessation of the fuel supply from the mother.
2. Such rapid hormonal adaptation fails to occur in infants of diabetic women.
    a. Chronic intrauterine oversupply of glucose induces fetal pancreatic islet cell hypertrophy and hyperinsulinemia, which persists after birth and often causes neonatal hypoglycemia (blood sugar less than 30 mg per deciliter).
    b. Twenty-five percent to 40% of infants of diabetic mothers will experience hypoglycemia, with macrosomic and preterm infants at the highest risk.
3. Infants of diabetic mothers also secrete less glucagon and fewer catecholamines in response to spontaneous hypoglycemia, resulting in the inability of the liver to produce glucose in response to stress.
4. Other neonatal metabolic derangements of both IDDM and GDM include hyperbilirubinemia, acidosis, hypocalcemia, and hypomagnesemia.

Respiratory Distress Syndrome

1. Respiratory distress syndrome (RDS) is a common cause of neonatal morbidity and mortality.
2. Recent obstetric advances, including frequent evaluations of fetal lung maturity, have helped to decrease the incidence of RDS dramatically.
3. Fetal hyperinsulinemia may interfere with surfactant production and delay lung maturity, leading to a five- to sixfold greater risk of RDS in the premature infant of the inadequately controlled diabetic mother.

CHANGES IN UTEROPLACENTAL CIRCULATION AND FETAL OXYGENATION

1. Diabetes significantly impairs uteroplacental perfusion.
2. In addition, the structure of the placenta itself is modified by diabetes. The villi are enlarged, intervillous spaces are smaller, and effective uterine blood flow is reduced.
3. The presence of increased maternal glycosylated hemoglobin (HbA_{1c}) also may compromise fetal oxygenation.
    a. When glucose covalently binds to the two β chains in the adult Hb (HbA), it creates HbA_{1c}, which interferes with oxygen uptake.
    b. In insulin-dependent diabetic women, HbA_{1c} interferes with oxygen transport and compromises fetal oxygenation.
    c. Serial measurements of HbA_{1c} concentration provide valuable information on the quality of maternal blood sugar control and the effectiveness of therapy.

DIABETIC KETOACIDOSIS (DKA)

1. DKA is a serious and often preventable cause of maternal and fetal morbidity and mortality. It affects up to 0.7% of

pregnancies complicated by GDM and 1.7% to 9.3% of gravidae with IDDM.

   a. Perinatal mortality ranges from 22% to 65%, depending on the presence of coma, gestational age, serum glucose and osmolality, blood urea nitrogen (BUN), insulin requirements, and duration of the acidotic state. Fortunately, monitoring and therapy can resuscitate the fetus *in utero* and prevent fetal death.

   b. Maternal mortality from DKA during pregnancy is comparable to the mortality of ketoacidosis in the general population (approximately 5%).

2. The etiology of DKA is often multifactorial. Common precipitating factors include:

   a. Poor patient compliance.
   b. Undiagnosed diabetes.
   c. Administration of β-mimetic agents.
   d. Emesis.
   e. Poor physician management.

3. Regardless of the etiology, ketoacidosis may occur in gravid diabetics with a lesser degree of hyperglycemia (150 to 300 mg per deciliter) than in nongravid diabetics.

4. Symptoms include:

   a. Nausea and vomiting.
   b. Malaise.
   c. Altered mental status (ranging from drowsiness to lethargy and coma).
   d. Polydipsia.
   e. Polyuria.
   f. Abdominal pain.

5. Classic signs include hyperventilation (Kussmaul respiration), a fruity or acetone breath odor, dehydration, and, occasionally, hypotension. Although serum sodium, potassium, and BUN may be low, normal, or high, virtually all patients have total body sodium and potassium deficits.

6. The diagnosis of DKA is confirmed by:

   a. Plasma glucose greater than 300 mg per deciliter.
   b. Plasma HCO_3 less than 15 mEq per liter.
   c. pH less than 7.30.
   d. Serum acetone at 1:2 dilutions.

7. Once the diagnosis of DKA is confirmed, prompt treatment and continuous fetal monitoring are imperative (Table 5.2).

   a. Fluid deficits of up to 10 L are not uncommon.

      i. Approximately half of the deficit should be replaced in the first 5 hours, using warmed, isotonic fluids (normal saline).

      ii. Intravascular volume expansion improves organ and peripheral perfusion, lowers serum osmolarity, dilutes hyperglycemia, prevents metabolic acidosis, and allows peripheral uptake of exogenously administered insulin.

   b. Total body potassium deficit ranges from 3 to 10 mmol per kilogram and must be replaced following initiation of rehydration and concurrently with intravenous insulin.

Table 5.2. Treatment of diabetic ketoacidosis

1. Monitor: Electrolyte, blood glucose, arterial blood gases, fluid intake/out each hour. Consider intraarterial catheter for continuous measurement of blood pressure and blood sampling. Also consider central venous catheter to evaluate response to fluid therapy. Continuously monitor fetal heart rate and uterine activity.
2. Fluids: 1–2 L of isotonic saline in the first hour; 300–500 mL/h of 0.45% or 0.9% saline thereafter, determined by the serum sodium via a large peripheral vein or central venous catheter.
3. Insulin: 10–20 U of regular insulin IV, then continuous infusion of 5–10 U/h until plasma glucose reaches 200 mg/dL. Then decrease to 1–2 U/h.
4. Potassium: 40 mEq KCl/L of fluid after 2–4 h of insulin therapy and establishment of urine output >0.5 mL/kg/h.
5. Sodium bicarbonate: Administer for pH <7.1.
6. Glucose: Begin administering IV glucose when plasma levels decline to 200–250 mg/dL.

Source: After Whiteman VE, Homko CJ, Reece EA. Management of hypoglycemia and diabetic ketoacidosis in pregnancy. *Obstet Gynecol Clin North Am* 1996;23:87.

    i. Both urinary losses and the intracellular shift of potassium in the presence of glucose and insulin may lead to dramatic declines in plasma potassium.
    ii. Electrocardiographic monitoring is essential because the fluctuating potassium gradient can cause cardiac dysrythmias.
  c. Begin insulin therapy after starting volume replacement.
    i. An intravenous bolus of 10 to 20 U of regular insulin is followed by an infusion of 5 to 10 U per hour.
    ii. Aim to decrease serum glucose concentration by 30% to 40% in the first 4 hours of therapy.
    iii. When serum glucose levels reach approximately 250 mg per deciliter, start an intravenous dextrose infusion at 150 mg per hour and decrease the insulin infusion to 1 to 2 U per hour.
    iv. Normoglycemia (80 to 120 mg per deciliter) is the goal of therapy.
  d. Sodium bicarbonate is reserved for patients with an arterial pH less than 7.1.
    i. Sodium bicarbonate may cause paradoxic intracerebral acidosis and hinder oxygen delivery to tissues.
    ii. Limit the dosage to 100 mEq (2 amps) per liter of intravenous fluid (0.45% saline), to minimize hyperosmolarity and pain with injection.
    iii. Discontinue use of sodium bicarbonate when the pH reaches 7.20 and change fluid to 0.9% saline.

TIMING OF DELIVERY

1. Both maternal and fetal conditions must be considered when planning delivery of the fetus of the diabetic mother.
   a. The parturient who has maintained normoglycemia and is carrying a healthy fetus may be allowed to progress to term and experience spontaneous labor. Fetal maturation should be confirmed before delivery.
   b. Premature labor should be treated with bed rest, intravenous fluids, and magnesium sulfate.
      i. β-Sympathomimetic agents are contraindicated because they have direct antiinsulin effects and induce hyperglycemia and ketoacidosis.
      ii. The use of corticosteroids for fetal lung maturation may be justified, provided glucose homeostasis is maintained.
   c. If fetal surveillance suggests a compromised pregnancy, prompt delivery may be necessary, even without evidence of fetal lung maturity.
2. Method of delivery
   a. Fetal intolerance to labor or macrosomia may make successful vaginal delivery unlikely.
   b. The obese parturient with GDM is at substantially increased risk of fetal macrosomia and operative delivery.
   c. Even when all factors are ideal and labor is allowed to occur, the diabetic parturient is more likely to require cesarean delivery.
   d. GDM patients with excellent glycemic control and normosomic infants are at equal risk of cesarean section as poorly controlled parturients with macrosomic infants.

INTRAPARTUM MANAGEMENT OF THE DIABETIC PARTURIENT

1. Preoperative evaluation of the diabetic parturient should be directed at those organ systems most commonly affected by chronic diabetes mellitus.
   a. The presence of renal insufficiency, cardiac disease, or long-standing diabetes increases the incidence of peripartum complications.
      i. Coexisting hypertension significantly increases morbidity and mortality.
      ii. Renal insufficiency is associated with a lower hematocrit, greater urinary protein loss, and higher serum creatinine.
   b. Look for peripheral or autonomic neuropathy and document the extent of any sensory or motor deficits.
2. Physical examination
   a. Thoroughly evaluate the airway for signs of stiff joint syndrome and the potential for difficult intubation (see following).
   b. Look for signs of cardiac decompensation. The older parturient or one with suspected or documented cardiac disease should have a recent ECG.

3. Baseline laboratory evaluation includes electrolytes, BUN, creatinine, and glucose.
4. Intrapartum glucose control
   a. Hypoglycemia is the most common complication in neonates of diabetic mothers. Antenatal maternal hyperglycemia also can produce neonatal acidosis.
   b. Maintaining maternal plasma glucose at a normal concentration (70 to 120 mg per deciliter) during labor significantly reduces the incidence of neonatal acidosis and hypoglycemia.
   c. Commonly used insulin–glucose protocols can attain this goal (Table 5.3A–E).
      i. Glucose requirement during labor is constant at 2.55 mg per kilogram per minute.
      ii. Insulin requirements vary.
         (1) Frequently, insulin is not needed during the first stage of labor due to the fasting state and increased glucose utilization.
         (2) Usual insulin requirements range from 0 to 5 U of regular insulin per hour.
   d. Glucose and insulin infusions should be maintained on separate mechanical pumps.
   e. Although preventing hyperglycemia is important, avoiding hypoglycemia with attendant ketosis also is essential, as these metabolic imbalances significantly prolong labor and induce neonatal hypoglycemia.

Table 5.3A.   Management of women with insulin-dependent diabetes mellitus for elective cesarean delivery or scheduled labor induction

1. Give the usual insulin dose the evening before surgery and a small meal before midnight. In the morning, give one-fourth to one-half of the usual dose of intermediate-acting insulin. Titrate 5% glucose infusion to maintain blood glucose at 70–120 mg/dL.
2. Measure fasting glucose on the morning of surgery and obtain a finger stick glucose every 1–2 h thereafter. If fasting glucose is >120 mg/100 mL or if the surgery is delayed, start 5% glucose at 2.55 mg/kg/min and insulin at 1–5 U/h to maintain blood sugar at 70–120 mg/dL. Delay surgery until euglycemia is maintained for 4 h.
3. If fasting glucose level is <120 mg/100 mL, start intravenous fluids without dextrose. Hold additional insulin.
4. Treat any blood glucose >120 mg/dL with sliding scale, intermittent, IV boluses of insulin. Dose 1–10 U of insulin for each 50 mg/dL increment >120 mg/dL.
5. Immediately postpartum, decrease insulin to 60% of prepregnancy dose or one-third to one-half of antepartum dose. Continue frequent blood glucose monitoring.

Source: Homko CJ, Khandelwal M. Glucose monitoring and insulin therapy during pregnancy. *Obstet Gynecol Clin North Am* 1996;23:47.

Table 5.3B.   Management of women with insulin-dependent diabetes mellitus for elective cesarean delivery or scheduled labor induction: insulin and glucose infusion

1. Withhold all subcutaneous insulin. Measure blood sugar.
2. Begin continuous infusion insulin at 1–2 U/h and glucose at 150 mg/kg/h. Measure blood glucose each hour and modify insulin infusion.
3. Adjust insulin from 0.5–2.0 U/h. Treat >140 mg/dL with IV bolus insulin 2 U and increase infusion. Blood sugar <70 mg/dL, administer 2–5 g of glucose.

Source: Ramanathan S, Khoo P, Arismendy J. Perioperative maternal and neonatal acid-base status and glucose metabolism in patients with insulin-dependent diabetes mellitus. *Anesth Analg* 1991;73:105.

Table 5.3C.   Management of women with insulin-dependent diabetes mellitus for elective cesarean delivery or scheduled labor induction: low-dose constant insulin infusion for the intrapartum period

1. Finger stick blood glucose every hour.
2. Blood glucose <100 mg/dL, insulin 0 U, IV 5% dextrose lactated Ringer's solution.
3. Blood glucose 100–140 mg/dL, insulin 1.0 U/h, IV 5% dextrose lactated Ringer's solution.
4. Blood glucose 141–180 mg/dL, insulin 1.5 U/h, IV normal saline.
5. Blood glucose 181–220 mg/dL, insulin 2.0 U/h, IV normal saline.
6. Blood glucose >220 mg/dL, insulin 2.5 U/h, IV normal saline.

Source: Committee on Technical Bulletins of the American College of Obstetricians and Gynecologists. ACOG technical bulletin. Diabetes and pregnancy. Number 200—December 1994. *Int J Gynaecol Obstet* 1995;48:331.

Table 5.3D.   Management of women with insulin-dependent diabetes mellitus for elective cesarean delivery or scheduled labor induction: intermittent insulin bolus

1. No morning insulin.
2. Use non–dextrose-containing fluids.
3. Measure blood sugar frequently.
4. Treat blood glucose >120 mg/dL with 1–2 U of IV insulin.

Source: Datta S. *Common problems in obstetric anesthesia,* 2nd ed. St. Louis: Mosby–Year Book, 1994:373.

Table 5.3E. Insulin management in labor

1. Blood sugar <120 mg/dL: Give one-third the usual daily dose of insulin subcutaneously (intermediate acting). Measure blood sugar every 1–2 h. If blood sugar increases to >120 mg/dL, begin insulin infusion of 0.5–2.0 U/h.
2. Blood sugar >120 mg/dL on arrival: Give one-third the usual daily dose of insulin subcutaneously (intermediate acting). Measure blood sugar every 1–2 h. Begin intravenous insulin infusion immediately. Monitor as above and treat blood sugar >140 mg/dL with 1–2 U of IV insulin bolus.

Source: Datta S. *Common problems in obstetric anesthesia,* 2nd ed. St. Louis: Mosby–Year Book, 1994:373.

5. Management of diet-controlled, gestational diabetics is simpler. Usually, intravenous fluids without dextrose provide adequate control of maternal plasma glucose concentration while monitoring is continued, as in the IDDM parturient.
6. Immediately postpartum, insulin requirement drops to approximately 60% of the prepregnancy requirement. The dose will return to baseline in about 5 to 6 days.

THE AIRWAY AND DIABETES IN PREGNANCY

1. The airway of the gravida with either IDDM or GDM presents several potential problems.
2. IDDM seen in parturients frequently begins in childhood as juvenile-onset diabetes mellitus (JODM) and is associated with the syndrome of limited joint mobility (LJM).[1]
   a. Nonfamilial short stature; thick, tight, waxy skin; delayed sexual maturation; early microvascular complications; and limited mobility of the small joints
   b. LJM is found in 28% of JODM patients within 5 years of diagnosis.
   c. One-third of patients with LJM will have severe manifestations, including significant involvement of the cervical spine.
      i. Impaired cervical spine movement, especially limited movement at the atlantooccipital joint, impairs the ability to intubate the trachea.
      ii. There is a 26% to 41% incidence of difficult intubation in diabetic patients undergoing general anesthesia.
         (1) Difficult intubation correlates with inflexibility of the joints of the hand.
         (2) An easy bedside test for joint abnormalities is to have the patient oppose the palms of the hands and see if the proximal interphalangeal joints of the fourth and fifth fingers will touch (Fig. 5.1).
3. The gravida with GDM also is at risk for difficult intubation, but for different reasons.

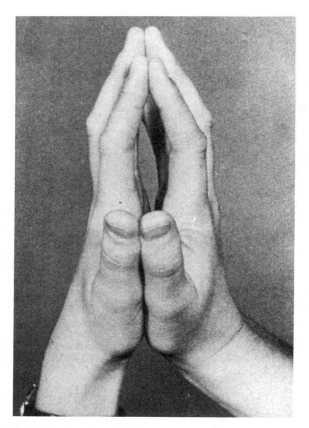

Fig. 5.1.   Limitation of small joint mobility evidenced by inability to approximate the interphalangeal joints, "the prayer sign." Patients with this manifestation of diabetes frequently present difficulties with direct laryngoscopy and tracheal intubation. (Source: Kennedy L, Archer D, Campbell S, Beacom R, Carson D, Johnston P. Limited joint mobility in type I diabetes mellitus. *Postgrad Med J* 1982;58:481, with permission.)

    a. The majority of gestational diabetic women are obese (body mass index greater than 30 or greater than 150% ideal body weight).

    b. Obesity plus pregnancy increase the likelihood of difficult intubation by tenfold.

NEUROPATHY AND REGIONAL ANESTHESIA

Autonomic Neuropathy

1. Occurs within 15 years of onset of insulin treatment in up to 30% of diabetics. About 23% of gravidae with IDDM have autonomic dysfunction.

2. Manifestations include:
   a. Orthostatic hypotension or lightheadedness.
   b. Diarrhea or constipation.
   c. Bladder complaints.
   d. Resting tachycardia. (Diabetic parturients experience less of an increase in resting heart rate with pregnancy than do nondiabetics. Resting tachycardia is not an appropriate marker of autonomic dysfunction in pregnancy.)
   e. Decreased heart rate variability with deep breathing or vagal stimulation.
   f. Diabetic gastroparesis is extremely rare in pregnancy, and gastric function is not significantly different than that of the nondiabetic pregnant woman.
3. General anesthesia in the parturient with autonomic neuropathy
   a. Hypotension and a significant decline in heart rate occur during induction.
   b. Less rebound follows tracheal intubation.
   c. Thirty-five percent of diabetics require vasopressor treatment.
   d. The fetus of the IDDM mother tolerates hypotension poorly.
4. Regional anesthesia
   a. Sympathetic blockade may induce a greater degree of hypotension than in the nondiabetic.
   b. Cardiac and vasoconstrictive responses to hypotension are blunted by autonomic neuropathy because the sympathetic nerves are less well supplied with norepinephrine.
   c. Ephedrine or phenylephrine are appropriate treatment choices, as determined by the heart rate.

Peripheral Neuropathy
1. Up to 50% of diabetics have some evidence of peripheral neuropathy.
   a. Distal sensory and motor lesions are most common.
   b. Symptoms include paresthesias, pain, or hypesthesia of the distal extremities.
   c. Small fiber neuropathy is less common and presents as distal burning pain or hyperalgesia. Autonomic neuropathy is more commonly associated with small fiber disease.
2. If contemplating regional analgesia–anesthesia, document the extent and type of peripheral neuropathy.
3. Changes in nerve structure and blood supply inherent to diabetes mellitus may place the affected parturient at increased risk of all types of peripartum nerve injury.
   a. Assure careful and proper positioning during both general and regional anesthesia.
   b. The ulnar nerve, as it passes through the cubital tunnel, is most commonly affected during general anesthesia.

   c. Passage of the fetus through the pelvis, placement of forceps, and the lithotomy position may cause nerve injury during vaginal delivery. Commonly affected are the lumbosacral trunk, and sacral, femoral, lateral femoral cutaneus, and lateral popliteal nerves.

REFERENCE

1. Grgic A, Rosenbloom A, Weber F, Giordano B, Malone I, Shuster J. Joint contracture—common manifestation of childhood diabetes mellitus. *J Pediatr* 1976;88:584.

Perinatal Physiology and Pharmacology

Of necessity, there is a close relationship between a mother and her fetus. The fetus receives all its nourishment and oxygen from the mother. In addition, this intimate connection exposes the fetus to almost any substance to which the mother is exposed. Any drug given during gestation can potentially affect the fetus and the newborn.

PLACENTA
Structure

1. The placenta is a disc-shaped organ.
   a. It is the interface between the mother and her fetus.
   b. It serves as a fetal lung, a gastrointestinal system, and an excretory system.
   c. It permits passage of some substances while acting as a barrier to others.
   d. At term, the placenta weighs about 500 g.
2. The basic structural unit of the placenta is the chorionic villus.
   a. Villi are highly vascular projections of fetal tissue surrounded by the chorion, the outermost layer of fetal tissue.
   b. The chorion has two layers:
      i. The syncytiotrophoblast, which lies in direct contact with maternal blood within the intervillous space.
      ii. The cytotrophoblast (Fig. 6.1).
   c. No continuous direct communication exists between maternal and fetal circulations.
3. Substances travel in maternal blood to the intervillous space. There, they cross
   a. The two layers of trophoblast.
   b. Fetal connective tissue.
   c. Fetal capillary wall into the fetal blood stream (Fig. 6.2).
4. Occasionally a delicate villus may break.
   a. Fetal cells enter the intervillous space and the maternal circulation.
   b. Maternal sensitization to fetal red blood cells (isoimmunization) may occur.

Uteroplacental Circulation

1. The blood supply to the placenta is maternal in origin.
   a. Uteroplacental blood flow near term is approximately 600 mL per minute.
   b. Maternal blood spurts into the intervillous space with each heart beat.
   c. Blood is forced upward and laterally, bathing the chorionic villi.
   d. Venous openings ultimately drain through uterine and pelvic veins (see Fig. 6.1).

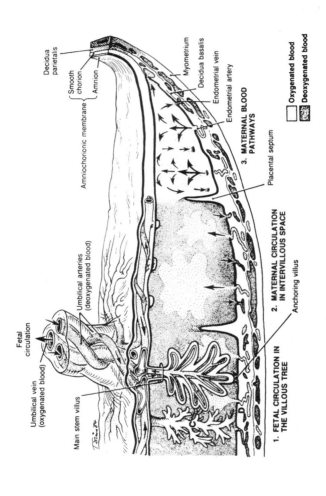

Fetal
circulation

Umbilical vein
(oxygenated blood)

Main stem villus

Umbilical arteries
(deoxygenated blood)

Decidua
parietalis

Smooth
chorion

Amnion

Amniochorionic membrane

Myometrium

Decidua basalis

Endometrial vein

Endometrial artery

3. MATERNAL BLOOD
PATHWAYS

Oxygenated blood

Deoxygenated blood

Placental septum

2. MATERNAL CIRCULATION
IN INTERVILLOUS SPACE

Anchoring villus

1. FETAL CIRCULATION IN
THE VILLOUS TREE

2. At term, the uteroplacental circulation appears maximally vasodilated.
   a. Flow depends mostly on maternal blood pressure.
   b. Changes in intrauterine pressure and the pattern of uterine contractions can interfere with placental blood supply.

Function

Synthesis and Metabolism

1. The placenta can synthesize hormones, including estrogen, progesterone, chorionic gonadotropin, and placental lactogen.
2. Placental lactogen
   a. Abundant in the mother but not the fetus
   b. Promotes insulin resistance in the mother by blocking the peripheral uptake and utilization of glucose
   c. Also promotes maternal mobilization and use of free fatty acids
   d. These actions ensure a ready glucose supply for the fetus and placenta.
3. Placental cellular receptors
   a. Insulin
   b. β-Adrenergic receptors
4. Placental enzymes
   a. Adenylate cyclase, alkaline phosphatase, and pseudocholinesterase
   b. Catechol-*O*-methyl transferase and monoamine oxidase impede the transplacental passage of catecholamines.
5. The placental barrier
   a. Allows the mother to accept the fetus (nonself).
   b. Acts as a filter, permitting selective transport of maternal antibodies to the fetus.
      i. Some of these antibodies help provide fetal immunity.

◄ ───

Fig. 6.1. Schematic drawing of a section through a full-term placenta. 1: The relation of the villus chorion (*C*) to the decidua basalis (*D*) and the fetal placental circulation. 2: The maternal placental circulation. Maternal blood flows into the intervillous spaces in funnel-shaped spurts, and exchanges occur with the fetal blood as the maternal blood flows around the villi. 3: The inflowing arterial blood pushes venous blood into the endometrial veins, which are scattered over the entire surface of the decidua basalis. Note that the umbilical arteries carry deoxygenated fetal blood to the placenta and that the umbilical vein carries oxygenated blood to the fetus. Note that the cotyledons are separated from each other by placenta (decidual) septa of the materna portion of the placenta. Each cotyledon consists of two or more main stem villi and their many branches. (Source: Cunningham FG, MacDonald PC, Gant NF, et al. The placenta and fetal membranes. In: Cunningham FG, Gant NF, MacDonald PC, et al., eds. *Williams' Obstetrics*, 20th ed. Stamford: Appleton & Lange, 1997:116, with permission.)

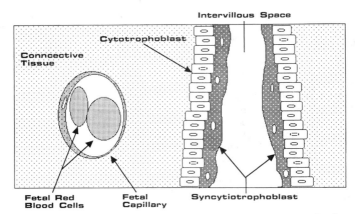

Fig. 6.2. Schematic representation of a fetal villous, showing the tissue layers that separate fetal and maternal blood in the human placenta. The cytotrophoblast layer is much less distinct in the third trimester than depicted here.

      ii.   Others can cause fetal disease.
          (1) In Rh isoimmunization, maternal antibodies specific for fetal red blood cells cross the placenta and produce fetal hemolytic anemia.
          (2) Antibodies producing maternal autoimmune disease (e.g., thyrotoxicosis, idiopathic thrombocytopenic purpura, myasthenia gravis, and systemic lupus erythematosus) also can attack fetal tissue.

Placental Exchange
1. Functionally, the placenta is a complex organ of exchange. Nutrients, waste products, and toxins continuously cross (Table 6.1).
    a. Most substances traverse the trophoblast by simple diffusion, also known as flow-limited transfer.
    b. Polar (hydrophilic) substances (e.g., metabolic wastes, nutrients, and some drugs) need special help to cross the lipid membranes of the placenta. Specialized transport processes include facilitated diffusion, active transport, and pinocytosis. Unlike simple diffusion, these methods of transfer expend energy.
3. Most drugs and respiratory gases cross the placenta by *simple diffusion,* which uses no energy. The rate at which substances pass from mother to fetus depends only on the difference in concentration of the substance in maternal and fetal blood.
4. Compounds that cross the placenta through *facilitated diffusion* also travel down a concentration gradient.
    a. Here, however, the speed of transfer is faster than predicted for simple diffusion.

Table 6.1. Mechanisms of placental exchange

Mechanism	Example
Simple diffusion	Oxygen
	Carbon dioxide
	Sodium
	Chloride
	Fatty acids
Facilitated diffusion	Glucose
	Lactate
Active transport	Amino acids
	Calcium
	Phosphorus
	Iron
	Vitamins A and C
Pinocytosis	IgG

    b.   Substances occurring in low concentration in maternal plasma that are essential to the fetus (e.g., glucose and lactate) traverse the placenta by facilitated diffusion.

5. *Active transport* involves transferring compounds against a concentration gradient. Substances actively transported include some amino acids, calcium, phosphorus, iron, and vitamins A and C.

6. The placenta acts as a barrier to most proteins, the most notable exception being immunoglobulin G (IgG).

    a.   IgG probably crosses the placenta by pinocytosis (endocytosis), which involves specific receptors located on the trophoblast.

    b.   Once IgG attaches to the receptor, it is enclosed in small vacuoles. These vacuoles then pinch off and cross to the fetal side of the trophoblast. There, they release their contents.

Respiratory Exchange

Respiratory gases pass to the fetus by simple diffusion. At the tissue level, respiratory exchange also depends on the interaction of oxygen and carbon dioxide with hemoglobin and on the nature of blood flow in the maternal and umbilical circulations.

OXYGEN

1. Multiple factors enhance fetal oxygenation.

    a.   Fetal hemoglobin binds oxygen tightly, favoring oxygen uptake from maternal blood.

    b.   The high concentration of fetal hemoglobin and a greater cardiac output per unit of body weight than in the adult favor efficient uptake and distribution of oxygen within the fetus.

2. Oxygen transfer across the placenta is blood flow limited and not related to the thickness or surface area of the placenta.

    a.   The difference between the maternal and fetal partial pressures of oxygen determines the gradient for oxygen diffusion across the placenta.

b.   Relative differences in the affinity of maternal and fetal hemoglobins for oxygen account for most of the difference between maternal and fetal pO_2.
    i.   The oxyhemoglobin dissociation curve of fetal hemoglobin lies to the left of the dissociation curve of adult hemoglobin.
    ii. Fetal blood binds oxygen more tightly and has a higher oxygen content at a given pO_2 than adult blood.

CARBON DIOXIDE

1. Diffuses readily across the placenta
2. Factors accounting for difference between maternal and fetal pCO_2
    a.   Shunting or unequal distribution of maternal and fetal blood flow within the placental vasculature
    b.   Placental metabolism produces carbon dioxide.
3. Factors favoring transfer of carbon dioxide from fetus to mother
    a.   Fetal hemoglobin has a lower affinity for carbon dioxide than does maternal hemoglobin.
    b.   The hyperventilation of pregnancy lowers maternal pCO_2.
    c.   Both oxygen and carbon dioxide influence the binding of the other to hemoglobin. Placental transfer of one gas enhances the exchange of the other.

FETAL OXYGENATION

1. The umbilical vein, carrying oxygenated blood to the fetus, empties into the portal sinus.
    a.   Then, most of the blood bypasses the liver by flowing through the ductus venosus to the inferior vena cava.
    b.   The remainder passes through the liver via the portal and hepatic veins.
2. The oxygen-rich blood in the ductus venosus enters the right atrium and traverses the foramen ovale into the left atrium.
    a.   There it mixes with pulmonary venous blood and travels through the left ventricle to the aorta.
    b.   This arrangement ensures well-oxygenated blood for the coronary and cerebral circulations.
3. Blood returning from the head, brain, and upper body via the superior vena cava enters the right atrium.
    a.   Then, with blood from the inferior vena cava, it flows from the right ventricle to the pulmonary artery.
    b.   Most of the blood entering the pulmonary artery skips the lungs by flowing through the ductus arteriosus directly into the descending aorta.
    c.   The umbilical arteries, arising from the internal iliac arteries, carry desaturated blood out of the fetus and back to the placenta.

PHYSIOLOGIC CHANGES OF PREGNANCY THAT ALTER PHARMACOKINETICS

1. Hyperventilation and decreased functional residual capacity increase the maternal uptake of inhalation anesthetics during pregnancy.

2. Progesterone and motilin concentrations increase during gestation. These compounds slow gastrointestinal motility, potentially altering the absorption of oral medications.
3. Hormonal changes are thought to be responsible for the decrease in minimum alveolar concentration (MAC) seen during gestation and the increased susceptibility of nerves to local anesthetics.
4. During pregnancy, total body water increases by up to 8 L, and plasma volume increases by 50%, expanding the volume of drug distribution.
5. Serum albumin concentration falls.
   a. Free fatty acids and acidic drugs (i.e., salicylates, anticonvulsants, and benzodiazepines) compete for a reduced number of albumin binding sites.
   b. As the affected drugs are less protein bound, they may be more potent than in nonpregnant women.
6. The serum concentration of α_1-acid glycoprotein remains stable. The free fraction of basic drugs, including local anesthetics and opioids that bind primarily to α_1-acid glycoprotein, does not change during gestation.
7. Hepatic metabolism may increase during pregnancy, as enzyme induction by progesterone speeds elimination of some drugs.
8. Renal plasma flow and glomerular filtration rise during gestation. Clearance of drugs that are primarily renally excreted, such as pancuronium, will increase.

Transfer of Drugs

1. Drugs that readily cross the blood–brain barrier also freely cross the placenta.
2. The concentration of drugs on the maternal side of the placenta determines the degree of fetal exposure.
   a. Maternal drug delivery to the placenta depends on:
      i. Dose and duration of administration.
      ii. Route of administration.
      iii. Rate of absorption.
      iv. Uteroplacental blood flow.
      v. Maternal metabolism and excretion.
      vi. Maternal protein binding.
      vii. Maternal pH and the pKa of the drug.
3. Drug concentration in fetal plasma depends on:
   a. Fetal protein binding.
   b. Cardiac output.
   c. Tissue uptake.
   d. Metabolism.
   e. Excretion.

FETAL PHYSIOLOGY AND PHARMACOKINETICS

1. Differences from the adult:
   a. Uptake into the fetus begins as drug passes through the placenta and enters the fetal circulation by way of the umbilical vein.
   b. Drug distribution depends on several factors.
      i. The drug may undergo considerable metabolism within the liver. This "first-pass" metabolism by

the fetal liver can significantly lower the amount of drug delivered to highly perfused organs such as the heart and the brain.

   ii. However, most drug bypasses the liver via the ductus venosus and directly enters the arterial circulation.

   iii. Shunts within the fetal circulation (i.e., foramen ovale and ductus arteriosus) also alter fetal drug distribution.

2. Determinants of fetal blood drug concentration:
   a. Maternal dose.
   b. Placental transfer.
      i. The rate of transfer depends primarily on differences in maternal and fetal protein binding and acid-base status.
      ii. Maternal protein binding limits the amount of free (unbound) drugs available for placental transport. This mechanism significantly limits fetal exposure to highly bound drugs (e.g., bupivacaine).
   c. The pH gradient between maternal and fetal blood also can influence the transfer of weakly acidic or basic compounds.
      i. Normally, a slight (0.1) pH gradient exists between the maternal and fetal circulation.
      ii. Only non-ionized drugs cross the lipid barrier of the placenta.
      iii. With acidic drugs (salicylates, anticonvulsants, barbiturates), the pH gradient limits transfer.
      iv. Basic drugs (local anesthetics and opioids)
         (1) The lower fetal pH favors drug transfer to the fetus (more drug exists in the ionized state in the lower pH of the fetal tissues).
         (2) "Ion trapping" of basic drugs can occur if fetal pH falls.
            (a) As un-ionized drug enters the fetal circulation, it becomes ionized and cannot diffuse back to the maternal circulation.
            (b) Both local anesthetics and opioids can become "trapped" in the fetus by this mechanism.

3. Fetal drug elimination
   a. Metabolism
      i. By term, most hepatic microsomal enzyme systems are present, but they are often less effective than adult enzymes.
      ii. The premature infant has even more limited metabolic capabilities.
   b. Urinary excretion
      i. Drug enters the amniotic fluid, where it may be swallowed by the fetus.
      ii Once reingested, drug may reenter the systemic circulation after being absorbed from the gastrointestinal tract.
   c. Diffusion back to the mother

Measuring Fetal Drug Effect

Drug Measurement

1. To determine the effects of a drug on the fetus or newborn, one must know the plasma concentration of drug at the time the reputed drug effect occurs.
2. Before birth, maternal plasma concentration of drug provides an indirect measurement of fetal plasma concentration.
3. The human placental perfusion model can indirectly provide additional help to quantify fetal drug exposure.

Testing for Intrapartum Drug Effects

1. Fetal heart rate patterns provide indirect information about the fetal effects of maternally administered drugs.
2. Radioactive tracers (xenon[133] or indium[113]) and Doppler ultrasonography can measure placental, fetal umbilical, and aortic blood flow.
3. *In utero* drug concentrations can be measured by cordocentesis.

Postpartum (Newborn) Testing

1. At birth, blood from the maternal vein, umbilical vein, and umbilical artery can be analyzed for the presence of specific drugs and their metabolites.
2. These data can provide some information about the amount of drug transferred to the fetus and its uptake by fetal tissues.
   a. The umbilical venous (UV) concentration of drug represents drug delivered to the fetus via the placenta.
   b. The ratio of umbilical venous to maternal venous drug levels (UV/MV) reflects the rate and extent of placental transfer.
   c. Umbilical arterial (UA) drug concentration is the portion of drug remaining after tissue uptake and metabolism.
   d. The ratio of drug concentration in the umbilical artery to the umbilical vein (UA/UV) shows the extent of uptake by fetal tissues.
   e. These measurements do not, however, indicate the total amount of drug present in the infant. To quantify fetal drug exposure accurately, one must repeatedly sample and analyze neonatal blood and urine.
3. Other methods of testing neonatal drug effects
   a. Nonspecific tests
      i. Apgar scores
      ii. Acid-base status
   b. Neurobehavioral tests
      i. Designed to look for subtle behavioral drug effects
      ii. These tests examine the neonate's muscle tone and ability to:
         (1) Alter the state of arousal.
         (2) Suppress responses to repetitive or intrusive stimuli.
         (3) Respond appropriately to external events.
         (4) Initiate complex motor acts and the appropriateness of reflex motor responses.

iii. Tests include:
   (1) The Brazelton Neonatal Behavioral Assessment Scale (BNBAS).[1]
      (a) Looks explicitly at the mother-infant interaction
      (b) Requires specific training and considerable time to perform
   (2) Early Neonatal Neurobehavioral Scale (ENNS).[2]
      (a) Designed to examine the effect of anesthetic drugs
      (b) Done 2 to 8 hours after birth, a time that theoretically correlates with the maximum effect of prenatally administered drugs
      (c) Requires less time than the BNBAS
      (d) Focuses on muscle tone and the infant's response to repetitive stimuli
   (3) The Neurologic and Adaptive Capacity Score (NACS).[3]
      (a) Takes less time to do than the ENNS
      (b) Has gained favor with many anesthesiologists
      (c) Examines muscle tone closely; differentials between different muscle groups (i.e., flexors and extensors of the neck)
      (d) Authors believed these variables could distinguish between the effects of maternal drugs and birth trauma.
iv. Many anesthesiologists consider the transient neurobehavioral changes detected by these tests to be clinically insignificant.
v. However, controversy still surrounds this subject.
   (1) In nonhuman primates, postnatal behavioral maturation may be altered by drug exposure at birth.
   (2) Milestones in brain development may be delayed, but complex cognitive processes such as learning, memory, and attention are not substantially affected.
   (3) Other researchers suggest that exposure to obstetric analgesia (opioids and nitrous oxide) may lead to future substance abuse.[4]
vi. Hopefully, future research will help resolve this controversy.

Specific Drugs
INDUCTION AGENTS

1. Thiopental
   a. Highly lipid-soluble drug
   b. Passes readily from mother to fetus. Equilibrium between maternal vein and umbilical vein occurs within 3 minutes.

    c. Pregnancy prolongs half-life, probably because of an increased volume of distribution.

    d. In early pregnancy (7 to 13 weeks), the dose for hypnosis is 17% less and for anesthesia is 18% less than in nonpregnant women.

    e. Thiopental undergoes rapid distribution in the fetus. The UA/UV ratio is 0.46 by 4 to 7 minutes after induction and 0.87 after 8 to 22 minutes.

    f. Some drug undergoes "first-pass" metabolism in the fetal liver.

    g. It produces neonatal depression only in large doses (8 mg per kilogram).

2. Ketamine

    a. Often used for its ability to ablate awareness and provide profound analgesia

    b. At a dose of 1 mg per kilogram, ketamine does not commonly cause maternal dreaming.

    c. It causes maternal tachycardia and hypertension on induction. Thus, it is unsuitable for use in women with preeclampsia.

    d. It rapidly crosses the placenta. Umbilical cord drug concentration exceeds maternal blood concentration within 2 minutes.

3. Propofol

    a. Produces less maternal hypertension than thiopental

    b. Attenuates the catecholamine response to laryngoscopy and tracheal intubation

    c. There is rapid placental transfer of this drug.

        i. The UV/MV ratio at delivery following an induction dose of 2 mg per kilogram is about 0.65.

        ii. A UA/UV ratio of 1.07 after a single maternal bolus of propofol suggests rapid fetal tissue uptake and equilibration.

        iii. Both fetal and maternal blood concentrations fall rapidly after induction.

        iv. When using a continuous infusion of propofol to maintain anesthesia, the UA/UV ratio is lower (0.70) than after a single bolus, suggesting continued fetal tissue uptake of drug.

    d. It is rapidly cleared from the fetal circulation.

        i. Fetal blood concentration falls to 0.078 ng per milliliter by 2 hours after birth.

        ii. Some propofol can be detected in breast milk.

    e. Neonatal effects of propofol are unclear. Larger induction doses (greater than 2.5 mg per kilogram) and use of a continuous propofol infusion to maintain anesthesia may transiently depress neurobehavioral scores.

4. Benzodiazepines

    a. Diazepam and midazolam are the two most thoroughly studied benzodiazepines.

    b. Both are used for maternal sedation and to induce general anesthesia.

    c. Both are highly protein bound but readily cross the placenta and induce neonatal to mother effects.

        i. Oral administration produces poor sucking in infant.

        ii. Intravenous administration may cause hypotonia and hypothermia.

    d. In addition, their onset is too slow to be useful during a rapid sequence induction of general anesthesia.

    e. Diazepam

        i. Highly lipid soluble

        ii. Molecular weight of 285 daltons.

        iii. In labor, it can decrease beat-to-beat fetal heart rate variability.

        iv. The maximum fetal blood concentration occurs 5 to 10 minutes after maternal administration.

        v. Neonatal plasma concentrations are higher than maternal concentrations at birth, possibly reflecting more rapid distribution of the drug in the mother.

    f. Midazolam

        i. Shorter half-life and less tissue irritation than diazepam

           (1) Water soluble in its injectable formulation

           (2) At physiologic pH, its structure changes and it becomes lipid soluble.

        ii. Readily crosses the placenta and can cause neonatal depression

           (1) Neonates exposed to midazolam have lower ENNS scores for body temperature, general body tone, and arm recoil for the first 2 hours of life compared with those exposed to thiopental.

           (2) Placental transfer is extensive with both drugs.

           (3) The neonatal elimination half-life of midazolam averages 6.3 hours.

INHALATION AGENTS AND MUSCLE RELAXANTS

1. All the inhalational agents freely cross the placental barrier.

    a. The UV/MV ratio for nitrous oxide is 0.79 after 10 to 14 minutes. Fetal uptake also occurs rapidly, with a UA/UV ratio of 0.89 after an average of 36 minutes.

    b. The halogenated agents are highly lipid soluble, nonionized, and low in molecular weight; thus, they cross the placenta rapidly.

        i. The UV/MV ratio for 0.65% halothane is 0.35; for 1% enflurane, it is 0.6.

        ii. Fetal uptake of isoflurane is more rapid than halothane.

        iii. Pregnancy decreases the MAC of isoflurane. At 8 to 12 weeks' gestation, isoflurane MAC is 28% less than isoflurane MAC in nonpregnant women.

        iv. There are no measurable maternal or neonatal differences among sevoflurane and desflurane or isoflurane.

2. Muscle relaxants
   a. Highly polar
   b. Do not cross the placenta easily
   c. Fetal blood concentrations of nondepolarizing muscle relaxants are 5% to 20% of maternal blood concentrations.
   d. Succinylcholine transfers rapidly to the fetus. However, the resulting fetal concentration is low.
   e. Rocuronium is an alternative to succinylcholine for rapid sequence induction and intubation in the parturient.
      i. In parturients, the effect of 0.6-mg per kilogram rocuronium peaks 98.1 seconds after injection, a time comparable to that in nonpregnant patients.
      ii. In one study, increasing the dose of thiopental from 4 to 6 mg per kilogram improved the intubating conditions (decreased patient movement and allowed earlier intubation).
      iii. Ketamine allows easier tracheal intubation at 50% neuromuscular block than does thiopental.
      iv. Increasing the dose of rocuronium to 0.9 mg per kilogram speeds its onset, but prolongs its duration.
      v. Postpartum, succinycholine, vecuronium, and rocuronium have a prolonged duration.

LOCAL ANESTHETICS

1. Basic drugs that principally bind to α_1-acid glycoprotein
2. Placental transfer depends on:
   a. pKa (pH at which 50% of a drug is ionized).
   b. Maternal and fetal pH.
   c. Extent of protein binding.
3. Fetal effects
   a. Fetal hypoxia and acidosis accentuate the transfer of these weak bases, yielding higher fetal-to-maternal ratios ("ion trapping").
   b. Neurobehavioral studies show varying results depending on the test used. Any effects are subtle and must be diligently sought.
4. Bupivacaine
   a. More than 80% protein bound
   b. Placental transfer is limited compared with lidocaine (70% protein bound).
      i. Mean UV/MV ratio is approximately 0.3.
      ii. The ratio is similar whether the drug is administered in the epidural or the subarachnoid space.
      iii. High lipid solubility encourages rapid uptake by fetal tissues, which may account for the increase in bupivacaine elimination half-life in pregnancy.
      iv. Metabolized to the inactive 2,6-pipecolylxylidine. Both bupivacaine and 2,6-pipecolylxylidine can be detected in the newborn urine for at least 36 hours after delivery.
   c. Toxicity
      i. Greater than lidocaine
      ii. Cardiac depression more profound and prolonged.

        iii.   Peak maternal arterial bupivacaine concentrations do *not* approach unsafe levels during epidural anesthesia for cesarean section.[5]

5. Lidocaine
   a. Less highly protein bound than bupivacaine
   b. Higher UV/MV ratios
   c. Unlike bupivacaine, the route of administration influences the UV/MV ratio of lidocaine. With local perineal infiltration, the ratio is higher (1.32) than after epidural administration.
   d. Lidocaine lacks adverse neonatal neurobehavioral effects.
   e. Placental transfer of lidocaine hydrocarbonate is similar to that of lidocaine hydrochloride.

6. 2-Chloroprocaine
   a. An ester local anesthetic
   b. Rapid hydrolysis by plasma cholinesterase
      i. *In vivo* half-life after epidural anesthesia is measured in minutes.
      ii. *In vitro* half-life is measured in seconds.
      iii. Metabolites, 2-chloroamino-benzoic acid and 2-diethylaminoethanol are inactive.
      iv. Because of this rapid clearance from maternal plasma, only small amounts cross the placenta and appear in the fetal circulation.
   c. When choosing a drug for perineal infiltration, 2-chloroprocaine is a better option than lidocaine because little, if any, pharmacologically active drug reaches the fetus.

7. Ropivacaine
   a. Amino amide local anesthetic
   b. Structurally related to mepivacaine and bupivacaine
   c. In contrast to bupivacaine (a racemic mixture of R and S enantiomers), ropivacaine is marketed as the pure S-enantiomer.
   d. Placental transfer is similar to that of bupivacaine.
      i. After epidural injection, ropivacaine is cleared from plasma more slowly than bupivacaine.
      ii. As a result, the free concentration of ropivacaine in maternal and umbilical cord plasma is twofold higher than that of a similar dose of bupivacaine.
   e. Ropivacaine has a similar duration, but it has less cardiotoxicity than equal concentrations of bupivacaine.
   f. Most clinical trials suggest equipotency with bupivacaine.
   g. Potential advantages over bupivacaine
      i. Less motor block
      ii. Less urinary retention
      iii. Less toxicity

8. Levobupivacaine
   a. The pure S-enantiomer of bupivacaine
   b. Early studies indicate that its sensory profile is similar to that of bupivacaine.

9. Cocaine
   a. Aminoester
   b. Widely abused
   c. Rapidly crosses the placenta

d. Its metabolites, norcocaine and cocaethylene, also are rapidly transferred.
e. Cocaine impairs placental permeability and could inhibit the transplacental exchange of nutrients and metabolites, which may explain associated fetal growth retardation.

OPIOIDS

1. Although systemic opioids have long been used, they are not particularly effective for labor analgesia and cause marked maternal sedation.
2. Opioids also can cause neonatal respiratory depression.
   a. The infant is more sensitive than the adult to the central nervous system actions of opioids.
      i. Lower brain myelin content
      ii. Higher cerebral blood flow
      iii. Altered protein binding
      iv. Different respiratory control mechanisms
3. Morphine
   a. More extensively metabolized in parturients than in nonpregnant patients
   b. Peak plasma concentrations occur within 15 minutes of intramuscular administration.
   c. Placental transfer is rapid.
   d. A pseudoequilibrium occurs in 5 minutes, and the fetal-to-maternal ratio is close to 1.
4. Meperidine
   a. Less likely than morphine to induce neonatal respiratory depression (depresses the newborn's respiratory response to carbon dioxide less than does morphine).
   b. Very lipid soluble and readily crosses the placenta
      i. Following intravenous injection, the drug appears in fetal plasma within 2 minutes.
      ii. Maternal-fetal equilibrium occurs by 6 minutes.
      iii. After intramuscular injection, UV/MV ratio rises as the time to delivery increases.
      iv. After 2 to 3 hours, the concentration of meperidine is higher in fetal than in maternal blood.
      v. Larger maternal doses and repeated injections increase the fetal concentration of drug.
      vi. With multiple doses, a concentration gradient persists between maternal and fetal blood, maximizing fetal exposure.
   c. The neonate can metabolize meperidine, although not as efficiently as can the adult.
      i. Normeperidine, the principal metabolite of meperidine, can be recovered from neonatal urine for 2 to 6 days after birth.
      ii. In animals, normeperidine depresses respiration as much as does meperidine.
   d. Like other opioids, meperidine decreases fetal heart rate variability during labor.
      i. Most likely, this effect is secondary to central nervous system depression and does not warrant obstetric intervention.
      ii. Variability is not affected during stimulating events such as fetal movement or uterine contractions.

e.   Meperidine and probably normeperidine cause changes in the neonatal electroencephalogram and behavior.

i.   Maternal meperidine exposure also may alter infant behavior. If given shortly before birth (1.5 to 5.3 hours), meperidine may interfere with neonatal breastfeeding.

ii.   Even low doses of meperidine (25 mg) depress BNBAS scores.

(1)   Infants exposed to meperidine *in utero* have more abnormal reflexes and altered regulation of state scores.

(2)   The longer the drug-to-delivery interval, the greater the impact of meperidine on neurobehavior.

iii.   Naloxone reverses meperidine-induced respiratory depression but only partly reverses the neurobehavioral changes.

5.   Fentanyl

a.   More lipophilic and more protein bound (69%) than meperidine

b.   Fentanyl provides labor analgesia after intravenous, epidural, or subarachnoid administration.

c.   Intravenous injection

i.   Pain relief begins within 5 minutes and lasts less than 1 hour.

ii.   Rapid tissue uptake ensures a short plasma half-life.

iii.   Fetal–neonatal effects:

(1)   Provokes a brief decrease in fetal heart rate variability.

(2)   Rapidly crosses the placenta and appears in fetal blood within 1 minute.

(3)   UV/MV ratios range from 0.05 to 0.7.

(4)   Umbilical venous concentrations correlate linearly with maternal fentanyl dose.

(5)   No effect on Apgar scores, incidence of respiratory depression, and NACS.

iv.   Patient-controlled intravenous fentanyl can be used for labor analgesia.

v.   Bolus injection of large doses of fentanyl (i.e., 2.5 μg per kilogram) near delivery can produce significant neonatal respiratory depression.

d.   Fentanyl potentiates epidural bupivacaine.

i.   Prolonged epidural infusion (up to 15 hours) of bupivacaine plus fentanyl 2 μg per milliliter lacks a measurable effect on Apgar scores, neurobehavioral testing, and umbilical artery blood gas values.

ii.   UV/MV fentanyl ratio approaches 1.0 within 2 hours.

iii.   Epidural fentanyl lacks an effect on fetal heart rate variability.

e. When given during epidural anesthesia for cesarean section, fentanyl improves the quality of lidocaine and bupivacaine anesthesia without producing detectable changes in neonatal respiratory rate, minute ventilation, pulmonary compliance, or neurobehavior.

6. Sufentanil
   a. Increasingly used for spinal and epidural labor analgesia
   b. In pregnant sheep, sufentanil 50 μg lacks effects on maternal mean arterial pressure, heart rate, and uterine blood flow; fetal mean arterial pressure and heart rate; and maternal and fetal acid–base status.
   c. After epidural injection, maternal arterial plasma concentration peaks within 30 minutes.
   d. Sufentanil is rarely detected in the fetal plasma or umbilical cord blood.

7. Alfentanil
   a. A highly protein-bound (88.7%), rapidly acting opioid analgesic with a short elimination half-life
   b. These properties suggest that it may be an ideal labor analgesic.
      i. Rapid elimination should guard against long-term neonatal effects.
      ii. Unfortunately, animal and human studies have not confirmed these advantages.
         (1) The pharmacokinetics of alfentanil are similar in pregnant and nonpregnant women.
         (2) After 30 μg per kilogram, the UV/MV ratio of is 0.31.
         (3) Unbound alfentanil readily crosses the placenta.
         (4) The fraction of unbound alfentanil is higher in the fetus than in the mother (the fetus has a lower serum concentration of α_1-acid glycoprotein).
         (5) In newborn monkeys, alfentanil produces longer-lasting behavioral effects than does meperidine.

8. Butorphanol and nalbuphine
   a. Narcotic agonist-antagonist drugs often are used for maternal labor analgesia.
   b. These drugs may present less risk of respiratory depression than do pure agonists.
   c. The impact of butorphanol and nalbuphine on fetal heart rate pattern, Apgar scores, and neurobehavioral scores is similar to that produced by meperidine. However, these effects are minimal and transient.
   d. Epidural butorphanol prolongs the duration of local anesthetics. However, a dose of 3 mg produces maternal sedation and a sinusoidal fetal heart rate pattern.

OTHER DRUGS

1. Anticholinergic agents
   a. Atropine

        i.   Readily crosses the placenta and produces a fetal tachycardia.

        ii. A fetal-to-maternal ratio of 1.0 is seen 4 hours after injection.

  b. Glycopyrrolate

        i.   Is a quaternary ammonium compound.

        ii. Undergoes only limited placental transfer.

        iii. Unlike atropine, produces no change in fetal heart rate.

        iv. One case report suggests that this failure to increase fetal heart rate could be detrimental when neostigmine (which readily crosses the placental barrier) is given with glycopyrrolate.[6]

2. Sympathomimetic agents

  a. Ephedrine

        i.   Readily crosses the placenta.

        ii. Increases fetal heart rate and beat-to-beat variability.

        iii. Has transient, subtle effects on the newborn electroencephalogram.

3. Antihypertensive agents

  a. Labetalol

        i.   Blocks both α- and β-adrenoreceptors.

        ii. Lowers blood pressure mostly through blockade of α-adrenoreceptors in peripheral arterioles.

        iii. Reflex tachycardia does not occur because of β-adrenoreceptor blockade.

        iv. Crosses the placenta with a UV/MV ratio of 0.5.

        v. In mature newborns, maternal administration of labetalol produces no clinically significant sympathetic blockade.

  b. Esmolol

        i.   A water-soluble β_1-adrenoreceptor antagonist

        ii. Has a rapid onset and a short duration.

          (1) Distribution half-life is 2 minutes.

          (2) Elimination half-life averages 9 minutes in nonpregnant patients.

          (3) Because of its low lipid solubility and rapid metabolism, placental passage should be minimal. However, it produces dose-dependent β-adrenergic blockade in the fetus during maternal administration.[7]

        iii. Case reports underline potential problems with the use of this drug during pregnancy. Fetal bradycardia, decreased neonatal muscle tone, weak cry, and and apneic spells have been reported in association with maternal esmolol administration.

4. Antiarrhythmics

  a. Adenosine is being used increasingly to terminate narrow complex tachycardias of supraventricular origin in nonpregnant patients.

  b. In pregnant ewes, bolus injection of adenosine transiently produced maternal bradycardia followed by tachycardia and decreased diastolic and mean arterial pressures.[8] Adenosine lacked effect on maternal and fetal arterial blood gas tension, fetal heart rate, and arterial pressure.

   c. Case reports describing its use in terminating supraventricular tachycardias confirm this lack of effect on the fetal heart rate.

5. H_2-Receptor agonists

   a. Cimetidine and ranitidine are commonly used to reduce the volume and raise the pH of maternal gastric secretions.

   b. Cimetidine has a low lipid solubility and a pKa of 6.8, and might be expected to have limited placental transfer.

      i. However, the UV/MV ratio is 0.84 at 90 to 120 minutes after intravenous injection.

      ii. Peak umbilical venous concentrations occur at 60 minutes.

      iii. When given orally the night before cesarean section and again intramuscularly 1 to 3 hours before surgery, cimetidine has a UV/MV ratio of 0.6.

      iv. Rapid renal excretion plays a role in elimination from the fetus.

   c. Exposure during the first trimester of pregnancy does not increase the frequency of major malformations.[9]

6. Metoclopramide

   a. Has a low molecular weight and high lipid solubility.

   b. Has rapid placental transfer (less than 1 minute after intravenous injection).

   c. The mean fetal-to-maternal ratio is 0.6 in humans.

   d. Apgar scores and NACS are unchanged.

REFERENCES

1. Brazelton TB. *Neonatal behavioral assessment scale,* 2nd ed. Philadelphia: JB Lippincott Co, 1984.
2. Scanlon JW, Brown WU, Weiss JB, Alper MH. Neurobehavioral responses of newborn infants after maternal epidural anesthesia. *Anesthesiology* 1974;40:121.
3. Amiel-Tison C, Barrier G, Shnider SM, Levinson G, Hughes SC, Stefani SJ. A new neurologic and adaptive capacity scoring system for evaluating obstetric medications in full-term newborns. *Anesthesiology* 1982;56:340.
4. Jacobson B, Nyberg K, Eklund G, Bygdeman M, Rydberg U. Obstetric pain medication and eventual adult amphetamine addiction in offspring. *Acta Obstet Gynecol Scand* 1988;67:677.
5. Downing JW, Johnson HV, Gonzalez HF, Arney TL, Herman NL, Johnson RF. The pharmacokinetics of epidural lidocaine and bupivacaine during cesarean section. *Anesth Analg* 1997;84:527.
6. Clark RB, Brown MA, Lattin DL. Neostigmine, atropine, and glycopyrrolate: does neostigmine cross the placenta? *Anesthesiology* 1996;84:450.
7. Eisenach JC, Castro MI. Maternally administered esmolol produces fetal β-adrenergic blockade and hypoxemia in sheep. *Anesthesiology* 1989;71:718.

8. Mason BA, Ogunyemi D, Punla O, Koos BJ. Maternal and fetal cardiorespiratory responses to adenosine in sheep. *Am J Obstet Gynecol* 1993;168:1558.
9. Magee LA, Inocencion G, Kamboj L, Rosetti F, Koren G. Safety of first trimester exposure to histamine H2 blockers. A prospective cohort study. *Dig Dis Sci* 1996;41:1145.

Surgery during Pregnancy

Only for the parturient must an anesthesiologist personally give anesthesia to more than one patient simultaneously. This unique circumstance requires a thorough understanding of the anatomic and physiologic changes associated with pregnancy and the current developmental state and drug sensitivity of the embryo or fetus. As many as 2.2% of pregnant patients undergo surgery during pregnancy. This number may be an underestimate, as surgery may be performed before a woman recognizes she is pregnant.

FETAL SAFETY: DEVELOPMENTAL EFFECTS OF ANESTHETICS

1. Virtually all anesthetic given to the mother are rapidly shared with her unborn child.
2. Neuromuscular blocking drugs are notable exceptions to this generalization. They cross the placenta with difficulty because they are quaternary ammonium salts.
3. This ready drug transfer leads to important questions concerning the safety of these agents in the developing embryo or fetus.
   a. The Food and Drug Administration (FDA) has an established risk-classification system to help physicians weigh risk and benefit when contemplating the use of therapeutic drugs during pregnancy (*Federal Register* 1980; 44:37434) (Table 7.1).
   b. Other sources of information, especially about older, generic drugs, are texts such as *Drugs in Pregnancy and Lactation*[1] or *Drugs: Facts and Comparisons,*[2] which classify therapeutic drugs on the basis of a thorough review of the current literature.
      i. Sometimes the risk category in *Drugs in Pregnancy and Lactation* differs from that in the package insert.
      ii. This discrepancy usually occurs because of availability of new information after the original FDA approval.

Changes in Risk throughout Gestation

1. Many texts divide the risk of drug administration during pregnancy into problems in early gestation (direct fetal effects, mainly toxicity) and late gestation (maternal effects that indirectly produce fetal injury). Although this demarcation separates the injurious effects of drugs during early and late gestation, drugs can be directly toxic to a fetus after organogenesis, and hypotension and hypoxia can be just as harmful to an embryo.
2. Teratogenicity
   a. Exposure to a teratogen during gestation can bring about significant changes in the form or function of an infant.

Table 7.1.   FDA fetal-risk categories for therapeutic agents

Category A   Controlled studies have shown no risk to the fetus during the first trimester, and later trimesters as well. Risk is remote (e.g., water).

Category B   Animal studies have demonstrated no fetal risk, but no controlled studies have been performed in humans. Animal studies have shown adverse fetal effects, but these results were not confirmed in controlled human studies. No risk is evident after the first trimester.

Category C   Either studies have shown fetal risk in animals (teratogenic or embryocidal), but no controlled human studies have been performed, or there are no available data in humans or animals for an agent. Drugs of this class should be given only if the benefits outweigh the risks.

Category D   Confirmed evidence exists for human fetal risk, but benefits are acceptable despite known risk (i.e., life-or-limb situations or serious disease for which no safer drugs exist [e.g., diazepam]).

Category X   Agents of this class are contraindicated in pregnant patients for any reason because animal or human studies have displayed teratogenicity or there is evidence of fetal risk from prior human experience. Fetal risk clearly outweighs any clinical benefit of their use in pregnancy (e.g., thalidomide).

Source: *Federal Register* 1980;44:37434–37436, with permission.

     b. Of most concern is exposure during organogenesis, a phase of critical differentiation and development, which occurs between 3 and 8 weeks after conception.
     c. Because the brain continues to develop, even after birth, the duration of central nervous system susceptibility probably extends well beyond the first trimester.
     d. Teratogenic effects may be structural anomalies, functional disorders (including behavior), growth retardation, or death.
     e. Timing, dosage, and duration of treatment are the most critical factors that determine whether a given drug exposure will be teratogenic.
     f. Any agent given in the right dosage at the right time probably can be teratogenic. Still, despite conflicting animal data, very few drugs have proved to be teratogenic in humans.
  3. Later in pregnancy, any prolonged disruption of placental oxygen delivery (by either impaired maternal oxygenation or uterine hypoperfusion) can induce fetal asphyxia and its resultant effects (including death). Anesthetic complications that may produce fetal asphyxia include:
     a. Intubation difficulties with or without gastric acid aspiration.
     b. Unrecognized esophageal intubation.
     c. High or complete spinal block during regional anesthesia.
     d. Unintended deep inhalational anesthesia.

Induction Agents
1. Thiopental
   a. Teratogenic to chicken embryos
   b. In mice and rats, up to 100 mg per kilogram had no teratogenic effect, although some mice exhibited retarded growth after very large doses.
   c. No specific studies have directly investigated teratogenicity or fetal toxicity in humans.
   d. Thiopental is classified as a pregnancy category C agent. Its long history of safe administration in pregnant patients justifies its continued use.
2. Methohexital
   a. Category B
   b. Reproductive studies in rats and rabbits at four and seven times the recommended human dose, respectively, revealed no teratogenic or embryo/fetal toxic effect.
   c. Human studies are lacking.
3. Ketamine
   a. In rats, 120 mg per kilogram IM lacked teratogenic effects.
   b. In contrast, large doses produced neural tube defects in chick embryos.
   c. No specific reproductive studies have been performed in humans.
   d. Ketamine did not receive pregnancy risk classification by its manufacturer before expiration of its patent, so a risk-assessment category is not noted in *PDR Generics.*
   e. The pharmaceutical compendium, *Drugs: Facts and Comparisons,* has given ketamine a category C rating.
4. Etomidate
   a. Etomidate is embryotoxic in rats when administered at one and four times the normal human dose.
   b. Doses from 0.3 to 5.0 mg per kilogram markedly decreased birth survival in rats and rabbits.
   c. Well-controlled studies in pregnant women are absent.
   d. Category C
5. Propofol
   a. Rats and rabbits given 15 mg per kilogram of propofol (six times the recommended induction dose in humans) daily throughout pregnancy showed no reproductive effects.
   b. Developmental effects of propofol in humans are unknown.
   c. Category B

Inhaled Agents
Potent Agents
   There are no controlled studies of the safety of any of these anesthetics in pregnant surgical patients. Their FDA pregnancy risk classification comes from animal studies.

1. Halothane
   a. The most studied of the currently available potent agents
   b. Rats exposed to 1 minimum alveolar concentration (MAC) in 25% oxygen for 12 hours during organogenesis developed skeletal abnormalities.

      c. Shorter exposures (1 hour) in rats rabbits during different times of development lacked an effect on pregnancy outcome.

      d. Long-term exposure to subanesthetic concentrations resulted in growth retardation but no anomalies.

      e. No adequate reproductive studies have been performed in humans.

      f. Category C

2. Enflurane

      a. In mice, exposure to 0.01%, 0.1%, or 1.0% for 4 hours on 6 consecutive days during major organogenesis resulted in an increased incidence of cleft palate (1.9%), fused vertebrae, bent and fused ribs, and renal abnormalities in the highest dose group.

      b. In rats, exposures to 1 MAC (1.68%) of enflurane for 6 hours on 3 succeeding days during organogenesis revealed no teratogenic effect.

      c. Long-term subanesthetic administration to rats before conception (female and male) and through pregnancy was associated with lower birth weights but no defects.

      d. No controlled studies have been performed in humans.

      e. Category B

3. Isoflurane

      a. Mice

            i. Embryotoxic at doses six times greater than normally used in humans.

           ii. No reproductive effects after trace (0.006%) and subanesthetic (0.06%) exposures

         iii. A dose of 0.6% induced significant growth retardation, decreased ossification, renal abnormalities, and a high incidence of cleft palate (12%).

      b. In rats, 6-hour exposures to 1.05% on 3 successive days during major organogenesis produced no evidence of teratogenicity.

      c. No controlled investigations have been done in parturients.

      d. Category C

4. Desflurane

      a. Rats exposed to 1 MAC-hour per day from the critical development period to birth had no anomalies.

      b. No well-controlled studies have been performed in humans.

      c. Category B

5. Sevoflurane

      a. No embryotoxic or teratogenic effects in rats and rabbits exposed to 1 MAC without the use of a carbon dioxide absorber

      b. Reproductive effects have not been investigated in parturients.

      c. Category B

      d. Studies of the reproductive effects of Compound A, formed by the degradation of sevoflurane in the strongly alkaline environment of the carbon dioxide absorber (soda lime or barium hydroxide lime), have not been done. Maintain at least 3 L per minute fresh gas flow when giving sevoflurane to parturients to minimize the inhaled concentration of Compound A.

Nitrous Oxide

1. Has a long history of apparent safe use for both anesthesia and analgesia in obstetrics
2. However, recent information about the metabolic effects of nitrous oxide fueled controversy over use in early pregnancy.
3. Rats exposed to 50% nitrous oxide for 2 to 6 days, or to 70% nitrous oxide for 24 hours during critical phases of early development had skeletal abnormalities and resorption (abortion). Exposure to subanesthetic doses throughout pregnancy induced resorption, small birth weight, and minor skeletal abnormalities.
4. Possible mechanisms
   a. Inhibition of methionine synthetase
      i. Nitrous oxide impairs deoxyribonucleic acid (DNA) synthesis through its inhibition of methionine synthetase, an important intermediate enzyme in the production of deoxythymidine.
      ii. Nitrous oxide oxidizes the cobalt of the vitamin B12 cofactor in the methionine synthetase enzyme complex, which inhibits the conversion of 5-methyl tetrahydrofolate and homocysteine into tetrahydrofolate and methionine. This effect appears to be the origin of the pernicious anemia-like condition seen in some patients who receive nitrous oxide.
      iii. There is evidence of depressed activity of methionine synthetase and DNA content in fetal rats exposed to nitrous oxide.
      iv. Tetrahydrofolate deficiency from the disruption of methionine synthetase does not fully explain the embryo and fetal toxicity associated with nitrous oxide.
         (1) Developmental toxicity occurs at doses of nitrous oxide far higher than that required to inhibit methionine synthetase maximally.
         (2) Toxicity is not prevented by administration of folinic acid, as is the case with the pernicious anemia-like syndrome.
   b. α_1-Adrenergic activity
      i. α_1-Adrenergic antagonists prevent embryo resorption and situs inversus.
      ii. Nitrous oxide, like ketamine, is an N-methyl-D-aspartate (NMDA) receptor antagonist. Both have similar analgesic and hemodynamic effects. GABA agonists (i.e., most other anesthetics) block NMDA receptor effects of nitrous oxide.[3] Potent anesthetics (halothane and isoflurane) also prevent nitrous oxide teratogenicity in rats.
5. Human data
   a. Much of the reproductive safety data regarding nitrous oxide in humans comes from epidemiologic studies in female employees in operating rooms and dentist's offices, who could be exposed to trace amounts of this gas

for extended periods. Unfortunately, these types of exposures also are not comparable to those of pregnant patients undergoing surgery with a short-duration nitrous oxide-containing anesthetic.

b. Studies of embryo/fetal toxicity of nitrous oxide in pregnant patients undergoing surgery are limited.

   i. Patients undergoing cervical cerclage with either general anesthesia including nitrous oxide or conduction block had no difference in the rate of spontaneous abortions.[4]

   ii. A large Swedish registry study provides the most reassuring data about the safety of nitrous oxide in patients having surgery during pregnancy. Here 2,252 women underwent surgery in the first trimester; 2,929 under general anesthesia. No significant increase in birth abnormalities was detected in those receiving general anesthesia, 98% of whom received nitrous oxide.[5]

6. Although a conservative approach would be to avoid nitrous oxide, a wealth of clinical data support the safe and continued use of it as part of a balanced anesthetic during all aspects of pregnancy.

Local Anesthetics

1. Local anesthetics may have direct neurotoxic effects, but most data suggest that they lack embryo or fetal toxic actions.

2. Procaine, lidocaine, and tetracaine exposure in early chick embryo and lidocaine exposure in mice embryo preparations affected neural tube closure.

3. However, no data exist suggesting teratogenicity in intact animals for any local anesthetic.

4. 2-Chloroprocaine and tetracaine (category C): No intact animal studies have been performed, and human data are lacking.

5. Bupivacaine (category C): There was increased fetal and embryo loss in rats and rabbits at five to nine times the maximal clinical dose, although there was no evidence of teratogenicity. Human data are lacking.

6. The package insert for lidocaine states that no animal or human studies report adverse embryo or fetal effects: therefore, it has been given a category B classification.

7. The recently released local anesthetic ropivacaine lacked teratogenic effects in rats and rabbits at up to five times the recommended maximal dose in humans. However, because no definitive controlled studies have been performed in humans, ropivacaine has been classified category B.

SPECIFIC COMMON PROCEDURES
Cervical Cerclage
Definition

1. Used to prevent second-trimester fetal loss from cervical incompetence

2. Diagnosis

   a. Repeated history of painless cervical dilation in the second or early third trimester

b. Prolapse of the membranes through the cervix or spontaneous rupture of membranes and expulsion of the fetus typically follow.

c. Making the diagnosis of cervical incompetence is often difficult.

   i. Painless cervical dilation of 2 to 4 cm occurs in 24% to 34% of otherwise asymptomatic gravidae who go on to deliver at term.

   ii. No single pathognomonic physical finding or test confirms a precise diagnosis.

   iii. It is therefore a diagnosis of exclusion after the obstetrician rules out the other causes of midtrimester effacement (e.g., preterm labor).

Methods and Types of Cervical Cerclage

1. Shirodkar was first to develop an intravaginal method of encircling the internal cervical os.

   a. The Shirodkar procedure involves the incision of the cervix at the level of the internal os, elevating the vaginal mucosa and bladder, and placing a Mersilene 5-mm band (braided Dacron) around the cervix.

   b. The complex nature of the Shirodkar method makes it difficult to perform during pregnancy and places the urinary tract at risk.

   c. A modification of the Shirodkar procedure has been described with fewer cervical incisions and a nylon ligature instead of the 5-mm band. This modification is equally effective and easier to remove than the original procedure.

2. The McDonald procedure

   a. Uses a purse-string suture as high as possible around the exocervix, at approximately the level of the internal os.

   b. With four to five bites, the suture is placed deeply into the cervix and pulled tightly enough to close the cervical os completely.

3. A far less common procedure is the Würm procedure.

   a. This approach uses criss-crossing, heavy, double-mattress sutures across the cervical opening at the level of the internal os.

   b. The Würm procedure reportedly can delay delivery until at or near term. It can be used in conjunction with amniocentesis to reduce bulging membranes and as a method for repeated cerclage when either the Shirodkar or McDonald cerclage has failed.

4. The transabdominal cervicoisthmic cerclage is by far the most complex and difficult procedure for the surgical treatment of cervical incompetence.

   a. It is reserved for women in whom vaginal cerclage has either failed or is impossible.

   b. It involves the intraabdominal placement of a ligature around the cervix above the cardinal and uterosacral ligaments.

   c. It is recommended for patients in whom the cervix is congenitally short, amputated, or scarred from an extensive cone biopsy or unsuccessful prior cerclage, when

the fornices are lacerated, or in the presence of subacute cervicitis.
d. Disadvantages
  i. Requires two abdominal procedures (the cerclage and a subsequent cesarean section)
  ii. Has a higher complication rate, related to the high vascularity and proximity of ureters to the surgical site
5. Timing
  a. Cerclage done between weeks 16 and 19 of gestation has the greatest chance of success.
  b. Before 14 weeks, pregnancy losses frequently are due to genetic anomalies or imperfect implantation.
6. Contraindications to cervical cerclage include:
  a. Bleeding.
  b. Active labor or significant uterine contractions.
  c. Ruptured membranes (although this is becoming a relative contraindication, as studies have investigated use of cerclage in patients with premature rupture of membranes).
  d. Cervical dilation greater than 4 cm.
  e. Intrauterine infection.
  f. Fetal abnormalities.
  g. Abruptio placenta.

Elective Cervical Cerclage
1. The procedure requires adequate analgesia and vaginal wall relaxation. The surgeon must retract the vagina enough to expose the cervix for surgical manipulation.
2. Cerclage has been performed under general (with and without a potent inhalation agent), regional (epidural or spinal), local (a paracervical block or pudendal nerve block), and no anesthesia.
3. As for any other surgical procedure, the best technique is the one with which the anesthesiologist has the most experience and feels most comfortable. No anesthetic technique is a substitute for diligent intraoperative and postoperative monitoring of uterine activity and use of appropriate tocolytic agents.

Emergency Cerclage
1. The woman with bulging hour-glass membranes protruding through a dilated cervix is more problematic. This tenuous circumstance requires emergency reduction of the presenting amniotic sac (with or without fetal presenting parts) and subsequent cervical cerclage.
2. General anesthesia with potent inhalation agents provide uterine relaxation and may allow return of the presenting parts to the uterus. Coughing and bucking on intubation and extubation may risk membrane rupture.
3. Growing experience suggests that regional anesthesia is safe and effective for emergency cerclage. When a tocolytic agent is used (e.g., terbutaline, ritodrine, indomethacin, or nitroglycerin), the choice of anesthetic technique makes little difference.

4.   Suggested technique of spinal anesthesia for emergency cerclage
   a.   Place the patient in a lateral decubitus position (with head-down tilt if requested by the obstetrician).
   b.   Identify the subarachnoid space with a small-gauge pencil-point needle.
   c.   Drug:
      i.   Three milliliters 0.25% bupivacaine, or
      ii.   One and a half to 2.0 mL 0.5% bupivacaine.
      iii. Both drugs are slightly hypobaric and will not produce extensive sensory block, even if the patient is positioned with a head-down tilt.

OTHER GYNECOLOGIC SURGERY

Ovarian Surgery

1.   Surgery for ovarian cysts accounts for up to 39% of operations during pregnancy.
2.   Adnexal masses complicate 1 in 556 pregnancies. About one-third are persistent corpus luteal cysts, and another third are benign cystic teratomas. Two percent to 5% are cancerous.

Ectopic Pregnancy

1.   Implantation outside of the uterus is by far the most important surgical complication of pregnancy. The incidence of ectopic pregnancy has tripled through the 1970s to 1987 to a rate of 16.8 per 1, 000 reported pregnancies. Better diagnosis, increased incidence in pelvic inflammatory disease, advanced maternal age, use of intrauterine contraception devices, tubal reanastomosis surgery, and *in vitro* fertilization techniques may have some role in this increase.
2.   Ectopic pregnancy is the second leading cause of maternal mortality, accounting for 6% to 7% of pregnancy-related deaths. The risk of dying of an ectopic pregnancy is ten times greater than that of dying of complications of a term pregnancy.
3.   Increasingly sensitive pregnancy tests and high-resolution transvaginal ultrasonography have made possible early detection, before rupture and hemorrhage. Early diagnosis and improved treatment modalities have dramatically changed the management of ectopic pregnancy.
   a.   Traditionally, ectopic pregnancy was treated with emergency laparotomy to remove the ruptured fallopian tube.
   b.   With earlier, accurate diagnosis, more than 50% of ectopic pregnancies are unruptured at the time of surgery. Earlier diagnosis also has allowed the development of new treatment modalities (e.g., methotrexate and ultrasound-guided transvaginal aspiration).

Laparotomy Versus Laparoscopic Surgery

1.   Until recently, traditional management of both ovarian masses and ectopic pregnancies was exploratory laparotomy. Because of concern about ovarian cancer, adnexal masses still may require open exploration for proper staging and excision.

2. Laparoscopy has become common during pregnancy. As operator skills and instruments have improved, progressively more laparoscopic operative procedures are attempted. Advantages of laparoscopic surgery during pregnancy include:
    a. Reduced pain and limited fetal exposure to postoperative opioids.
    b. Consumption of fewer resources and shorter hospital stay.
    c. A panoramic view of the abdominal contents with minimal uterine manipulation.
    d. More rapid return to mobility, reducing incidence of thrombophlebitis.

Carbon Dioxide Pneumoperitoneum

1. Whereas the maternal advantages of laparoscopic surgery are clear, its effects on the embryo/fetus are controversial.
2. Laparoscopy requires intraabdominal insufflation of carbon dioxide to provide adequate exposure. Despite several non-reassuring animal studies, a growing human experience suggests that laparoscopy is safe during pregnancy, and this technique will likely see progressively wider use.[6]
3. Potential problems with carbon dioxide pneumoperitoneum.
    a. Carbon dioxide insufflation induces maternal hypercapnia and respiratory acidemia. In animals, fetal hypercarbia and acidosis follow without delay.
    b. Also in animals, carbon dioxide insufflation increases the p_aCO_2-end-tidal carbon dioxide ($ETCO_2$) gradient. Increasing maternal ventilation improves the fetal acidemia, but capnography still underestimates the degree of maternal hypercarbia.
4. Consider the following when providing anesthesia for laparoscopic surgery:
    a. Continuously monitor fetal heart rate (FHR), if possible.
    b. Limit abdominal insufflation pressure to 15 to 20 mm Hg.
    c. Increase maternal minute ventilation in response to a rising $ETCO_2$.
    d. If signs of fetal compromise develop (i.e., tachycardia or bradycardia), measure maternal blood gas tensions to guide further therapy.
    e. Consider converting to an open procedure if worrisome FHR changes accompany pneumoperitoneum.

NONGYNECOLOGIC SURGERY
Common Operations
Appendectomy

1. The most common non-obstetrical problem that leads to surgical intervention in the parturient is appendicitis, accounting for more than two-thirds of all surgery for gastrointestinal disease during pregnancy.
2. The incidence of pathologically confirmed appendicitis is between 1 in 833 and 1 in 6,600 deliveries.

DIAGNOSIS

1. Pregnancy can alter the signs and symptoms of acute appendicitis.
2. Classic localizing right lower quadrant pain is uncommon after the first trimester, probably the result of the displacement of the appendix upward and laterally by the expanding uterus.
3. In addition, the gravid uterus isolates the inflamed appendix from the parietal peritoneum, removing the classic peritoneal signs of guarding and rebound.
4. The closer to term, the more difficult the symptoms become to unravel.
   a. Appendicitis may be mistaken for early labor.
   b. Pain may not even be the chief complaint.
   c. Patients may be afebrile or with only low-grade temperature elevation.

TREATMENT

1. Appendicitis is a surgical condition.
2. Delay can mean death; appendiceal rupture increases both maternal and fetal mortality.
3. Pregnancy is not a contraindication to appendectomy, and neither should it be a reason for delay.
4. The type and location of surgical incision for antepartum appendectomy is determined by the operating surgeon, particularly because the position of the appendix changes over the course of pregnancy. The most common location is a right midtransverse incision over the site of maximal tenderness. However, because other entities are included in the differential diagnosis of abdominal pain during pregnancy, some surgeons will use either a low midline incision or a transverse muscle-cutting incision at the level of the umbilicus to allow optimal abdominal exposure if the appendix is normal.

ANESTHESIA

1. Appendectomy during pregnancy has been performed under both regional and general anesthesia.
2. Both techniques are safe and effective throughout pregnancy. They provide adequate analgesia and operating conditions.

Cholecystectomy

1. Gallbladder disease is the second most common non-obstetric abdominal condition found during pregnancy, with as many as 1 in 1,259 parturients undergoing cholecystectomy.
2. Pregnancy appears to predispose to gallstone formation.
   a. Progesterone relaxes gallbladder smooth muscle and decreases its responsiveness to cholecystokinin.
   b. The between-meal and after-meal residual volume within the gallbladder almost doubles.
   c. Both estrogen and progesterone hypersaturate the bile with cholesterol.
   d. The combination of gallbladder stasis and increased bile cholesterol causes sludging and ultimately stone formation, particularly in multiparous women.

3. Many surgeons advocate conservative management of these patients with intravenous hydration, antibiotics, analgesia, fasting, and nasogastric suction.
    a. Risks of conservative management
        i.   Nutritional problems requiring total parenteral nutrition can develop.
        ii. Gallbladder disease can progress to gallstone pancreatitis. When pancreatitis complicates cholecystitis, maternal mortality, which is negligible for uncomplicated cholecystectomy, increases to 15%, and fetal mortality is 60%.
    b. The safest time for open cholecystectomy may be during the second trimester, when the risk of abortion and premature labor is lowest.
4. Surgical intervention is usually indicated when:
    a. Biliary colic is repetitive or fails to respond to 4 days of conservative therapy.
    b. Perforation is suspected.
    c. Significant obstructive jaundice is present.
    d. Uncontrolled diabetes coexists.
    e. Whenever other intraabdominal emergency conditions cannot be ruled out (e.g., perforated peptic ulcer, appendicitis).
5. During the last decade, laparoscopic cholecystectomy has become the primary technique for removing the diseased gallbladder in the nonpregnant population.
    a. Laparoscopic cholecystectomy has been successfully performed during the first, second, and third trimesters.
    b. To avoid uterine and fetal trauma during trocar placement, many surgeons use an open Hasson trocar-introduction technique before insufflation, or they place the Veress insufflation needle into an alternative site far from the uterus.
6. Anesthetic considerations
    a. Most would choose general anesthesia for cholecystectomy (open and laparoscopic).
    b. Epidural anesthesia has been described with the following caveats:
        i.   Limit intraabdominal insufflation pressures (approximately 10 mm Hg).
        ii. Have a highly motivated patient and surgeon.
    c. Regardless of anesthetic technique, questions about the fetal effects of carbon dioxide pneumoperitoneum remain.
    d. At a minimum, assess FHR preinduction, postinduction, and after surgery.

Neurosurgery

Hemorrhage

1. Intracranial hemorrhage from rupture of an aneurysm or arteriovenous malformation (AVM) is a devastating complication of pregnancy, with a maternal mortality rate of up to 50%.
2. Although rare, occurring in 0.01% to 0.05% of pregnancies, intracranial hemorrhage accounts for 4.0% to 8.5% of maternal deaths.

3. The majority of the pregnancy-related intracranial hemorrhages occur antepartum (92%), with only 8% arising after delivery.
4. The decision to operate to correct intracranial aneurysms or AVMs should be made based on neurosurgical, not obstetric, indications. Both the mother and fetus benefit from appropriate repair during pregnancy.

Tumors
1. There is no difference in the incidence of primary intracranial tumors between pregnant and nonpregnant women of similar ages.
2. Pregnancy may speed the progression and worsen the symptoms of these tumors, especially meningiomas, which can have progesterone or estrogen receptors.
3. The management of intracranial tumors first seen during pregnancy should be individualized.

Trauma
1. Trauma is the number one cause of death in women of childbearing years.
2. The incidence of trauma, particularly head trauma, during pregnancy is no different from that in the nonpregnant population.

Anesthetic Considerations
1. Balance
   a. Cerebral perfusion.
   b. Optimal operating conditions.
   c. Fetal well-being.
   d. Uterine relaxation.
2. Increased intracranial pressure or the presence of aneurysm or AVM mandates a smooth induction of anesthesia with a controlled intubation.
   a. Aspiration risk and high oxygen consumption favor rapid-sequence induction and intubation.
   b. Rapid-sequence induction including intravenous lidocaine, fentanyl, β-blockade, or sodium nitroprusside to control responses to laryngoscopy is a reasonable compromise.
3. Controlled hypotension may be lifesaving. Sodium nitroprusside has been used effectively in pregnancy, but requires continuous fetal monitoring to evaluate the effects of maternal hypotension on FHR.

HYPERVENTILATION
1. Controlled hyperventilation is commonly used in the treatment of increased intracranial pressure.
2. In the parturient hyperventilation may:
   a. Decrease uterine blood flow.
   b. Impair placental oxygen transfer by shift of the oxyhemoglobin dissociation curve.
   c. Decrease fetal oxygen tension.
3. Most fetuses will tolerate mild-to-moderate maternal hypocapnia. A target p_aCO_2 of 30 mm Hg appears safe. FHR

monitoring may aid in diagnosis of fetal compromise due to excessive maternal hyperventilation.

Cardiac Surgery

1. The physiologic demands of pregnancy may cause acute decompensation of previously compensated valvular, congenital, or ischemic heart disease.
2. The incidence of heart disease of all types during pregnancy is less than 1%, and severe cardiac dysfunction is very uncommon.
3. When medical management of cardiac disease fails, surgery may be the only treatment option.
4. Valvular surgery is still the most common cardiac procedure performed during pregnancy.
5. Although still uncommon, cardiac surgery has become a safe and effective treatment modality during pregnancy.
6. Fetal survival has increased from 50% to 80% in the modern cardiac operating room.[7]

Cardiopulmonary Bypass

1. Cardiopulmonary bypass places mother, placenta, and fetus at risk by exposing them to a nonphysiologic environment. Some of the deleterious changes include:
   a. Hypotension.
   b. Hypothermia.
   c. Altered coagulation.
   d. Release of vasoactive factors.
   e. Rheologic changes in blood.
   f. Nonpulsatile blood flow.
   g. Potential air or particulate emboli.
2. Pregnant women tolerate cardiopulmonary bypass as well as nonpregnant women of similar age.
   a. This, unfortunately, is not the case for the embryo or fetus.
   b. Bypass, maternal instability, and the emergency circumstances surrounding cardiac surgery probably contribute to fetal mortality.
3. Cardiopulmonary bypass and uterine blood flow
   a. Because of higher oxygen consumption and cardiac output, increased bypass flow rates may be required to maintain fetal well-being.
   b. Adequate perfusion pressure also is necessary to maintain flow in the low-resistance uteroplacental circulation.
      i. Blood pressure decreases precipitately with initiation of bypass.
      ii. Hypotension can decrease placental perfusion.
         (1) Fetal tachycardia or bradycardia may arise in response to hypoxemia and acidemia.
         (2) Fetal bradycardia is especially common during hypothermic cardiopulmonary bypass in parturients.
4. Current recommendations for managing cardiopulmonary bypass in the parturient include the following[8]:
   a. Maintain adequate pump flow and systemic pressure: that is, a cardiac index of 2.0 to 2.7 L per minute per square meter and a mean arterial pressure of 60 mm Hg.

b. Avoid hypothermia. If possible, keep temperature at 32°C
c. Monitor FHR.
d. Increase pump flow and systemic pressure if fetal bradycardia follows the institution of bypass.
e. Minimize the length of bypass.
f. Avoid systemic hyperkalemic cardioplegia because of its damaging effects on the fetus and placenta. Retrograde delivery is the method of choice for cardioplegia.

Vasoactive Drugs and Inotropes
1. Epinephrine
   a. A potent α- and β-adrenoreceptor agonist
   b. Has an important role in vascular support in cardiac surgery, shock, and for bronchodilatation in acute asthma
   c. Concern with use in pregnancy: α-Agonist action may decrease uterine blood flow. However, initial indication for epinephrine therapy usually poses a greater threat to uterine blood flow. Do not hesitate to use epinephrine when clinically indicated.
2. Norepinephrine
   a. In the doses typically used to treat hypotensive shock, norepinephrine is a mixed α- and β_1-adrenoreceptor agonist.
   b. The α-agonist effects can decrease uterine blood flow and increase uterine resting tone as well as the frequency and intensity of contractions.
3. Ephedrine
   a. Both a direct-acting α- and β-adrenergic agonist and an indirect sympathomimetic (through its enhanced release of norepinephrine from adrenergic nerve terminals)
   b. In animals, it seems to selectively spare uterine vessels, thereby enhancing uterine perfusion.
4. Phenylephrine
   a. A selective α_1-adrenergic agonist
   b. Causes marked vaso- and venoconstriction
   c. Decreases uterine blood flow in animals
   d. Has been used safely to treat regional anesthesia-induced hypotension in humans
5. Dopamine
   a. Both a direct-acting α- and β-adrenergic agonist and an indirect-acting sympathomimetic that stimulates the release of norepinephrine from sympathetic nerve terminals
   b. At low dose (1 to 5 μg per kilogram per minute), it is an agonist at vascular D_1-dopamine receptors, which enhance renal function.
   c. At higher doses, dopamine increases uterine vascular resistance in a dose-dependent fashion.
6. Dobutamine
   a. A synthetic catecholamine that is a racemic mixture, which predominantly activates β_1- and β_2-adrenoreceptors with minimal α-receptor activity.
   b. The net cardiovascular effect is an increase in cardiac output with a concomitant decrease in vascular tone.

       c. Dobutamine is ideal for the treatment of cardiac failure associated with increased systemic vascular resistance.

       d. In animals, dobutamine increases in uterine vascular tone were less than those produced by comparable doses of dopamine.

7. Amrinone and milrinone
   a. These agents have both inotropic and vasodilatory activity and appear to act by enhancing intracellular cyclic adenosine monophosphate (cAMP) concentrations through their selective inhibition of type III phosphodiesterase.
   b. Milrinone has a shorter half-life and fewer side effects. It also shows greater selectivity for the type III phosphodiesterase, making it the drug of choice in this class.
   c. In animals, both drugs do not decrease uterine blood flow, and even increase it in some studies.[9]

8. Sodium nitroprusside
   a. A potent, short-acting dilator of both arterioles and venules, used to treat severe hypertension
   b. Sodium nitroprusside effectively controls hypertension associated with severe preeclampsia, without evidence of either maternal or fetal toxicity.
   c. It also can be useful when deliberate hypotension is required, as in intracranial aneurysm clipping.
   d. Because of its potency, it should be used only by experienced personnel and with appropriate maternal and fetal monitoring.

9. Nitroglycerin
   a. A potent direct-acting vaso- and venodilator
   b. When used as a vasodilator in preeclamptic parturients, it effectively reduces arterial pressure without changes in uterine blood flow.
   c. With evidence of comparable efficacy between nitroglycerin and sodium nitroprusside, the absence of toxicity and tachyphylaxis with nitroglycerin warrants its choice as the first-line vasodilator for rapid treatment of most hypertensive crises.

Other Operations

Ureterolithotomy and Percutaneous Nephrostomy

1. About 1 in 1,500 pregnancies is complicated by kidney or urinary tract stones.
2. Even though the risk of renal calculi is no different between pregnant and nonpregnant women, determining the origin of acute abdominal pain in a pregnant woman is a challenge.
3. Stones may predispose a parturient to premature labor.
4. Management
   a. Almost two-thirds of stones pass spontaneously.
   b. Most of the remainder can be managed conservatively and definitive therapy delayed until after pregnancy.
   c. Persistent obstruction causing declining kidney function, obstruction in a patient with a solitary kidney, intractable pain, frequent infection proximal to the stone, or refractory premature labor may mandate intervention.

    d. Recent advances in ureteroscopy have made basket or forceps extraction a more viable option during pregnancy.

    e. Extracorporeal shock-wave lithotripsy is *absolutely contraindicated* during pregnancy because of the risk of disrupting developing fetal tissues.

Pheochromocytoma

1. A rare tumor of the sympathetic nervous system that is very uncommon during pregnancy
2. When present, it carries a devastatingly high maternal and fetal mortality.
3. If unrecognized before labor, more than 50% of mothers and their children may die of complications of uncontrolled hypertension.
4. Diagnosis rests on the presence of increased levels of catecholamines or their metabolites in blood and urine. Magnetic resonance imaging has been suggested as a powerful tool to assist in localizing the tumor.
5. Preoperative management requires control of the hypercatecholamine state with the α-adrenergic blocker phenoxybenzamine (a pregnancy risk category C agent).
   a. It allows restoration of normal vascular tone and intravascular volume.
   b. β-Blockade, particularly with propranolol, also is an important part of blood pressure control.
6. Resection may occur during pregnancy, immediately after cesarean section or, laparoscopically, shortly after vaginal delivery.
7. Anesthetic considerations
   a. Maintain an adequate depth of anesthesia to prevent vascular responses to noxious stimuli. This challenge requires modifying the normal rapid-induction sequence to include opioids, intravenous lidocaine, or a potent agent to blunt a hypertensive response to intubation.
   b. Intraoperative invasive hemodynamic monitoring is important for prompt recognition and treatment of hypertension before and hypotension after tumor removal.

ANESTHETIC CONSIDERATIONS
Fetal Monitoring
1. Continuous fetal monitoring allows assessment of fetal well-being throughout anesthesia and surgery.
2. Fetal heart rate
   a. Detectable by transabdominal ultrasound after week 16 of pregnancy and by vaginal ultrasonography even earlier
   b. Begins to exhibit beat-to-beat variability after weeks 25 to 27 of gestation.
   c. Monitoring
      i. An FHR transducer can easily be positioned and left in place (unless it would interfere with the sterile surgical field).
      ii. External Doppler transducers have a poor signal-to-noise ratio and cannot detect subtle changes in beat-to-beat variability.

iii.   Gross alterations in FHR variability (e.g., loss of beat-to-beat variability) give fairly reliable indications of changes in fetal status.
iv.   Besides heart rate variability, changes in baseline FHR are an indication of fetal condition.
   (1)   Moderate degrees of hypoxemia can produce transient-to-prolonged fetal tachycardia (FHR greater than 160 beats per minute).
   (2)   If fetal tachycardia arises intraoperatively, search for maternal hypoxemia, hypovolemia, or any other factors that could interfere with gas exchange at the placental interface.
   (3)   Fetal bradycardia (FHR less than 110 beats per minute) may arise under conditions of profound hypoxemia.
3.   Uterine activity
   a.   Most anesthetics depress uterine activity, so intraoperative monitoring is rarely needed.
   b.   Monitoring in the recovery room may help detect early signs of preterm labor.

Regional Versus General Anesthesia
1.   Local, regional, and general anesthesia can provide suitable surgical conditions in pregnant women.
2.   The ultimate choice of anesthetic should be based on maternal status, extent and anatomic region of the planned surgery, and the expertise of the anesthesiologist.
3.   Regional anesthesia has the following theoretical advantages:
   a.   Reduces the risk of maternal aspiration, as long as supplemental sedation is kept to a minimum.
   b.   Decreases fetal drug exposure, particularly if a subarachnoid block is used.
   c.   Uses local anesthetics, which unlike inhalational agents, are not known teratogens.
   d.   Allows the use of intrathecal or epidural opioids for intraoperative and postoperative pain relief.
4.   A carefully performed general anesthetic presents no greater maternal risk than does either local or regional anesthesia.

Premature Labor
1.   Parturients undergoing anesthesia and surgery are at significant risk for premature labor and spontaneous abortion.
2.   Surgery during the second trimester increases the risk of spontaneous abortion fivefold.
3.   These data point to the need for postoperative uterine monitoring and aggressive tocolytic management if contractions are associated with cervical change.

ANESTHETIC TECHNIQUE
1.   Aspiration prophylaxis
   a.   A nonparticulate antacid (0.3 M sodium citrate, 30 mL) shortly before induction will increase the pH of any existing gastric contents.

b. H_2-Receptor antagonists (cimetidine, famotidine, nizatidine, or ranitidine) will reduce gastric acid secretion (both acidity and volume).

c. Metoclopramide, 10 mg orally or intravenously, enhances gastric emptying.

2. To avoid aortocaval compression, no woman at more than 25 weeks of gestation should be transported to or placed on the operating room table supine.

3. If FHR and uterine-contraction monitoring are feasible (greater than 17 weeks' gestation) and not within the surgical field, place external transducers before induction.

4. If fetal monitoring is impossible, assess FHR before and after induction of anesthesia and then again at the end of surgery. Because the reading and interpretation of continuous FHR and uterine-contraction patterns are not part of the day-to-day job of an anesthesiologist, close consultation with an obstetrician may be necessary if unusual changes occur intraoperatively.

5. For general anesthesia, remember the following:

a. Carefully denitrogenate the patient by using 100% oxygen by mask before induction to reduce the risk of maternal and fetal hypoxemia.

b. Even with adequate gastric acid prophylaxis therapy, do a rapid-sequence induction and intubation with a cuffed endotracheal tube and cricoid pressure.

c. Aspiration is as great a problem on extubation as on intubation. Delay extubation. Look for objective signs of intact airway reflexes and motor strength (e.g., adequate tidal volumes, train-of-four without a decrement, head lift for 5 seconds).

d. Proper ventilation is very important during general anesthesia in the parturient.

   i. Mechanical hyperventilation markedly reduces uterine blood flow.

   ii. Monitor end-tidal capnography closely, and sample arterial blood gases, if necessary, to maintain p_aCO_2 within normal pregnancy limits (30 to 35 mm Hg).

   iii. Remember, pregnancy decreases the arterial-to-$ETCO_2$ gradient. $ETCO_2$ approximates p_aCO_2.

REFERENCES

1. Briggs GG, Freeman RK, Yaffee SJ. *Drugs in pregnancy and lactation: a reference guide to fetal and neonatal risk,* 4th ed. Baltimore: Williams & Wilkins, 1994.

2. Kastrup EK, Hebel SK, eds. *Drugs: facts and comparisons.* St. Louis: Facts and Comparisons, 1997.

3. Jevtovic-Todorovic V, Todorovic SM, Mennerick S, et al. Nitrous oxide (laughing gas) is an NMDA antagonist, neuroprotectant and neurotoxin. *Nat Med* 1998;4:460.

4. Crawford JS, Lewis M. Nitrous oxide in early human pregnancy. *Anaesthesia* 1986;41:900.

5. Mazze RI, Källén B. Reproductive outcome after anesthesia and operation during pregnancy: a registry study of 5405 cases. *Am J Obstet Gynecol* 1989;161:1178.

6. Nezhat FR, Tazuke S, Nezhat CS, Seidman DS, Philips DR, Nezhat CR. Laparoscopy during pregnancy: a literature review. *J Soc Laparoendosc Surg* 1997;1:17.
7. Pomini F, Mercogliano D, Cavalletti C, Caruso A, Pomini P. Cardiopulmonary bypass in pregnancy. *Ann Thorac Surg* 1996;61:259.
8. Strickland RA, Oliver WC Jr, Chantigian RC, Ney JA, Danielson GK. Anesthesia, cardiopulmonary bypass, and the pregnant patient. *Mayo Clin Proc* 1991;166:411.
9. Santos AC, Baumann AL, Wlody D, Pedersen H, Morishima HO, Finster M. The maternal and fetal effects of milrinone and dopamine in normotensive pregnant ewes. *Am J Obstet Gynecol* 1992;166:257.

Mechanisms of Labor Pain

During labor, pain is felt in the dermatomes supplied by the spinal cord segments that receive input from the uterus, cervix, pelvis, and perineum. In the absence of therapeutic intervention, these stimuli cause spinal sensitization, activating adjacent segments, extending the field of pain.

STAGES OF LABOR

1. Labor is characterized by painful, progressive uterine contractions that cause dilation and effacement of the cervix. Descent and delivery of the fetus and placenta through the birth canal follow.
2. There are four stages of labor:
   a. The first stage, which must overcome cervical resistance, is divided into latent and active phases.
   b. During the second stage of labor, descent continues, and the fetus is finally born. Episiotomy is often done at the end of the second stage, although by this time, damage to the pelvic musculature has already occurred.
   c. The third stage of labor begins with the birth of the fetus and ends with complete expulsion or extraction of the placenta.
   d. The fourth stage ends 1 hour postpartum.

First and Second Stages of Labor

1. Pain of the first stage of labor comes from uterine contractions that cause effacement of the cervicovaginal angle and dilatation, distention, stretching, and tearing of the cervix and perineum.
   a. The force of uterine contractions against the closed or dilating cervix and perineum places pressure on nerve endings among the muscle fibers of the body and fundus of the uterus and induces inflammatory changes within uterine muscle.
   b. Other sources of pain: contraction of an ischemic myometrium and cervix, and vasoconstriction from sympathetic hyperactivity.
   c. Tissue injury and uterine contractions enhance the responsiveness of both the peripheral and central nervous systems (sensitization).
      i. Peripheral sensitization reduces the firing threshold of nociceptor afferent nerve terminals.
      ii. Central sensitization produces an activity-dependent increase in the excitability of spinal neurons.
   d. The resulting pain is felt between the umbilicus and pubes and across the back at the level of the top of the sacrum. It is a summation of:
      i. Acute deep and superficial somatic pain from the pelvic joints, vagina, and perineum.
      ii. Acute visceral pain from the uterus and cervix.
      iii. Pain referred to skin and muscle of the abdominal wall and the back.

2. During the second stage of labor, the nociceptive stimulation from the fully dilated cervix decreases, but the presenting part of the fetus distends pain-sensitive structures in the pelvis and perineum, adding to the ongoing pain.
   a. Progressively greater distention stretches and tears fascia and subcutaneous tissue of the vagina and adjacent structures (urethra, bladder, fascia and muscle of the pelvic cavity, peritoneum, and uterine ligaments).
   b. Some patients also report aching, burning, or cramping in the thighs or legs, probably reflecting secondary hyperalgesia involving the L1 to L3 and S2 dermatomes.
3. Acute tissue destruction, such as occurs during labor, induces both primary and secondary hyperalgesia.
   a. *Primary hyperalgesia* occurs at the site of injury and results from sensitization of peripheral sensory receptors of Aδ and C fibers. Central sensitization has only a small role in primary hyperalgesia.
   b. *Secondary hyperalgesia* occurs distant from the site of injury, and is mediated by central sensitization, enabling Aβ-fiber activation to produce pain.
4. Repeated C-fiber input or central summation of C and Aδ nociceptive activity facilitates nerve activity within the dorsal horn and induces *central sensitization.* This enhanced responsiveness of dorsal horn neurons, also called "wind up," is due partly to the interaction of three mediators released by the C-fiber terminals:
   a. Glutamate, which acts on 9-amino-3-hydroxy-5-methylisoxazole (AMPA) and *N*-methyl-D-aspartate (NMDA) receptors.
   b. Substance P, which acts on neurokinin-1 receptors.
   c. Neurokinin A, which acts on neurokinin-2 receptors and appears to play a major role in acute nociception.
5. Central sensitization then alters the spatial extent, responsiveness, and threshold of the receptive fields of the dorsal horn neurons.
   a. NMDA antagonists (i.e., ketamine) can block central hypersensitive states.
   b. Opioids bind to presynaptic inhibitory receptors on C-fiber terminals and can delay or block wind-up by reducing or stopping C-fiber input into dorsal horn nociceptive neurons.

Third and Fourth Stages of Labor
1. Pain during the third and fourth stages of labor reflects the noxious stimuli that have previously accompanied fetal descent and the separation of the placenta.
2. The central and peripheral hyperalgesic state present by delivery normally diminishes as the damaged visceral and somatic tissue recuperates.
3. Mechanical hyperalgesia (conducted by Aβ fibers) may persist for several days after the incision or cutting of tissue, such as the episiotomy.

PAIN PATHWAYS
Afferent Pain Pathways
Superficial and Deep Somatic Pain Pathways

1. Dilation, distention, and stretching of the muscles, pelvic joints, and vagina during labor produces somatic pain.
   a. Deep somatic pain follows activation of nociceptors in muscle, nerves, or joints.
   b. Cutaneous activation of nociceptors produces superficial somatic pain.
2. Nociceptive information is conveyed from the periphery to the central nervous system (CNS) via myelinated (Aδ) and unmyelinated (C) primary afferent fibers.
   a. These nerves have average conduction velocities of 15 m per second and less than 1 m per second, respectively.
   b. Aδ fibers are the major peripheral source of information on the more discriminative aspects of pain. This pain, known as first pain, is well localized, sharp, and pricking in nature and provides early warning of tissue damage. Aδ fibers respond most strongly to noxious heat and pressure and less strongly to chemical stimulation.
   c. C fibers have been implicated in tonic pain perception, often described as dull, burning, or aching. This pain is known as second pain and is preferentially attenuated by opioids. Nociceptors, associated with the free nerve endings of C fibers, are most strongly activated by chemical mediators.
3. Central sensitization from a noxious stimulus, such as incisional pain, also can activate other nerve fibers, such as the large, low-threshold mechanoreceptive Aβ-primary sensory neurons, which are not usually involved in pain.
4. Nociceptors are polymodal: They respond to thermal, mechanical, and chemical noxious (or painful) stimuli. Under normal circumstances, most are inactive and unresponsive (" silent" or "sleeping"). Inflammation can sensitize these nociceptors. They develop spontaneous discharges and become more responsive to peripheral stimulation.
   a. Inflammatory mediators, released in damaged tissue, sensitize nociceptors by activating second-messenger systems.
   b. After peripheral injury, many afferent fibers also express newly formed nocireceptors.
5. After leaving the periphery, the afferent nerve fibers accompany the sympathetic nerves, passing to the uterine plexus, then to the inferior, middle, and superior hypogastric plexus, and finally to the aortic plexus of the celiac plexus.
   a. The nociceptive afferents then travel to the lumbar sympathetic chain and run cephalad with the lower thoracic sympathetic nerves. They leave the sympathetic chain through the rami communicantes associated with the T10, T11, T12, and L1 (occasionally L2 and L3) spinal nerves.
   b. The cell bodies of these afferent fibers lie within the dorsal root ganglia. The afferent fibers pass through the posterior spinal nerve roots and make synaptic contact in the dorsal horn of the spinal gray matter.

Visceral Pain Pathways

1. Acute pain after visceral injury is often intense, vaguely localized, referred to distant regions of the body (referred pain), and accompanied by powerful motor and autonomic reactions, including spasms of the abdominal musculature and increased sympathetic outflow.

2. The area of referral is segmental and superficial (muscle or skin) and corresponds to the spinal segments that innervate the involved viscera.

3. Stimulation of visceral nerves at low intensities produces a vague feeling of fullness and nausea. Higher intensities cause a sensation of pain.

4. The viscera are innervated by vagal and spinal afferent pathways comprising thinly myelinated Aδ fibers and unmyelinated C fibers.

5. Silent nociceptors have been described in visceral nerves. These nociceptors are found in mucosal, muscle, and serosal layers of viscera and exhibit chemosensitivity, thermosensitivity, and mechanosensitivity.

6. Spinal visceral nerve cell bodies are located in dorsal root ganglia.
   a. On their route to the spinal cord, these nerves typically pass through or near prevertebral ganglia (where they can give off collateral axons to autonomic ganglion cell bodies) and paravertebral ganglia.
   b. Visceral afferent nerve fibers display a consistent pattern of central termination throughout the spinal cord. Areas of projection include laminae I and V, but not the intermediate dorsal horn.
      i. Visceral afferent nerve fibers reach the dorsal horn via Lissauer's tract and join medial and lateral bundles of fine fibers that run along the edges of the dorsal horn.
      ii. Somatic neurons are located mainly in laminae II, III, and IV of the dorsal horn, whereas viscerasomatic neurons are located in laminae I, V, and in the ventral horn.

7. The viscera are sparsely innervated, and many C fibers respond to stimuli from more than one organ.
   a. Consequently, visceral pain is vague and poorly localized, whereas somatic input is promptly localized.
   b. Some compensation for the low number of visceral afferents is provided by the significantly greater rostrocaudal intraspinal spread of visceral afferent nerve terminals.

8. The spinal neurons on which visceral afferents terminate typically receive convergent cutaneous and deep input.

9. Most mechanosensitive afferents innervate muscle, but two populations of mechanosensitive afferents innervate viscera:
   a. Seventy percent to 80% of fibers have a low response threshold.
   b. Twenty percent to 30% have a high threshold.
   c. The uterus is innervated by a population of afferent fibers that do not begin to respond until the distending stimulus intensity is in the range of pressures associated with pain.

10. Opioid receptors also play a role in activating sympathetic and parasympathetic low-threshold visceral nerves.
11. Visceral afferents undergo peripheral and central sensitization, which produces visceral hyperalgesia, felt mainly as discomfort and pain associated with visceral disorders.
    a. Sensitization of afferent visceral fibers increases afferent neural input to the spinal cord.
    b. Spinal cord release of neurotransmitters, including glutamate and peptides, such as substance P, follows activation of silent nociceptors. These compounds alter the excitability of spinal neurons.
    c. Thus, visceral hyperalgesia produces central sensitization by a mechanism similar to cutaneous models.

Spinal Pain Modulation
1. Peripheral nociceptive afferents terminate in an ordered way in the dorsal horn of the spinal cord.
   a. The thinly myelinated Aδ fibers end in laminae I and V.
   b. The unmyelinated C fibers enter outer lamina I and lamina II. These high-threshold sensory fibers activate a large number of second-order interneurons within the dorsal horn.
      i. There are two main functional groups of dorsal horn cells:
         (1) The "nociceptive-specific."
         (2) The "multireceptive" (also called "wide dynamic range" or "convergent").
      ii. The former respond solely to noxious stimuli, whereas the latter also are activated by innocuous stimuli.
2. Interneuronal networks in the spinal gray matter modulate nociceptive information and transmit it to neurons that project to the brain.
   a. While certain stimuli sensitize these projection neurons and increase nociceptive transmission, other inputs produce inhibition.
   b. The balance between the excitatory and inhibitory processes is the basis of the gate theory of pain transmission.

Spinal Neurotransmitters and Neuromodulators
1. The spinal neurotransmitters come from afferent nerve fibers, intrinsic neurons, and descending fibers and include:
   a. Excitatory amino acids, particularly glutamate.
   b. Neuropeptides, such as substance P.
   c. Calcitonin gene-related peptide.
   d. Vasoactive intestinal polypeptide.
   e. Prostaglandins.
   f. Dopamine.
   g. Serotonin.
   h. GABA.
   i. Catecholamines.
   j. Somatostatin.
   k. Acetylcholine.
   l. Histamine.
   m. Nitric oxide.

2. As with peripheral nociceptors, sensitization of dorsal horn nociceptive neurons is the result of activation of second-messenger systems.
3. Inhibitory neurotransmitters in the nociceptive circuits of the dorsal horn include:
   a. Opioid agonists.
   b. Enkephalins.
   c. GABA.
   d. Glycine.
   e. Noradrenaline.
4. The analgesia produced by spinal opioids comes from binding to specific receptors located on the primary afferents and second-order neurons.
   a. Opioid binding inhibits nociceptive transmission to the thalamus and cortex.
   b. There are μ-, ∂-, and κ-opioid receptors in the substantia gelatinosa (laminae II and III) and nucleus proprius (laminae IV, V, and VI) of the dorsal horn.
   c. Stimulation of both spinal and supraspinal opioid-sensitive sites may be essential for the production of analgesia by spinally administered opioids.
      i. Morphine produces analgesia by binding at supraspinal μ_1-receptors and the spinal μ_2-receptors.
      ii. Respiratory depression is secondary to binding at supraspinal μ_2-receptors.
5. The $GABA_A$ and $GABA_B$ receptors have both pre-and post-synaptic inhibitory actions.
6. Glycine acts postsynaptically to inhibit nociceptive transmission.
7. Norepinephrine diminishes substance P release from primary A∂ and C afferents and reduces response of dorsal horn neurons to noxious stimuli. It also modulates pain by stimulating acetylcholine release by binding to α_2-adrenoreceptors on spinal cholinergic interneurons.

Ascending Pain Pathways

1. After processing in the dorsal horn, nociceptor input travels directly, or via brainstem relay nuclei, to the thalamus and then into the cortex, where the conscious sensation of pain is generated. Simultaneously, output from the dorsal horn activates flexor motor neurons in the ventral horn, generating the withdrawal reflex. Both the sensation of physiologic pain and the flexion withdrawal reflex occur together.
2. Nociceptive projection neurons in the spinal cord transmit information to a number of regions of the brainstem and diencephalon.
   a. These projection neurons travel in the spinothalamic, spinomesencephalic, spinoreticular, and spinolimbic tracts, which lie in the anterolateral quadrant of the spinal cord.
   b. A large fraction of spinothalamic and spinomesencephalic tract cells are concentrated in the lumbar and sacral laminae I, IV to VI, and X.
   c. Spinothalamic neurons with a dominant input from viscera or muscle are situated in segments just rostral and

caudal to segments containing spinothalamic tract cells with a dominant cutaneous input from the distal part of an extremity.
3. Uterine and vaginal distention induces nociceptive activity in neurons of the dorsal column nuclei.
   a. This visceral information is relayed together with cutaneous somatic pain (conducted by Aδ fibers) information in the medial lemniscus to the thalamus.
   b. Most neurons (85%) in the ventral posterior lateral nucleus of the thalamus respond to both cutaneous and visceral stimuli. Although the cutaneous input is somatotopic, the visceral input is not viscerotropic.

Descending Pain Pathways
1. The sensation of pain is subject not only to modulation during its ascending transmission from the periphery through the medulla to the cortex, but also to segmental modulation and descending control from higher centers.
   a. This control is manifested via pathways that originate at the level of the cortex, the thalamus, and the brainstem (the periaqueductal gray, the raphe nuclei [raphe dorsal nucleus and raphe magnus], and locus coeruleus and subcoeruleus complex).
   b. Other structures involved include limbic structures, the Kölliker-Fuse nuclei, and several nuclei of the bulbar reticular formation.
   c. Descending inhibition from the thalamus is in part mediated via relay stations in the brainstem.
2. The main neurotransmitter systems implicated in descending pain control are:
   a. Serotonin (5-HT1A and 5-HT3 receptors).
   b. α_2-Adrenoreceptors.
   c. $GABA_A$ receptors.
   d. Glycine receptors.
   e. Acetylcholine receptors.
   f. Opioid receptors.

FACTORS INFLUENCING THE SEVERITY OF LABOR PAIN
1. Pain is a subjective phenomenon commonly characterized as a multidimensional experience, varying in quality and intensity.
   a. Pain-intensity scales can be used clinically to guide the provision of analgesia and to quantify pain.
   b. They consist of a line with two opposites that can be numeric (varying from 0, "no pain at all," to 10 cm, "worst possible pain"), or categoric (varying from "no pain" to "worst possible pain").
   c. Pain-descriptor questionnaires, such as the McGill Pain Questionnaire, assess both the quality and intensity of pain.[1]
2. The severity of labor pain varies widely, with many factors influencing its severity.

Neurohumoral Changes
1. Pregnancy is associated with an increased nociceptive tolerance related to increased plasma β-endorphin concentrations. The opioid antagonist naltrexone reverses this effect.

2. Lower plasma substance P concentration also may contribute to the altered pain tolerance in pregnancy. In addition, progesterone modifies deactivation of substance P by an endopeptidase.

3. Clinically, pregnant women need approximately 30% less local anesthetics for epidural analgesia than do nonpregnant women. Although some of this effect may be related to increased sensitivity to local anesthetics (see later), some also may be related to changes in pain tolerance associated with pregnancy.

4. Pregnancy also is associated with an increased sensitivity to both regional and general anesthetics. This altered susceptibility may be due to:
   a. A direct effect of progesterone on membrane excitability.
   b. Indirect actions of neurotransmitters.
   c. Increased permeability of the neural sheath.
   d. Potentiation of the analgesic effect of endogenous opioids.
   e. Pharmacokinetic and pharmacodynamic differences between pregnant and nonpregnant women.

5. The hormonal changes of pregnancy may influence pain neuropeptides in the spinal cord.
   a. The increase in pain threshold is likely to be maximal toward the end of gestation, possibly related to opioid activity in the spinal cord.
   b. Both somatic and visceral antinociceptive effects of epidural lidocaine are potentiated in near-term pregnant rats. However, smaller doses of epidural lidocaine are more effective for visceral than for somatic pain.[2]

Obstetric Factors

1. Women having their first labor complain of more intense pain, have longer labors, and consume more analgesics than do multiparous patients.

2. The frequency of contractions and cervical dilatation predict pain for primigravid women, but only the amount of cervical dilatation predicts pain in multiparae.

3. Regardless of parity, untreated parturients report the highest pain scores at 8- to 10-cm cervical dilatation. Advanced cervical dilation requires an increased concentration of epidural bupivacaine for analgesia.

4. Histories of severe menstrual and low-back pain also correlate with pain scores in labor, whereas the roles of fetal position and oxytocin are controversial.

Physical and Chemical Factors

1. Both physical and chemical factors may alter a patient's response to epidural labor analgesia.
   a. Pregnancy alters the distribution of local anesthetics within the spinal canal and enhances the sensitivity of nerves to local anesthetic blockade.
   b. Reduced thoracic kyphosis and caudad position of the apex of the lumbar lordosis may enhance cephalad spread of spinal analgesia in late pregnancy.

    c. Increased spread of spinal and epidural blockade in early pregnancy is unlikely to be related to changes in posture, but instead may be related to enhanced neural sensitivity.
2. Cerebrospinal fluid (CSF) pH is higher in the second and third trimesters of gestation (7.33 to 7.34) compared with that in nonpregnant patients (7.30).
    a. Higher pH increases the amount of local anesthetic in the non-ionized base form, which should enhance the rate of diffusion across the nerve sheath and nerve membrane, contributing to faster onset of block in pregnant patients.
    b. However, clinical studies showed that pregnancy-induced changes in acid-base state of CSF (CSF pH, pCO_2, HCO_3) have little effect on the spread of spinal anesthesia.

Demographic Variables
1. There are marked differences in pain beliefs among different cultures.
    a. Each patient has a unique background, personality, religion, previous experience, and expectation, all of which can influence the pain experience.
    b. For example, American women expect labor to be more painful than do Dutch women,[3] and Catholic women report less pain during active labor than either Protestant or nonreligious parturients.[4]
2. Aging impairs pain perception.
    a. Although both Aδ and C fibers are clearly affected, preferential loss of myelinated fibers occurs with aging.
    b. Vibrotactile sensitivity, which is subserved by Aβ fibers, seems to provide the earliest detectable evidence of age-related disturbance of sensory function.
    c. Older women have less painful labors than do younger women.

Anxiety
1. Untrained primigravidae reported more severe labor pain than those attending childbirth classes.
    a. Neurons from the spinothalamic tract that project to the central lateral nucleus in the median thalamus have large receptive fields and may have a role in the motivational-affective aspects of pain.
    b. Motivational-affective circuits can mimic pain states, most notably in patients with anxiety (i.e., an untrained primigravida).
2. Although the available data suggest that a prepared mother will be less anxious and cope better with labor pain, the mechanism of anxiety's impact on pain is controversial.
    a. Anxiety shows a strong correlation with visual-analog scale (VAS) ratings of pain and unpleasantness. The higher the levels of anxiety, the higher the VAS scores of pain and unpleasantness.

      b. In addition, anxiety and stress induce release of epinephrine, which may sensitize or directly activate peripheral nociceptors.

3. Conversely, anxiety also may release endogenous opioids, and there are strong suggestions that anxiety can inhibit pain perception, not directly, but by diverting attention from the painful stimulus. Anxiety focused on pain may increase pain, whereas anxiety focused on other sources may reduce pain.

ANALGESIA AND LABOR

1. Little is known of the effects of epidural analgesia on the progress of labor, method of delivery, and neonate.
      a. In the second stage of labor, there is evidence that epidural analgesia attenuates endogenous oxytocin production (Ferguson's reflex) and reduces uterine contractility.
      b. It is assumed that the motor block associated with epidural analgesia reduces maternal effort during pushing and causes relaxation of the pelvic floor, which predisposes to malrotation of the fetal head.
      c. In first-stage labor, epidural analgesia does not reduce uterine contractility, but may slow cervical dilatation.
2. Fluid infused before regional analgesia transiently decreases uterine activity.
      a. A liter of normal saline decreases uterine activity for 10 to 20 minutes.
      b. Rapid volume expansion may cause a sudden release of the atrial natriuretic peptide (ANP) or have a direct mechanical effect on the uterine vasculature, producing local release of endothelial vasoactive peptides.
      c. ANP is directly secreted by the atrium. It causes vasodilatation, natriuresis, and diuresis, and inhibits the secretion and action of angiotensin II and noradrenaline. It is also a potent inhibitor of the uterine contractility.

IMPLICATIONS

1. Pain can be therapeutically approached at the supraspinal, spinal, and peripheral levels.
      a. Supraspinal structures such as the ventral posterior lateral nucleus or the spinal dorsal column nuclei could be specifically stimulated to produce labor analgesia.
      b. Peripherally, the observation that most nociceptors are normally "silent" or "sleeping" but become sensitized by inflammation suggests that blocking peripheral sensitization or the respective spinal field can minimize pain.
      c. Central sensitization requires that temporal or spatial summation of postsynaptic excitatory potentials exceeds the action-potential threshold of the cell.
            i. The receptive field of a dorsal horn neuron is divided into the firing zone and the subliminal zone, which surrounds the former and does not respond to the initial repetitive stimuli.
            ii. In this subliminal zone, an increase in excitability can convert a previously subthreshold stimulus to

a suprathreshold stimulus and generate a hyper-excitable state.

    iii.   This phenomenon can be reduced or avoided by preadministration of various agents, such as opioids, local anesthetics, nonsteroidal antiinflammatory drugs, clonidine, nitric oxide, or ketamine (preemptive analgesia).

    iv.   Unfortunately, postinjury analgesia has a much-diminished effect on an established state of hyperexcitability. Low doses of morphine prevent central sensitization, but once it is established, high doses are necessary to suppress it.

2.   An alternative approach to labor analgesia should involve searching for a synergistic combination of drugs that would enhance pre- and postsynaptic inhibition of dorsal horn nociceptive circuits.

3.   The ideal method of analgesia would relieve pain before and during tissue injury and last until complete tissue healing occurs. Intrathecal, but not epidural, local anesthetics inhibit temporal summation of repeated electric stimuli. These data may provide a rationale for the use of combined spinal-epidural or continuous spinal techniques in laboring women.

RATIONALE FOR PAIN RELIEF

1.   The pain of labor serves no useful purpose. Women neither want nor need to experience labor pain.

    a.   Unfortunately, some still believe that the experience of labor pain enhances a parturient's birth experience.

    b.   Others fear that adequate analgesia will impair the progress of labor.

2.   Although the severity of labor pain may decrease with subsequent pregnancies, its characteristics remain constant.

3.   By using our growing understanding of pain processing and the mechanisms of analgesia, we can strive to provide safe, effective labor analgesia that does not adversely effect the progress or outcome of labor.

REFERENCES

1. Melzack R. The McGill Pain Questionnaire: major properties and scoring methods. *Pain* 1975;1:277.
2. Kaneko M, Saito Y, Kirihara Y, Kosaka Y. Pregnancy enhances the antinociceptive effects of extradural lidocaine[KS1] in the rat. *Br J Anaesth* 1994;72:657.
3. Senden IPM, Wetering MD, Eskes TKAB, Brerkens PB, Laube DW, Pitkin RM. Labor pain: a comparison of parturients in a Dutch and an American teaching hospital. *Obstet Gynecol* 1988;71:541.
4. Wuitchick M, Hesson K, Bakal D. Perinatal predictors of pain and distress during labor. *Birth* 1990;17:186.

9

Alternatives to Conduction Analgesia

NONPHARMACOLOGIC PAIN RELIEF

Concern for maternal–fetal safety and the desire for a satisfactory birth experience have fostered an "antianesthesia" atmosphere in some obstetric suites. Some claim that "intervention" is unnecessary in the "natural" process of parturition. To them, the use of anesthesia represents patient failure and risks disastrous fetal outcome. This sentiment has led some patients and obstetricians to seek alternative methods of labor pain relief. These methods avoid exogenous drugs; however, most leave the parturient with considerable pain. The birth experience may still be unsatisfactory (or at least very painful).

Prepared Childbirth

Natural Childbirth

THE DICK-READ METHOD

1. Grantly Dick-Read
   a. Coined the term *natural childbirth*.
   b. Suggested that labor pain arose from socially induced expectations about parturition.
   c. Asserted that childbirth is not an inherently painful process.
   d. Outlined the "fear-tension-pain syndrome."
      i. Fear incites tension in the circular muscle fibers of the lower part of the uterus.
      ii. This tension produces pain perception.
   e. To eliminate labor pain:
      i. Correct faulty expectations (i.e., that labor will be painful).
      ii. Use progressive muscle relaxation.
      iii. Dick-Read also introduced breathing exercises:
         (1) Deep breathing during early stages of labor.
         (2) More rapid breathing during contractions toward the end of the first stage.
         (3) Panting during a contraction if bearing down is undesirable.
         (4) Breath-holding when bearing down.
2. This method of natural childbirth has its limitations; even Dick-Read admitted that normal labor could involve some pain.

PSYCHOPROPHYLAXIS

1. Developed in the Soviet Union in 1954 by A. Nikolayev
2. Presented to Western scientists by Velvovsky
3. Stated that perceived pain was "conditioned reflex labor pain."
   a. Pain came from neural impulses arising in labor that were experienced as painful because of disruption of

excitatory-inhibitory processes in the cortex and sub-cortex.
b. Psychoprophylaxis would prevent excitatory-inhibitory imbalance through:
    i. Deep breathing during each contraction.
    ii. Stroking of sections of the abdomen combined with deep breathing.
    iii. Pressure applied to "pain-prevention points" along the small of the back and the medial surface of the anterior superior ilia.

FERNAND LAMAZE
1. A French obstetrician
2. He became acquainted with the teaching of Velvovsky while touring Russia in 1951.
3. Upon returning to France, he began using the techniques, with some of his own variations:
    a. Rapid breathing during the second stage of labor.
    b. Panting during crowning and delivery.
    c. Controlled neuromuscular relaxation during labor.
    d. Deletion of stroking, pain-prevention points, and timing of contractions from Velvovsky's technique.
4. The Lamaze method is the most popular approach to pre-pared childbirth in the United States, although it is often modified with parts of the Dick-Read method.
    a. Differences in preparatory techniques reflect variance in trainers, treatment settings, and theoretical orienta-tions.
    b. Most programs, however, include three distinct compo-nents:
        i. Information about normal anatomy and physio-logy of pregnancy, labor, and delivery.
        ii. Relaxation training.
        iii. Breathing techniques that usually follow varia-tions of the format outlined by Dick-Read.
        iv. Many instructors add husband participation:
            (1) Timing contractions.
            (2) Delivering reminders about breathing tech-niques.
            (3) Providing support.

Bradley
1. The second most popular form of childbirth education in the United States
2. Originates from the work during the 1940s of Robert Bradley, M.D.
    a. Believed women could be taught to cope with labor pain as animals did
    b. Introduced husbands into the labor room
    c. Argued against the "meddlesome interference with nature's instinctual conduct and plans" and the "terri-ble indignities of drugs"
3. Today, proponents of the Bradley method continue to emphasize unmedicated childbirth, arguing that with the

proper preparation and a supportive coach, nine of ten women can give birth without medication.

Duola

1. Reassurance and support are important aspects of natural childbirth regimens.
2. A *duola,* or supportive lay companion, significantly improves labor outcome.
3. Compared with no support person, duola patients may have
   a. Shorter labors (8.8 hours compared with 19.3 hours in one study).
   b. Fewer perinatal problems.
   c. Better interactions with their newborns.
   d. More vaginal deliveries.
   e. Fewer requests for epidural analgesia.[1]

LeBoyer

1. The French obstetrician
2. Developed the concept of "childbirth without violence"
   a. Newborn suffers psychological trauma from
      i. Noise.
      ii. Bright lights.
      iii. Other stimulation associated with a traditional delivery.
   b. He advocated
      i. Delivery in semidarkness.
      ii. Minimal noise to avoid disturbing the neonate.
      iii. Immediately after delivery:
         (1) The baby lifted onto mother's abdomen.
         (2) Then lowered into a warm bath after the umbilical cord stops pulsating.
3. Among the objections to LeBoyer's methods:
   a. Subdued lighting may hinder assessment of the baby's condition and color.
   b. Hypothermia may develop while the baby is on the mother's abdomen or in the bath.
   c. Placing the baby on the mother's abdomen, which is higher than the placenta, until the cord stops pulsating can allow a serious loss of blood from baby to placenta.
   d. Placental transfusion to the neonate can result in volume overload, increased hematocrit and blood viscosity, and pulmonary hypertension.
4. LeBoyer technique versus conventional delivery
   a. Hypothermia did not occur in babies who had skin-to-skin contact with their mother at birth.
   b. Immersion in the water bath had no adverse effects.
   c. No baby suffered from treatable jaundice.
   d. No baby suffered from anemia due to delayed clamping of the cord.
   e. The quiet and subdued lighting did not interfere with communication or observation of the mother's or baby's condition.
   f. The LeBoyer babies cried less.
   g. LeBoyer mothers' memories of the birth experience were always positive.

- h.   There is probably no infant or maternal advantage compared with a gentle, conventional delivery.
5.   Placental-to-neonate blood transfusion
  - a.   Occurs when the umbilical cord clamping is delayed for more than 5 seconds after delivery.
  - b.   Neonate is at or below the level of the placenta.
  - c.   Up to 35 mL per kilogram of blood flows to the neonate.
  - d.   Transfusion may still occur with the infant above the level of the placenta (i.e., on the mother's abdomen).
  - e.   Blood volume may increase rapidly by 50%.
    - i.   Most infants respond with compensatory vasodilation.
    - ii.   Some may suffer marked volume overload.
    - iii.   Hematocrit and blood viscosity increase.
      - (1)   Transient (several days) pulmonary hypertension is possible.
  - f.   The amount of placental transfusion during LeBoyer deliveries varies.
    - i.   Full placental transfusion (35 mL per kilogram)
      - (1)   Acute vascular distention
      - (2)   High risk of:
        - (a)   Cardiac failure.
        - (b)   Respiratory problems.
        - (c)   Central nervous system problems.
    - ii.   Twenty milliliters per kilogram may be optimal for oxygen transport.
    - iii.   Infants delivered according to the LeBoyer method should be examined carefully for signs and symptoms of hyperviscosity.[2]

Efficacy
1.   Prepared childbirth techniques provide some degree of pain relief.
  - a.   Lamaze-trained primiparae may use fewer narcotics and neuraxial blocks and have a higher frequency of spontaneous vaginal deliveries compared with "matched" controls.
  - b.   Primiparae who had prepared childbirth training
    - i.   Lower pain scores than those with no training.
    - ii.   However, 81% still requested epidural anesthesia.
2.   Relaxation training is the most therapeutically active component of the Lamaze regimen.
  - a.   Lamaze classes teach women breathing, pushing, and relaxation techniques.
  - b.   They hope to instill in mothers the confidence to use these techniques to successfully manage labor.
  - c.   Self-evaluation of performance during labor is one of the most important components of the childbirth experience.
3.   Many women will still request additional analgesia.
  - a.   Childbirth classes should include reliable information about anesthetic options.
  - b.   Regional anesthesia can be a reasonable compromise that minimizes pain and stress but still allows participation of the mother and father in the birth of their infant.

Hypnosis
1. Hypnosis has long been used to lessen or relieve the pain of labor and delivery.
2. Advantages
   a. Does not obtund airway reflexes, impair the sensorium, or produce hypoventilation
   b. Produces neither hypotension nor decreased uteroplacental perfusion
   c. Does not cause itching or nausea and vomiting
   d. Circumvents neonatal depression
3. Reported benefits
   a. Shorter first stage of labor
   b. Causes better neonatal acid–base status (versus general anesthesia)
   c. More rapid recovery from birth asphyxia with hypnosis (versus general or regional anesthesia)
4. Hypnosis plus childbirth education
   a. Significantly increased pain threshold in susceptible parturients
   b. Shorter first stage of labor
   c. Less medication
   d. More frequent spontaneous deliveries
   e. Infants had higher Apgar scores.
   f. Highly susceptible, hypnotically treated women had lower depression scores after birth.
   g. Possible causes of superior outcomes in the hypnosis group
      i. Reduced pain perception
      ii. Higher pain tolerance
   h. Study subjects were highly motivated volunteers.
      i. Willing to try hypnosis
      ii. Participated in twice the typical amount of childbirth training[3]
5. Patient selection and preparation
   a. Evaluate for suggestibility by using the eye roll test.
   b. Preparation
      i. A series of 30-minute conditioning sessions
      ii. With each session, a greater degree of trance is obtained.
      iii. One technique consists of
         (1) Induction, counting down from 10 to 0 while descending a flight of stairs.
         (2) By imagining peaceful scenes, suggestions of arm levitation, glove anesthesia, and, finally, abdominal anesthesia.
6. Hypnosis, however, is not for everyone.
   a. Of any random group, only 25% are easily hypnotized.
   b. Reported complications range from acute anxiety to frank psychosis.
   c. Strong contraindications to hypnosis:
      i. Evidence of psychosis.
      ii. Evidence of a strong unconscious wish to regress.

        iii.   History of psychoneurotic hysterical conversion reactions.

        iv.   Evidence of strong fear or ambivalence regarding birth or motherhood.

        v.   Hyperemesis gravidarum during the first trimester.

        vi.   Nightmares in the last trimester.[4]

7. Other obstetric uses of hypnosis
   a. An adjunct to the medical treatment of premature labor
   b. Treatment of acute pregnancy-associated hypertension

Acupuncture

1. Background
   a. Chi (qi) energy runs along 12 meridians (channels).
   b. Two forms of energy, yin and yang, must be in balance.
   c. Imbalance causes disease and pain.
   d. Inserting needles into acupuncture points, which lie on the meridians, and gently vibrating them can reestablish balance.
      i. Traditionally, vibrations were generated by hand, but today electrical stimuli are more common.
2. Acupuncture has been used to help control labor pain in China and the Far East for many years.
   a. In China, acupuncture produces surgical analgesia in only 60% to 70% of patients.
   b. It is least effective for pain in the lower part of the body.
   c. Success depends on
      i. Patient selection.
      ii. Motivation.
      iii. Deeply embedded cultural conditioning.
3. Acupuncture
   a. Can produce a state of hypoalgesia that varies with a given patient's pain threshold.
   b. Does not provide complete pain relief.
   c. This hypoalgesic state may be mediated by endogenous opioids (endorphins).
4. Clinical studies
   a. Some pain relief
   b. Forty percent to 80% of laboring women still request additional analgesia.
   c. Occasionally associated with shorter stage one labor.
   d. Maternal response is usually positive.
5. Acupuncture analgesia is incomplete, unpredictable, inconsistent, and time consuming. Needles may become dislodged, patients' movements are restricted, and electroacupuncture can interfere with electronic monitoring of mother and fetus.

Transcutaneous Electrical Nerve Stimulation (TENS)

1. The use of TENS in modern medicine derives from the gate-control theory of pain.
   a. Cells in the posterior horn of the spinal gray matter have a gating function.

    b. Activity in low-threshold, large afferent fibers (not conducting pain) "closes the gate" and blocks conduction in afferent pain fibers to the pain pathways.

    c. TENS is thought to work by a combination of increasing the release of endogenous opiates and closing the pain gate.

  2. The TENS stimulator is a dual-output device.

    a. Each output can be varied in both amplitude and rate.

      i. The amplitude varies from 0 to 220 V.

      ii. Frequency ranges from 40 to 150 Hz.

    b. Two pairs of silicon electrodes are placed paravertebrally.

      i. T10 to L1 spinal levels

      ii. S2 to S4 spinal levels

    c. Upper level

      i. The amplitude and frequency are adjusted until the patient is aware of a tingling or tickling sensation.

      ii. This background stimulation is maintained continuously.

    d. Lower level

      i. The amplitude and frequency are set higher than the upper level.

      ii. Electrodes are stimulated from the beginning until 30 seconds after each contraction.

    e. As labor progresses, the frequency and amplitude of stimulation are varied to achieve the best results.

  3. Efficacy

    a. Usually provides some relief of pain during the first stage of labor.

      i. Decreases the need for narcotic analgesics

      ii. May shorten the first stage of labor

    b. Less effective in the second stage

    c. Some patients find TENS especially helpful with "back labor."

    d. Over 70% of parturients find TENS helpful enough to request it for a subsequent labor.

  4. TENS has certain advantages over other forms of labor analgesia.

    a. It is safe, noninvasive, and instantly reversible.

    b. It can easily be administered by a trained midwife.

    c. Although TENS appears to be of minimal benefit in the second stage of labor, it can complement conventional methods of analgesia.

Biofeedback

  1. Biofeedback has been used for more than a decade to help patients cope with chronic pain.

  2. Two methods

    a. The autonomic or skin conductance level (SCL) method

      i. Electrodes are placed on the patient's second and third fingers of the left hand.

      ii. The patient wears earphones.

      iii. SCL is detected by the electrodes and is indicated to the patient by a series of clicks heard through the earphones.

        iv. An increase in SCL, heard as an increase in the rate of clicks, indicates increased arousal.

   b. The voluntary muscle relaxation or electromyographic (EMG) method
        i. Seems to be more effective.
        ii. Electrodes are applied 5 cm apart in the midline of the abdomen.
        iii. The ground electrode is placed above the umbilicus and the two active electrodes are placed below.
        iv. The patient also wears earphones.
        v. As with the SCL method, increased EMG activity (decreased relaxation) is indicated by a faster rate of clicks through the earphones.

3. Effects
   a. Decreased tension of voluntary muscles may reduce perineal trauma associated with delivery.
   b. Concentration on relaxation may distract the woman from her pain.
   c. Relaxation also may enhance descending modulatory pain pathways.

4. Efficacy
   a. More effective in early than active labor
   b. Women using EMG biofeedback report lower levels of pain both by a visual analog scale and by a verbal descriptor scale than do controls.
   c. It may shorten first stage of labor.
   d. It may decrease use of other analgesics.

5. Biofeedback is easily taught.
   a. Instruction can be given in group format.
   b. There are four to six weekly training sessions
   c. The patient can practice daily at home.

SYSTEMIC ANALGESICS IN OBSTETRICS

1. Systemic drugs have been used for labor pain since 1847.
2. Their use is still very common for several reasons:
   a. They are simple to use and do not require anesthesia personnel.
   b. They require minimal monitoring.
   c. They have a low incidence of complications.
   d. Neuraxial analgesia may not be available in all hospital settings.
   e. Regional analgesia may be contraindicated in certain conditions.
   f. Some women fear regional analgesia.
3. Systemic medications do have their disadvantages.
   a. They seldom provide complete analgesia.
   b. They cause sedation and possibly respiratory depression in parturients and neonates.
   c. They delay gastric emptying in parturients and may precipitate nausea and/or vomiting.
   d. They have been associated with adverse fetal and neonatal effects (loss of beat-to-beat variability, neonatal respiratory depression).

Opioid Analgesics

1. Parenteral opioids may be given by intermittent bolus or by patient-controlled analgesia (PCA).
   a. The route and timing of administration influence maternal uptake and placental transfer.
   b. Intermittent bolus
      i. Subcutaneous (SC) injection
      ii. Intramuscular (IM) injection
         (1) The SC and IM injections are simple but painful.
         (2) The resultant analgesia is delayed in onset and is variable in quality and duration.
      iii. Intravenous (IV) injection
         (1) More uniform quality and onset
         (2) Drugs are easier to titrate.
2. PCA
   a. Better pain relief with lower drug doses
   b. Less risk of maternal respiratory depression
   c. Less placental transfer of drug
   d. Less nausea and/or vomiting
   e. Greater patient satisfaction
   f. Smaller, more frequent dosing
      i. More stable plasma drug concentrations
      ii. More consistent analgesia
   g. The intermittent and intensifying episodes of pain that occur during labor unfortunately limit the efficacy of systemic opioids.

Morphine

1. The most important alkaloid of opium
2. Binds in a stereospecific manner to saturable sites (μ-receptors) in the brain, spinal cord, and other tissues
3. The usual doses for maternal analgesia:
   a. Two to 5 mg IV
   b. Five to 10 mg IM
4. Onset
   a. Three to 5 minutes after IV injection
   b. Twenty to 40 minutes after IM injection
5. Metabolized in the liver to morphine-3-glucuronide and then excreted by the kidneys
6. Rapidly crosses the placenta and the blood–brain barrier of the immature fetus
   a. Maternal morphine decreases fetal heart rate (FHR) variability and also may lower baseline FHR.
   b. Neonates are very susceptible to the respiratory depressant effects of morphine.
      i. Neonates are more sensitive to morphine than to meperidine, possibly due to a greater permeability of the infant brain to morphine.
      ii. This sometimes profound newborn respiratory depression and excessive maternal sedation has caused morphine to fall into disfavor as a labor analgesic.

Meperidine
1. Qualitatively similar to morphine
   a. A 60- to 80-mg IV dose is approximately equianalgesic with 10 mg of morphine.
   b. Because of its potency and lipophilicity (which speed onset), meperidine is one of the most widely used opioids for labor analgesia.
2. Doses (every 2 to 4 hours)
   a. Twenty-five to 50 mg IV
   b. Fifty to 100 mg IM
3. Onset
   a. Within 5 minutes after IV injection
   b. Forty-five minutes after IM injection
4. Usually given with a phenothiazine because meperidine can cause significant nausea and vomiting.
5. Pharmacokinetics (IV injection)
   a. Maternal plasma concentration peaks within 1 minute.
   b. Meperidine remains detectable throughout labor.
   c. It appears in fetal blood within 90 seconds.
   d. It equilibrates between maternal and fetal compartments in 6 minutes.
   e. Half-life
      i. About 2.5 hours in the mother
      ii. Eighteen to 23 hours in the neonate
6. It is metabolized in the liver to three compounds:
   a. Meperidic acid.
   b. Normeperidic acid.
   c. Normeperidine (pharmacologically active)
      i. First detectable in maternal plasma 10 minutes after meperidine injection
      ii. Plasma concentration rises rapidly for 20 minutes.
      iii. Concentration continues to increase slowly throughout labor.
      iv. It readily crosses the placenta.
         (1) Its half-life in the neonate is about 60 hours.
         (2) Neonatal concentrations may be further increased by its own metabolism of placentally transferred meperidine.
7. Maternal meperidine can cause neonatal respiratory depression.
   a. Incidence is related to:
      i. The time between injection and delivery.
      ii. The quantity of drug administered.
      iii. The rate of maternal metabolism.
   b. Maximal risk occurs 2 to 3 hours after maternal injection.
   c. If given within 1 hour of birth, neonatal depression is rare.
   d. The variable neonatal response to maternal meperidine correlates with the drug's fetal kinetics.
      i. In the first 2 hours, fetal tissue uptake limits plasma meperidine concentrations.
      ii. After 3 hours, the fetus is clearing the drug from its tissues.

          iii. Normeperidine is a potent respiratory depressant.
- (1) It may be responsible for neonatal depression.
- (2) This may be especially important after multiple maternal meperidine doses.
- (3) Or neonatal depression is related not to normeperidine, but to the amount of unmetabolized meperidine passing from mother to fetus.
- (4) Both compounds accumulate in fetal tissues.

          iv. Pharmacologically, the best time to be born following maternal meperidine is within 1 hour, or more than 4 hours, after a single, small IV dose.

8. Fetal effects of maternal meperidine
   a. Diminished FHR variability for up to 1 hour
   b. Long-term variability is impaired more than is short-term variability.
   c. Meperidine decreased the frequency and duration of fetal movements.
      i. This effect is maximal in the first 20 minutes after injection.
   d. These two issues may cause confusion when trying to assess fetal condition.

Fentanyl

1. A very lipid-soluble and highly protein-bound drug
2. One hundred times as potent as morphine
3. Seven hundred fifty times as potent as meperidine
4. Onset
   a. Almost immediate when given IV
   b. Seven to 8 minutes following IM injection
   c. Maximal analgesia and respiratory depression may not occur immediately.
5. Duration
   a. Thirty to 60 minutes after a single IV dose of up to 100 µg
   b. One to 2 hours after IM injection
   c. As with all opioid analgesics, the respiratory depressant effects may outlast analgesia.
6. Advantages for labor analgesia
   a. Rapid onset
   b. Short duration
   c. Absent active metabolites
   d. Low emetic activity
7. Fentanyl rapidly crosses the placenta.
   a. It is detected in fetal blood within 1 minute of maternal IV injection.
   b. Peak fetal blood concentrations occur at 5 minutes.
8. Clinical effects
   a. Produces a temporary mild analgesia but fails to completely eradicate uterine contraction pain, especially in late labor.

b. FHR variability is decreased for 30 minutes, but maternal fentanyl does not impair newborn respiratory function.
c. No effect on:
   i. Newborn respiratory function
   ii. Apgar scores
d. In an unblinded comparison, meperidine caused more maternal nausea, vomiting, sedation, and neonatal respiratory depression than did fentanyl.
e. PCA administration more effective than nurse administered boluses.

Nalbuphine

1. A synthetic opioid agonist-antagonist of the phenanthrene series
2. Chemically related to both the opioid analgesic oxymorphone and the narcotic antagonist naloxone
3. Equipotent with morphine on a milligram basis
4. The usual dose is 10 to 20 mg every 4 to 6 hours.
5. Onset
   a. Within 2 to 3 minutes of IV administration
   b. Less than 15 minutes after SC or IM injection
6. The plasma half-life is 5 hours.
7. The duration of analgesia ranges from 3 to 6 hours.
8. Nalbuphine-induced respiratory depression peaks after a dose of 10 to 20 mg.
9. Repeated doses
   a. Prolonged analgesia without cumulative respiratory effects
   b. Larger doses do not increase the intensity of pain relief.
10. Nalbuphine delivered by PCA may produce better pain relief than meperidine in primiparous patients in the first stage of labor

Butorphanol

1. A synthetically derived opioid agonist-antagonist of the phenanthrene series
2. Analgesic potency
   a. Five to eight times that of morphine
   b. Thirty to 50 times that of meperidine
3. The usual dose in labor is 1 to 2 mg IV or IM every 3 to 4 hours.
4. Onset
   a. Within a few minutes after IV injection
   b. Ten to 15 minutes after IM injection
   c. Peak analgesic activity occurs in 30 to 60 minutes.
5. The analgesic dose of butorphanol (2 mg) depresses respiration to a similar degree as equivalent analgesic doses of morphine (10 mg) or meperidine (70 mg). However, doubling the dose (4 mg) does not produce appreciably greater depression.
6. Comparison with meperidine
   a. Butorphanol provides similar or significantly more analgesia at 30 minutes and 1 hour after administration.

   b. Fetal effects (Apgar scores, time to sustained respiration, umbilical venous pH, FHR, neonatal neurobehavioral scores) also are similar.
   c. Maternal side effects, although infrequent, are more common after meperidine.
7. Comparison with fentanyl
   a. Both drugs were equally safe.
   b. Both lacked an effect on active labor.
   c. Butorphanol provided better initial analgesia, with fewer patient requests for more medication.[5]

Pentazocine
1. A member of the benzazocine series (also known as the benzomorphan series).
2. It has both agonist and weak antagonist properties.
3. A 30-mg dose of pentazocine is usually as effective an analgesic as morphine (10 mg) or meperidine (75 to 100 mg).
4. Analgesia and sedation usually occur
   a. Within 15 to 20 minutes after IM injection.
   b. Two to 3 minutes after IV administration.
5. The plasma half-life of pentazocine is 2 to 3 hours.
6. Antagonist actions
   a. Weakly antagonizes the analgesic effects of morphine and meperidine
   b. Partially reverses meperidine's cardiovascular, respiratory, and behavioral depressant effects
   c. Has about one-fiftieth the antagonistic activity of nalorphine, another agonist-antagonist.
7. Dosage
   a. Most commonly, a single IM 30-mg dose
   b. An IV 20-mg dose may be adequate.
      i. This dose may be repeated two to three times at 2- to 3-hour intervals.
8. Respiratory depression can be seen with pentazocine but with a ceiling at 40 to 60 mg.
9. Side effects
   a. Sedation (most common)
   b. Sweating
   c. Dizziness or lightheadedness
   d. Nausea occurs, but vomiting is less common than with morphine.
   e. Psychotomimetic effects
      i. Anxiety
      ii. Nightmares
      iii. Weird thoughts
      iv. Fear of impending death
      v. Hallucinations
      vi. These effects are seen with increasing frequency when doses approach and exceed 60 mg.
      vii. These have limited pentazocine's use in obstetrics.

Nonnarcotic Analgesics and Tranquilizers
Phenothiazines
1. Sometimes combined with opioids in labor
   a. Produce sedation

     b. Decrease the potential for opioid-induced nausea and vomiting

2. Rapid placental transfer may decrease FHR beat-to-beat variability.

3. Neonatal depression is rare.

4. Chlorpromazine, promazine, and prochlorperazine may cause maternal hypotension via α-adrenergic blockade.

5. Promethazine (Phenergan)
    a. Most commonly used phenothiazine
    b. In early labor, 50 mg provides sedation and anxiolysis.
    c. In active labor, 25 to 75 mg IM or IV can be combined with an appropriately reduced dose of opioid (usually meperidine).
        i. This drug combination can be repeated once or twice at 4-hour intervals.
    d. The maximum recommended dose of promethazine during labor is 100 mg in 24 hours.
    e. Promethazine also is a mild respiratory stimulant and may counteract opioid respiratory depression.

Hydroxyzine (Vistaril)

1. An antihistamine
2. Provides sedation
3. Prevents nausea and vomiting
4. Is usually combined with a reduced dose of an opioid
    a. Potentiates the action of opioids and barbiturates
    b. The usual dose in labor is 25 to 50 mg IM (IV injection is very irritating to the veins).
5. No neonatal respiratory depression

Scopolamine

1. Historically used for amnesia and sedation in laboring women
2. No respiratory depression
3. In combination with an opioid, scopolamine produces "twilight sleep."
4. A high incidence of agitation and excitement has reduced its use to virtually zero.
5. It crosses the placenta
    a. Increases FHR
    b. Obliterates beat-to-beat variability
    c. Is reversed by maternal physostigmine

Barbiturates

1. Pentobarbital, secobarbital, amobarbital
2. Produce sedation and anxiolysis, not analgesia
3. May increase pain perception when given without an opioid
4. Most common use: sedation/hypnosis during latent labor, when delivery is remote
5. Also used for sleep in women in false labor
6. Dosage
    a. Pentobarbital: 100 to 200 mg
    b. Secobarbital: 100 mg
    c. Both drugs are given by mouth or IM.

7. All barbiturates are lipid soluble and readily cross the placenta.
   a. When administration is limited to early labor, a single dose rarely results in neonatal depression.
   b. Secobarbital plus meperidine is labor analgesia.
      i. Increased incidence of neonatal depression
      ii. Prolonged time before birth in which the infant is at risk of opioid-induced depression

Ketamine
1. A phencyclidine derivative
2. Induces a dissociative state
   a. Intense analgesia
   b. Inconsistent amnesia
3. Has rapid onset and a short duration after IV injection.
4. Dosage
   a. Can be given IM or IV
   b. One mg per kilogram IV produces unconsciousness.
   c. Ten to 20 mg can provide analgesia for vaginal delivery.
      i. Can be repeated every 2 to 5 minutes
      ii. Should not exceed 1 mg per kilogram in 30 minutes
      iii. Total dose: 100 mg
5. Side effects
   a. Ketamine stimulates the sympathetic nervous system and can exacerbate hypertension in preeclamptic patients.
   b. There are no significant maternal or newborn complications with low doses (less than or equal to 1 mg per kilogram)
   c. Larger doses (1.5 to 2.0 mg per kilogram) have been associated with:
      i. Maternal laryngospasm.
      ii. Increased uterine tone.
      iii. Low Apgar scores.
      iv. Neonatal depression.

Nonsteroidal Antiinflammatory Drugs
1. Ketorolac
   a. A member of the pyrrolo-pyrrole group of nonsteroidal antiinflammatory drugs
   b. Inhibits the synthesis of prostaglandins by inhibiting the enzyme prostaglandin synthetase
   c. Lacks effect on opiate receptors
   d. Is *not* recommended in obstetric analgesia
      i. May suppress uterine contractions
      ii. Crosses the placenta, causing closure of the fetal ductus arteriosus

Benzodiazepines
1. Mechanism of action
   a. Bind to specific postsynaptic receptors in the central nervous system
   b. Increase the efficacy or availability of the inhibitory amino acid, glycine

c. Also increase the effect of γ-aminobutyric acid (GABA), an inhibitory neurotransmitter
d. Provide
   i. Anxiolysis
   ii. Sedation
   iii. Muscle relaxation
2. Benzodiazepines have never been used extensively in obstetric patients because of significant side effects.
3. Diazepam
   a. Readily crosses the placenta
      i. May accumulate in the fetus
      ii. Fetal blood concentration may exceed maternal concentration.
   b. Has a long maternal half-life (24 to 48 hours).
   c. Metabolized in the liver
   d. Active metabolites
      i. Desmethyldiazepam
      ii. Oxazepam
      iii. Half-lives are greater than 50 hours.
   e. Neonatal effects
      i. Hypotonicity
      ii. Hypoactivity
      iii. Larger doses can produce:
         (1) Low Apgar scores.
         (2) Apneic spells.
         (3) Reluctance to feed.
         (4) Impaired temperature regulation and metabolic responses to cold stress.
      iv. Can displace bilirubin from albumin-binding sites, increasing the risk of kernicterus
      v. Can hinder maternal recall of labor and delivery
4. Midazolam
   a. Is water soluble.
   b. Is rapidly metabolized to minimally active compounds.
   c. Is two to five times as potent as diazepam.
   d. Neonatal effects
      i. Rapidly crosses the placenta
      ii. The umbilical vein-maternal vein ratio is approximately 0.65.
      iii. Neonatal elimination half-life is 6.3 hours.
      iv. Exposure to induction doses
         (1) High incidence of neonatal respiratory depression
         (2) May have decreased temperature.
         (3) May have decreased tone.
   e. A potent amnestic effect may reduce maternal recall of labor and delivery.

Inhalational Analgesia

Although uncommon in the United States, inhalational analgesia is still an acceptable form of labor pain relief. Inhalational analgesia is used frequently in Europe and Canada if regional analgesia is unavailable. Nitrous oxide remains the agent of choice. In Great Britain, it may be administered by unsupervised midwives. Inhalational analgesia does not usually provide complete relief of severe labor pain, but it can provide substantial analgesia and a cooperative mother.

Nitrous Oxide

1. Throughout the world, nitrous oxide continues to be a commonly used inhalational labor analgesic.
2. Questionable efficacy
   a. There is no difference in pain scores compared with placebo (air).[6]
   b. Still, a concentration of 50% or more provides satisfactory labor analgesia in about 50% of parturients.
3. Drug delivery
   a. A nitrous oxide-oxygen blender or a premixed 1 : 1 cylinder limits the delivered concentration of nitrous oxide. These devices must be checked frequently to prevent unintentional administration of high concentrations of nitrous oxide and hypoxic gas mixtures.
   b. The parturient inhales the gas mixture with a face mask.
      i. She begins breathing gas as soon as she feels a contraction.
      ii. Continuous administration via nasal cannulae, in addition to a face mask, may improve the analgesic efficacy.
4. Limitations
   a. Limited efficacy
   b. Pollution of the labor suite
      i. Nitrous oxide concentrations above 25 ppm
      ii. Potential effects
         (1) Reduces methionine synthase activity
            (a) May interfere with the synthesis of deoxythymidine and deoxyribonucleic acid
            (b) Can produce megaloblastic bone marrow changes and neurologic abnormalities
         (2) May increase the risk of spontaneous abortion, infertility, and other health problems among exposed health care workers
   c. Hypoxemia
      i. Theoretical causes
         (1) Hypoventilation between contractions
         (2) Diffusion hypoxemia
      ii. In clinical studies, breathing 50% nitrous oxide and oxygen intermittently produced higher oxygen saturations after a contraction than breathing compressed air.
5. Side effects
   a. No change uterine activity
   b. Mild myocardial depression
   c. Sympathetic stimulation may increase peripheral resistance.
   d. In humans, inhalation of nitrous oxide lacks a measurable effect on maternal blood pressure and heart rate, or uterine artery pressure.

    e. It may increase cerebral blood flow in both mother and baby.

6. Neonatal effects

    a. Nitrous oxide is eliminated via the lungs within a few minutes of birth.

    b. Very little metabolism

    c. No effect on neonatal respirations or neurobehavior

Potent Halogenated Agents

1. Produce dose-related uterine muscle relaxation
2. At 0.5 minimum alveolar concentration (MAC), halothane, enflurane, or isoflurane diminish spontaneous uterine activity, but the uterine muscle still responds to oxytocin.
3. Greater concentrations impair the uterine contractile response to oxytocin.

METHOXYFLURANE

1. A popular inhaled agent for labor analgesia in the late 1960s and early to mid-1970s
2. Better pain relief, less restlessness, and a less pungent odor than trichloroethylene
3. Better pain relief but more sedation than 50% nitrous oxide in oxygen
4. The potential for nephrotoxicity after long exposure sharply limited its use.

ENFLURANE

1. Better labor analgesia than 50% nitrous oxide
2. More sedation than nitrous oxide
3. No impact on estimated blood loss, Apgar scores, or umbilical cord blood acid–base balance
4. No maternal or fetal renal dysfunction (fluoride toxicity)
5. No adverse neonatal neurobehavioral effects

ISOFLURANE

1. Advantages
    a. Low blood–gas solubility
    b. It produces anesthesia rapidly without significant accumulation.
    c. No adverse effects on maternal or fetal renal function, newborn Apgar scores, or neonatal neurobehavioral scores
    d. Maternal amnesia is rarer than with enflurane.
2. Disadvantages
    a. Mild drowsiness
    b. Pungent odor

DESFLURANE

1. Blood–gas solubility coefficient of 0.42 (similar to nitrous oxide)
2. MAC of between 6.0% and 7.25%
3. Effect dissipates rapidly
4. When used during the second stage of labor, it lacks effect on Apgar scores, neonatal acid–base and blood gas data.

5. No signs of maternal renal dysfunction
6. Amnesia and breath holding are common.

SEVOFLURANE
1. Advantages
   a. Blood–gas partition coefficient of 0.69
   b. MAC about 2%
   c. Less pungent than other agents
2. No published studies using sevoflurane for labor analgesia exist to date.

PERIPHERAL NERVE BLOCKS
1. Alternatives to lumbar epidural analgesia include:
   a. Paracervical, lumbar sympathetic, and sterile water blocks for the pain of the first stage of labor.
   b. Pudendal block for the second stage.

Paracervical Block
1. First reported in 1926
2. Stops afferent nerve transmission at the paracervical or Frankenhäuser's plexus
   a. Lies lateral and posterior to the junction of the uterus and cervix, at the base of the broad ligament
   b. A local anesthetic solution bathes the parametrial tissues, blocking nerve transmission and alleviating pain during the first stage of labor.

Technique
1. Place the patient in the lithotomy position with left uterine displacement.
2. Timing
   a. Acceleration phase of labor
   b. After the cervix is dilated 8 cm, the risk of intrafetal injection of local anesthetic increases greatly.
   c. Second-stage pain is not relieved.
3. Use a 12- to 14-cm, 22-gauge needle.
   a. A needle guide prevents injury to the birth canal and fetus and precisely defines the depth of local anesthetic injection.
   b. The most popular guides are the Kobak needle and guide and the Iowa trumpet.
4. The index and middle fingers of the right hand introduce the needle guide into the lateral fornix of the cervix for the right side of the pelvis and vice versa for the left side.
   a. Diverts the needle laterally into Frankenhäuser's plexus
   b. Lowers the risk of intrafetal or intramyometrial injection
   c. Excessive pressure during needle placement will decrease the distance to the uterine vessels.
5. Aspirate.
6. Inject increments of local anesthetic.
7. Limit the depth of the injection to 3 mm.
   a. Deposits local anesthetic just below epithelium.
   b. Limits risk of injection into paracervical venous plexus.

8. After drug injection:
    a. Place the parturient in the left lateral position.
    b. Monitor heart rate, blood pressure, and FHR for at least 30 minutes.
9. Site of injection
    a. Two 10-mL injections at the 3 and 9 o'clock cervical positions
    b. Or, further from uterine vessels at 4 and 8 o'clock
    c. Or, 3- to 5-mL injections at four sites around the cervix (4, 5, 7, and 8 o'clock)
        i. Less risk with IV injection
        ii. Fewer failures
    d. Or, 3 mL at six different sites
        i. Faster onset
        ii. More consistent analgesia
    e. Radiologic studies show that local anesthetic spreads uniformly regardless of injection site(s).
10. Timing of contralateral injections
    a. Some recommend a 10- to 15-minute delay.
    b. There is no increase in complications when injecting the contralateral side immediately.
    c. Most now recommend waiting for approximately two maternal contractions, or 5 minutes.
11. Efficacy
    a. Pain relief usually begins within 5 minutes.
    b. Success depends on operator experience and timing.
    c. Complete relief: 62% to 80% of parturients
    d. Partial relief: 10% to 25%
    e. No relief: 5% to 13%
    f. Block can be repeated in 30 minutes if the parturient still uncomfortable.
    g. Most obstetricians do not exceed four blocks.
    h. Duration
        i. Is related to choice of anesthetic.
        ii. Correlates with parturient's cervical dilation.
        iii. Epinephrine prolongs the duration of lidocaine and 2-chloroprocaine, but not bupivacaine or mepivacaine.
        iv. Phenylephrine increases the duration of mepivacaine, but not lidocaine.
        v. Epinephrine
            (1) Fetal hypoxemia from uterine artery vasoconstriction
            (2) Longer first stage of labor from decreased uterine activity

Choice of Local Anesthetic
1. Use small volumes of dilute solutions of local anesthetic.
2. There is no need to inject more than 10 mL of local anesthetic on each side.
3. The choice of local anesthetic remains controversial.
    a. Aminoesters (2-chloroprocaine)
        i. Rapid metabolism and low toxicity
        ii. Only traces persist in fetal blood at delivery.

      iii. Risk of post-block fetal bradycardia may be lower with 2-chloroprocaine than with lidocaine.

      iv. Short duration is a major disadvantage.

b. Amide local anesthetics

    i. Metabolized in the liver

    ii. Fetal metabolism

      (1) The immature fetal liver clears these drugs slowly.

      (2) Significant concentrations of unmetabolized drug are found in the fetus.

      (3) Most drug leaves fetal circulation by diffusion through the placenta to maternal blood.

      (4) Unmetabolized mepivacaine has been blamed for perinatal death following paracervical block.

    iii. Prilocaine

      (1) Undergoes significant extrahepatic metabolism.

      (2) May be less likely to produce fetal bradycardia (10.9%) than lidocaine (22.1%) or mepivacaine (21.9%).

      (3) However, it may produce methemoglobinemia in the infant following a single paracervical block.

    iv. Lidocaine

      (1) Increased FHR beat-to-beat variability

      (2) No change in maternal or fetal acid–base status

    v. Bupivacaine

      (1) Not approved for paracervical block in the United States

      (2) Several studies demonstrate safety.

        (a) Analgesia lasts about 2 hours.

        (b) Reported incidence of fetal bradycardia is low (2.0%).

      (3) Fetal–neonatal effects

        (a) No neurobehavioral changes after paracervical block with 0.25% bupivacaine

        (b) Local anesthetic is used in over half of perinatal deaths associated with paracervical block.

Effect on Labor

1. Individual responses vary greatly.
2. In aggregate, only small, variable changes in uterine activity occur after block.
3. Any changes most likely represent the normal progress of labor.

Maternal Complications

1. Uncommon
2. Anaphylaxis is very rare.
3. Pain and maternal fright can trigger neurogenic syncope.

4. Most other complications stem from either error in technique or infection.
   a. Systemic toxic reactions
      i. Intravascular injection
      ii. Overdose of local anesthetic
      iii. Toxicity usually presents as central nervous system irritability.
         (1) Palpitations
         (2) Metallic taste
         (3) Tinnitus
         (4) Dysarthria
         (5) Drowsiness
         (6) Confusion
         (7) Convulsions
      iv. Symptoms are usually transient.
      v. Occasionally, hypotension and cardiovascular collapse occur.
   b. Hematoma of the broad ligament
      i. Laceration of uterine vessels
      ii. Superficial laceration of the vagina with the tip of the needle
   c. Sciatic nerve block
      i. Unilateral sensory disturbances of the lower extremities
      ii. These resolve with resolution of the block.
   d. Infection
      i. Postpartum parametritis
      ii. Subgluteal and retropsoal abscesses
         (1) Can spread laterally to the hip joint.
         (2) Symptoms
            (a) Occurrence is a few hours to several days after block.
            (b) Severe pain
            (c) Limitation of motion
            (d) Fever
         (3) Treatment
            (a) Antibiotics for gram-negative and anaerobic organisms
            (b) Large abscesses require surgical debridement.
   e. Neuropathy
      i. One per 2,000 blocks
      ii. Symptoms
         (1) Severe buttock pain that radiates down the posterior surface of the ipsilateral leg
         (2) As pain worsens, the patient cannot walk.
         (3) Onset ranges from 12 hours to 10 days after block.
         (4) Symptoms may worsen over 1 to 10 days, followed by progressive improvement and complete recovery.
      iii. Etiology
         (1) Direct trauma to the sacral plexus
         (2) Hematoma formation around the sacral plexus

   iv. A palpable sacroiliac mass without fever is suggestive.
   v. Treatment
     (1) Analgesics
     (2) Early assisted ambulation

Fetal Complications
 1. Fetal bradycardia
   a. Reported incidence: 2% to 70%
     i. Reasons for variable rate
      (1) Different definitions
      (2) Methods of fetal monitoring
      (3) Drug dosage
      (4) Local anesthetic
      (5) Patient selection
   b. Begins 2 to 10 minutes after injection
   c. Usually resolves within 20 minutes
   d. Is more common in parturients with preexisting, non-reassuring FHR tracings
 2. The etiology is unclear. There at least four theories.

REFLEX BRADYCARDIA
 1. Due to manipulation of the fetal head, uterus, or the uterine blood vessels
 2. Thought to be harmless
 3. Usually resolves promptly

DIRECT FETAL CENTRAL NERVOUS SYSTEM AND MYOCARDIAL DEPRESSION
 1. Local anesthetic rapidly crosses the placenta.
   a. It may directly produce central nervous system and myocardial toxicity.
 2. Local anesthetic may reach fetus by a more direct route than maternal systemic absorption.
   a. Diffusion across the uterine arteries
   b. Fetuses with bradycardia after paracervical block have higher plasma concentrations of mepivacaine than do their mothers.
   c. Fetal acidosis would worsen this effect through ion trapping.
 3. Others report that fetal local anesthetic concentrations are consistently lower than maternal concentrations.
 4. Thus, fetal hypoxemia, not direct myocardial depression, is more likely the explanation of bradycardia after paracervical block.

INCREASED UTERINE ACTIVITY
 1. Decreases uteroplacental perfusion
   a. The resultant fetal hypoxemia can produce bradycardia.
 2. Direct injection of bupivacaine into the uterine arteries of gravid ewes increases uterine tone.
 3. Lidocaine intermediately increases uterine tone.
 4. 2-Chloroprocaine has no effect.
 5. Uterine activity can increase after paracervical block.

UTERINE ARTERY VASOCONSTRICTION

1. Currently, the most likely explanation
2. Local anesthetics produce a direct, nonadrenergic, or vaso-constrictive effect.
   a. Local anesthetic concentrations comparable to those that occur during paracervical block can significantly decrease uterine blood flow in animals.
   b. Decreased uterine blood flow produces fetal hypoxemia, which causes sinoatrial node suppression and narrow QRS complex fetal bradycardia.
   c. One study found a fivefold increase in fetal bradycardia after paracervical block in parturients with evidence of preexisting uteroplacental insufficiency.
3. Fetal pO_2 decreases after paracervical block.
   a. Uterine artery vasoconstriction
   b. Decreased fetal perfusion
   c. Effect independent of advancing labor and uterine contractions
4. The significance of fetal bradycardia varies.
   a. The fetus develops a transient metabolic acidosis only when bradycardia lasts longer than 10 minutes.
   b. The fetus needs time *in utero* to recover.
      i. Apgar scores are better in fetuses delivered more than 30 minutes after a bradycardic episode.
      ii. Fetuses experiencing bradycardia may have depressed 1-minute Apgar scores, but should have normal scores by 5 minutes.
      iii. Meperidine analgesia is more commonly associated with neonatal compromise (umbilical artery pH less than or equal to 7.15 and a 1-minute Apgar score less than or equal to 7) than paracervical block.
5. Treatment
   a. Optimize uteroplacental perfusion.
      i. Maintain uterine displacement.
      ii. Assure adequate maternal blood pressure.
      iii. Give supplemental oxygen.
   b. Avoid immediate delivery to allow time for intrauterine resuscitation.
   c. Bradycardia longer than 10 minutes
      i. Fetal scalp pH sampling may help determine the need for rapid delivery.
   d. Bradycardia longer than 45 minutes
      i. Severe fetal hypoxemia
      ii. Intrauterine death
   e. Postnatal exchange transfusion has been used to treat local anesthetic toxicity when immediate delivery is unavoidable.

Summary

1. Although epidural analgesia for labor is very popular in academic obstetric practices, community use of the paracervical block is significant.

2. Most experts agree on the following recommendations:
   a. Avoid it in parturients with preterm or stressed fetuses.
   b. Avoid it in complicated deliveries such as breech or multiple gestations.
   c. Do not place the block when the cervix is more than 8 cm dilated.
   d. Maintain uterine displacement during and after placement of the block.
   e. Limit the depth of injection to 3 mm. Aspirate frequently.
   f. After injecting the local anesthetic on one side, wait 5 to 10 minutes and observe FHR before injecting the other side.
   g. Use small volumes (10 mL on each side) of dilute local anesthetic without epinephrine.
   h. Monitor the FHR continuously after the block.
   i. Have resuscitative equipment available.

Lumbar Sympathetic Block
1. Lower uterine and cervical afferent sensory fibers join the sympathetic chain at L2 to L3.
2. Paravertebral lumbar sympathetic block interrupts the transmission of pain impulses before the nerves enter the spinal cord.
3. It was first described in parturients in 1927.
4. It was first used in the United States in 1933.
5. Block may be useful in the
   a. Parturient with previous back surgery.
   b. Parturient who refuses lumbar epidural analgesia.

Technique
1. The parturient sits to provide maximal flexion of the spine.
2. Identify the spinous process of L2.
3. After sterile preparation, make a skin wheal 5 to 8 cm laterally from the mid-point of the L2 spinous process on each side of the back.
4. Introduce a 10-cm, 22-gauge needle at a 20-degree angle cephalad until it touches the transverse process of L2.
   a. Withdraw the needle to the skin and redirect it to pass below the transverse process.
   b. With the needle directed medially, advance approximately 4.5 cm to contact the vertebral body.
   c. Attempt to "walk off" the vertebral body by redirecting the needle laterally 5 to 10 degrees.
      i. The needle will then be located anterolateral to the vertebral body, at the medial attachment of the psoas muscle.
      ii. A loss of resistance syringe may help determine when the needle is beyond the psoas muscle fascia.
         (1) There is resistance to injection of air in the muscle.
         (2) A "pop" may be felt and resistance is lost when the needle advances through the psoas fascia and into the area of the lumbar sympathetic trunk.

iii. Inject local anesthetic in two 5-mL aliquots, with frequent aspiration.
      (1) The inferior vena cava lies on the right and the aorta on the left of the vertebral body.
      (2) The needle also is close to the subarachnoid and epidural spaces.
5. Repeat the procedure on the opposite side.
6. Local anesthetic
   a. Lidocaine
      i. Without epinephrine: 60 to 90 minutes of analgesia
      ii. With epinephrine: 120 minutes of pain relief
   b. Tetracaine 0.5% lasts up to 4 hours.
   c. Bupivacaine 0.5% with epinephrine 1:200,000 lasts about 4 hours.
   d. A catheter technique allows repeated injections.

Effect on Labor

1. It may accelerate the first stage of labor.
   a. Five to 15 minutes of uterine hypertonus may follow lumbar sympathetic block.
   b. It may convert an abnormal uterine contractile pattern to a normal one.
2. In a recent randomized clinical trial, lumbar sympathetic blocks were associated with more rapid cervical dilation, shorter first and second stages of labor, and fewer cesarean sections for dystocia than epidural analgesia.[7]

Maternal Complications

1. The most common side effect is hypotension (15% to 20%).
   a. Local anesthetic spreads to the celiac and splanchnic plexi, producing splanchnic vasodilation and hypotension.
   b. A smaller volume of drug may decrease the magnitude of the hemodynamic changes.
   c. A 500-mL fluid bolus may help offset this hypotension.
2. Other complications
   a. Systemic toxicity with seizures
   b. Injection into an intervertebral foramen can cause subarachnoid or epidural block
   c. Rarely, parturients may suffer retroperitoneal hemorrhage.
   d. Other complications include:
      i. Paraesthesia and pain on injection.
      ii. Motor paralysis of the lower extremities, possibly due to anterior spinal artery ischemia.
      iii. Transient lower extremity motor block from local anesthetic spread to the genitofemoral nerve.
      iv. Total spinal anesthesia.
      v. Postdural puncture headache.
      vi. Horner's syndrome.
      vii. Intralymphatic injection with possible lymphocele formation.

Fetal Complications

1. There are no direct fetal complications reported with lumbar sympathetic block.

2. Increased uterine activity after the block could transiently decrease fetal heart rate. However, there are no reports of fetal asphyxia related to uterine tetany.

Summary
1. Lumbar sympathetic block is used infrequently in labor and delivery.
2. It is technically difficult to place.
3. Parturients may be more uncomfortable during placement than they are during induction of epidural analgesia.
4. It provides a finite duration of analgesia unless one places catheters.
5. It does not relieve the pain of the second stage of labor.
6. Lumbar sympathetic block does not produce motor blockade and may speed labor.

Sterile Water Block
1. Low back pain during labor
   a. Continuous in about one-third of women
   b. More common with an occipitoposterior presentation of the fetus
   c. Pain impulses from the posterior part of the cervix and uterus are transmitted to spinal cord segments T11 to L1.
   d. Cutaneous branches from these segments supply the skin over the low back area.
2. Intradermally injected hypotonic sterile water
   a. Causes local irritation.
   b. Stimulates the surrounding tissues, inducing analgesia.
   c. Analgesia may originate in the mid-brain centers or be caused by gate control at the spinal level.
   d. Intradermal injection of 0.1 mL sterile water at four different spots in the low back area, approximately corresponding to the borders of the sacrum, may relieve low back pain during labor.

Pudendal Block
1. First described in 1908
2. First American article published in 1916
3. Transvaginal block described in 1954
4. The pudendal nerve is the major source of sensation in the lower vagina, vulva, and perineum.
   a. This nerve is the largest branch of the pudendal plexus.
   b. This nerve also carries somatic fibers to the anterior divisions of the second, third, and fourth sacral nerves.
   c. It provides the motor innervation of the perineal muscles.
   d. Anatomy
      i. The nerve travels through the lower part of the greater sciatic foramen and enters the gluteal region.
      ii. It passes posterior to the ischial spine and continues into the lesser sciatic foramen.
      iii. It enters Alcock's canal, where it lies along the lateral border of the ischiorectal fossa. The pudendal nerve then divides into:

(1) The perineal nerve.
(2) The dorsal nerve to the clitoris.
(3) The inferior hemorrhoidal nerve.
5. Pudendal block provides pain relief during:
   a. The second stage of labor.
   b. Low forceps delivery.
   c. Repair of vaginal and perineal lacerations.

Technique
1. It is most commonly performed transvaginally.
2. A transperineal approach also is possible.
3. Place the parturient in the lithotomy position.
   a. Use an Iowa trumpet or Kobak needle and guide to protect the vaginal mucosa and the fetal presenting part.
   b. To block the patient's right pudendal nerve, hold the needle between the middle and index fingers of the right hand and palpate the ischial spine. (The left hand holds the needle for the left side.)
      i. The sacrospinous ligament lies 1 cm medial and posterior to the ischial spine.
      ii. Direct the needle through the sacrospinous ligament to a depth of about 1 cm.
      iii. Aspirate for blood and inject 10 mL of local anesthetic on each side.
4. Analgesia begins in 2 to 10 minutes and lasts 20 to 60 minutes, depending on the local anesthetic used.

Choice of Local Anesthetic
1. Lidocaine 1%
   a. Appears in maternal and fetal blood within 5 minutes.
   b. Peak concentrations occur within 10 to 20 minutes.
   c. Epinephrine
      i. Prolongs the block.
      ii. Lowers the maternal and fetal blood concentrations of lidocaine.
   d. Maternal lidocaine concentrations are lower than those reported after epidural blockade with the same dose of drug.
2. 2-Chloroprocaine
   a. Short duration
   b. Block may be repeated
3. Regardless of local anesthetic, use dilute drug solutions for pudendal nerve block.
   a. Limits maternal absorption
   b. Decreases risk of maternal or fetal systemic toxicity if repeat blocks are necessary

Effect on Labor
1. Pudendal block may slightly prolong the second stage of labor but does increase the risk of operative delivery.

Maternal Complications
1. The most frequent complication: failure
2. Local anesthetic toxicity

      a. Rapid absorption
      b. Intravascular injection
      c. Overdose
  3. Retroperitoneal hematoma
      a. Vascular injury to the internal pudendal artery
      b. Temperature elevation in a parturient with a decreasing hematocrit heralds an infected retroperitoneal hematoma.
      c. Treatment
         i. Broad-spectrum antibiotics
        ii. Blood replacement, if necessary
  4. Retropsoal or subgluteal abscesses have been reported after pudendal and paracervical blocks.

Summary
  1. Effective
      a. Second stage of labor
      b. Vaginal delivery
      c. Operative vaginal delivery (vacuum or outlet forceps)
      d. Repair of vaginal and perineal damage
  2. Ineffective
      a. Midforceps application
      b. Intrauterine manipulation

CONCLUSIONS

This chapter has explored various nonpharmacologic methods of pain relief and coping available to the parturient, as well as some common systemic medications, inhalational analgesic techniques, and peripheral nerve blocks used as alternatives to neuraxial analgesia. Not all methods are suitable for every patient. Some may still leave the mother with considerable pain. Neuraxial techniques remain the most reliable, effective methods of maternal pain relief.

REFERENCES

1. Scott KD, Berkowitz G, Klaus M. A comparison of intermittent and continuous support during labor: A meta-analysis. *Am J Obstet Gynecol* 1999;180:1054
2. Nelle M, Krause M, Bastert G, Linderkamp O. Effects of LeBoyer childbirth on left and right systolic time intervals in healthy term neonates. *J Pernat Med* 1996;24:513.
3. Harmon TM, Hynan MT, Tyre TE. Improved obstetric outcomes using hypnotic analgesia and skill mastery combined with childbirth education. *J Consult Clin Psychol* 1990;58:525.
4. Wahl CW. Contraindications and limitations of hypnosis in obstetric analgesia. *Am J Obstet Gynecol* 1962;84:1869.
5. Atkinson BD, Truitt LJ, Rayburn WF, Trunbull GL, Christensin HD, Wlodaver A. Double-blind comparison of intravenous butorphanol (Stadol) and fentanyl (Sublimaze) for analgesia during labor. *Am J Obstet Gynecol* 1994;171:993.
6. Carstoniu MA, Levytam S, Norman P, Daley D, Katz J, Sander AN. Nitrous oxide in early labor. *Anesthesiology* 1994;80:30.
7. Leighton BL, Halpern SH, Wilson DB. Lumbar sympathetic blocks speed early and second stage induced labor in nulliparous women. *Anesthesiology* 1999;90:1039.

10

Anatomy of the Epidural Space

1. Proper placement of neuraxial needles and catheters is an exercise in applied anatomy and requires a clear mental image of locations and relations of various structures.
2. Three aspects of spinal anatomy emerge as recurring themes.
   a. Many published accounts of the soft tissues of the vertebral canal are inaccurate. Possible reasons for this shortcoming include:
      i. Study of preserved and distorted material.
      ii. Examination by methods that create artifact (i.e., epiduroscopy or radiologic imaging after contrast injection).
      iii. The inherent challenges of scrutinizing frail tissues hidden within very sturdy walls.
      iv. The imagination of medical illustrators.
   b. Variability is part of nature, and anatomic features display expected interindividual differences.
   c. It is impossible to know too much anatomy.
      i. The images we carry in our minds of the objects a needle strikes, the location of the catheter tip, or the pattern of solution spread are the basis on which we plan redirection of the needle or speculate on the cause of unexpected anesthetic distribution.
      ii. Text and images are an imperfect means of instruction in anatomy.
         (1) Frequent examination of a skeleton is helpful in mastering the intricate topography of the vertebrae.
         (2) Dissection is invaluable in gaining an appreciation of actual anatomy and can usually be arranged at medical schools, refresher courses, or in the autopsy lab.

SURFACE LANDMARKS

1. The level of needle insertion is inferred from palpable bony landmarks.
   a. In obstetrics, Tuffier's line, or the line between the iliac crests, is the most common reference (Fig. 10.1).
      i. Accuracy is less than 50%.
      ii. Reasons
         (1) Variations in the amount of subcutaneous fat, resulting in a more rostral apparent site in obese patients
         (2) The level of the iliac crests is widely variable (Fig. 10.2).
            (a) The line between them crosses the vertebral column with a maximal incidence at the L4–L5 disc (perhaps higher on average in men than in women).

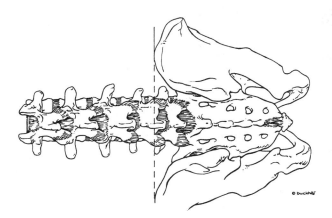

Fig. 10.1. The most common reference for level of insertion of lumbar epidural or spinal needles is the line between the iliac crests, or Tuffier's line. (Source: Reproduced from Covino BG, Scott DB. *Handbook of epidural anesthesia and analgesia.* Orlando: Grune & Stratton, 1985, with permission.)

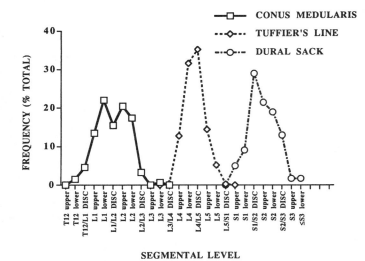

Fig. 10.2. Anatomic features show interindividual variation in a normal distribution. The level at which the line between the iliac crests (Tuffier's line) crosses the vertebral column is most often the L4–5 disc but may be as high as the L3–4 disc and as low as the L5–S1 disc. The caudal tip of the dural sac and the end of the spinal cord (the conus medularis) show similar variability.

(b) The range is from as low as the L5–S1 disc to as high as the L3–L4 disc (4).
2. Identification of the mid-line
   a. Palpation of spinous processes may be impeded by abundant subcutaneous tissue.
   b. Sitting patient (positioned squarely on the bed and without deformity)
      i. Symmetry
      ii. Mid-line skin crease
   c. Lateral position
      i. Visible landmarks are not useful.
      ii. Palpation may be deceptive.
         (1) Apparent location of the vertebral column can be more dependent than the location at which the mid-line structures are ultimately found.
   d. A 2-in., 22-gauge needle can be used to locate spinous processes while anesthetizing superficial tissues.
      i. In the obese subject, a 22-gauge spinal needle might be necessary.
   e. A mid-line tuft of hair or dimple is a superficial indication of a possible partial spinal bifida. In this setting, a normal epidural space may not exist, and the nerve roots cannot be assumed to be free in the cerebrospinal fluid (CSF).
3. Sacral hiatus
   a. Widely patent in children
   b. Unpredictable in adulthood
      i. Palpation often fails to identify the sacral crurae on either side of the hiatus.
      ii. Fusion of the posterior roof of the sacral vertebral canal is typically complete down to the S5 level, where the sacral hiatus remains open.
         (1) Absence of any posterior bony roof, or virtually complete closure or the sacral vertebral canal, is found in about 8% of subjects.
      iii. In 5% of adult sacral bones, the anterior-posterior diameter of the canal at the hiatus is less than or equal to 2 mm.

POSTERIOR LIGAMENTS
1. The supraspinous ligament
   a. Joins the tips of the spinous processes.
   b. May be felt as a heavy mid-line band in thin individuals (Fig. 10.3).
   c. Thins and vanishes in the lower lumbar region to allow greater flexion.
2. The interspinous ligament
   a. Narrow mid-line web between the spinous processes
   b. Fibers run in a posterocranial direction.
   c. False "loss of resistance"
      i. Slitlike cavities filled with fat may develop in this ligament.

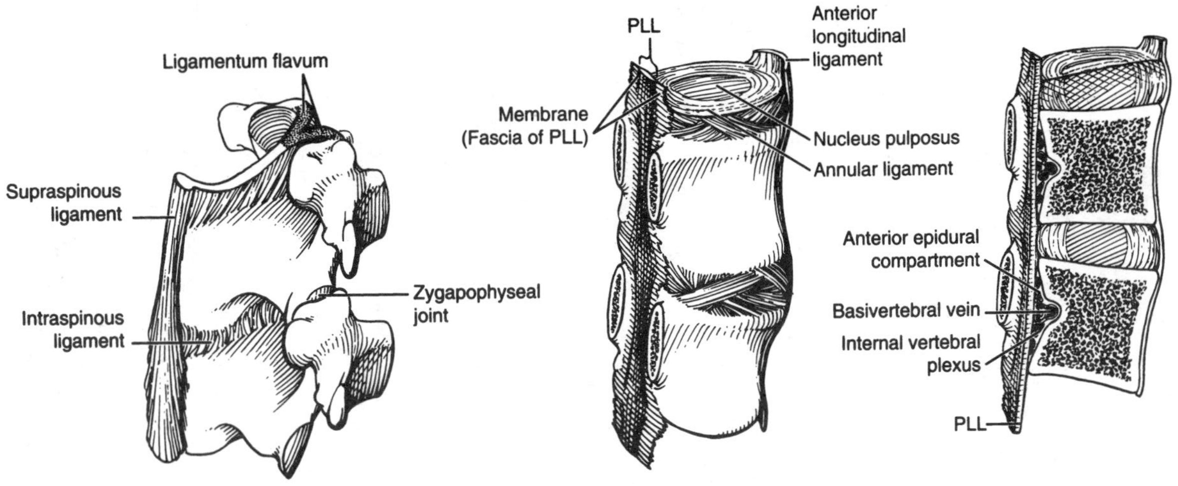

Fig. 10.3. Ligaments of the lumbar vertebral column. The supraspinous ligament joins the tips of the spinous processes, and the interspinous ligaments form a web between them. The posterior longitudinal ligament (*PLL*) runs behind the vertebral bodies joining the discs and extends laterally as a membrane, whereas the broad anterior longitudinal ligament reinforces the front of the column. Veins occupy the area anterior to the PLL. The annular ligament surrounds the nucleus pulposus of the intervertebral disc. (Source: Reproduced from Hogan QH. A reexamination of anatomy in regional anesthesia. In: Brown D, ed. *Regional anesthesia.* Philadelphia: WB Saunders, 1996:50, with permission.)

      ii. A slightly oblique needle may pass out of the side of this narrow ligament (Fig. 10.4).
- d. At its anterior margin, the interspinous ligament blends into the ligamentum flavum.
3. Both supraspinous and interspinous ligaments are composed largely of fibrous collagen.
    - a. A needle passing through them generates a characteristic snapping sensation as the fibers are severed.
4. Ligamentum flavum
    - a. Is 80% elastin, which gives its characteristic yellow color.
    - b. Its dense homogenous texture is readily appreciated during needle passage.
    - c. It is under tension and retracts to half its length when cut.
    - d. It spans from the anterior surface of the rostral lamina of an adjacent pair of vertebrae to the posterior aspect of the lower lamina.
    - e. The right and left halves meet at an angle of less than 90 degrees, and a gap may be present in the mid-line.
    - f. The lateral edges wrap anteriorly around the medial margin of the facet joints, reinforcing the joint capsule.
    - g. Bone may grow into its margins, even in young patients.
    - h. It is usually between 2 and 5 mm thick. This dimension is not a useful parameter in judging the placement of an epidural needle.

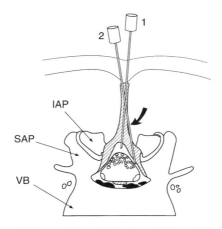

Fig. 10.4. A needle inserted exactly in the mid-line will travel in the interspinous ligament and then into the ligamentum flavum (shown together as *cross-hatched* in this drawing). The epidural space is thickest from posterior to anterior (between the ligamentum flavum and dura) in the mid-line. A needle inserted slightly at an angle (in this image, about 13 degrees from the sagittal plane) may exit the interspinous ligament (*arrow*) before reaching the ligamentum flavum, creating the impression of a loss of resistance. Also, when not in the mid-line, a needle will encounter the ligamentum flavum at a greater depth and will travel a longer course through the ligamentum flavum before reaching the epidural space. Finally, the thickness of the epidural space decreases away from the mid-line so that the dura is encountered immediately on piercing the ligamentum flavum.

    i. If the needle passes through the mid-line slit it may enter the epidural space without engaging the ligamentum flavum.

    j. The pathway of a needle through the ligamentum flavum may be substantially longer because the ligament is not in a coronal plane, but is steeply angled, and the needle will not engage it at right angle (see Fig. 10.4).

VERTEBRAL BONES

1. The lumbar vertebral column often has more or less than five vertebrae.
   a. The L5 vertebra is fused to S1 in 6.2% of normal subjects.
   b. The S1 vertebra shows incomplete fusion to S2 in 5.3%.
   c. Developmental defects in a lumbar vertebral arch occur in 3.9% of subjects. In the paramedian approach to the epidural space, the posterior bony elements are contacted first as a reference point, so absent bone could result in uncertain needle placement.
2. The lumbar vertebral bones (Fig. 10.5) are complicated structures that can best be appreciated as elements encircling the central vertebral canal, combined with processes extending from them.
   a. Vertebral body
      i. Is anterior to the vertebral canal
      ii. Is the largest part of the vertebral bone
      iii. Carries a large part of the load supporting the body
      iv. Is markedly wider at the endplates than in the middle, resulting in an hourglass shape
      v. Has articulation with adjacent vertebral bodies
         (1) Intervertebral discs
         (2) Heavy anterior longitudinal ligament in the front
         (3) Band of posterior longitudinal ligament behind
   b. The pedicles
      i. Arise from the posterior aspect of the vertebral bodies.
      ii. Form the lateral walls of the vertebral canal.

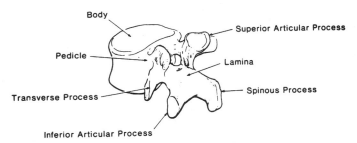

Fig. 10.5. Components of a lumbar vertebra.

     c. The laminae
       i. Platelike
       ii. Close the circle and form the posterior boundary
          of the vertebral canal
     d. The transverse processes extend laterally from the junction of the pedicle and lamina.
     e. The spinous process extends from the mid-line fusion of the laminae but may not remain in the mid-line as it continues posteriorly.
     f. Superior and inferior articular processes
       i. Attach to either side of the lateral laminae.
       ii. Form the zygapophyseal (facet) joints with their corresponding members from the adjacent vertebra.

3. Must identify the gap between the spinous processes during mid-line epidural and spinal needle placement
     a. The inferior edge of the spinous processes are somewhat concave downward (Fig. 10.6).
     b. The space between the interspinous processes lies at an angle of about 63 to 83 degrees from the axial plane (13).
     c. Flexion of the spine widens the space.
     d. Loss of disc height
       i. May narrow or obliterate the space.
       ii. May diminish the interlaminar gap through which the needle must ultimately pass.
     e. The lamina is the bone most commonly encountered by the needle, which usually indicates a need for a more rostral needle direction.
     f. *By far the most common anatomic error in needle placement is mistaken identification of the mid-line.*

EPIDURAL SPACE

1. Lies inside the vertebral canal but outside the dural sac
2. Artist's depictions
     a. Uniform width
     b. Completely encircling the dura

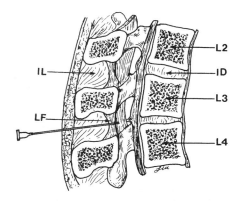

Fig. 10.6. Sagittal view of the course of an epidural needle into the epidural space.

3. In reality, the lumbar vertebral canal is mostly filled by the
    dural sac.
    a. The epidural space is empty (a "potential space") in
        large areas where dura contacts the bone and ligament
        of the vertebral canal wall.
    b. Epidural contents are contained in a series of metameri-
        cally and circumferentially discontinuous compartments
        separated by zones where the dura contacts the canal
        wall (Fig. 10.7).
    c. Inferior to the L4–L5 disc and in the sacral canal.
        i.   Mostly epidural fat.
        ii. The dural sac.
             (1) Tapers to a smaller diameter.
             (2) Does not fill the canal as completely.
        iii. The variability of sacral anatomy is reflected in the
             highly unpredictable sacral canal volume (12 to 65
             mL in adults).

Posterior Epidural Space

1. In the sagittal plane, this compartment has a "saw-tooth"
    appearance (see Fig 10.7).
2. Filled by a fat pad.
    a. Triangular in axial section.
    b. Confined between the dura and ligamenta flava.
    c. Longitudinally the fat extends slightly under the caudal-
        most portion of the lamina above.
    d. For the most part, this fat is not adherent to adjacent
        structures.[1]
        i.   Allows movement of the dura within the canal
             during spinal flexion.

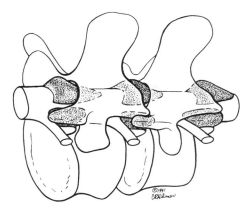

**Fig. 10.7. Drawing of the distribution of the contents of the epidural
space. The *stippled areas* represent posterior (toward the top of the
image) and lateral epidural compartments, separated by areas in
which the dura contacts the canal wall and there are no contents.
The anterior epidural space is not shown.**

      ii.   Allows air or solution entry during loss of resistance technique as the needle tip first advances from ligamentum flavum into the vertebral canal.

     iii.   Permits catheters or fluid to pass between the surfaces of the fat, canal wall, and dura.

  e.   Average is 4.5 to 5.5 cm.

  f.   Range from 3 to 9 cm.

  g.   Less than 3 cm in 0.2% of parturients.

  h.   Greater than 6 cm in 11% of parturients.

  i.   Not easily predicted.

  j.   Slightly greater at L1–L2 than at L3–L4.

  k.   Weakly correlates with weight.

  l.   Sources of variability.

      i.   Natural differences between individuals.

     ii.   The geometry of the posterior epidural compartment.

        (1)   The epidural space is closest to the skin at the posterior apex of the triangular area under the ligamentum flavum.

        (2)   Near the mid-line, a needle may pass through the ligamentum flavum perhaps 1 cm less deep than off the mid-line near the facet joint where the ligamentum flavum is less superficial (see Fig. 10.4).

3.   Posterior epidural fat pad.

  a.   Attached along its posterior mid-line by a vascular pedicle that enters through the gap between the right and left ligamenta flava.

      i.   This mesentery-like attachment and the accompanying fat pad may be seen as a mid-line filling defect in radiologic contrast studies and as an incomplete "membrane" during epiduroscopy.

     ii.   Cryomicrotome or histologic examinations.

        (1)   No mid-line fibrous septum.

        (2)   Epidural fat is unique in the body in having virtually no fibrous content.

    iii.   Asymmetric development of cutaneous anesthesia after epidural local anesthetic injection.

        (1)   Often attributed to the hypothetical median septum.

        (2)   A technical error of needle or catheter insertion is more likely: Reinsertion results in complete block.

4.   The rigid enclosure of the posterior epidural space allows the tissues to generate a subatmospheric tissue fluid pressure.

  a.   Lymphatic drainage

  b.   Balance of osmotic and hydrostatic forces across the capillary endothelium (Starling forces).

  c.   This, and deformation of fat and dura as the needle advances further, produce the force that aspirates a hanging drop into the needle hub as the tip enters the compartment.

5.   Lateral epidural compartment.

  a.   Medial to each intervertebral foramen.

  b.   Filled with segmental nerves, vessels, and fat.

    c. The pedicles are an incomplete lateral wall for the vertebral canal (see Fig. 10.7).

        i. Except in advanced degenerative disease, the intervertebral foramina are widely open.

        ii. This allows the free egress of solution injected within the vertebral canal.

    d. Because of the lack of a rigid barrier at the intervertebral foramina, the pressure within the epidural space closely reflects intraabdominal pressure.

        i. Increased abdominal pressure (i.e., during a cough or pregnancy).

            (1) Readily transmitted to the epidural space.

            (2) Should press structures together under greater force.

            (3) Permits more extensive spread of injected solution injected between the structures.

            (4) Probably contributes to the greater spread of epidural anesthesia in parturients.

6. Epidural veins

    a. May enlarge with vena caval obstruction; diverts venous blood flow.

    b. This effect also may alter the distribution of injected solution.

Anterior Epidural Space

1. Separated from the rest of the vertebral canal by a fine membrane that stretches laterally from the posterior longitudinal ligament.

2. Almost entirely filled by a nearly confluent internal vertebral plexus, from which the mid-line basivertebral vein originates as it penetrates into the vertebral body.

    a. In most subjects, this is the only epidural site with large veins and is the most common place where epidural catheters encounter veins.

    b. If a more cephalad needle angle is used, as is done with thoracic epidural catheterization or during a paramedian approach, the catheter may be less apt to advance anteriorly toward these veins.

Clinical Correlations

1. A posterior mid-line or median approach to the epidural space passes sequentially through the supraspinous and interspinous ligaments and the ligamenta flava.

2. A paramedian approach traverses the paraspinal soft tissues and the ligamenta flava only.

3. The behavior of solutions and catheters within the epidural space can be explained by anatomic findings.

4. Needle tip traverses the ligamentum flavum.

    a. Injected air or saline enters the plane between the nonadherent posterior fat pad and vertebral canal wall.

    b. This is the loss of resistance noted when the syringe plunger suddenly yields to pressure during needle advancement.

    c. Less commonly, the needle might pass into the substance of the posterior fat pad, making catheter passage difficult.

5. Solution or air injected into the epidural space.
    a. Readily distributes between the surfaces of the various structures.
    b. Encircles the dura.
    c. Occasionally spread is limited in the posterior mid-line where the dura may adhere to the lamina or fat.

6. Distance a needle travels after entering the epidural space before penetrating the dura.
    a. About 7 mm.
    b. Range from 2.0 mm to as much as 2.5 cm.
    c. This measurement in part reflects indentation of the dura by the needle; larger needles require greater advancement to reach CSF.
    d. Magnetic resonance imaging measurements show a range of 4 to 9 mm.
    e. In clinical practice, there is great variability in this dimension
       i. Posterior epidural compartment has a complex shape (see Fig. 10.7).
       ii. Anterior-posterior dimension will depend on exactly where the space is traversed.
       iii. When the needle enters the spinal canal away from the mid-line.
          (1) May encounter the dura with no further advancement.
          (2) The posterior epidural fat pad thins toward its lateral margin (see Fig. 10.4).

7. The largest lumbar space is at the L3–L4 level.

8. Catheters and injectate.[2]
    a. As a catheter is passed through the needle, there may be a brief resistance to advancement as the tip impinges on the dura.
    b. A catheter tip inserted 3 cm into the vertebral canal after a mid-line skin puncture.
       i. Most commonly travels to a site in the lateral epidural space.
       ii. Injected solution still surrounds the dura.
    c. Distribution of injected fluid.
       i. Uneven distribution can occur with small volumes (e.g., 4 mL).
       ii. Larger volumes (e.g., 10 mL) consistently show uniform distribution.
    d. If the catheter tip lies exterior to the intervertebral foramen in the paravertebral space, the distribution of the injectate is preferentially back into the vertebral canal (Fig. 10.8).
       i. The muscular confines of the perivertebral space produce high pressures with injection.
       ii. The adjacent spinal canal has a maximum pressure equal to the CSF pressure (about 15 cm of water) and accepts flow by displacing CSF.

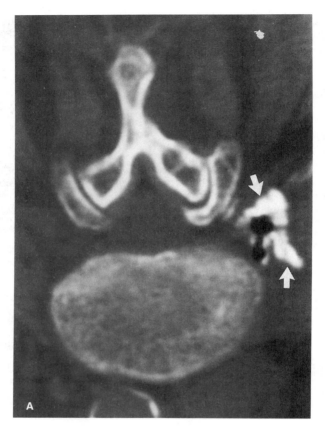

Fig. 10.8. Axial computerized tomography images of contrast injection through a lumbar epidural catheter that provided good postoperative analgesia. Injection of 4 mL of solution (A) distributes only in the area of the catheter tip beyond the intervertebral foramen (*arrows*), but injection of an additional 10 mL (B) encircles the dural sac and even exits the contralateral foramen (*arrows*). Small amounts of air appear black.

MENINGES AND CEREBROSPINAL FLUID

1. Spinal anesthesia
    a. Place the tip of the needle through the dural and arachnoid membranes.
    b. Within the CSF of the subarachnoid space.
2. The spinal dura mater
    a. Connective tissue sac.
    b. From the skull, where its fusion with the foramen magnum terminates the epidural space.

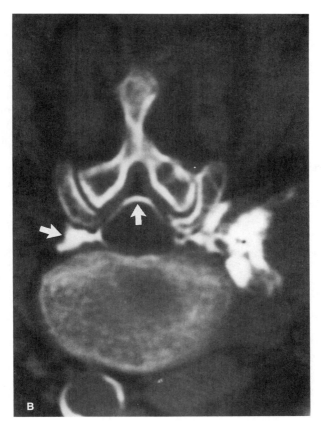

Fig. 10.8. (continued)

   c. To the caudal terminus at about the S2 level (see
       Fig. 10.2).
   d. Other attachments
      i. Weak
     ii. Except
         (1) Fibrous slips to the posterior longitudinal
            ligament, particularly in the lumbar region.
         (2) The dural nerve root sleeves are anchored to
            the epineural tissue in the intervertebral
            foramen.

Dura Mater

1. A posterior fold, termed the *plica dorsalis medianalis,* has
   been observed when epidural injectate (air or solution) compresses the dural sac.

   a.   Scattered attachments
        i.   Tether the dura to the posterior epidural fat and
             lamina.
        ii. Form a fold as adjacent dura is pressed inward.
   b.   In the undisturbed state, the dura is circular or oval in
        axial section.
2. The dura is thickest in the posterior mid-line, where it is
    tough enough to prevent puncture by epidural catheters.
    a.   CSF can rarely be aspirated from previously normally
         functioning catheters, or massive spinal anesthesia can
         follow injection of an epidural dose after previous doses
         performed normally.
    b.   These reports are almost certainly *not* due to migration
         of the epidural catheter tip through intact dura.
3. Composition
    a.   Lamellae
         i.   Predominantly collagen.
         ii. Some elastin.

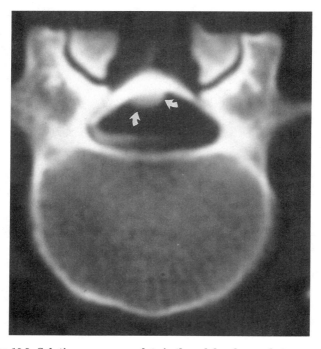

**Fig. 10.9. Solution may accumulate in the subdural space between
the dura and arachnoid membranes (*arrows*) without evidence of
excessive anesthesia. Rupture of a bleb such as is shown, for
instance, during an epidural top-off injection, would release a collection of local anesthetic into the subarachnoid space, resulting in sudden extensive block and the appearance of catheter migration.**

b. Clefts filled with ground substance account for dural permeability.
4. Because there are no rigid elements, the dural sac is freely compressible.
   a. Valsalva maneuver
      i. Dramatically and immediately collapses the lumbar and thoracic dural sac, displacing CSF rostrally.
      ii. By this mechanism, coughing after spinal anesthetic injection may produce a greater than expected anesthetic distribution.
   b. Increased abdominal pressure (i.e., obesity and pregnancy).
      i. Freely transmitted to the epidural space through the intervertebral foramina.
      ii. Compresses the dural sac.
      iii. Decreases CSF volume.
      iv. Decreased dilution of anesthetic then causes greater anesthetic effect.
   c. Longitudinal oscillation of CSF with the heartbeat is accentuated with elevated abdominal pressure and may contribute to greater anesthetic spread of spinal anesthesia during pregnancy.

Arachnoid Mater
1. A thin membrane within the dura
2. Encloses the subarachnoid space and the CSF

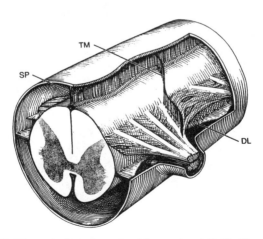

Fig. 10.10. The posterior subarachnoid space is subdivided by membranous partitions. The septum posticum (*SP*) runs down the mid-line and gives off transverse membranes (*TM*), which span to the posterior roots, which are themselves enmeshed in a membrane. The dentate ligaments (*DL*) attach the cord to the lateral dura. (Source: Reproduced from Hogan QH. A reexamination of anatomy in regional anesthesia. In: Brown D, ed. *Regional anesthesia.* Philadelphia: WB Saunders, 1996:50, with permission.)

3. Forms a physiologically active barrier
4. Only loosely attached to the inner aspect of the dura
    a. May recede from an advancing needle
    b. Clean puncture may be uncertain.
    c. Partial subdural injection is possible.
        i.   Local anesthetic injected during attempted spinal anesthesia will have a much diminished effect.
        ii. Epidural doses may produce extensive, sometimes unilateral anesthesia.

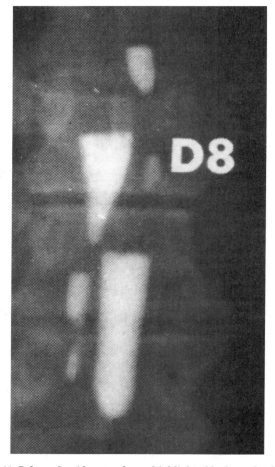

Fig. 10.11. Subarachnoid cysts, shown highlighted by hyperbaric contrast in an upright subject, are most common at thoracic levels but may be a cause for failed spinal anesthesia. (Source: Reproduced from Scott WG, Furlow LT. Myelography with pantopaque and a new technique for its removal. *Radiology* 1944;43:241, with permission.)

iii.   An epidural catheter placed in the subdural space
(or perhaps with some of the holes of a multiholed
catheter in the subdural space)
(1)   May produce a bleb of loculated anesthetic
(Fig. 10.9), which will only break free into
the CSF after repeated dosing.
(2)   This event will create the appearance of
catheter migration, because initial aspiration is negative for CSF, and the first or second anesthetic dose may have minimal or
expected performance.

Subarachnoid Space

1.   Anterior subarachnoid space is empty of structures.
2.   The posterior subarachnoid space is crowded with membranous elements (Fig. 10.10).
a.   A mesh of trabeculae spans the space from arachnoid to
join the pia mater, the meningeal layer that envelops
the surface of the cord and nerve roots.
b.   Denticulate ligaments extend laterally from the sides of
the cord to suspend it within the dural sac.
c.   Usually, a fenestrated partition the subarachnoid septum or septum posticum, extends from the posterior
mid-line of the cord to the inner aspect of the arachnoid
at the cervical and thoracic levels and often at lumbar
levels.
i.   The degree to which it affects distribution of anesthetic solutions is unknown.
3.   Cysts can occur within the subarachnoid space (Fig. 10.11).
a.   These saccular dilatations of the septum posticum are
present in 45% to 84% of normal subjects.
b.   Injection into them is a potential cause of inadequate
spinal anesthesia because local anesthetic will not dis-
tribute into the CSF.

REFERENCES

1.   Hogan Q, Toth J. Anatomy of the soft tissues of the spinal cord. *Reg Anesth Pain Med* 1999;24:303.
2.   Hogan QH. Epidural catheter tip position and distribution of injectate evaluated by computed tomography. *Anesthesiology* 1999;90:964.

Neuraxial Analgesia for Labor: Techniques

Both epidural and combined spinal—epidural (CSE) techniques can be used to provide effective labor analgesia. Both approaches begin by placing a needle in the epidural space. While this task is often easily accomplished, controversy surrounds many aspects of the techniques of epidural and CSE labor analgesia.

THE PROCEDURE

1. Carefully prepare a sterile work surface.
2. Neatly lay out all necessary equipment.
3. Prepare the skin at the back widely.
4. Place a sterile towel beneath the patient (or a sterile fenestrated drape over the patient's back).

Approach to the Epidural Space

Mid-line

1. Raise a skin wheal over the chosen interspace.
2. Infiltrate the subcutaneous layers with local anesthetic (while probing for a spinous process if palpation has been equivocal).
3. Insert the epidural needle through the skin, subcutaneous tissue, supraspinous and interspinous ligaments, and into the ligamentum flavum.
4. Keep the needle in the mid-line and in the sagittal plane, but angle it slightly cephalad (Fig. 11.1). Penetrating the skin in the rostral portion of the interspace, just below the caudad tip of the cephalad spinous process, will minimize the cephalad angle needed (Fig. 11.2).
5. The tissues (especially the ligamentum flavum) exert significant resistance both to advance of the needle and to injection of fluid.

Paramedian

1. Raise a skin wheal 1.5 cm from the mid-line, opposite the spinous process (whether the center, the cephalad, or the caudal end matters little).
2. Infiltrate the subcutaneous tissues, paravertebral muscles, and periosteum of the lamina (the latter is particularly sensitive) with about 5 mL dilute local anesthetic.
3. Insert the epidural needle
   a. Initially perpendicular to the skin until it reaches lamina.
   b. Then, withdraw and redirect the needle cephalad until it reaches either the upper border of the lamina or ligamentum flavum.
   c. Alternatively
      i. Insert the needle at an angle of 15 degrees to the sagittal plane and 135 degrees to the long axis of the patient (see Fig. 11.1).

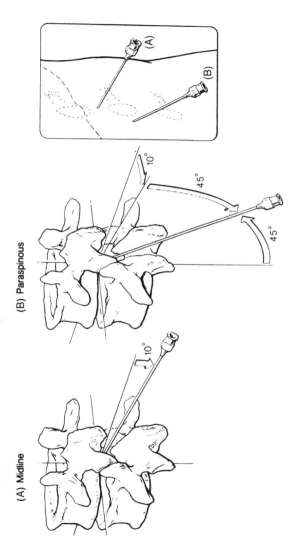

(A) Midline

(B) Paraspinous

Fig. 11.1. Sites of needle insertion for lumbar epidural block. A: Mid-line. Note insertion closer to the superior spinous process and the slight upward angulation. B: Paraspinous (paramedian). Note insertion beside caudad edge of "inferior" spinous process, with 45-degree angulation. (Source: Reproduced from Cousins MJ, Bromage PR. *Epidural neural blockade in clinical anesthesia and management of pain*, 2nd ed. Philadelphia: JB Lippincott Co, 1987:323, with permission.)

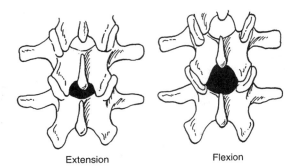

Extension   Flexion

Fig. 11.2.   Extension and flexion of the lumbar spine significantly affect the size and shape of the interlaminar space. Inserting the needle just below the upper spinous process provides the straightest path to the epidural space. (Source: Reproduced from Bonica JJ, McDonald JS. *Principles and practice of obstetric analgesia and anesthesia,* 2nd ed. Baltimore: Williams & Wilkins, 1995:404, with permission.)

> ii.   This method requires fewer passes of the needle, but a better understanding of spatial geometry.

Which Approach?
1. With a mid-line approach, needle angles are restricted by the spinous processes to 90 to 110 degrees.
2. The paramedian technique allows much steeper needle angles.
   a. The oblique angle may decrease the risk of dural puncture and ease catheter insertion.
   b. Other purported advantages of the paramedian approach include:
      i.   Use of a bony landmark (lamina) to identify the depth of the ligamentum flavum.
      ii.   Less need for lumbar flexion during needle insertion.
      iii. Excellent patient comfort if adequate local anesthetic infiltration is used.
      iv.   Avoidance of interspinous ligament pathologies such as calcifications or cysts.
      v.   Fewer catheter paresthesias due to improved threading conditions.
      vi.   The catheter more likely to be directed cephalad.
   c. Clinical studies have failed to prove a definitive advantage of the paramedian technique.
3. At this point, the data do not permit a clear choice of approach to the lumbar epidural space. Familiarize yourself with the technical aspects of both techniques.

Vertebral Level
1. For lumbar epidural anesthesia, accurate identification of the individual lumbar vertebrae is helpful for at least two reasons.

    a. First, the posterior approach may be blocked by the sacrum if the needle is inserted below the lumbar region.

    b. Second, placing the needle caudad to the conus medullaris limits the potential for spinal cord trauma.

       i. The spinal cord terminates at the conus medullaris.

      ii. The mean level of spinal cord termination is the L1–L2 disc.

         (1) In 95% of patients, the spinal cord terminates above the L2 vertebrae.

         (2) The level of the conus medullaris may be one-third of a vertebra lower in nonpregnant women than in men.

      iii. The dural sac ends at S1 or S2 in 83% of men and nonpregnant women.

      iv. Distally, a thin strand of pia covered with dura, known as the filum terminale, continues to the coccyx.

       v. Neural elements continue within the dural sac as the cauda equina.

         (1) Comprises approximately 15% of the lumbosacral subarachnoid space (7.1 to 7.3 mL).

         (2) Has a consistent spatial organization

            (a) Progressive rostrocaudal layering of roots from lateral to medial

            (b) The caudal sacral roots occupy a dorso-central position.

            (c) This spatial organization is maintained in part by strands of arachnoid mater.

2. Three interspaces are commonly used for lumbar epidural and spinal anesthesia:

    a. L4–L5.

    b. L3–L4.

    c. L2–L3.

    d. A line drawn between the bony iliac crests (Tuffier's line) intersects with the L4 vertebra or the L4–L5 interspace in 79% of supine, nonpregnant patients.

       i. In the lateral decubitus position,

         (1) A vertical line from the upper iliac crest will intersect the vertebral column one-half to one segment rostral to a line drawn between the iliac crests.

         (2) One factor that probably contributes to this phenomenon is pelvic tilt, which will be accentuated in patients with disparate hip and trunk widths.

      ii. Additional variability in the location of Tuffier's line

         (1) Soft tissue overlying the iliac crests

         (2) Expected variance in anatomic elements among individuals

    e. Alternative methods suggested for accurate identification of lumbar vertebral levels

       i. Count downward from the most prominent cervical spinous process (C7) or the intersection with the twelfth rib (T12).

      ii. Count upward from the L5–S1 interspace.

Posture
1. Sitting position
   a. Have the patient hang her legs over the side of the bed (while sitting as far from the edge as the length of her thighs will allow).
   b. Place a pillow on her lap.
   c. Encourage her to slouch forward at the waist, not the hips, with her arms folded in front of her on the pillow.
   d. An attendant or partner should stand in front of the patient and support her shoulders.
   e. Alternative sitting positions.
      i. Have the patient sit cross-legged in the middle of the bed. (This position provides good stability and lumbar flexion, but is not comfortable for all patients.)
      ii. Have the patient rest her arms and head on a bedside table.
2. Lateral position
   a. Have the patient move to the edge of the bed closest to the anesthetist.
   b. Place a pillow under her head, not her shoulder.
   c. Have the patient flex her lumbar spine as much as possible.
      i. Most women are unable to comply with this request unless they bend their knee up and their head down.
      ii. Neither move is strictly necessary, except as an aid to lumbar flexion.
3. Anesthetists vary in their preference for the sitting or lateral position.
   a. Most prefer the position in which they were initially taught to perform epidurals.
   b. Anesthetists trained to use the lateral position can more readily adapt to the sitting position than vice versa.
4. Patient preference
   a. Thin patients (body mass index less than 25) often prefer the lateral position.
   b. Obese patients (body mass index greater than 30) often prefer to sit.[1]
5. Flexion of the lumbar spine
   a. Increases the size of the interlaminar space.
   b. Eases posterior access to the lumbar epidural space (see Fig. 11.2).
   c. Increases the capacity of the vertebral canal.
   d. In nonpregnant women, lumbar spine flexion changes neither posterior epidural space depth nor the distance from skin to posterior epidural space.

Epidural Needles
1. Styles available for lumbar epidural anesthesia include Tuohy, Hustead, Crawford, Weiss, Cheng, and Crawley needles (Fig. 11.3).
2. Commercially available epidural needles are made of stainless steel with decreasing percentages of iron, chromium, nickel, manganese, and molybdenum/silicon.

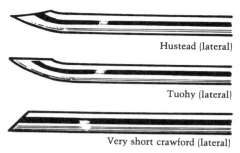

Hustead (lateral)

Tuohy (lateral)

Very short crawford (lateral)

Fig. 11.3.   Selected epidural needle tips. (Source: Reproduced from Mulroy MF. *Regional anesthesia: an illustrated procedural guide*. Boston: Little, Brown and Company, 1989, with permission.)

3.   Available Tuohy needles vary in length from 8 to 15 cm.
4.   Many epidural needles have alternating 1-cm opaque and polished zones to facilitate depth measurement.
5.   Many epidural needles have wings or other hub grip aids to help with control during insertion.
6.   The diameter or gauge of an epidural needle is a compromise between maximizing needle strength and space for catheter threading and minimizing local tissue trauma and the risk of postdural puncture headache (PDPH).
7.   Epidural and spinal needles can be deflected from their intended path of insertion (Fig. 11.4).
     a.   The magnitude of epidural needle deflection is intermediate between that occurring with pencil point and beveled spinal needles.
     b.   An 18-gauge Tuohy needle bends an average of 3 mm toward the orifice for every 5 cm of tissue traversed.
8.   Redirecting an epidural needle
     a.   Withdraw it into the subcutaneous tissues each time.
     b.   This maneuver minimizes lateral forces on the needle and reduces the risk of needle fracture, particularly in obese patients.

Identifying the Epidural Space
1.   The operator should be able to identify the epidural space as soon as the tip of the needle passes through the ligamentum flavum.
2.   Two commonly used approaches to identify the epidural space:
     a.   Hanging-drop technique
     b.   Loss of resistance (LOR) technique
     c.   Currently, the hanging-drop technique is the less popular approach.

Hanging-Drop Technique
1.   Relies on the negative pressure that develops on first entry into the epidural space.
     a.   A drop of fluid on the hub of the epidural needle is drawn into the needle on entering the epidural space.

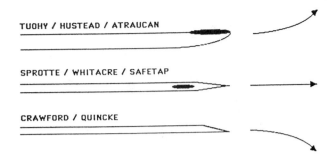

Fig. 11.4.   Deflection of epidural and spinal needles by tissue during placement. Direction of deflection depends on the design of the needle tip. (Source: Reproduced from Kopacz DJ, Allen HW. Comparison of needle deviation during regional anesthetic techniques in a laboratory model. *Anesth Analg* **1992;75:1050, with permission.)**

2. The pressure in the epidural space is affected by several physiologic variables, including:
   a. Arterial pulse.
   b. Respiration.
   c. Hypercarbia.
   d. Intrathoracic or intraabdominal pressures.
   e. Painful uterine contractions and maternal expulsive efforts raise lumbar epidural pressure.
      i.   Skeletal muscle activity
      ii. Increased intraabdominal pressure
      iii. Effective analgesia blunts these responses.
   f. Pressure in the undisturbed epidural space is positive, not negative.
   g. The initial entry pressure may be negative if the ligamenta flava bow forward and snap back along the epidural needle, or the tip of the needle indents or "tents" the dura.

Loss of Resistance Technique

1. There is almost complete resistance to injection through an epidural needle as it traverses the dense interspinous ligament or ligamentum flavum.
2. As the needle tip enters the epidural space, resistance to injection disappears abruptly.
3. The LOR technique can be done using air or saline within the syringe.
4. If saline is used, the epidural needle can be advanced directly by pressure on the shaft or hub, or indirectly by pressure on the plunger of the syringe.

Basic Technique

1. Attach an air-filled (or air/saline) syringe to the needle hub.
2. Brace both hands against the patient's back.
3. Hold the wings of the needle and advance it in a series of quantal steps.

4.   Pause between each step to apply pressure on the plunger.
5.   If the plunger bounces, advance the needle another step before testing again for LOR.

Alternatives

1.   Some anesthesiologists use a hybrid technique in which they hold and advance the needle using one hand and hold the syringe in the other. This is slightly less tedious, as bounce may be elicited repeatedly without having to pause between advances.
2.   Alternately, apply continuous pressure to the plunger of the syringe while advancing the needle with the nondominant hand (Fig. 11.5)
3.   Using a liquid-filled syringe, the epidural needle may be advanced solely by pressure on the plunger of the syringe.
     a.   Advance the syringe slowly and steadily by using the dominant hand to push on the plunger.
     b.   Apply inertia or breaking force by bracing the nondominant hand against the patient's back and holding the hub of the needle.
     c.   Once you reach the epidural space, injection of fluid becomes possible, and forward movement of the barrel of the syringe and needle stop automatically.

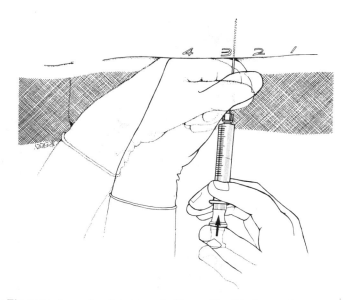

Fig. 11.5.   Loss of resistance: grip the needle with the nondominant hand. Extend the wrist and rock forward on the knuckles to drive the needle forward under rigid control. The thumb of the dominant hand applies constant pressure to the plunger of the syringe. (Source: Reproduced from Bromage PR. *Epidural analgesia.* **Philadelphia: WB Saunders, 1978:329, with permission.)**

    d.   As soon as LOR occurs, release the pressure on the plunger, so that you inject only a minimal amount of saline.

    e.   Then detach the syringe; any drip-back of saline is transient and is readily distinguished from CSF.

    f.   A modification of this technique may be necessary in the very occasional patient whose ligaments do not provide absolute resistance to injection of saline.

        i.   As before, the nondominant hand prevents sudden movement.

        ii.   Now, however, provide forward motion by gripping the barrel of the syringe with the fingertips of the dominant hand.

        iii.   Simultaneously, use the palm of that hand to apply more modest pressure to the plunger.

        iv.   You will feel and see the plunger move forward on entry into the epidural space.

        v.   This technique also prevents the inappropriate injection of saline into ligaments and paravertebral muscles.

  4.   Occasionally, LOR can be equivocal.

    a.   Attach an air-filled syringe to the hub of the epidural needle.

    b.   Tilt the needle in the direction opposite its bevel.

    c.   Attempt to inject.

        i.   If the needle is in ligament or soft tissue, resistance to injection will increase.

        ii.   If the needle is in the epidural space, resistance will not change (Fig. 11.6).

Air or Saline?

  1.   Air may increase the risk of unblocked segments.

    a.   Additional local anesthetic is usually effective treatment.

    b.   Other data suggest that blocks are identical after either air or saline.

  2.   Other potential complications of using air for the LOR technique include pneumocephalus, nerve root or spinal cord compression, subcutaneous emphysema, and venous air embolism.

    a.   Pneumocephalus

        i.   Typically presents as an immediate headache after dural puncture and intrathecal air injection.

        ii.   Computed tomography or magnetic resonance imaging can document intracranial air.[2]

        iii.   Treatment is primarily supportive and may include supplemental oxygen administration and avoiding nitrous oxide.

    b.   Case reports of lumbar root compression or paraplegia following the use of air in the LOR syringe have unusual clinical circumstances (i.e., very large air volumes) that limit their implications for routine clinical practice.

  3.   Neither air nor saline is associated with a greater risk of accidental dural puncture.

    a.   Dural puncture with air is more likely to produce a headache.

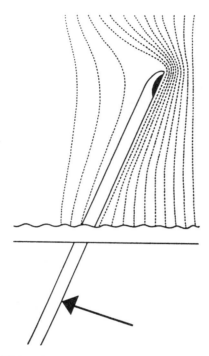

Fig. 11.6. **Tilting the needle during insertion compresses soft tissue, increasing resistance to injection. (Source: Modified from Brandstater B. The needle tilt test: an aid to epidural needle insertion.** *Anesthesiology* **1989;70:366.)**

  b. Headaches related to intrathecal air are faster in onset and shorter in duration than those related to dural trauma.[2]

 4. The volume of saline initially injected into the epidural space may affect the spread of a subsequent local anesthetic dose.

The Syringe

 1. Glass and plastic syringes are commercially available to use with the LOR technique.

 2. The ideal LOR syringe would have low inherent resistance, low cost, and no instances of the plunger sticking inside the barrel.

 3. Glass syringes

  a. Less inherent resistance

  b. Sticking sometimes occurs.

  c. "Dry polishing" a glass syringe produces less inherent resistance than wetting the same syringe with saline.

Epidural Needle Bevel Orientation
1. Primary clinical concerns
   a. Dural puncture and PDPH
   b. Epidural catheter threading
   c. Needle deflection during placement
2. Dural puncture and PDPH
   a. Orienting the bevel of a cutting-tipped spinal needle parallel to the longitudinal axis of the back markedly decreases the incidence of PDPH in nonpregnant patients.
   b. Identifying the epidural space with the needle bevel parallel to the longitudinal axis of the back decreases the risk of moderate-to-severe headache after accidental dural puncture (24% versus 70%).
3. Once the epidural space is located with a longitudinal-oriented needle bevel, should the needle be rotated 90 degrees to a transverse bevel position (cephalad or caudad) before threading the epidural catheter?
   a. Needle bevel direction has little or no effect on the spread of injected local anesthetic.
   b. It is easier to thread a catheter through a transverse needle bevel (cephalad or caudad) than through a laterally directed one.
4. Rotating the needle within the epidural space will orient its bevel cephalad and allow easier passage of the catheter.
   a. This practice has stimulated a lively debate.
   b. The argument against needle rotation rests almost entirely on a perceived increased risk of dural puncture.
      i. The dura can be readily punctured if the epidural needle is advanced while being rotated.
      ii. However, if the needle is held in position while being rotated, the risk of dural puncture does not increase.

Epidural Catheters
1. Currently, most epidural catheters are 18-, 19-, or 20-gauge and composed of nylon, polyurethane, or Teflon.
2. Some catheters contain removable wire stylets, which may increase the risk of paresthesia and venous or dural puncture. In the absence of a stylet, epidural catheters are unlikely to pierce intact dura.
3. A small needle hub insert that minimizes catheter buckling can markedly ease the threading of an epidural catheter.
4. On occasion, the catheter will not thread because only the tip of the needle has entered the epidural space. Here, advancing the epidural needle a few millimeters will allow the catheter to clear the bevel.

Single Hole Versus Multihole
1. Current epidural catheters have two basic designs:
   a. Single lumen (open end).
   b. Multi-orifice (blunt tip).
   c. Both have been used safely.
   d. Each type of catheter has theoretical advantages and disadvantages.

2. Multi-orifice catheters
    a. Disadvantages
        i.   Ports may lie in adjacent anatomic compartments (i.e., subarachnoid, subdural, epidural)
        ii. Multicompartment block has been reported
    b. Advantages
        i.   Better clinical performance
        ii. Fewer one-sided blocks
        iii. Fewer replaced or manipulated catheters
    c. Injection pressure determines the port from which drugs will exit.
        i.   With low injection pressures, drug exits primarily through the most proximal port.
        ii. With more vigorous injection, drug exits more uniformly from all ports.

Catheter Threading

1. Several techniques have been proposed to help insert the catheter into the tissues of the lumbar posterior epidural space.
2. Injecting 10 mL of air or liquid into the epidural space
    a. May decrease catheter paresthesiae.
    b. May decrease the risk of vessel puncture.
    c. Smaller volumes of air or saline lack an effect on either complication.

Depth of Insertion

1. Current epidural catheters usually have permanent markings that allow measurement of the length of catheter within the epidural space.
2. The length of catheter inserted into the epidural space may influence its efficacy and risks.
    a. Five to 6 cm may be the optimal insertion depth (Table 11.1)
    b. Catheters inserted only a few centimeters may dislodge.
    c. Those inserted more deeply are more likely to enter a vein.
    d. These depths may need to be modified for individual patients.
    e. Deeper insertion (i.e., 7 to 8 cm) may be appropriate for ambulatory or obese patients.
3. The distance from the skin to the epidural space
    a. Often increases as the patient moves from the upright, flexed position to a relaxed sitting posture to the lateral position.
    b. This change can be as much as 4 cm.
    c. It is greater in obese women than in thin women.
    d. If a catheter is taped to the skin with the patient in the upright, flexed position, it may be pulled out of the epidural space as she lies down.

Removal

1. Usually, epidural catheters are easily removed.

Table 11.1.   Insertion depth and frequency of complications and inadequate analgesia

Insertion depth (cm)	3	5	7
Number of patients	35	32	33
Intravenous catheters	2.8%	3.0%	17.5%[a]
Inadequate analgesia	31.4%	6.3%[a]	33.3%

[a] $p < .05$ vs. other groups.
Laboring women had multiorifice catheters inserted 3, 5, or 7 cm into the epidural space. All patients initially received 13 mL of 0.25% bupivacaine in divided doses.
Source: Data from Beilin Y, Bernstein HH, Zucker-Pinchoff B. The optimal distance that a multiorifice epidural catheter should be threaded into the epidural space. *Anesth Analg* 1995;81:301.

2. Normally, there is a considerable margin between the force needed to remove an epidural catheter and that needed to break it.
3. Occasionally, an epidural catheter is very difficult to remove due to "trapping" by vertebrae or ligaments. Suggested maneuvers include:
   a. Return to the original epidural placement position.
   b. Lateral decubitus position.
   c. Spinal flexion.
   d. Spinal extension (most likely to succeed).
   e. Injection of saline through the catheter during withdrawal.
   f. Leaving the catheter in place until the next day. Repeat the above maneuvers with the patient in bed or standing.
4. Rarely, epidural catheters knot *in situ*. The relationship between knot formation and depth of epidural catheter insertion remains conjectural.

Faulty Equipment
1. Manufacturing errors have reportedly occurred with
   a. Epidural needles.
   b. LOR syringes.
   c. Epidural catheters.
2. Correctly manufactured equipment may be incorrectly assembled into epidural kits with incompatible contents.
3. Briefly inspect each epidural kit before using it.

THE COMBINED SPINAL–EPIDURAL TECHNIQUE
1. Began as an anesthetic curiosity
2. In the 1980s, several authors described the currently popular needle-through-needle technique.
3. In many centers, this technique is widely used to provide labor analgesia.
4. As with any new technique, much remains to be learned about combined spinal–epidural anesthesia. As our experience grows, so will our understanding of the risks and benefits of this unique approach to neuraxial analgesia.

Why Combined Spinal–Epidural Technique?

1. Intrathecal injection can rapidly provide profound clinical effects with minimal amounts of drug. Unfortunately, current intrathecal techniques are limited to a single injection and, hence, a finite duration.
2. Multiple drugs can be injected over prolonged periods using an epidural catheter. However, safe and effective epidural blockade requires more time and more drug than do intrathecal techniques.
3. The CSE technique provides the rapid onset and greater drug potency of spinal anesthesia with the flexibility of epidural blockade. This combination has proved especially useful when providing labor analgesia.

Advantages of Combined Spinal–Epidural Technique for Labor Analgesia

1. The greatest advantage of CSE labor analgesia is the rapid onset of pain relief obtained with intrathecal injection of small amounts of opioids and local anesthetics (see Chapter 12).
2. A CSE technique that uses intrathecal opioids and epidural administration of dilute local anesthetic and opioid mixtures affords effective labor analgesia with a high degree of patient satisfaction.
    a. Patients like both the rapid onset of analgesia and the minimal degree of motor blockade that this approach provides.
    b. Some studies also suggest that CSE labor analgesia is associated with fewer forceps deliveries than is traditional epidural analgesia.

COMBINED SPINAL–EPIDURAL TECHNIQUES

1. There are four main varieties of CSE technique, each requiring different equipment and offering different advantages and limitations:
    a. The single-needle–single-interspace technique
        i. A needle is placed in the epidural space and local anesthetic is injected.
        ii. Then, the needle is advanced through the arachnoid and dura, and additional local anesthetic is injected intrathecally.
    b. The double-needle–double-interspace technique
        i. The epidural needle and catheter are inserted at one interspace.
        ii. Spinal injection at another interspace.
    c. The needle-through–needle-single-interspace technique
        i. The most popular variety of CSE
        ii. Requires a longer than usual spinal needle to protrude past the tip of the epidural needle (see following).
    d. The needle-beside-needle–single-interspace technique. Several devices are available with a spinal needle guide attached to, or incorporated into, the shaft of the epidural needle.

The Needle-through-Needle Technique

Equipment
1. The spinal needle must extend beyond the tip of the epidural needle.
    a. Too short or too long a protrusion may lead to failure.
    b. Factors that determine the length of protrusion
        i. The lengths of both the spinal and epidural needles
        ii. The design of the needle hubs
    c. The ideal length of protrusion is unknown.
        i. Manufacturers provide matching spinal and epidural needles for this technique.
        ii. Most have settled on a maximum protrusion of 10 to 15 mm.

Technique
1. Identify the epidural space.
2. Insert the spinal needle through the epidural needle.
    a. You will often feel a "pop" as the spinal needle penetrates the dura.
        i. The spinal needle may perforate the dura before it is fully extended beyond the tip of the epidural needle.
        ii. Stop advancing the spinal needle as soon as you feel the pop.
        iii. Continuing to advance the spinal needle past the pop will increase the likelihood of paresthesiae.
        iv. If the spinal needle has traversed the dura lateral to the mid-line, or tangentially, it may pass out of the subarachnoid space if inserted further (Fig. 11.7).
    b. Remove the stylet from the spinal needle and observe for CSF.
        i. If using the saline LOR technique to identify the epidural space, clear liquid in the hub of the spinal needle may be CSF or saline.
        ii. Usually, CSF appears promptly and will fill and drip from the hub of the spinal needle. Saline appears more slowly and in smaller quantities.
3. Fix the position of the spinal needle. (Pinch the hubs of the spinal and epidural needles together using the thumb and index finger of your nondominant hand.)
    a. The ligamentum flavum helps prevent excessive movement of a spinal needle inserted by itself.
    b. With the needle-through-needle technique, the epidural needle traverses the ligamentum flavum, and the spinal needle moves freely.
    c. The hub design of some needle-through-needle combinations allows the spinal needle to seat securely within the epidural needle.
4. Inject the appropriate drug (see Chapter 12).
    a. Although many experts recommend aspiration of CSF to confirm needle location before, during, or after intrathecal drug injection, I usually skip this step when using the CSE technique for labor analgesia for two reasons:
        i. First, the needle manipulation with aspiration may cause additional dural trauma.

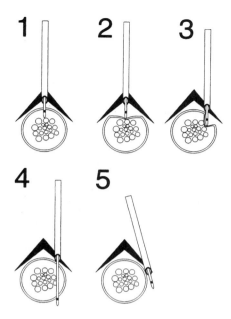

Fig. 11.7. Diagrammatic representation of different needle positions in vertebral canal. 1: Ideal situation; mid-line epidural needle guides spinal needle into subarachnoid space. 2: Spinal needle too short; indents but does not pierce dura. 3: Spinal needle too short and too lateral; longer needle might have produced successful dural puncture. 4: Spinal needle too long; has passed through dural sac and out again anteriorly. 5: Spinal needle too lateral; epidural needle in epidural space but guides spinal needle lateral to dural sac. (Source: Reproduced from Carrie LES. Combined spinal-epidural anesthesia for cesarean section. *Tech Reg Anesh Pain Manage* 1997;1:118, with permission.)

  ii. Second, the results of aspiration rarely change my management.
    (1) If initial aspiration is positive, I inject the drug.
    (2) If initial aspiration is negative, I inject the drug anyway.
      (a) The primary advantage of CSE labor analgesia is its rapid onset; it makes little sense to me to spend additional time trying to perform the technique.
      (b) If CSF appears spontaneously in my spinal needle, at least part of my injection will enter the subarachnoid space.
      (c) If the patient does not obtain adequate pain relief, I inject additional drug through the epidural catheter, regardless of my ability to aspirate CSF.

       iii.   Aspirating midway through injection strikes me as a good way to dislodge an appropriately placed needle.

       iv.   Aspiration at the end of injection does nothing other than reassure or upset the operator.

5. Remove the spinal needle and insert the epidural catheter.

Problems (Real and Imagined)

FAILURE TO OBTAIN CEREBROSPINAL FLUID

Patient Position

1. Initial success may be greater if the patient is sitting rather than lying on her side.
2. The ultimate ability to obtain CSF does not depend on the patient's position.
   a. The higher initial success rate in sitting patients presumably relates to the greater lumbar CSF pressure and narrower epidural space in that position.
   b. Alternatively, epidural needles placed with the patient in the lateral position may more likely be directed away from the mid-line, thus aiming the spinal needle away from the dura (see Fig. 11.7).

Needles

1. The spinal needle must penetrate the dura.
2. The dura is not a fixed structure; a needle will first tent, then perforate it (hence, the "pop" as the needle traverses the tensed dura).
3. The likelihood that a properly aimed needle will penetrate the dura depends on both tip configuration and the extent of protrusion.
   a. Cutting-point needles require less protrusion (but produce more headaches) than do pencil-point needles.
   b. Most pencil-point needles designed for use with the CSE technique protrude 10 to 15 mm beyond the tip of the epidural needle.
   c. Although needles that extend 15 mm past the tip of the epidural needle theoretically would increase the frequency of dural puncture, such an advantage remains unproven.

Technique

1. If the epidural needle is not in the epidural space, it is extremely unlikely that the spinal needle will find the subarachnoid space.
2. The epidural needle may be in the epidural space but (see Fig. 11.7).
   a. The spinal needle may be too short and its tip may indent, but not pierce, the dura mater.
   b. It may be too long and it may transfix the dural sac, passing out anteriorly.
   c. The spinal needle may be directed laterally and may pass the dural sac tangentially without piercing it.
3. If the epidural needle is properly cited, the spinal needle will sometimes "bounce" off the dura (especially if the patient is

lying on her side). Rotating the spinal needle 360 degrees or advancing the epidural needle 1 to 2 mm often solves this problem.

METALLIC PARTICLES

1. Passing spinal needles through Tuohy or Hustead needles creates a small groove on the inside of the tip of the epidural needle.
2. This groove, and concern about the possibility of depositing intrathecal metallic fragments, spurred the development of the needle-beside-needle–single-interspace technique.
3. But, there is no scientific evidence to suggest that the needle-through-needle CSE technique deposits metal fragments intrathecally.[3]

SUBARACHNOID CATHETER

1. An epidural catheter may pass into the subarachnoid space through the hole made by the spinal needle.
2. This risk is negligible.[4]
   a. It is impossible, even under direct vision, to pass a 16- or 18-gauge catheter through the dural puncture made by a 25-gauge Quincke needle.
   b. A catheter may be inserted with difficulty if multiple dural punctures are made.
   c. Catheters passed readily through dural punctures made by 17-gauge needles.
   d. In clinical practice, frequency of subarachnoid catheters is the same after both epidural and combined spinal-epidural techniques.

FACILITATED SPREAD

Spinal Anesthesia

1. Small amounts of epidural local anesthetic can significantly and rapidly increase the level of sensory blockade.
2. Several factors contribute to this increased spread.
   a. Merely injecting normal saline (10 mL) into the epidural space shortly after (5 minutes) the spinal anesthetic can increase the level of sensory blockade.
   b. If the level of spinal anesthesia has stabilized by the time of injection, epidural saline produces a small (2.0 ± 2.0 segment) rise in sensory level.
   c. Epidural saline no longer increases the level of sensory blockade once the level of spinal anesthesia begins to regress.

Epidural Drugs

1. The presence of a 24- or 27-gauge dural hole allows enhanced intrathecal passage of drugs injected into the epidural space.
2. The degree of this effect correlates with the size of the dural hole (Fig. 11.8)
3. In laboring women, epidural local anesthetic will block one to two more dermatomes in the presence of a small gauge dural hole versus no puncture.
4. Given the degree of interpatient variation, these small differences are not clinically significant.

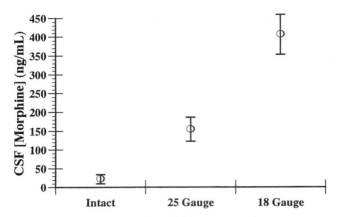

Fig. 11.8.   Cerebrospinal fluid morphine concentration measured at the cisternal magna 6 hours after lumbar epidural injection of 0.2-mg per kilogram morphine in sheep. Dural puncture was performed one interspace above the insertion site of the epidural catheter, 1 hour before morphine injection. (Source: Data from Swenson JD, Wisniewski M, McJames S, Ashburn MA, Pace NL. The effect of prior dural puncture on cisternal cerebrospinal fluid morphine concentrations in sheep after administration of lumbar epidural morphine. *Anesth Analg* 1996;83:523.)

EFFICACY

1. The needle-through-needle CSE technique is an effective way to deliver intrathecal drugs.
2. It also is an effective way to ensure placement of a catheter in the epidural space.
3. In a large clinical study, catheters placed as part of a CSE technique in laboring women were at least as reliable as those placed as part of epidural labor analgesia (Table 11.2).

HEADACHE

1. The incidence of headache after uncomplicated CSE labor analgesia is low.
2. Fewer than 8% of parturients report any headache.
3. Fewer than 3% have positional headaches.
4. The incidence of epidural blood patch is no different than after labor epidural analgesia.

INFECTION

1. Both meningitis and epidural abscess have been reported after CSE anesthesia.
2. These rare complications also are reported after spinal or epidural anesthesia.
3. Viridans streptococci, a common oropharyngeal bacteria, have emerged as major pathogens of meningitis after spinal anesthesia.
4. Routinely wearing a face mask during dural puncture may decrease the risk of this serious complication.

Table 11.2.   Efficacy of catheters placed for labor with the combined spinal–epidural technique (CSE) or after only attempting to identify the epidural space (epidural)

	Untestable[a]	Positive[b]	Negative	Equivocal[c]
CSE	56	935	2	11
Epidural	6	537	7	3

[a] Sixty-two catheters could not be adequately evaluated. Fifty-five CSE patients delivered within 2 hours of the start of the epidural infusion. Five patients delivered before any local anesthetics were injected, one catheter was accidentally removed, and one patient was not in labor.
[b] $p < .05$ CSE vs. epidural.
[c] Six of the 11 "equivocal" CSE catheters were one-sided, two produced bilateral but inadequate analgesia, and three produced adequate labor analgesia but failed to provide adequate anesthesia for cesarean section, postpartum tubal ligation, or manual removal of retained placenta. One "equivocal" epidural catheter was one-sided, one produced some sensory change but was inadequate for labor, and one was probably in the subdural space.
Data from Norris MC. Are combined spinal-epidural catheters reliable? *Int J Obstet Anesth* 1999 (*in press*).

REFERENCES

1. Vincent RD, Chestnut DH. Which position is more comfortable for the parturient during identification of the epidural space? *Int J Obstet Anesth* 1991;1:9.
2. Aida S, Taga K, Yamakura T, Endoh H, Shimoji K. Headache after attempted epidural block. The role of intrathecal air. *Anesthesiology* 1998;88:76.
3. Holst D, Mollmann M, Schymroszcyk B, Ebel C, Wendt M. No risk of metal toxicity in combined spinal-epidural anesthesia. *Anesth Analg* 1999;88:393.
4. Albright GA, Forster RM. The safety and efficacy of combined spinal and epidural analgesia/anesthesia (6,002 blocks) in a community hospital. *Reg Anesth Pain Med* 1999;24:117.

12

Neuraxial Analgesia for Labor: Intrathecal Drugs

1. The ideal labor analgesic should have:
   a. A localized site of action.
   b. No effects on motor function or the progress of labor.
   c. A small dose requirement.
   d. Low maternal–fetal drug exposure.
   e. Minimal maternal–fetal side effects.
   f. Reversibility.
2. Drugs injected into the intrathecal space fulfill many of these criteria.

RATIONALE FOR SPINAL ANALGESIA IN OBSTETRICS

1. Advantages of the intrathecal approach
   a. Reliable identification of the subarachnoid space
   b. Small drug requirement, which greatly decreases the chance of systemic drug toxicity
   c. Rapid, bilateral analgesia
   d. Increased efficacy of nonlocal anesthetic agents, minimizing maternal motor blockade
2. Currently, opioids and local anesthetics, alone or in various combinations, are the most commonly used intrathecal analgesics in laboring women.
   a. Intrathecal opioids
      i. Produce analgesia without significant changes in autonomic function, voluntary motor function, or response to innocuous stimuli.
      ii. Naloxone antagonizes subarachnoid opioid analgesia.
   b. Small doses of intrathecal isobaric local anesthetics
      i. Adequate but brief labor analgesia
      ii. Little hypotension or motor blockade
      iii. Excellent analgesia for the second stage of labor
      iv. Potentiate the action of intrathecal opioids
3. Bilateral analgesia develops more rapidly after intrathecal injection of a lipid soluble opioid (i.e., fentanyl or sufentanil) than after epidural injection of local anesthetics (Fig. 12.1).

MECHANISMS OF SPINAL ANALGESIA

1. Multiple spinal receptor systems are involved in nociceptive processing.
   a. These include opioid, α-adrenergic, serotonergic, cholinergic, γ-aminobutyric, and adenosine receptor agonist systems. *N*-methyl-D-aspartate (NMDA) receptor antagonists inhibit behavior induced by a noxious stimulus.
2. Acetylcholine, calcitonin, neurotensin, serotonin, somatostatin, neuropeptide Y, and ketamine have antinociceptive effects after intrathecal administration in animals.

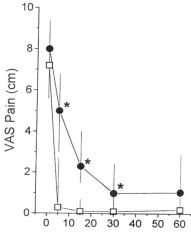

Fig. 12.1. Maternal pain relief following intrathecal sufentanil 10 µg (*open square*) versus epidural bupivacaine 30 mg (*closed circle*). (Source: Reproduced from D'Angelo R, Anderson MT, Philip J, Eisenach JC. Intrathecal sufentanil compared to epidural bupivacaine for labor analgesia. *Anesthesiology* 1994;80:1209, with permission.)

3. Modulation of the synapse between the primary afferent and the second-order neuron can alter the central passage of painful information. This control can be exercised at several points:
   a. Inhibition of afferent neurotransmitter release.
   b. Blockade of the effector mechanism by which the neurotransmitters released from primary afferents act.
   c. Alteration of the excitability of the second-order link.

Opioids
1. Act at sites before and after the synapse between the primary afferent and the second-order neuron
   a. A∂- and C-fiber stimulation releases substance P, a putative nociceptive neurotransmitter.
   b. Presynaptic actions of intrathecal opioids inhibit the release of substance P.
   c. Intrathecal opioids also hyperpolarize the postsynaptic cell membrane by increasing potassium conductance, thereby decreasing the excitability of the neuron.
2. Other mechanisms
   a. Morphine stimulates the release of adenosine from primary afferent nerves. Occupation of adenosine receptors produces mild analgesia.
   b. Additionally, high concentrations of morphine, fentanyl, meperidine, and sufentanil produce a weak local anesthetic effect on isolated nerves.

α_2-Adrenergic Agonists

1. α_2-Adrenergic receptors are found
   a. On primary afferent terminals at both peripheral and spinal nerve endings.
   b. On neurons in the superficial laminae of the spinal cord.
   c. Within several brainstem nuclei.
2. α_2-Adrenergic agonists
   a. Produce analgesia by spinal cholinergic activation.
      i. Descending noradrenergic pathways release norepinephrine.
         (1) Produces analgesia directly
         (2) Stimulates acetylcholine release, also causing analgesia
      ii. Epidural clonidine increases acetylcholine concentrations in lumbar cerebrospinal fluid (CSF).
   b. Epidural clonidine analgesia is increased in an additive fashion by intrathecal neostigmine.[1]

Local Anesthetics

1. The physiologic effects of local anesthetics are well known.
2. Small intrathecal doses of dilute local anesthetic solutions block mainly the small A∂ and C fibers, resulting in decreased pain perception but little motor blockade or hypotension.

PHARMACOKINETICS

1. Once injected into the subarachnoid space, analgesic drugs undergo redistribution via three mechanisms:
   a. Diffusion.
   b. Vascular transport.
   c. Bulk flow within the CSF.
2. Initially, drug moves by diffusion into the spinal cord, nerve roots, perineural fat, and across the dura into the epidural space.
   a. Drug is absorbed from these areas into the systemic vasculature.
   b. Drugs also undergo rostral–caudal movement within the CSF.
3. The predominant mechanism of redistribution for each drug depends on:
   a. Lipid solubility.
   b. Ionization.
   c. Molecular weight.

Lipid Solubility

1. The most important characteristic of a drug
   a. Effects uptake, clearance, and likelihood of rostral spread of both opioids and local anesthetics
   b. Increasing opioid lipid solubility
      i. Rapid uptake into the spinal cord
      ii. Faster analgesic onset
         (1) A somewhat lipid-insoluble drug, such as morphine, has an analgesic latency ranging from 15 to 60 minutes.

(2) The more lipid soluble opioids, such as fentanyl or sufentanil, begin to produce analgesia within minutes.

c. High lipid solubility also results in rapid redistribution within the CSF.

d. Clearance through systemic vascular absorption also is rapid, reducing the duration of a lipid-soluble drug.

2. Because spinally injected drugs avoid the blood–brain barrier, the intrathecal potency ratio of two drugs may not correlate with their systemic potency ratio.

a. High lipid solubility, which implies high systemic potency, results in a less potent intrathecal drug.

b. Intravenous sufentanil (octanol:water partition coefficient 1,757) is 12 to 15 times more potent than intravenous fentanyl (octanol:water partition coefficient 816).

c. Intrathecal sufentanil is only five to seven times more potent than intrathecal fentanyl.

Ionization and Molecular Weight

1. In their nonionized form, opioids and local anesthetics cross membranes and interact with specific receptors.

a. Commonly used opioids and local anesthetics have a pKA of 7.5 or greater.

b. Therefore, these drugs will exist mainly in the ionized form within the CSF.

2. Movement of molecules across the dura and into tissues is inversely related to the molecular weight and molecular configuration.

a. Opioids and local anesthetics used for labor analgesia have similar molecular weights but different molecular configurations.

b. Both types of drugs readily cross dural and tissue membranes.

NONANALGESIC PHYSIOLOGIC EFFECTS OF INTRATHECAL OPIOIDS

1. Besides analgesia, stimulation of intrathecal opioid receptors also can affect bladder, motor, gastrointestinal, and respiratory function and cause pruritus.

2. Most side effects are brief in duration and easily treated (Table 12.1).

a. Opioids can cause urinary retention by suppressing the micturition reflex through an action on both bladder contractility and sphincter tone.

b. High doses of μ-receptor agonists can induce skeletal muscle rigidity due to a receptor-specific interaction in brainstem centers.

3. Nausea and vomiting

a. Mechanism related to an action on the chemoemetic trigger zone in the dorsal medulla.

b. Fairly rare with the lipid-soluble opioids (except meperidine).

Table 12.1. Side effects of intrathecal opioids and their treatment

Problem	Treatment	Comment
Pruritus	Nalbuphine 5–10 mg IV, naloxone 40 µg IV, ondansetron 4 mg IV, diphenhydramine 25 mg IV	Pruritus is usually self-limited, but may be severe with morphine
	Pruritus is usually self-limited, but may be severe with morphine	
Nausea and vomiting	Metoclopramide 5–10 mg IV, nalbuphine 5–10 mg IV, naloxone 40 µg IV mg IV, propofol 10 mg IV	Nausea is most frequent after meperidine, usually self-limited
	Nausea is most frequent after meperidine; usually self-limited	
Urinary retention	Catheterization prn	
Hypotension	Intravenous fluids, ephedrine 5–10 mg IV	Resolves as analgesia diminishes
Respiratory depression	Naloxone 100 mg IV; may need to repeat	Significant hypotension is rare, most likely with meperidine or when opioids are used in combination with intrathecal local anesthetics
Postpartum prophylaxis	Naltrexone 25 mg PO	Consider after morphine

    c. More frequent, prolonged, and severe with morphine.

    d. If using intrathecal morphine for labor analgesia, consider giving postpartum naltrexone, 25 mg by mouth, to parturients who deliver within 12 hours of its injection.

Respiratory Depression

1. Respiratory effects of spinally administered opioids:
   a. Act at the chemosensitive anterolateral surface of the medulla.
   b. Decreased minute ventilation (decreased respiratory rate and tidal volume).
   c. Rightward shift of the carbon dioxide response curve.
   d. Decreased response to hypoxia.
2. Respiratory depression can occur with either the lipid-soluble or lipid-insoluble opioids. The time course, however, is very different.
   a. Intrathecal injection of a lipid-soluble opioid (fentanyl or sufentanil)
      i. Rapid redistribution of drug within the CSF
      ii. Early respiratory effects
      iii. Respiratory depression or arrest can occur within 5 to 10 minutes.
      iv. Risk is approximately 1 per 5,000, and probably greater if the patient has previously received systemic or neuraxial opioids.
   b. Treatment
      i. Oxygen
      ii. Stimulation
      iii. Naloxone
      iv. Intubation
   c. Delayed respiratory effects are seen following the injection of a lipid-insoluble opioid such as morphine. In this case, rostral spread of drug is slow, and effects may not be seen until 6 to 9 hours after injection.

Pruritus

1. The most common side effect
   a. Occurs, in varying degrees of severity, in 50% to 90% of patients
   b. With solely a lipid-soluble opioid, the pruritus is transient.
   c. Intrathecal morphine, when used for labor analgesia, produces severe, prolonged pruritus, which can persist postpartum.
2. Treatment (see Table 12.1).
   a. Antihistamines
      i. Anecdotally effective
         (1) Histamine release is not the mechanism of pruritus.
         (2) Facial pruritus results from a direct opioid receptor effect in the medulla.
         (3) Pruritus in other locations
            (a) Segmental in distribution

(b)   Correlates with degree of analgesia
(c)   Most likely, specific, opioid-mediated effect

b. Opioid-receptor antagonist
    i.   Effective therapy
    ii. Titrate to effect; excessive dose will reverse analgesia.

Do Intrathecal Opioids Cause Hypotension?

1. Maternal blood pressure often decreases after induction of intrathecal opioid labor analgesia.
2. The severity of this change depends on
    a. Timing of baseline blood pressure.
        i.   *Hypotension* is often defined as a percentage decrease from "baseline."
        ii. Pain and anxiety can increase maternal blood pressure.
        iii. Frequency of hypotension is greater if "baseline" blood pressure is an admission or preinduction value than if it is an antenatal value.
    b. Site of blood pressure measurement
        i.   Parturients often nursed in the lateral position.
        ii. Blood pressure in the dependent arm is more reflective of supine blood pressure than is the measurement in the nondependent arm.
        iii. Measurements in the nondependent arm after induction may overestimate the frequency of "hypotension."[2]
    c. Drug(s) injected
        i.   Fentanyl and sufentanil lack effect on maternal blood pressure in nonlaboring women.
            (1)   Produce afferent (i.e., light touch, temperature) but not efferent (i.e., sympathetic) block.
        ii. Meperidine and local anesthetics produce efferent conduction blockade and impair sympathetic tone.
            (1)   Significant hypotension can occur in these circumstances.

Fetal and Neonatal Effects

1. Transient fetal heart rate changes
    a. Reported after both intrathecal fentanyl and sufentanil
    b. Frequency varies from 3% to 30%
    c. Possibly related to uterine hyperactivity or rapid progression of labor
    d. Most studies suggest that the frequency of fetal bradycardia is the same after epidural or intrathecal labor analgesia.
    e. Treatment
        i.   Maternal position
        ii. Tocolysis
            (1)   Terbutaline

  (2) Nitroglycerin
  (3) Ephedrine
  iii. Surgical intervention is rarely indicated.
  f. Etiology
   i. Most likely, bradycardia following either intra-thecal or epidural drug administration is related to the onset of analgesia.
   ii. The intensity of uterine contractions depends on the balance between
    (1) Forces that encourage contraction (i.e., oxy-tocin)
    (2) Forces that inhibit contraction (i.e., β-adrenergic agonists, catecholamines).
   iii. The rapid fall in plasma catecholamines associated with the onset of analgesia may transiently upset this balance in favor of uterine contractile forces, resulting in uterine hyperactivity and potentially decreased blood flow to the fetus.
 2. Neonatal welfare
  a. Maternal–fetal sufentanil transfer is minimal.
  b. Neonatal outcome is unaffected by a single dose of intra-thecal fentanyl and subsequent epidural bupivacaine fentanyl infusion.

PATIENT SELECTION

 1. Patients who are candidates for neuraxial labor analgesia are candidates for intrathecal opioid administration.
 2. Specific indications
  a. Early labor: Intrathecal opioids can provide good labor analgesia without maternal motor blockade. Patients can continue to ambulate. Obstetricians worried about the impact of "early" epidural analgesia on labor outcome can be reassured.
  b. Advanced labor: A mixture of opioid and local anesthetic can rapidly provide profound maternal analgesia and perineal anesthesia with minimal motor blockade.
 3. Specific contraindications
  a. Patient refusal, infection at the puncture site, and sig-nificant coagulation defects
  b. I avoid this technique in women who have a history of a severe headache after minimal dural trauma. (Previous postdural puncture headache increases the risk of a subsequent postdural puncture headache.[3])

CHOICE OF AGENT

  Intrathecal opioids alone can provide good analgesia for the first stage of labor. However, their side-effect profile limits their usefulness as single agents.

Opioids

 1. Morphine
  a. Dose: 0.5 to 2 mg
  b. Onset: 30 to 60 minutes
  c. Duration: 2 to 10 hours
  d. Side effects

           i.   Pruritus, nausea, vomiting, urinary retention,
                somnolence
          ii.   May persist long after delivery
  2. Morphine–phenylpiperidine combinations
      a. Fentanyl–morphine
            i.   Dose
                 (1)   Fentanyl: 25 μg
                 (2)   Morphine: 0.25 mg
           ii.   Onset: minutes
          iii.   Duration: 2 to 4 hours
           iv.   Side effects
                 (1)   Pruritus, nausea, vomiting, urinary reten-
                       tion, somnolence
                 (2)   May persist long after delivery
      b. Sufentanil 10 μg plus morphine 0.25 mg
            i.   As above, more pruritus
  3. Sufentanil
      a. Dose: 5 to 10 μg
      b. Onset: minutes
      c. Duration: 90 to 120 minutes (larger dose does *not* pro-
          duce longer analgesia)
      d. Side effects
            i.   Pruritus
           ii.   Sedation
          iii.   Respiratory depression
           iv.   *Not* dose dependent (neither is analgesia)
  4. Fentanyl
      a. Dose: 25 to 50 μg (about 25% to 30% as potent as sufen-
          tanil)
      b. Onset: minutes
      c. Duration: 60 to 90 minutes
      d. Side effects
            i.   Pruritus
           ii.   Sedation
          iii.   Respiratory depression
  5. Meperidine
      a. Dose: 10 to 20 mg
      b. Onset: minutes
      c. Duration: 60 to 90 minutes
      d. Side effects
            i.   Sedation
           ii.   Nausea and vomiting (30%)
      e. Provides anesthesia as well as analgesia

Local Anesthetics
  1. Bupivacaine
      a. Formulation
            i.   I use the preservative-free solution that is mar-
                 keted for use with epidural anesthesia. These bot-
                 tles are usually labeled "not for spinal use."
           ii.   Although these solutions are considered isobaric,
                 they are, in fact, hypobaric and clearly behave
                 that way.
      b. Dose: 2.5 to 5.0 mg
      c. Duration: 60 minutes

    d. Side effects (dose dependent)
       i. Motor weakness
      ii. Hypotension
2. Ropivacaine
    a. Dose: 2 to 4 mg
    b. Indistinguishable from bupivacaine
3. Neither drug alone reliably relieves labor pain in a dose that does not produce motor blockade.

Local Anesthetic Opioid Combinations

1. Animal studies suggest that these combinations are synergistic.
2. Human dose–response studies are not yet published.
3. Clinical experience suggests that the addition of a local anesthetic will markedly decrease the dose of opioid needed to provide good labor pain relief.
4. Current recommendation
    a. Sufentanil: 1 to 2 µg
    b. Bupivacaine: 2.0 to 2.5 mg
    c. Onset: less than 5 minutes
    d. Duration: 60 to 120 minutes
    e. Side effects (mild)
       i. Decreased blood pressure
      ii. Itching (considerably less severe than that associated with 5 to 10 µg sufentanil)
     iii. Altered proprioception (legs feel numb and heavy, but motor function usually normal)

PROLONGING DURATION

1. Local anesthetic plus opioid: longer duration than either alone.
2. Epinephrine (200 µg) prolongs the duration of local anesthetic plus opioid, and has a minimal effect on the duration of opioid alone.
3. Clonidine (50 µg) prolongs duration of local anesthetic plus opioid.
4. None of these combinations will reliably provide analgesia for the duration of labor. I use these drugs for their rapid onset. I begin an epidural infusion immediately after induction of intrathecal analgesia. Thus, I am not specifically concerned about the duration of the intrathecal drug combination.

CONTINUOUS SPINAL ANALGESIA

1. A continuous technique overcomes many of the limitations of single injections.
    a. It allows repeated opioid injection during labor.
    b. It offers the option of using local anesthetics for vaginal or cesarean delivery.
    c. Other potential advantages of continuous spinal analgesia include:
       i. Dependable catheter placement.
      ii. The ability to provide analgesia and anesthesia rapidly.
     iii. Minimal drug requirement.
     iv. Symmetric, bilateral sensory blockade.

2. The unfortunate reports of cauda equina syndrome that followed the widespread introduction of small-gauge spinal catheters led the Food and Drug Administration to mandate their removal from the market.
3. Clinical and laboratory studies support two mechanisms for this serious complication:
    a. Use of a neurotoxic drug (lidocaine).
    b. Maldistribution of drug (Hyperbaric drug injected through a caudally directed catheter will pool in the dependent regions of the cord, exposing the cauda equina to higher than usual concentrations of local anesthetic.)
4. Current use
    a. Eighteen- to 20-gauge catheters
    b. Often discovered to lie in the subarachnoid space after accidental dural puncture
    c. *No* lidocaine
    d. Labor analgesia
        i. Intermittent injection of opioids or opioid-local anesthetic mixtures
            (1) Tachyphylaxis common
        ii. Continuous infusion
            (1) Local anesthetic–opioid mixtures
            (2) I infuse the same solution that I routinely use for epidural labor analgesia (0.083% bupivacaine plus 0.4 µg per milliliter sufentanil) at 2 mL per hour.
    e. Cesarean section
        i. Bupivacaine (isobaric or hyperbaric) is probably appropriate.
            (1) Pay attention to the dose of drug injected.
            (2) Suspect maldistribution if the level of sensory blockade is inadequate or uneven.
                (a) Inject a drug of different baricity.
                (b) Reposition the patient.
                (c) Abandon the technique.

CLINICAL ISSUES

1. Intrathecal opioids and the "test dose"
    a. Intrathecal opioids alone or in combination with local anesthetics will produce some sensory change, which may complicate the interpretation of a subsequent intrathecal "test dose."
    b. Other signs of intrathecal injection
        i. Hypotension
        ii. Motor block
2. Baricity of injectate
    a. In the absence of dextrose, all commonly used intrathecal opioid and local anesthetic solutions are hypobaric relative to CSF.
    b. Thus, maternal posture can influence spread of sensory block.
        i. After intrathecal injection of a local anesthetic-opioid mixture, parturients who sit during induction will develop a higher level of sensory blockade than will those who lie on their side.

      ii. When a parturient lies on her side during induction, more extensive block often develops on the nondependent (upper) side. Having the patient move to the opposite side will equalize the distribution of injected drug.

  c. Making injectate hyperbaric will limit its cephalad spread, but also will limit its efficacy.

Ambulation

1. Parturients have safely ambulated after intrathecal opioids alone or in combination with small doses of bupivacaine and epinephrine.
2. Despite its current popularity, ambulation lacks demonstrable impact on obstetric outcome, but it may improve maternal feelings of well-being and self-control.
3. The hemodynamic changes that follow intrathecal local anesthetics usually stabilize within 30 minutes.
4. If a patient wants to walk:
  a. Measure her blood pressure while she is sitting and while she is standing.
  b. Tests for motor weakness.
      i. Have her perform a partial deep knee-bend
      ii. Have her step up on a small stool without assistance.
  c. She should walk with an accompanying person and be wearing nonslip footwear.

REFERENCE

1. Hood DD, Mallak KA, Eisenach JC, Tong C. Interaction between intrathecal neostigmine and epidural clonidine in human volunteers. *Anesthesiology* 1996;85:315.
2. Kinsella SM, Black AMS. Reporting of "hypotension" after epidural analgesia during labour: effect of choice of arm and timing of baseline readings. *Anaesthesia* 1998;53:131–135.
3. Lybecker H, Moller JT, May O, Nielsen HK. Incidence and prediction of postdural puncture headache. A prospective study of 1,021 spinal anesthesias. *Anesth Analg* 1990;70:389.

Neuraxial Analgesia for Labor: Epidural Drugs

1. Although intrathecal opioids can provide good analgesia with no motor block, they have their limitations:
   a. Their duration is usually 1 to 2 hours.
   b. Repeated dural puncture or intrathecal catheter is needed for repeat doses.
   c. Opioids alone are often inadequate for the second stage of labor.
2. A lumbar epidural catheter can be used to provide analgesia throughout labor and, should the need arise, anesthesia for surgical delivery. Continuous infusion techniques, neuro-selective local anesthetics, and dilute local anesthetic—opioid solutions and other adjuvants provide excellent maternal analgesia without significantly impairing maternal motor function or fetal and neonatal physiology.

PHARMACOLOGY OF CONDUCTION BLOCKADE

1. Local anesthetics injected into the epidural space produce analgesia by inhibiting conduction in nerve fibers transmitting painful stimuli to the spinal cord.
2. Most available evidence suggests that this effect occurs at the level of the nerve root.
3. Pharmacology
   a. In the normal state, resting nerve cells are polarized, with a slightly negative transmembrane potential.
   b. When an action potential travels along a nerve, voltage-gated sodium channels open and allow nerve cell depolarization.
   c. Once a threshold transmembrane potential is reached, the action potential is propagated.
   d. Local anesthetics slow depolarization and block propagation of the action potential by binding to the voltage-gated sodium channels.
   e. Local anesthetics act inside the axon.
      i. Local anesthetics must initially assume a lipophilic (uncharged) form to cross the axonal membrane
      ii. Then, the molecule must assume its hydrophilic (charged) form to bind to the sodium channel.
      iii. Clinically useful local anesthetics
         (1) Weak bases
            (a) Lipophilic benzene ring
            (b) Tertiary amine (two forms) (Fig. 13.1).
               (i) Charged (hydrophilic)
               (ii) Uncharged (lipophilic)
   f. In solution, local anesthetic molecules exist in both charged and uncharged states.
      i. The balance between these two forms is determined by the relationship between the pKa of the local anesthetic and the pH of the solution.

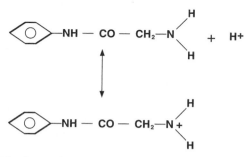

Figure 13.1. A generic amide local anesthetic in equilibrium between the charged quaternary amine form and the uncharged tertiary amine form. To diffuse into the nerve, the molecule must be in the uncharged tertiary amine configuration, but then is active in the receptor as a quaternary amine.

    ii.   The pKa of a given compound is the pH at which there are equal amounts of charged and uncharged drug. The pKa of clinically useful local anesthetics, which are weak bases, is above 7.0.

    iii.   Commercially available local anesthetic solutions are buffered to a low (acidic) pH.

        (1)   In these solutions, the vast majority of local anesthetic molecules are charged (the ratio of charged to uncharged molecules is 10^3 to $10^4 : 1$).

        (2)   One approach to speeding the onset of local anesthetic blockade is to raise the pH (i.e., with $NaHCO_3$) of the injected solution.

        (3)   As the pH of the solution approaches the pKa of the drug, more local anesthetic is in its uncharged, diffusible form.

g. Differential blockade

    i.   Clinically, pain transmission is more susceptible to local anesthetic blockade than light touch sensation, which in turn is more susceptible than motor function.

        (1)   The mechanism of this phenomenon is poorly understood, but axon size may have some role.

           (a)   Smaller nerve fibers are more susceptible to local anesthetic blockage than are larger fibers.

           (b)   Small-diameter Aδ (1 to 4 mm) and C fibers (0.4 to 1.2 mm) that conduct pain sensation are more easily blocked than are large Aα fibers (6 to 22 mm) that transmit motor impulses and proprioceptive information.

        (2)   Other possible mechanisms include anatomic site of blockade, location of the fibers

within the nerve bundle, and frequency-dependent blockade.

    ii. Local anesthetics also differ among themselves in the relative amounts of sensory and motor blockade they produce. Of the commonly used drugs, bupivacaine and ropivacaine produce less motor block than equianalgesic concentrations of lidocaine or 2-chloroprocaine.

  h. Lipid solubility and protein binding are important factors in determining a local anesthetic's potency, onset, and duration.

    i. Increased lipid solubility allows the drug to diffuse rapidly into the axon and then to its site of action.

    ii. Increased protein binding leads to a stronger bond between drug and receptor.

LOCAL ANESTHETICS

1. Theoretically, the best local anesthetic for labor analgesia will:
   a. Have a fast onset.
   b. Have a long duration.
   c. Be rapidly titratable.
   d. Preferentially block pain, compared with motor function.
   e. Have low toxicity.
2. In practice, no local anesthetic fulfills all of these requirements.
   a. One must prioritize among these categories.
   b. Most often, minimizing motor blockade takes precedence over onset.
   c. Unlike epidural anesthesia for cesarean section, toxicity is less important during labor because of the very low doses of drug used in this setting.

Bupivacaine

1. Currently, the most commonly used local anesthetic for labor analgesia.
   a. Produces relatively less motor blockade than most other local anesthetics.
   b. Is widely available.
   c. Has a relatively long duration.
2. Dose
   a. Bolus
      i.   Concentration: 0.125% to 0.25%
      ii. Volume: 10 to 20 mL
   b. Infusion: 0.125% at 10 to 20 mL per hour
3. Toxicity: At these doses (12.5- to 25.0-mg bolus and 12.5- to 25.0-mg per hour infusions), maternal systemic toxicity is unlikely.

Lidocaine

1. Produces more intense motor block and less analgesia than bupivacaine

Table 13.1. Relative potency of epidural local anesthetics in laboring women

Drug	EC_{50}[a]	EC_{95}[b]
Bupivacaine	0.065%	0.129%
Lidocaine	0.37%	0.52%
2-Chloroprocaine	0.43%	0.83%
Ropivacaine	0.111%	0.143%

[a] Concentration of local anesthetic (20 mL) that provided adequate labor analgesia (pain score less than 10 on a scale of 0 to 100) in 50% of patients.
[b] Concentration of local anesthetic (20 mL) that provided adequate labor analgesia (pain score less than 10 on a scale of 0 to 100) in 95% of patients.
Source: Data from Columb MO, Lyons G. Determination of the minimum local analgesic concentrations of epidural bupivacaine and lidocaine in labor. *Anesth Analg* 1995;81:833; Polley LS, Columb MO, Lyons G, Nair SA. The effect of epidural fentanyl on the minimum local analgesic concentration of epidural chloroprocaine in labor. *Anesth Analg* 1996;83:833; and Polley LS, Columb MS, Naughton NN, et al. Relative analgesic potencies of ropivacaine and bupivacaine for epidural analgesia in labor. *Anesth Analg* 1998;86:S384.

2. Is one-fourth to one-sixth as potent as bupivacaine (see Table 13.1)
3. Has a more rapid onset than bupivacaine

2-Chloroprocaine
1. Currently the only ester local anesthetic used for epidural anesthesia
2. Little toxicity
3. Rapid onset
4. Often used to provide epidural anesthesia for emergency operative delivery
5. Limitations
   a. Short acting; unless used as a continuous infusion, requires frequent reinjection.
   b. Doses that provide adequate labor analgesia are accompanied by significant motor block.
   c. Impairs the action of epidural bupivacaine and opioids.
      i. Although epidural 2-chloroprocaine rapidly provides labor analgesia, it markedly shortens the duration of subsequently injected epidural bupivacaine.
      ii. Epidural 2-chloroprocaine inhibits the effect of subsequent epidural fentanyl.
         (1) After cesarean delivery, epidural fentanyl provides a shorter and lesser degree of analgesia after 2-chloroprocaine than after lidocaine.
         (2) When injected together for labor analgesia, fentanyl appears to potentiate 2-chloroprocaine. Epidural fentanyl (60 μg) decreases the EC_{50} of epidural 2-chloroprocaine by 40% (Fig. 13.2).

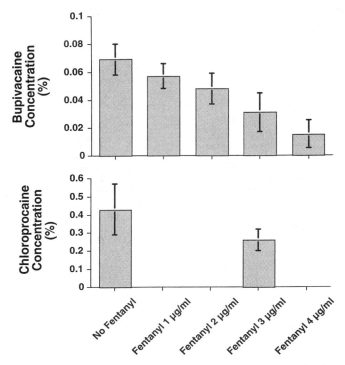

Figure 13.2.   The effect of epidural fentanyl on the minimum local anesthetic concentration for labor analgesia (*bars* are the 50% effective concentration and the *error bars* are the 95% confidence intervals). (Source: Data from Polley LS, Columb MO, Lyons G, Nair SA. The effect of epidural fentanyl on the minimum local analgesic concentration of epidural chloroprocaine in labor. *Anesth Analg* 1996;83:833; and Lyons G, Columb M, Hawthorne L, Dresner M. Extradural pain relief in labour: bupivacaine sparing by extradural fentanyl is dose dependent. *Br J Anaesth* 1997;78:493.)

6. Toxicity
   a. The *in vivo* half-life of 2-chloroprocaine in maternal plasma is 3 minutes.
   b. In most cases, this rapid destruction by plasma esterases limits the risk of systemic toxicity.
   c. However, in patients with atypical pseudocholinesterase, 2-chloroprocaine can cause prolonged block and toxicity after systemic absorption.
   d. 2-Chloroprocaine is historically associated with nerve injury and back pain.
      i. This is probably related to the preservatives, not to the drug itself.

ii. Neurologic damage was reported after accidental intrathecal injection of 2-chloroprocaine containing sodium bisulfite.

iii. In 1987, sodium bisulfite was replaced with disodium ethylenediaminetetraacetic acid (EDTA).

(1) This additive caused back pain, probably from muscle spasm related to hypocalcemia (EDTA chelates calcium).

(2) Currently, 2-chloroprocaine (Nesicaine™) is marketed without preservatives, and shelf life is prolonged by using dark bottles to protect the drug from light.

Ropivacaine

1. Structurally similar to bupivacaine
2. Lipid solubility, pKa, and protein binding also resemble that of bupivacaine.
3. Possible advantages versus bupivacaine
   a. Less cardiotoxicity
   b. Less motor blockade
   c. The lack of cardiotoxicity has little impact on ropivacaine's use for labor analgesia. The small bolus injections and dilute infusion mixtures that currently are used in laboring women make cardiac toxicity from unrecognized intravenous bupivacaine very unlikely.
   d. Less motor blockade may be advantageous. Small studies suggest that ropivacaine produces less maternal motor blockade than clinically equivalent doses of bupivacaine. No data suggest that this difference changes outcome.

Meperidine

1. Has local anesthetic-like properties
2. Is an effective spinal anesthetic for labor analgesia, tubal ligation, cesarean section, and other surgical procedures.
3. Epidural meperidine 100 mg provides effective labor analgesia, but produces significant sedation, itching, and nausea.

ADJUVANTS

Opioids

1. Epidural opioids alone (with the exception of meperidine) do not provide adequate labor analgesia.
2. Epidural opioids potentiate epidural local anesthetics (Figs. 13.2 and 13.3).
3. Dilute local anesthetic–opioid mixtures provide good labor analgesia with minimal maternal motor blockade.
4. The lipid-soluble opioids (fentanyl, sufentanil, and alfentanil) are most effective. Morphine's slow onset limits its use during labor.
5. Multiple studies have shown that commonly used doses of epidural opioids during labor have few detrimental maternal or fetal side effects.
6. Dose (Table 13.2)
   a. Fentanyl

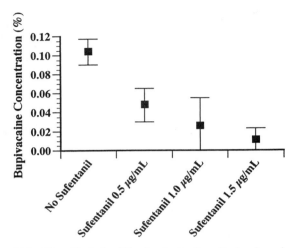

Figure 13.3. The effect of epidural sufentanil on the bupivacaine minimum local anesthetic concentration for labor analgesia (*bars* are the 50% effective concentration and the *error bars* are the 95% confidence intervals). (Source: Data from Polley LS, Columb MO, Wagner DS, Naughton NN. Dose-dependent reduction of the minimum local analgesic concentration of bupivacaine by sufentanil for epidural analgesia in labor. *Anesthesiology* 1998;89:626.)

Table 13.2. Recommended doses of epidural opioids for labor analgesia

Drug	Bolus Injection[a]	Continuous Infusion[b]
Fentanyl	50–100 µg	2–4 µg/mL
Sufentanil	10–15 µg	0.3–0.4 µg/mL

[a] Mix with 10–20 mL of 0.125% bupivacaine.
[b] Mix with 0.0625%–0.083% bupivacaine and infuse at 10–20 mL/h.

      i. One to 4 µg per milliliter progressively decreases the EC_{50} of bupivacaine in laboring women (see Fig. 13.2).
      ii. There is more itching with 4 µg per milliliter.
   b. Sufentanil
      i. Clinically, 0.3 to 0.4 µg per milliliter is effective.
      ii. There is profound potentiation of bupivacaine with larger doses (see Table. 13.3A on page 272).
   c. There are few differences between fentanyl, and sufentanil as adjuvants to epidural local anesthetics. Because of sufentanil's larger volume of distribution, it will

have less effect on the fetus than equipotent doses of fentanyl.

Sodium Bicarbonate

1. Commercially available local anesthetic solutions are buffered to a low pH.
2. Adding sodium bicarbonate will raise the pH of these solutions and speed local anesthetic onset.
3. Unfortunately, raising the pH of a local anesthetic solution also may increase the intensity of (motor) blockade.
   a. I rarely use bicarbonate for labor analgesia.
   b. For rapid onset of labor analgesia, use intrathecal drugs.
4. Adding bicarbonate to epidural lidocaine or 2-chloroprocaine will speed the onset of anesthesia for operative delivery.
5. Dose
   a. Lidocaine or 2-chloroprocaine: 1 mEq per 10 mL
   b. Bupivacaine: 0.1 mEq per 10 mL
   c. Larger doses of sodium bicarbonate will cause local anesthetic to precipitate.

Epinephrine

1. Enhances analgesia and shortens onset when added to local anesthetic solutions
2. Epinephrine has little to offer as an adjuvant for labor epidural analgesia.
   a. Epidural epinephrine increases motor block associated with local anesthetics.
   b. The β-agonist action of epinephrine can inhibit uterine contractions and significantly slow labor.

Clonidine

1. Clonidine is now available for epidural use in the United States.
2. Epidural clonidine potentiates local anesthetics (improved pain scores, longer duration) without increasing motor block.
3. Maternal and neonatal hemodynamic side effects are minimal and not clinically significant.
4. Maternal sedation is common with even low doses (50 to 75 µg).

TEST DOSES

1. Unrecognized intrathecal or intravascular injection of large doses of local anesthetic could have devastating consequences. To minimize these risks, many experts recommend injecting a "test dose," usually containing lidocaine and 15 µg epinephrine before giving the therapeutic dose of epidural local anesthetic.
2. Currently, providing epidural analgesia for labor does not require the use of concentrated local anesthetics, and the risks of unrecognized intravascular drug injection have

changed significantly. So, many are rethinking the routine use of the epinephrine test dose.

3. Intrathecal test dose
    a. Give the initial bolus in small increments to safeguard against unrecognized intrathecal injection.
    b. The local anesthetic content of most test doses (45 to 60 mg of lidocaine or 7.5 to 12.5 mg of bupivacaine) approaches or exceeds the amount used to induce labor epidural analgesia.
    c. The extra local anesthetic (and epinephrine) included in the test dose increases the risk of a motor block.
4. Intravascular test dose
    a. Epinephrine 15 µg is the most commonly used intravascular test dose. Tachycardia, hypertension, or subjective symptoms following its injection suggest intravenous catheter location.
    b. The major risk of unrecognized intravenous injection or infusion of dilute local anesthetic–opioid mixtures for labor epidural analgesia is inadequate pain relief, not systemic local anesthetic toxicity. Thus, the potential risks of epinephrine (increased motor block and decreased uterine activity) may outweigh its benefits in this setting.
    c. If the initial bolus of local anesthetic and opioid does not provide adequate analgesia, suspect a misplaced catheter.
        i. Look closely for sensory changes.
            (1) If present, try more local anesthetic.
            (2) If absent, the catheter could be intravascular or simply not in the epidural space. In either case, replace it.
    d. By looking for signs and symptoms of epidural blockade, rather than simply injecting a test dose to rule out intrathecal or intravascular catheter location, one can safely provide labor epidural analgesia without unneeded local anesthetic or epinephrine.

AMBULATION

1. No effect on the progress of labor.[1]
2. Patients like the idea of being able to walk after receiving labor pain relief.
3. This may be compatible with any epidural technique that minimizes motor block.
4. Practical questions.
    a. How much motor block is acceptable? Only a trial of walking is sufficiently sensitive and specific.
    b. Does impaired sensation, especially proprioception, make walking unsafe? Despite detectable posterior column sensor impairment, patients can ambulate safely with epidural analgesia.
    c. Is hypotension a concern? Postural hypotension is rarely a problem.
    d. How badly do laboring women want to walk? Patients rarely want to walk. However, techniques that mini-

mize motor block allow women to move about in bed more easily and may improve satisfaction.

5. If a patient does want to ambulate after induction of labor epidural analgesia, strive to minimize motor block. Use the lowest effective concentration of local anesthetic (preferably either bupivacaine or ropivacaine). Avoid epinephrine. Check blood pressure for orthostatic changes. Assess motor function (patients should be able to do a modified deep knee-bend). Have an attendant walk with the patient.

CONTINUOUS INFUSIONS

1. Compared with intermittent bolus techniques, continuous techniques require fewer interventions and provide greater patient satisfaction.
2. Continuous infusions have a few potential limitations.
   a. Continuous epidural infusions deliver more drug than do intermittent bolus injections.
   b. Continuous infusion of relatively concentrated local anesthetic solutions may produce excessive maternal motor blockade.
      i. Diluted local anesthetic–opioid mixtures are as effective as more concentrated solutions.
      ii. Evaluate the extent of sensory and motor block every 2 to 3 hours and change infusion rate or concentration if necessary.

PATIENT-CONTROLLED EPIDURAL ANALGESIA

1. Patient-controlled epidural analgesia (PCEA) is a relatively new technique that allows the patient to self-medicate and titrate to a desired level of pain relief.
2. The usual practice (Table 13-3B on page 272)
   a. Induce epidural analgesia.
      i. Begin a "background" infusion of a dilute local anesthetic–opioid mixture (usually 6 to 8 mL per hour).
      ii. Allow patients to self-medicate with additional drug as needed (usually 3- to 6-mL boluses every 15 to 30 minutes).
   b. Currently, the interplay between drug concentration, background infusion, and bolus size remains undefined.
3. Compared with continuous infusion techniques, PCEA patients use less drug, have similar levels of analgesia and satisfaction, and no differences in labor outcome or need for physician intervention.
4. Compared with intermittent bolus techniques, pain control and satisfaction often are better with PCEA, but there are no differences in the amount of drug used.

SUGGESTED TECHNIQUES (TABLE 13.3A–C)

1. The technique of labor epidural analgesia should be tailored to each patient.
2. No single drug combination works in all clinical situations.

**Table 13.3A. Suggested techniques
for epidural labor analgesia**

Induction Clinical Situation	Epidural Analgesia/ Bolus	Combined Spinal Epidural Analgesia/ Intrathecal Injection
Very early labor (<3-cm cervical dilation)	10–15 mL 0.083% bupivacaine + 0.4 µg/mL sufentanil[a]	Sufentanil 5 µg or sufentanil 1.2 µg + bupivacaine 2.5 mg[b]
Labor (3- to 7-cm cervical dilation)	10-15 mL 0.125% bupivacaine + 1 µg/mL sufentanil or 5–10 µg/mL fentanyl	Sufentanil 1.2 µg + bupivacaine 2.5 mg[b]
Advanced labor (>7-cm cervical dilation)	15–20 mL 0.125% bupivacaine + 1 µg/mL sufentanil or 5–10 µg/mL fentanyl, or 10–15 mL 0.25% bupivacaine + 1 µg/mL sufentanil or 5–10 µg/mL fentanyl	Sufentanil 1.2 µg + bupivacaine 2.5 mg[b] or sufentanil 5 µg + bupivacaine 2.0–2.5 mg

Fentanyl 250 µg can be substituted for the sufentanil.
[a] Add 20 mL 0.5% bupivacaine and 50 µg sufentanil to 100 mL preservative-free normal saline.
[b] Inject 3 mL of above local anesthetic–opioid solution.

Table 13.3B. Maintenance

Continuous Infusion	Patient-Controlled Epidural Analgesia (PCEA)
0.083% bupivacaine + 0.4 µg/mL sufentanil at 12 mL/h	0.083–0.125% bupivacaine + 0.4 µg/mL sufentanil
PCEA Settings	
Bolus	4–8 mL
Lockout	5–20 min
Basal infusion	0–8 mL/h

Comments: Use higher concentration and shorter lockout if not using a basal infusion. With any settings, patients will consume little drug until they reach 7- to 8-cm cervical dilation. Then, pain and medication demand escalates rapidly.

Table 13.3C. Special situations

Clinical Situation	Response
Patient wants to walk	Change maintenance infusion to 0.4% bupivacaine + 0.8 µg/mL sufentanil[a] at 12 mL/h.
Breakthrough pain	
No analgesia, no sensory change	Replace catheter.
One-sided block, "hot spot"	Withdraw catheter 1 cm. Position patient with painful side down.Bolus with 5–10 mL 0.125% bupivacaine. If no relief in 15–20 minutes, replace catheter.
Inadequate density of block	Bolus with 5–10 mL 0.25% bupivacaine. Increase concentration of local anesthetic in infusion mixture.
Severe pain, unresponsive to above (assuming local anesthetic injection produces bilateral sensory change)	5–10 mL 0.5% bupivacaine
Perineal analgesia/anesthesia	
Delivery remote	10 mL 0.125% bupivacaine ± opioid
Delivery imminent	10 mL 0.25% bupivacaine, or 10 mL 1.5% lidocaine + 1:200,000 epi + NaHCO$_3$,[b] or 10 mL 2% 2-chloroprocaine[b]

[a] Add 20 mL 0.25% bupivacaine and 100 µg sufentanil to 100 mL preservative-free normal saline.
[b] May need repeat injection or longer duration drug to provide anesthesia for perineal repair.

3. Some important variables include:
    a. Stage of labor.
    b. Acceptable degree of motor block.
    c. Patient expectations.
    d. Drug cost and availability.
    e. Availability of qualified anesthetic personnel.

REFERENCE

1. Bloom SL, McIntire DD, Kelly MA, et al. Lack of effect of walking on labor and delivery. *N Engl J Med* 1998;339:76.

General Anesthesia
for Cesarean Delivery

1. In the United States, 15% to 22% of cesarean deliveries are accomplished under general anesthesia. The frequency of general anesthesia for cesarean delivery varies greatly among individual hospitals. Several of the factors that influence the use of general anesthesia are:
   a. Patterns of labor analgesia: A higher use of epidural analgesia for labor decreases the use of general anesthesia for cesarean delivery.
   b. Patient populations: High-risk obstetric centers with more stressed and distressed fetuses needing immediate delivery may use general anesthesia more commonly.
   c. Obstetrician and anesthesiologist practice patterns: The diagnosis of fetal distress and, therefore, the need for emergency delivery vary from institution to institution.

INDICATIONS

1. In modern practice, general anesthesia for cesarean delivery is reserved for limited situations (Table 14.1). Coexisting maternal diseases, which contraindicate regional anesthesia and rapid deterioration of fetal well-being, are the most common of these indications. In addition, not every regional anesthetic proves adequate for the entire surgical procedure.
2. Some women will specifically request general anesthesia. These patients tend to be slightly older, of higher parity, and of lower socioeconomic class, or have had a previous pregnancy loss.

ADVANTAGES

1. General anesthesia produces rapid, reproducible conditions for cesarean delivery.
2. General anesthesia has a long record of fetal and relative maternal safety.
3. Success of general anesthesia is independent of a patient's anxiety about remaining "awake."

DISADVANTAGES

1. Airway management
   a. Anatomic and physiologic changes of pregnancy increase the risk of failed intubation. Parturients are at increased risk for aspiration of gastric contents.
   b. The often hectic and tumultuous conditions surrounding emergent cesarean delivery may compromise preoperative evaluation of the parturient with a potentially difficult airway.
2. Equipment and medication errors
   a. Anesthesia machines on most labor floors are used less often than in the general surgical suite. They also may receive less frequent routine maintenance, increasing the possibility of undetected malfunction.

Table 14.1. Indications for general anesthesia for cesarean delivery

Acute severe fetal distress
    Epidural catheter not *in situ*
Relative and absolute contraindications to regional anesthesia
    Maternal hemodynamic instability
    Severe maternal hemorrhage
    Coexisting maternal cardiac disease (e.g., severe right-to-left shunt, fixed primary pulmonary hypertension, severe aortic stenosis)
    Maternal coagulopathy
    Maternal infection
    Superficial to the lumbosacral spine
    Sepsis
Patient refusal of regional anesthesia
Regional anesthesia inadequate for surgery

    b.   The obstetric suite is an ideal site for drug substitution or other misuse. Anesthetic medications often are prepared, labeled, and left unattended on an operating room anesthesia cart. Later, they may be used immediately to induce general anesthesia.
  3.   Finally, the physiologic consequences of the induction of general anesthesia and tracheal intubation may prove deleterious to the mother with coexisting medical conditions (e.g., cardiac or neurologic diseases).

PREPARATION FOR GENERAL ANESTHESIA

Airway Assessment

  1.   The following contribute to difficult tracheal intubation in the parturient:
    a.   The often emergent nature of cesarean delivery limits the time for preanesthetic evaluation and preparation.
    b.   Medical personnel who can help with a difficult airway are relatively scarce.
    c.   Anatomic airway changes in the gravida, perhaps exacerbated by poor positioning, obesity, or preeclampsia/eclampsia, increase the technical difficulty of tracheal intubation.
    d.   Inexperienced anesthesiology personnel are often assigned to the labor and delivery suite.

Importance of Airway Assessment

Maternal Mortality

  1.   While anesthetic-related maternal mortality has decreased considerably since the early 1980s, risk related to general anesthesia has remained stable. Maternal mortality associated with general anesthesia is 17-fold greater than that associated with regional anesthesia.[1]

2. Most maternal deaths are related to difficulties with airway management. Failed intubation is approximately ten times more frequent in parturients than in general surgical patients.

Identifying the Patient "At Risk"

1. Preanesthetic assessment can identify patients at high risk for cesarean section and those at high risk for airway complications. Communication with the patient's obstetrician and early anesthetic intervention should decrease the need for general anesthesia in these women.
2. Attempt to identify the parturient with a potentially difficult airway soon after her admission to the labor and delivery suite. Look for presence of the many different indicators of difficult airway (i.e., ability to open the mouth, mandibular length, and loose dentition). Attempt to visualize the normal oropharyngeal anatomy (soft palate, uvula, and tonsillar fossae).

Factors Associated with Difficult Airway

Anatomic Abnormalities

1. Many parturients who prove difficult to intubate have anatomic abnormalities that would make intubation problematic under any circumstances. Common anatomic findings include a receding jaw, limited mouth opening, and prominent teeth.
2. Large prospective trials have identified a variety of physical findings that correlate with increased difficulty at tracheal intubation (Table 14.2).

Obesity

1. Commonly complicates anesthetic-related maternal deaths
    a. Death is often directly due to failure to establish an adequate airway.

Table 14.2. Relative risk of difficulty at tracheal intubation compared with a Mallampati class 1 airway

Anatomic Feature	Relative Risk
Mallampati 4	11.30
Receding mandible	9.71
Protruding maxillary incisors	8.00
Mallampati 3	7.58
Short neck	5.01
Mallampati 2	3.23
Mallampati 1	1.00

Source: From Rocke DA, Murray WB, Rout CC, Gouwns E. Relative risk analysis of factors associated with difficult intubation in obstetric anesthesia. *Anesthesiology* 1992;77:67, with permission.

b. Obesity (body mass index greater than 23) doubles the incidence of partially obliterated oropharyngeal anatomy.
2. Obesity increases the risk of cesarean delivery. In the morbidly obese parturient (greater than 300 lb), the cesarean delivery rate may exceed 50%.

Pregnancy-induced Hypertension
1. Carries an increased risk of cesarean section
2. May predispose to difficult intubation

Avoiding Trouble with the Difficult Airway
Early Induction of Epidural Analgesia
1. Early induction of labor analgesia usually precludes the need for general anesthesia, should cesarean delivery later become necessary.
2. However, not every epidural anesthetic proves adequate for cesarean delivery. Intraoperative induction of general anesthesia may be required if unanticipated events delay closure of the abdomen and create distress in the awake (and aware) parturient.
3. Time constraints may limit the ability to use an epidural catheter placed during labor for emergency cesarean section. Routine use of rapidly acting local anesthetics (i.e., alkalinized 3% 2-chloroprocaine or 2% lidocaine with epinephrine) may further decrease the need for general anesthesia among these women.

Developing a Plan
1. Identifying the parturient with a potentially difficult airway helps ensure adequate time to plan and to communicate with the obstetrician before the need for general anesthesia.
2. Appropriate planning may include awake intubation, fiberoptic bronchoscopy-assisted intubation, surgical control of the airway, or retrograde intubation. Such intervention requires time to collect personnel and equipment.

Experienced Personnel
1. The experience of the anesthesiologist plays an important role in the incidence of anesthetic-related maternal mortality. Most failed intubations occur at night or on weekends when patients are cared for by less-experienced anesthetists.
2. In most failed intubations, the anesthetist has a partially obstructed view of the larynx. More experience in dealing with the difficult airway (e.g., use of gum elastic bougies, light wands, etc.) may convert a failed tracheal intubation into a successful one.

Acid-Aspiration Prophylaxis
1. Pharmacologic methods of acid-aspiration prophylaxis are part of the planning for every general anesthetic for cesarean delivery.
2. Drug trials in humans provide conflicting data on which regimen is best.
3. No one agent (or combination of agents) will ensure a nonfatal aspiration.

4. Acidity of the aspirate may be more crucial than volume.
5. Clinicians use antacids, H_2-receptor antagonists, and meto-clopramide in varying combinations in a search for the optimally prepared "full stomach."

Urgent or Emergent Cesarean Delivery

1. Labor significantly slows or eliminates physiologic gastric emptying, resulting in a true "full stomach."
2. No acid-aspiration prophylaxis regimen reliably reduces the volume and raises the pH of gastric contents in the laboring patient.

Antacid

1. Administration of 0.3 M of sodium citrate quickly and reliably increases the pH of intragastric contents.
2. Sodium citrate should be given shortly before surgery. Gastric pH may remain above 2.5 for as little as 15 minutes.

Ranitidine

1. The coadministration of single-dose ranitidine (50 mg) intravenously and 0.3 M sodium citrate orally maintains intragastric alkalinization longer than antacid alone; however, this effect becomes significant only 2 hours after treatment.
2. Regularly scheduled parenteral ranitidine doses do not adequately prepare the gastric contents of the laboring parturient presenting for emergent or urgent cesarean delivery under general anesthesia. Instead, give an oral antacid before inducing general anesthesia for urgent or emergent cesarean delivery.

Effervescent Cimetidine–Sodium Citrate

1. Effervescent cimetidine–sodium citrate (400 mg and 0.9 M, respectively, in 15 mL of water) effectively alkalinizes intragastric contents. This combination will maintain intragastric pH significantly higher than antacid alone at 1 hour after treatment and beyond.
2. These results are similar to those seen after the coadministration of intravenous ranitidine and oral sodium citrate.

Omeprazole

1. Omeprazole, which blocks the proton pump in the parietal cell, effectively reduces both intragastric volume and acidity after a double-dose oral regimen (40 mg at night and early morning) in women fasted before elective cesarean delivery.
2. Single-dose omeprazole provides inadequate preparation of gastric contents.

Metoclopramide

1. Metoclopramide often is given before the induction of general anesthesia for urgent cesarean delivery. It will increase lower esophageal sphincter tone and decrease gastric volume within minutes of parenteral administration.
2. Opioids inhibit the effects of metoclopramide. A dose of metoclopramide at induction or during general anesthesia in hope of emptying the stomach before extubation is, therefore, of questionable value.

Elective Cesarean Delivery

1. The patient scheduled for cesarean delivery should routinely fast for at least 6 hours before induction of general anesthesia.
2. Sodium citrate adequately alkalinizes gastric contents in these women.
3. Studies suggest that various regimens of H_2-receptor blockers, antacids, and metoclopramide may decrease the number of women "at risk" for acid-aspiration pneumonitis (i.e., gastric aspirate volume greater than 25 mL or pH less than 2.5). However, none will alter anesthetic management—all parturients still require a rapid sequence induction with cricoid pressure.

Positioning

Uterine Displacement

Always provide uterine displacement to avoid supine hypotension. Methods of uterine displacement are not as important as their routine and vigilant practice.

Optimal Airway Management

1. Before all cesarean sections, take time to ensure optimal alignment of the shoulders, neck, and head ("sniffing" position). This step will maximize the chances of successful intubation and help emergency airway management, should it become necessary.
2. Blankets are ubiquitous in the delivery suite. Even the extremely obese parturient can be optimally positioned using folded and stacked blankets to support the upper back and maternal occiput (see Chapter 19, Fig. 19.1).

Monitoring and Equipment

The parturient undergoing cesarean section requires the same types of intraoperative monitoring as any patient having emergency intraabdominal surgery.

Airway/Breathing

1. End-tidal gas analysis is essential in the management of the patient under general anesthesia.
   a. Measuring end-tidal nitrogen (or oxygen) can document adequate denitrogenation before rapid sequence induction of anesthesia.
   b. Capnography helps confirm proper position of the tracheal tube.
   c. Intraoperative capnometry aids in monitoring maternal ventilation. Maternal hyperventilation and hypocapnia may hinder uterine blood flow and placental gas exchange.
2. In the term parturient, decreased alveolar dead space and increased alveolar ventilation combine to lower the end-tidal to arterial carbon dioxide gradient toward zero.

Circulation

1. A freely flowing, securely fastened, large-bore (at least 18-gauge) peripheral intravenous catheter should be *in situ* before induction of general anesthesia for routine cesarean delivery. Certain high-risk conditions as well as changing

intraoperative surgical conditions may demand additional
intravenous access.
- a. Occasionally, peripheral intravenous access is impossible.
- b. Keep an adequate supply of disposable central venous
access kits immediately available.
2. Have equipment available for rapid infusion of warmed,
intravenous fluids.
3. The ability to transduce intraarterial and central venous
pressures, as well as to measure cardiac output, is vital in
the management of certain obstetric or coexisting medical
conditions.

Fetus
1. Monitor fetal heart rate electronically until surgical preparation of the abdomen or even induction of anesthesia (if an
internal scalp electrode is already in place).
2. Any change in fetal heart rate can be evaluated by the perinatal team.
- a. Signs of rapid intrauterine deterioration can increase
the urgency of delivery.
- b. The diagnosis of acute fetal distress can be reevaluated
on arrival in the operating room, sometimes eliminating
the need for immediate surgery.

Preoxygenation and Denitrogenation
1. Filling the lungs with oxygen prolongs the interval from
onset of apnea to hypoxemia and is a critical part of a rapid
sequence induction for any emergent surgical patient.
2. The gravida has a decreased apnea to hypoxemia time.
- a. Functional residual capacity is smaller (thus the reservoir of oxygen in the lungs after the onset of apnea is
smaller).
- b. At term, oxygen consumption increases 20% to 30%.
- c. Especially in the supine position, airway closure occurs
during tidal breathing, increasing shunt fraction and
producing hypoxemia.
3. Denitrogenation occurs more rapidly in parturients.
- a. Decreased functional residual capacity
- b. Increased minute ventilation
4. Two common methods of preoxygenation and denitrogenation:
- a. Four vital capacity breath hyperventilation.
- b. Three-minute tidal volume breathing.
- i. Both produce a similar rise in p_aO_2 and a similar
fall in oxygen saturation desaturation during
apnea (an average duration of 50 seconds).
- ii. Four vital capacity breath hyperventilation does
not wash out nitrogen as effectively as 3-minute
tidal volume breathing (5% end-tidal nitrogen vs.
1%). The extra margin of safety (10 to 15 additional seconds of apnea) provided before hypoxemia, however, is clinically insignificant.
- c. Unless a tight mask fit is ensured, room air (and, therefore, nitrogen) is entrained into the breathing circuit.
Alveolar oxygen concentration then becomes unpredictable.

Pretreatment/Defasciculation

Fasciculation

1. Pregnancy, as early as in the first trimester, decreases the incidence and severity of fasciculation.
2. At term, the incidence of fasciculation decreases to 9%.
3. Pretreatment with d-tubocurarine (0.05 mg per kilogram) does not further reduce this incidence.

Myalgia

1. At term, only 7.5% to 13% of women report postoperative myalgia.
2. Pretreatment with d-tubocurarine does not decrease the incidence of postoperative myalgia.

Action of Succinylcholine

1. In term parturients, pretreatment with d-tubocurarine does not alter the onset of succinylcholine neuromuscular blockade.
2. Paralysis lasts 120 to 150 seconds longer in non-pretreated patients.
   a. This prolongation of neuromuscular paralysis is of questionable clinical significance.
   b. The time to recovery is short enough to have the patient begin spontaneous (or assisted) ventilation before the end of surgery, but it is still far longer than a patient will tolerate during a difficult intubation.
3. I see no benefit to pretreatment. Omit it when inducing general anesthesia for cesarean delivery.

INTRAVENOUS INDUCTION AGENTS (TABLE 14.3)

Thiopental/Thiamylal

1. In the United States, thiopental (or its analog, thiamylal) is the most frequently used drug for induction of general anesthesia for cesarean delivery.
2. The mean dose of thiopental needed to induce general anesthesia (3.5 mg per kilogram pregnant body weight) is 35% less than the mean induction dose needed in nonpregnant patients.[2]
3. Fetal effects
   a. Kinetics
      i. Thiopental appears in fetal blood within 45 seconds of maternal administration.
      ii. Fetal drug concentrations peak 1.5 to 3.0 minutes after induction.
      iii. Rapid maternal redistribution and nonuniform intervillous blood flow lead to a wide variability in measured umbilical venous (UV) and maternal venous (MV) blood thiopental concentrations. Neither UV nor MV thiopental concentrations correlate with induction-to-delivery times.
      iv. Uptake by the fetal liver and dilution with systemic venous blood further decrease fetal arterial thiopental concentration.
      v. Barbiturate can still be measured in the maternal blood up to 9 hours after delivery, and minute concentrations are measurable in the colostrum.

Table 14.3.   General anesthesia for cesarean delivery: induction agents

Drug	Dose	Maternal Effects	Neonatal Effects
Thiopental/ thiamylal	4 mg/kg		Low Apgar scores with dose >7 mg/kg
Methohexital	1 mg/kg		Increased incidence of low Apgar scores, a prolonged time to sustained respiration
Ketamine	1.0–1.5 mg/kg	Hypertension, tachycardia, decreased recall, increased dreaming	>2 mg/kg increased neonatal depression
Etomidate	0.3 mg/kg	Pain on injection, myoclonus	Slightly increased umbilical venous base deficit, a possible neonatal adrenal suppression
Midazolam	0.2–0.3 mg/kg	0 (%) recall	± Increased incidence of low 1-min Apgar scores, a transient postdelivery hypotonus
Propofol	2.0–2.8 mg/kg	Cutaneous rash, pain on injection	± Transient neurobehavioral changes

b. A single 4- to 7-mg per kilogram bolus of thiobarbiturate does not affect Apgar scores. A maternal induction dose of 8 mg per kilogram will increase the number of Apgar scores less than 7.

4. I usually use thiopental/thiamylal 5 mg per kilogram to induce general anesthesia for cesarean delivery.

Methohexital

1. Methohexital is 2.5 to 3.0 times as potent as thiopental.
2. An induction dose of methohexital greater than 1 mg per kilogram has been associated with an increased number of low Apgar scores and a delayed time to sustained respiration.

Ketamine

1. Advantages
    a. Supports maternal blood pressure. This may be important in the face of significant maternal hemorrhage.
    b. It induces peripheral catecholamine release, which may improve or prevent bronchospasm in asthmatic patients.
    c. It appears to lower the incidence of intraoperative maternal awareness.
    d. Compared with thiopental, induction of general anesthesia with ketamine may decrease postoperative morphine requirements.
2. Disadvantages
    a. Dose-dependent maternal hypertension: Although perhaps best avoided in parturients who may not tolerate hypertension at induction (i.e., preeclampsia or coexisting neurosurgical disease), in elective cesarean delivery, ketamine 1 mg per kilogram does not increase maternal blood pressure at induction or intubation any higher than does thiopental 4 mg per kilogram.
    b. Dreaming/dysphoria
3. Fetal effects
    a. Ketamine concentrations in umbilical blood peak 1 to 2 minutes after maternal intravenous administration.
    b. Apgar scores are similar in neonates delivered abdominally after induction of anesthesia with ketamine 1 mg per kilogram or thiopental 3 mg per kilogram.
    c. Induction of general anesthesia with ketamine 2 mg per kilogram is associated with neonatal depression.

Etomidate

1. Advantages
    a. Rapid onset
    b. Short duration (quickly hydrolyzed to an inactive substance)
    c. Production of little cardiorespiratory change
2. Disadvantages
    a. Frequent pain on injection and myoclonus
    b. The incidence of myoclonus may be lower during rapid sequence induction due to succinylcholine paralysis.
3. Kinetics
    a. Readily crosses the placenta

b. The concentration in maternal blood is nil by 2 hours after induction.
c. Only a very small amount is found in the colostrum.
4. Fetal effects
    a. Compared with thiopental 3.5 mg per kilogram, etomidate 0.3 mg per kilogram is associated with a slight increase in umbilical vein base deficit versus thiopental (−6.5 versus −4.7). This effect has questionable clinical significance.
    b. Early neonatal adrenal suppression also has been reported after maternal etomidate.

Midazolam

1. Midazolam 0.2 to 0.3 mg per kilogram is an effective induction agent for cesarean delivery.
2. Comparison with thiopental 3.5 to 4.0 mg per kilogram
    a. A slightly greater (8 mm Hg) maternal diastolic blood pressure during induction
    b. No difference in induction time (time to loss of maternal lid reflex after injection of midazolam) or the duration of postanesthetic recovery
3. Fetal effects
    a. Midazolam crosses the placenta less rapidly than does thiopenta.
    b. Lower 1-minute Apgar scores versus thiopental induction. (Twenty percent of neonates [5 of 26] delivered after induction of general anesthesia with midazolam had low Apgar scores [and 3 of the 5 needed tracheal intubation and intermittent positive-pressure ventilation] versus 4% after thiopental.[3] This difference in 1-minute Apgar scores was not seen in another comprehensive study of midazolam.[4])
    c. Funic blood acid–base analysis and time to sustained respiration are similar in neonates delivered after induction of general anesthesia with either drug.
    d. Neurobehavioral scores may be transiently depressed compared with thiopental.
    e. The average elimination half-life in neonates is shorter for midazolam than for thiopental (6.3 versus 14.7 hours).

Propofol

1. Advantages
    a. Rapid induction
    b. Quick recovery
    c. Better suppression of airway reflexes that thiopental
2. Propofol 2.0 to 2.8 mg per kilogram versus thiopental 4.0 to 5.0 mg per kilogram.
    a. Blood pressure tends to fall more with thiopental.
        i.   This hypotension corrects with tracheal intubation.
        ii. Following intubation, maternal systolic arterial blood pressure rises higher and returns to baseline more slowly after thiopental.
        iii. After induction of general anesthesia with propofol, maternal blood pressure remains 10 to 12 mm

Hg below baseline during the remainder of the predelivery period.

b. There is more pain on injection (up to 37%) with propofol. Occasional patients develop a cutaneous rash.

c. There is no difference in postanesthetic recovery time.

3. Fetal effects
   a. Propofol readily crosses the placenta.
   b. Propofol is rapidly cleared from the neonatal circulation.
   c. The number of neonates with low 1-minute Apgar scores (less than 7) after induction of general anesthesia with propofol is similar to that reported after thiopental.
   d. Funic blood acid–base analysis is similar in neonates after induction of general anesthesia with propofol or thiopental.

4. Propofol does not justify its routine use for cesarean delivery. It may be a good choice for the parturient with asthma.

5. Propofol infusions have been used to maintain general anesthesia with or without nitrous oxide.

NEUROMUSCULAR RELAXANTS

All currently used neuromuscular blocking drugs cross the placenta, but their highly ionized, hydrophilic state greatly limits this transfer. The neonate is clinically affected only under unusual conditions.

Succinylcholine

1. Succinylcholine 1.0 to 1.5 mg per kilogram is the most commonly used drug to facilitate tracheal intubation in a rapid sequence induction of general anesthesia for cesarean delivery.

2. Although detectable neonatal concentrations of succinylcholine are possible after routine clinical maternal administration, neonatal paralysis has been reported only in an infant homozygous for atypical serum cholinesterase.

Nondepolarizing Neuromuscular Relaxants

1. Certain maternal conditions (i.e., malignant hyperthermia, cholinesterase deficiency, neurologic disease with upper motor neuron paresis) may contraindicate the use of succinylcholine.

2. Awake tracheal intubation without sedation can be difficult, unpleasant for both patient and anesthesiologist, and potentially deleterious in certain coexisting disease states.

3. Vecuronium
   a. A dose of 0.2 mg per kilogram given in a rapid sequence before thiopental will provide intubating conditions in 156 seconds.
   b. Paralysis lasted almost 2 hours.

4. Rocuronium
   a. A dose of 0.6 mg per kilogram will produce a 50% neuromuscular block within approximately 45 seconds. Latencies until 90% and 100% block are approximately 80 and 105 seconds. At this time, intubating conditions will be good to excellent in most patients.

      b. A dose of 1.2 mg per kilogram will produce a neuromuscular block in even less time.
      c. Either dose will produce neuromuscular paralysis for longer than succinylcholine, a fact to remember if there is any doubt as to the ability to intubate the trachea.
    5. After delivery, any muscle relaxant can be used to maintain paralysis.
    6. A peripheral nerve stimulator helps manage neuromuscular paralysis and reversal.

MAINTENANCE OF ANESTHESIA

Before delivery of the fetus, general anesthesia for cesarean delivery usually includes 50% nitrous oxide in oxygen plus 2/3 MAC volatile agent.

Volatile Agent
1. The specific choice of a volatile agent to maintain anesthesia before delivery is immaterial.
2. Isoflurane, enflurane, halothane, sevoflurane, and desflurane do not alter behavioral or biochemical markers of neonatal outcome.
3. Administering two-thirds of the minimum alveolar concentration (MAC) of the volatile agent ensures maternal amnesia and limits the maternal stress response better than lesser concentrations.
4. Higher concentrations of volatile agent (i.e., 2% halothane) may lower 1-minute Apgar score, umbilical vein pO_2, and pH, and increase umbilical vein base deficit.

Oxygen Concentration
1. Fetal p_aO_2 correlates with maternal F_iO_2.
2. When increasing maternal F_iO_2 above 0.5, a more potent agent must be substituted for the decreasing N_2O. Otherwise, the maternal catecholamine response to "light" anesthesia may decrease uterine blood flow and hinder fetal oxygen delivery.
3. In most cases a maternal F_iO_2 of 0.5 to 0.6 will provide reasonable fetal oxygenation.
4. Consider giving 100% oxygen in emergencies when fetal oxygenation may be compromised.
5. See Table 14.4 for a suggested method of general anesthesia for cesarean delivery.

BLOOD LOSS
1. Volatile anesthetics relax uterine muscle and may produce relative uterine inertia and hemorrhage.
2. In women who have delivered vaginally, oxytocin stimulation produces adequate uterine contraction despite the use of low-dose volatile anesthetic.
3. Clinically, the use of supplemental low-dose (less than 1 MAC) volatile anesthetic to help ensure amnesia does not increase intraoperative blood loss.
4. Several nonrandomized studies have reported more blood loss during cesarean section under general anesthesia com-

Table 14.4. Suggested technique for general anesthesia for cesarean section

Premedication
    Thirty milliliters of 0.3-M sodium citrate (or its equivalent) PO within 15 minutes of induction

Positioning
    Uterine displacement
    Arrange shoulders and neck in "sniffing" position

Monitors and special equipment
    Electrocardiography
    Noninvasive blood pressure
    Pulse oximetry
    Temperature
    Peripheral nerve stimulator
    Oxygen analyzer
    Capnometry
    Bladder catheter
    Forced warm air, warming blanket (for operations >1 h)

Induction (in delivery room, after surgeon ready to make incision)
    Preoxygenation (high-flow 100% oxygen, tight-fitting face mask)
    Three-minute tidal volume breathing, or
    Four vital capacity breaths
    Rapid sequence intravenous induction with cricoid pressure
    Thiopental 5 mg/kg pregnant body weight (PBW) IV
    Succinylcholine 1.5 mg/kg PBW IV
    Tracheal intubation and inflation of cuff, check breath sounds, and check far capnographic evidence of expired carbon dioxide
    Begin surgery

Maintenance
    Before delivery
    Nitrous oxide/oxygen 50:50 with 0.67 MAC volatile agent
    Nondepolarizing muscle relaxant, as needed
    After delivery
    Nitrous oxide/oxygen 70:30
    Intravenous opioid (i.e., morphine sulfate, 0.2–0.5 mg/kg, as tolerated according to maternal hemodynamics)
    Intermediate duration nondepolarizing neuromuscular blocker), as needed

Emergence and recovery
Extubation
Fully reactive and awake
Five-second headlift
Supplemental oxygen
Monitoring (recovery room)
Pulse oximetry

Table 14-4.   (*continued*)

Continuous electrocardiography

Blood pressure

Titrate intravenous analgesic to patient comfort, begin intravenous patient-controlled analgesia (PCA) infusion (i.e., morphine sulfate, 2-mg bolus; 10-min lockout; 1-h maximum of 10 mg), PCA protocol orders

Discharge from recovery room by usual criteria

Follow-up note the next day and thereafter, as indicated

---

pared with regional anesthesia. There are at least two possible explanations for these data:
   a. General anesthesia may increase blood loss.
   b. Patients who receive general anesthesia (i.e., emergency procedures, women with placenta previa) may be at increased risk of blood loss during surgery (selection bias).
5. Transfusion therapy has evolved as physicians (and the public) focus on the transmission of blood-borne pathogens.
   a. In some centers, the use of blood and blood products has decreased considerably.
   b. Massive transfusion (greater than 5 U of packed red cells) is usually complicated by coexisting obstetric conditions associated with hemorrhage (i.e., abnormal placentation, coagulopathy after abruption or with preeclampsia, and emergency surgery).

AWARENESS
1. Awareness, dreaming, and recall have been described in the parturient under general anesthesia.
   a. Maternal drug dose for general anesthesia during cesarean delivery is chosen to limit potential neonatal effects.
   b. The short induction-to-incision time often leaves the anesthesiologist with a "lightly" anesthetized mother.
   c. The incidence of dreaming varies between 0% and 25%. The incidence of dreaming seems to depend on the emergent nature of the delivery and perhaps the emotional state of the mother before induction of general anesthesia.
   d. The following may influence the incidence of awareness and recall:
        i.   Choice of induction agent.
        ii. Technique for anesthetic maintenance before delivery of the fetus.
        iii. Time from anesthetic induction to delivery.
        iv. The possible emergency nature of delivery.
        v.   The method of detection of intraoperative awareness.

Thiopental and Ketamine
1. Up to 60% of parturients will be aware (purposeful movements of an isolated limb) after thiopental 4 mg per kilo-

gram (plus 0.67 MAC volatile agent to and 50% nitrous oxide/oxygen or 100% oxygen for general anesthesia before delivery of the fetus). The addition of ketamine 0.5 mg per kilogram to thiopental 2 mg per kilogram for induction reduces the incidence of awareness by half. Ketamine 1.0- to 1.5-mg per kilogram induction reduces the incidence of awareness to 0% to 20%.

2. Maternal recall is potentially damaging to both the mother (psychologically) and the anesthesiologist (medico-legally, as well as psychologically).
    a. The incidence of recall is reported to be 0% to 18%.
    b. The incidence of recall is seemingly unaffected by the choice of ketamine or thiopental as the induction agent but may be more likely during emergency cesarean delivery.

Propofol

1. Anesthetic induction with propofol 2.3 to 2.5 mg per kilogram followed by maintenance with low-dose halothane in 50% nitrous oxide/oxygen is associated with a 40% incidence of intraoperative awareness.
2. Recall was reported by 0% to 20% of women after induction of general anesthesia with propofol 2.1 to 2.3 mg per kilogram followed by 50% nitrous oxide/oxygen and low-dose isoflurane.

Practical Considerations

1. Isolated limb techniques, lower esophageal contractility, and processed EEG monitors reveal awareness or "light" anesthesia but are poor predictors of maternal recall.
2. If light anesthesia is detected, there may not be any pharmacologic intervention that can "erase" the event.
3. Although explicit recall of stimuli under general anesthesia for cesarean delivery is rare, there is evidence of auditory processing of perioperative stimuli and learning.
4. Consider all parturients at least "aware" of the auditory environment in the operating room.
    a. Limit casual conversation.
    b. Quiet verbal reassurance of the anesthetized parturient is perhaps justified until delivery of the baby and the opportunity to "deepen" the anesthetic.

NEONATAL EFFECTS OF GENERAL ANESTHESIA
Neonatal Evaluation

1. In most prospective studies (with relatively small numbers of patients), general anesthesia produces a similar incidence of depressed neonates (reflected by low 1- and 5-minute Apgar scores) as regional anesthesia.
2. Neonates born to mothers under general anesthesia scored lower on the habituation and orientation items of the Early Neonatal Neurobehavioral Score (ENNS) at 3 hours, but not at 24 hours of life and beyond, compared with neonates born under regional anesthesia.

Preexisting Fetal Condition

1. At elective cesarean delivery, there is a higher frequency of fetal umbilical arterial blood pH less than 7.10 associated with *regional* anesthesia.
2. Very low (less than 4) 1-minute Apgar scores are more common *general* anesthesia.
3. Neonates born under general anesthesia after *nonelective* cesarean delivery are more likely to need oxygen and intubation.
4. Fortunately, anesthetic technique does not correlate with neonatal mortality.

Timing of Delivery

1. Obstetricians should not sacrifice technique for speed during cesarean section under general anesthesia.
2. There is no correlation between clinical or biochemical indices of neonatal outcome and the time between induction and delivery.
3. Increasing the uterine incision-to-delivery (U-D) interval may influence neonatal outcome. Possible reasons for deterioration in neonatal status with increasing U-D interval include:
   a. An acute decrease in uteroplacental perfusion due to uterine artery spasm or venocaval compression during uterine manipulation.
   b. Inhalation of amniotic fluid by the fetus during prolonged delivery.
   c. Fetal head compression during difficult delivery.
4. Fetal condition and maternal disease (i.e., preeclampsia) may be more important than U-D interval in determining neonatal condition at birth.

SUMMARY

1. The scientific basis of the practice of general anesthesia for cesarean delivery is based on human and animal data, but routine practice is more often dictated by tradition, cost, or the choice of the individual anesthesiologist.
   a. Choice of induction agent probably is based on cost and tradition.
      i. Thiopental and ketamine are inexpensive and have a long record of safety.
      ii. Development of newer drugs to induce general anesthesia has had little practical application in obstetric anesthesia.
   b. There is no alternative at present to the use of succinylcholine to facilitate rapid sequence induction and tracheal intubation.
   c. The volatile agents in routine use today are interchangeable.
2. Within the guidelines of routine anesthetic care, fetal outcome depends mostly on preexisting fetal status at the time of cesarean delivery; that is, a healthy term fetus can withstand anesthesia and delivery better than a distressed, preterm fetus.

REFERENCES

1. Hawkins JL, Koonin LM, Palmer SK, Gibbs CP. Anesthesia-related deaths during obstetric delivery in the United States, 1979–1990. *Anesthesiology* 1997;86:277.
2. Gin T, Mainland P, Chan GTV, Short TG. Decreased thiopental requirements in early pregnancy. *Anesthesiology* 1997;86:73.
3. Bland BAR, Lawes KG, Duncan PW, Warnell I, Downing JW. Comparison of midazolam and thiopental for rapid sequence induction for elective cesarean section. *Anesth Analg* 1987;66:1165.
4. Ravlo O, Carl P, Crawford ME, Bach V, Mikkelsen BO, Nielsen HK. A randomized comparison between midazolam and thiopental for elective cesarean section anesthesia. II. Neonates. *Anesth Analg* 1989;68:234.

Epidural Anesthesia
for Cesarean Delivery

1. Because of the growing popularity of epidural analgesia for labor, the use of epidural anesthesia for cesarean section has increased in recent decades.
2. Using an epidural block for cesarean section is a stringent test of the technique because deficiencies in analgesia cannot be covered by the free use of depressant drugs.
3. Despite its considerable popularity, epidural anesthesia has its limitations. Some key issues include:
   a. Maternal hypotension.
   b. Neonatal acidosis.
   c. Postdural puncture headache.
   d. Quality of anesthesia.
   e. Failure rate.

ADVANTAGES OF EPIDURAL ANESTHESIA FOR CESAREAN SECTION

1. Flexibility
   a. With an epidural catheter, the block can be adjusted, prolonged, and even reinitiated, as the clinical situation demands.
   b. The level and density of sensory block can be altered by the selection, volume, and concentration of injected drug(s).
      i. A parturient can receive labor analgesia with a dilute local anesthetic–opioid mixture.
      ii. Incremental injection of more concentrated local anesthetics can rapidly provide surgical anesthesia.
2. Ability to prolong the block
   a. The duration and extent of surgery may be uncertain.
      i. Repeat cesarean section
      ii. Potential cesarean hysterectomy
         (1) While cesarean hysterectomy may last more than 2 hours, parturients with a functioning epidural catheter rarely require intraoperative conversion to general anesthesia.
         (2) Repeated epidural injections of local anesthetic maintain maternal comfort throughout the operation.
3. In addition to intraoperative anesthesia, an epidural catheter also can be used for postoperative analgesia.
4. The gradual onset of epidural blockade may help limit the frequency and severity of maternal hypotension.
   a. Epidural anesthesia has proven safe for the woman with severe preeclampsia.
   b. Similarly, parturients with certain cardiac lesions (i.e., severe aortic stenosis) have a limited ability to respond to sudden hemodynamic changes. Slowly inducing epidural anesthesia while maintaining maternal blood pressure

with fluids and vasopressors is a very effective way to manage these potentially unstable patients.

CONTRAINDICATIONS
Absolute
1. Patient refusal
2. Infection at the site of needle insertion

Controversial
Neurologic Disease
1. Currently available evidence suggests that women with pre-existing neurologic disease can safely receive epidural anesthesia.
2. Deterioration after delivery is more likely related to the natural history of the disease.

Hypovolemia
1. Do not induce epidural anesthesia in a patient who is hypovolemic from acute blood loss.
   a. The combination of sympathectomy and hypovolemia can produce profound hypotension.
2. However, epidural anesthesia is a safe choice if intravascular volume can first be restored and then maintained.

Coagulopathy
1. Unchecked bleeding within the epidural space can cause permanent neurologic injury.
2. Think twice before inducing epidural anesthesia in a patient with a coagulopathy or thrombocytopenia.
3. Potential causes of coagulopathy during pregnancy include:
   a. Preeclampsia.
   b. Abruption.
   c. Fetal demise.
   d. Amniotic fluid embolus.
   e. Iatrogenic (maternal anticoagulation—heparin, coumadin, etc.).

Back Pain
1. Neither intervertebral disc herniation nor back pain precludes epidural anesthesia.
2. Epidural anesthesia does not increase severity of preexisting back pain or the incidence of new postoperative backache.

COMPARISON OF EPIDURAL AND SPINAL BLOCKADE
Although there are obvious similarities between epidural and spinal blockade, there are clinically important differences.

Mechanism of Blockade
1. Spinal blockade is achieved by injection of local anesthetic in the cerebrospinal fluid (CSF). Drug dose and baricity are the key determinants of the extent and duration of spinal anesthesia.
2. With epidural anesthesia, baricity is not a factor.

   a. The extent of block is related to the volume of the drug injected.
   b. The density of block is related to the total mass of drug.

Efficiency
1. Epidural anesthesia for cesarean section may require more time and resources than spinal block.
    a. The time from induction until skin incision is usually longer with epidural anesthesia.
    b. If this time is spent in the operating room, patient charges also may be greater.
2. Although safe induction of the dense sensory and motor block required for cesarean section does take longer with epidural than with spinal anesthesia, the two techniques have multiple similarities.
    a. Both require preanesthetic evaluation, patient consent, intravenous access, proper positioning, insertion of the needle, and injection of the local anesthetic.
    b. With careful selection of local anesthetic and adjuvant agents, the difference in onset can be as short as 10 minutes.

Complications
1. Complications unique to epidural anesthesia include:
    a. Accidental dural puncture and intrathecal catheter placement.
    b. Intravascular placement of needle or catheter.
    c. In some settings, the frequency of inadequate block also is greater with epidural than with spinal anesthesia.

Duration
1. Despite its many advantages, single-injection spinal anesthesia has one major limitation: its finite duration.
2. Because epidural anesthesia can be induced and maintained with an indwelling catheter, it remains the best choice when flexibility and prolonged duration are required.

PHYSIOLOGY OF EPIDURAL BLOCKADE
Mechanism of Action
1. Local anesthetics produce reversible neural blockade by preventing the passage of sodium ions through the nerve membrane.
2. Distribution after injection
    a. When injected into the epidural space, most drug diffuses into the circulation, where is it redistributed to other tissues for metabolism and eventual excretion.
    b. Some drug binds to fatty tissue within the epidural space.
    c. The rest reaches target nerve fibers within the spinal nerves and nerve roots.
3. Two mechanisms account for neural blockade during epidural anesthesia:
    a. Direct blockade at the spinal nerve root.
    b. Local anesthetic diffusion through the dura, arachnoid, and pia mater to reach the spinal cord itself. The concentrations of local anesthetic in the CSF during epidural

anesthesia are similar to those found during spinal anesthesia.

Cardiovascular

1. Sympathetic blockade
   a. A midthoracic level of sympathetic blockade causes vasodilation in both lower extremities and the splanchnic circulation.
      i. Reduction in venous return to the heart decreases cardiac output, which then reduces blood pressure.
      ii. Decreased arteriolar tone plays a lesser role.
   b. Blockade to T4 also impairs left ventricular contractility by inhibiting conduction in afferent cardiac sympathetic nerves. If the block extends to T1 (completely blocking cardiac sympathetic nerve fibers), heart rate may slow.

Pulmonary

1. No effect on inspiratory function
2. Expiratory pressures and flow rates are decreased in relation to the degree of impairment of abdominal muscle function.
   a. Midthoracic blockade by using 2% lidocaine with epinephrine decreases peak expiratory pressure by 45%.
   b. Bupivacaine decreases expiratory pressure by only 10%.
   c. Once cesarean section begins, expiratory flow rates decrease considerably.
3. Subjective dyspnea may develop if the level of sensory blockade exceeds T2.
   a. About 5% of women having epidural anesthesia for cesarean section report this symptom.
   b. Its etiology is probably the lack of proprioceptive input from the chest wall and intercostal musculature.
   c. Reassurance is the most appropriate treatment.

Endocrine

Epidural anesthesia blunts the endocrine stress response to cesarean section. Increases in plasma concentrations of cortisol, catecholamines, and blood glucose are less with epidural compared with general anesthesia.

Hematologic

1. In orthopedic patients, epidural anesthesia decreases the risk of venous thrombosis and postoperative pulmonary embolism.
2. Epidural anesthesia also decreases intraoperative blood loss compared with general anesthesia. Epidural anesthesia-related hypotension only partially explains this effect, as blood loss does not always correlate with intraoperative blood pressure.

Obstetric

Epidural anesthesia lacks any consistent effects on uterine, intervillous, or umbilical blood flow. Maternal hypotension and the use of epinephrine-containing local anesthetics are exceptions.

LOCAL ANESTHETIC
Amides
1. Although many local anesthetics are available for epidural anesthesia, not all are suitable for use in obstetrics.
   a. Mepivacaine and prilocaine rapidly induce profound anesthesia of moderate duration.
      i. Mepivacaine produces less vasodilation than does lidocaine. This effect delays its absorption from the epidural space and prolongs its duration.
      ii. Mepivacaine metabolism is markedly prolonged in the fetus, and significant neonatal neurobehavioral effects have been reported.
      iii. Large doses of prilocaine (greater than 600 mg) can cause methemoglobinemia, ruling out its use for cesarean section.
   b. Etidocaine rapidly produces long-lasting sensory and motor blockade, but profound motor block can long outlast sensory analgesia.

Lidocaine
1. Lidocaine's potency, rapid onset, and moderate duration make it one of the most commonly used drugs for epidural anesthesia. Both 1.5% and 2.0% concentrations are used for cesarean section.
2. Intrathecal lidocaine may be neurotoxic.
   a. Cauda equina syndrome has been reported after the subarachnoid injection of 2% lidocaine through a misplaced catheter.
   b. These cases emphasize the importance of intrathecal test doses and the need for careful management of recognized spinal catheters.

Bupivacaine
1. Advantages
   a. Provides anesthesia of slow onset and long duration
   b. Produces relatively greater-intensity sensory than motor blockade
2. Bupivacaine is more cardiotoxic than lidocaine.
   a. Both drugs depress intracardiac conduction by blocking sodium channels. However, bupivacaine binds to the open sodium channel for much longer than lidocaine, making it 16 times more potent than lidocaine in reducing cardiac contractility and conductivity.
   b. The high maternal mortality associated with unrecognized intravenous bupivacaine injection probably relates to the difficulties involved in resuscitating a parturient, not to the greater intrinsic toxicity of bupivacaine in parturients.
3. A 0.5% concentration is used for cesarean section. Although a 0.75% concentration is available, the Food and Drug Administration (FDA) rescinded its approval for use in obstetrics because of a high incidence of cardiac complications.

Ropivacaine
1. A new amide local anesthetic structurally similar to mepivacaine and bupivacaine (Fig. 15.1).

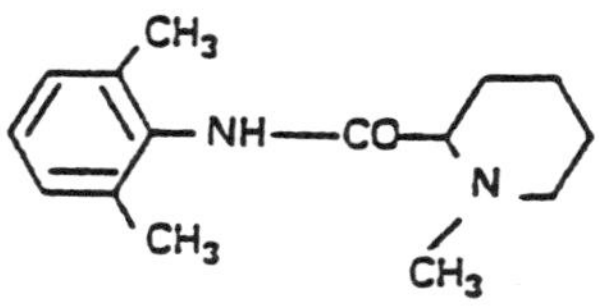

Mepivacaine

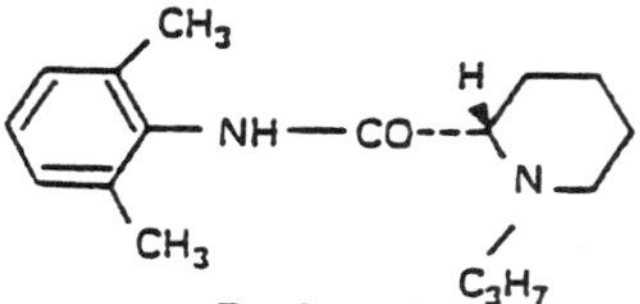

Ropivacaine

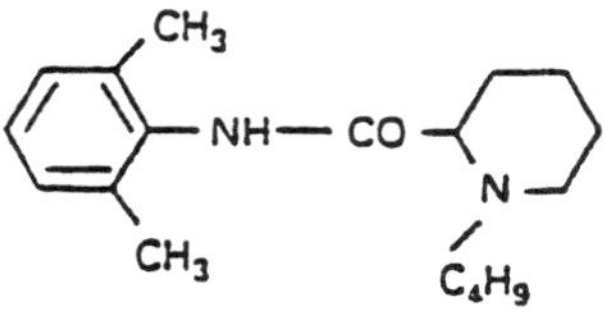

Bupivacaine

Figure 15.1. Ropivacaine is an amide local anesthetic in the same family as mepivacaine and bupivacaine. One basic structural difference is seen on the piperidine nitrogen of the respective molecules, as bupivacaine has a butyl group; mepivacaine, a methyl group; and ropivacaine, a propyl group. A second important distinction relates to the fact that this group of drugs is chiral, with an asymmetric carbon atom in the amine ring, resulting in two mirror-image forms of the compounds. Both mepivacaine and bupivacaine are racemic mixtures, containing equal amounts of the *r*- and *s*-enantiomers, whereas ropivacaine is produced solely as the *s* form.

2. It is the first local anesthetic prepared as the pure *s*-enantiomer.
    a. Previous amide local anesthetics have been prepared as racemic mixtures.
    b. Although both enantiomers of bupivacaine have similar local anesthetic actions, the *d*-enantiomer is considerably more cardiotoxic.
    c. The *s*-enantiomer preparation of ropivacaine is markedly less cardiotoxic than racemic bupivacaine.
3. Ropivacaine is available in 0.2%, 0.5%, 0.75%, and 1.0% concentrations. The FDA approved only the 0.5% concentration for cesarean section.

4. Ropivacaine 0.5% versus bupivacaine 0.5% at cesarean section
   a. Both produce similar sensory anesthesia.
   b. The duration of motor block is significantly shorter after ropivacaine.
   c. Neonatal outcome and umbilical cord blood–gas tensions are similar.

Esters

1. The only clinically useful ester local anesthetic for cesarean section under epidural anesthesia is 3% 2-chloroprocaine. This drug is short acting, not very potent, and unlikely to cause systemic toxicity. When used for elective cesarean section, 2-chloroprocaine has no detectable adverse maternal or neonatal effects. The *in vitro* maternal and fetal plasma half-lives of 2-chloroprocaine are 11 and 15 seconds, respectively. The *in vivo* half-life in maternal plasma is 3 minutes. Because fetal acidosis does not increase the placental transfer of 2-chloroprocaine, it may be a good choice for the mother with a possibly asphyxiated fetus.

2. In the 1980s, prolonged neurologic deficits were reported after unrecognized subarachnoid injection of large volumes of 2-chloroprocaine. 2-Chloroprocaine, at low pH, when combined with sodium bisulfite, produced irreversible conduction blockade in isolated nerve fibers. 2-Chloroprocaine alone or sodium bisulfite 0.2% at physiologic pH produced no signs of irreversible toxicity. Possibly, sulphur dioxide, liberated from the bisulfite at a low pH diffused into the nerve membrane and formed sulfurous acid, which caused the damage. Also, rapid administration of large volumes of fluid into the subarachnoid space, in the presence of systemic hypotension, decreased spinal cord perfusion and produced signs of cord ischemia.

3. The manufacturer replaced the sodium metabisulfite preservative with the calcium chelator, EDTA. Unfortunately, binding of calcium by EDTA produced hypocalcemic tetany in the paraspinous muscles and reports of severe spasmodic back pain after large doses of this preparation of 2-chloroprocaine. A new preservative-free preparation is now available.

4. 2-Chloroprocaine impairs the analgesic efficacy of subsequently administered epidural opioids. This effect is seen with both morphine and fentanyl. 2-Chloroprocaine prevents the analgesic effects of fentanyl, even after the local anesthetic-induced epidural block has receded. Although the mechanism of this effect is unclear, 2-chloroprocaine binds to, but does not activate, μ- and κ-receptors.

5. 2-Chloroprocaine also impairs the action of bupivacaine if the two agents are used together or sequentially. A mixture of 2-chloroprocaine and bupivacaine produces shorter acting epidural analgesia than does bupivacaine alone. In the isolated rat sciatic nerve, a metabolite of 2-chloroprocaine persists after recovery from neural blockade and interferes with the subsequent action of bupivacaine.

ADJUVANT AGENTS

Many anesthesiologists add a variety of compounds to the local anesthetic used for cesarean section epidural anesthesia. These drugs aim to speed the onset, enhance the quality, and prolong the duration of epidural local anesthetic blockade.

Epinephrine

1. A vasoconstrictor that decreases the rate of vascular absorption of some local anesthetics. This effect allows more anesthetic to reach sites of action within the nerve membrane and improves the density and duration of anesthesia.
2. In addition to its vasoconstrictor action, epinephrine enhances epidural local anesthetics by a direct action on α_2-adrenergic receptors in the dorsal horn of the spinal cord.
3. Epinephrine 2.5 to 5.0 µg per milliliter (1:400,000 to 1:200,000) will significantly improve the quality of anesthesia provided by 2% lidocaine.
4. Epinephrine has an inconsistent effect on the anesthesia provided by 0.5% bupivacaine.
5. Systemic absorption of epinephrine after epidural injection induces hemodynamic changes related to the drug's β-agonist action.
   a. Vasodilation decreases systemic vascular resistance and blood pressure.
   b. Heart rate increases in response to the decrease in blood pressure as well as to epinephrine's direct chronotropic action.
   c. α-Agonist actions also may occur.
      i. Epidural injection of epinephrine-containing local anesthetics in patients with underlying uteroplacental insufficiency increases placental vascular resistance.
      ii. In women with severe preeclampsia, epidural epinephrine may contribute to maternal hypertension.
6. Commercially available epinephrine-containing local anesthetic solutions are buffered to a pH of 3.5 to prevent oxidation of the epinephrine.
   a. Solutions without epinephrine are buffered to a higher pH (5.0) and have a shorter latency.
   b. The onset of lidocaine with epinephrine can be hastened either by adding epinephrine to the plain drug shortly before use or by increasing the pH of the commercial preparation with sodium bicarbonate.
7. Clinical recommendations
   a. Only add epinephrine to lidocaine.
   b. Use the lowest effective concentration (1:400,000).
   c. If using a commercially prepared solution, add $NaHCO_3$ to speed onset.

Other α_2-Agonists

1. Other α_2-agonists also produce analgesia after epidural injection.
2. The most extensively studied of these drugs is clonidine.
   a. Like epinephrine, epidural clonidine prolongs the duration of motor blockade associated with epidural local anesthetics.

   b. Epidural clonidine decreases maternal heart rate and blood pressure. With larger doses, maternal sedation, which can be associated with snoring, obstructive apnea, and episodes of arterial oxygen desaturation, occurs.

Opioids
Fentanyl and Sufentanil
1. Improve intraoperative analgesia and provide some post-operative analgesia
2. Animal studies suggest that visceral nociceptors are more sensitive than somatic ones to the synergistic interaction of local anesthetics and opioids.
3. Fentanyl
   a. The addition of fentanyl to epidural bupivacaine may hasten the onset of sensory blockade.
   b. Fentanyl 100 μg does not change the duration of sensory or motor blockade produced by 0.5% bupivacaine. However, fentanyl significantly improves the quality of intraoperative analgesia. Intravenous fentanyl may be equally as effective.
   c. Epidural fentanyl 100 μg lacks detectable adverse maternal or neonatal effects.
4. Sufentanil has similar effects. Large doses of sufentanil (i.e., greater than 50 μg) can produce mild neonatal neurobehavioral depression.

Morphine
1. Has a longer latency than fentanyl or sufentanil
2. Can provide prolonged postoperative analgesia
3. In some studies, morphine also improves intraoperative analgesia.

Clinical Recommendations
   I routinely add fentanyl 100 μg to the final dose of epidural bupivacaine when providing anesthesia for cesarean section. Lidocaine with epinephrine provides good intraoperative anesthesia without additional opioids. The ability of epidural fentanyl to improve the quality of 2-chloroprocaine anesthesia remains unproved.

Sodium Bicarbonate
1. Increasing the pH of the local anesthetic speeds the onset of bupivacaine, lidocaine, and 2-chloroprocaine neural blockade.
   a. 2-Chloroprocaine and lidocaine are readily alkalinized to near physiologic pH without precipitation by adding sodium bicarbonate.
   b. Bupivacaine precipitates with the addition of small amounts of sodium bicarbonate.
2. Sodium bicarbonate may speed the onset of local anesthetic blockade by increasing the acidity of the nerve cytoplasm. (Fig. 15.2).

SOME TECHNICAL CONSIDERATIONS
The Appropriate Sensory Level
1. The needed level of sensory blockade for cesarean section varies from T8 to T2.

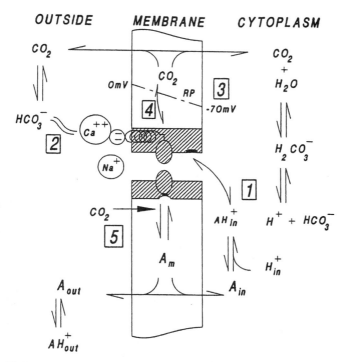

Figure 15.2. Sodium bicarbonate increases the speed of onset of local anesthetics not by increasing the pH of the solution closer to the pKa, as had been previously thought, but by increasing the acidity of the nerve cytoplasm, leading to trapping of the cationic form of local anesthetic. The carbon dioxide formed also modifies the sodium channel, influencing binding. Bicarbonate leads to sodium channel inactivation, a channel conformation known to bind local anesthetic more tightly. (Source: Reprinted from Wong K, Strichartz GR, Raymond SA. On the mechanisms of potentiation of local anesthetics by bicarbonate buffer: drug structure-activity studies on isolated peripheral nerve. *Anesth Analg* 1993;76:131, with permission.)

    a. Some of this variation is explained by operative technique (exteriorizing the uterus for repair requires a higher level of block).

    b. Pain sensations from pelvic organs enter the spinal cord at T10 to L1.

    c. Some pelvic nerves accompany sympathetic fibers through the various intraabdominal plexi and the greater splanchnic nerve to reach the spinal cord as high as T4.

    d. Visceral pain also arises from other intraabdominal structures, such as the peritoneum, which are innervated by sensory afferents that enter the spinal cord as far cephalad as T4.

2. The lower extent of sensory blockade also is important.
   a. Another cause of visceral pain during cesarean section is incomplete block of the large nerve roots of L5 to S2.
   b. Blocking of these roots is required to prevent pain from traction on the uterosacral ligaments or bladder.

Perioperative Management

1. Preoperative evaluation
   a. As with all anesthetics, evaluate parturients who are to receive epidural anesthesia preoperatively.
   b. A focused history and physical evaluation should include:
      i. Maternal health history.
      ii. Anesthesia-related obstetric and surgical history.
      iii. Evaluation of airway and back.
      iv. Baseline blood pressure.
   c. Explain the procedure and possible complications and obtain informed consent.
2. Aspiration prophylaxis
   a. All parturients are at high risk of regurgitation and aspiration of stomach contents. While choosing regional over general anesthesia will decrease this risk, it does not eliminate it.
      i. Blocks fail.
      ii. Excessive sensory blockade or profound maternal hypotension can impair airway reflexes and consciousness.
   b. Give 30 mL 0.3 M sodium citrate within 15 minutes of induction of epidural anesthesia for cesarean section.
3. Equipment and setting
   a. Have appropriate resuscitation equipment available.
      i. Essentials are a means of positive-pressure ventilation, an oxygen source, and suction.
      ii. Monitoring consists of blood pressure, heart rate, and pulse oximetry.
   b. Have a vasopressor, usually ephedrine, readily available.
4. Insert epidural catheter (see Chapter 11)
5. The test dose
   a. Unrecognized intrathecal or intravenous injection of local anesthetics can prove fatal.
   b. Inspection, aspiration, and incremental injection of the catheter are essential to prevent these complications.
      i. When using a multiorifice catheter, inspection and aspiration will detect the vast majority of intravenous catheters.
      ii. Incremental injection will ensure that patients do not suffer systemic toxicity from unrecognized intravenous injection.
6. Patient position
   a. Have the parturient lie supine with left uterine displacement.
   b. Provide left uterine displacement either with some type of wedge (a 1-L bag of IV fluid works well) or by tilting the operating table to the left (my preference).

  c. Rare patients will become hypotensive with *left* uterine displacement, but will recover with *right* uterine displacement.

7. Monitor the fetus
  a. Document fetal heart tones during induction of anesthesia but before preparation of the surgical site for incision.

8. Intravenous fluids
  a. Prophylactic intravenous fluids may not prevent or decrease the frequency of hypotension.
  b. Intravenous fluids remain the first treatment for hypotension.
  c. The intravenous solution should not contain dextrose. Rapid dextrose infusion produces maternal hyperglycemia, hyperinsulinemia, and an increase in blood lactate. Neonatal hyperglycemia and then hypoglycemia follow shortly after delivery.

9. Choose a local anesthetic
  a. For elective or urgent cesarean section
    i. 0.5% Bupivacaine, 0.5% ropivacaine, 3% 2-chloroprocaine, or 1.5% to 2.0% lidocaine with epinephrine.
    ii. Give one of these drugs in 3 to 5-mL aliquots until a T4 sensory level is achieved.
      (1) Bupivacaine and ropivacaine require 30 minutes to achieve a T4 sensory level.
      (2) Usually 20 to 30 mL of drug will produce an adequate level of sensory block for cesarean section.
      (3) For laboring patients, inject 10 to 15 mL of drug in the labor room while the patient is being prepared for surgery. Once the anesthetic level begins to rise, transport the patient to the operating room. Inject the final bolus shortly after transfer of the patient to the operating table.
  b. For emergent cesarean section
    i. Use either 1.5% to 2.0% lidocaine with epinephrine, or 3% 2-chloroprocaine.
    ii. Inject the drug in divided doses over 2 to 3 minutes, while constantly questioning the patient about symptoms of intravascular or intrathecal injection.
    iii. Always aspirate before each incremental injection.
    iv. In laboring women receiving a continuous epidural infusion of local anesthetic and opioid, 2% or 1.5% lidocaine with epinephrine produces surgical anesthesia in approximately 4 minutes. 3% 2-Chloroprocaine has a slightly faster onset, approximately 2 to 3 minutes.
  c. Adjuvant agents
    i. Epinephrine
      (1) Add to lidocaine to improve quality of block. (Epinephrine lacks clinically significant benefits when added to bupivacaine, ropivacaine, or 2-chloroprocaine.

(2) Commercially prepared epinephrine-containing local anesthetic solutions are buffered to a low pH and will have a delayed onset. To speed onset, either add epinephrine directly to plain solutions of local anesthetic or add $NaHCO_3$ to commercially prepared solutions.

ii. $NaHCO_3$ will speed the onset of lidocaine or 2-chloroprocaine

iii. Fentanyl

(1) Improves surgical anesthesia when added to bupivacaine or lidocaine. Efficacy when added to ropivacaine or 2-chloroprocaine is either unclear or not yet studied.

(2) Also effective when 100 μg to final bolus of local anesthetic.

iv. Morphine

(1) Provides prolonged postoperative analgesia.

(2) Inject 2 to 3 mg after delivery.

10. Supplemental oxygen

a. Giving supplemental oxygen to the mother before delivery will increase umbilical p_aO_2.

b. Using a nonrebreathing face mask will significantly increase maternal F_iO_2.

11. Intraoperative problems

a. Pain

i. Intraoperative discomfort occurs during 10% to 50% of cesarean section epidural anesthetics.

ii. Causes of intraoperative pain

(1) Breakthrough pain: pain that is perceived despite bilateral sensory blockade. Epidural local anesthetics do not completely block afferent nerve conduction. High-intensity stimuli may overcome otherwise adequate sensory blockade. Available local anesthetics vary in their ability to produce dense sensory block. Lidocaine requires the addition of epinephrine; 0.5% bupivacaine and ropivacaine are often inadequate as sole agents.

(2) Pain conducted through unblocked nerves: Both a T4 upper sensory level and excellent sacral anesthesia are important. In some individuals, peritoneal stimulation may require a sensory block up to T1.

(3) Referred pain: Subdiaphragmatic blood or amniotic fluid produces shoulder pain in up to 6% of patients. Because the sensory innervation of the diaphragm is via the phrenic nerve, it cannot be blocked safely. Placing the operating table in a 5- to 10-degrees head-up tilt (reverse Trendelenburg position) may reduce subdiaphragmatic pooling of blood and amniotic fluid.

(4) Inadequate or uneven sensory blockade: Inadequate block may be due to a misplaced

catheter or to an inadequate dose of local anesthetic. With anterior epidural catheter placement, medial spread of local anesthetic is inhibited by trabeculations between the ventral aspect of the dura and the posterior longitudinal ligament. In the event of unilateral anesthesia, the catheter should be removed and replaced. Unblocked segments are much less common than either unilateral block or a block that does not rise high enough. Additional local anesthetic usually produces anesthesia of these nerve roots.

(5) Unrecognized sensory block regression during surgery is another cause of intraoperative pain. Inject additional local anesthetic via the epidural catheter at regular intervals (every 30 to 45 minutes for lidocaine and 2-chloroprocaine, and every hour for bupivacaine or ropivacaine).

   iii. Prevention and treatment of intraoperative pain

(1) Provide and maintain dense sensory blockade extending from the sacral dermatomes to at least T4.

(2) Treatment depends on the duration and the intensity of pain.

   (a) Inject additional local anesthetic.

   (b) Intravenous or epidural fentanyl 100 μg improves intraoperative analgesia without affecting maternal ventilation or neurobehavior in healthy term infants.

   (c) Nitrous oxide in oxygen in a ratio of 50%:50% provides effective analgesia of rapid onset and offset.

   (d) Intravenous ketamine 0.2 to 0.4 mg per kilogram provides both analgesia and sedation.

   (e) If the epidural block is clearly inadequate, proceed directly to general or spinal anesthesia.

b. Shivering

   i. Approximately 30% of women shiver during cesarean section under epidural anesthesia.

   ii. Current work suggests that shivering is a normal thermoregulatory response to cooling.

(1) Cooling is initially due to redistribution of heat from the core to peripheral tissues.

(2) Later (after 1 hour) cooling is due to heat loss.

(3) Heat loss, but not redistribution, is prevented by forced warm air heating blankets.

c. Nausea and vomiting

   i. Nausea and vomiting from cerebral hypoperfusion are often the first symptoms of hypotension.

      ii.   Other causes of intraoperative nausea and vomiting include peritoneal manipulation, anxiety, and opioids.

     iii.   Preventing hypotension reduces the likelihood of nausea and vomiting.

     iv.   Pretreatment with metoclopramide 10 mg decreases the frequency of nausea and vomiting.

CONDITION OF THE NEWBORN

1. Epidural anesthesia for cesarean section requires the use of large doses of local anesthetic, which readily crosses the placenta and could have significant effects in the newborn.
   a. Most studies report that 1-minute Apgar scores are higher in infants born of mothers who received epidural anesthesia compared with those born of mothers who receive general anesthesia.
   b. Usually by 5 minutes, the difference in Apgar scores disappears.
   c. Most studies report no significant differences in neonatal acid–base status between epidural and general anesthesia for elective cesarean delivery. Maternal hypotension or ephedrine therapy may increase the risk of umbilical acidosis.
2. Maternal drugs may produce more subtle changes in newborn behavior.
   a. Studies usually report better neonatal neurobehavioral status in babies delivered by elective cesarean section under epidural rather than general anesthesia.
   b. These differences usually disappear by 24 hours.
   c. There are no differences in scores among babies whose mothers received epidural lidocaine, bupivacaine, 2-chloroprocaine, or ropivacaine.
3. Urgent cesarean section
   a. With fetal acidosis, blood is redistributed to vital organs such as the heart and brain, and other areas begin anaerobic metabolism.
   b. Local anesthetic concentrations may be higher in the acidotic fetus compared with the nonacidotic fetus.
      i.   The uncharged form of local anesthetic readily crosses the placenta, becoming positively charged in the acidotic fetus.
      ii.   As the local anesthetic is now in the charged form, it is unable to recross the placenta and return to the maternal circulation.
      iii.   The ionic form of the local anesthetic has become "trapped" within the placenta and fetus.

REFERENCE

1. Practice guidelines for obstetrical anesthesia. A report by the American Society of Anesthesiologist's task force on obstetrical anesthesia. *Anesthesiology* 1999;90:600.

Spinal Anesthesia
for Cesarean Delivery

Spinal anesthesia has seen intermittent use in obstetrics since 1900. In the past, a high incidence of hypotension and the risk of headache were serious limitations. Although hypotension is still common, use of intravenous fluids, left uterine displacement, and ephedrine have limited its severity and neonatal impact. The advent of pencil-point spinal needles has greatly reduced the risk of postdural puncture headache.

ADVANTAGES/DISADVANTAGES

Advantages

1. Spinal anesthesia has several advantages over epidural blockade for cesarean section.
   a. The technique is safe, simple, and quick.
      i. Spinal anesthesia produces extensive, profound blockade with a single injection of only 5% to 10% of the amount of drug required for epidural blockade.
         (1) Maternal systemic absorption produces blood drug concentrations of about 5% of those developing with epidural blockade.
         (2) The fetus is exposed to only minute amounts of drug.
      ii. Once you have located the subarachnoid space and injected an appropriate amount of local anesthetic, you are virtually assured of good, dense, bilateral sensory blockade.
      iii. Surgery can begin within 5 to 10 minutes of drug injection. Spinal anesthesia's inherent efficiency can save both time and money.
   b. Epidural anesthesia is a technically complex, potentially dangerous, and time-consuming procedure.
      i. Epidural anesthesia places the patient at risk of dural puncture with a large-gauge needle.
      ii. It involves the injection of potentially lethal doses of local anesthetic.
      iii. The safe induction of epidural anesthesia requires time.
         (1) Drugs are injected in small boluses at 2- to 3-minute intervals.
         (2) Onset of surgical anesthesia can take more than 30 minutes.
2. Spinal anesthesia usually produces better operating conditions than does epidural block.
3. Patients prefer spinal anesthesia.

Disadvantages

1. High block
   a. Sensory blockade occasionally ascends into the cervical region.

b. These high levels of block can impair maternal respiration.

c. Fortunately, diaphragmatic function usually remains intact, and only minor changes in respiratory function develop.

d. Only rarely do sensory and motor block extend high enough to warrant endotracheal intubation.

2. Spinal headache is inseparable from this anesthetic technique. The recent introduction of small-gauge, pencil-point spinal needles has markedly decreased this risk.

3. Maternal hypotension
   a. Frequent
   b. Profound, prolonged hypotension can harm both mother and infant.
   c. Intravenous fluids, careful attention to left uterine displacement, and the judicious use of ephedrine can minimize this problem.

4. Duration
   a. A single subarachnoid injection provides only a finite period of anesthesia.
   b. Sometimes surgery outlasts the anesthetic.
   c. Combined spinal epidural anesthesia is an alternative for possibly prolonged procedures.

INDICATIONS/CONTRAINDICATIONS

1. There are few absolute contraindications to spinal anesthesia:
   a. Maternal refusal.
   b. Uncorrected hypovolemia.
   c. Coagulopathy.
   d. Infection at the site of needle puncture.

2. Many also hesitate to induce spinal anesthesia in a variety of other situations.
   a. Nonreassuring fetal heart rate (FHR) tracing.
      i. Although some argue for the rapid induction of general anesthesia in this setting, spinal anesthesia is often a safe alternative and may have significant advantages.
         (1) General anesthesia offers speed, but induction and intubation impair uterine blood flow.
         (2) In laboring women, spinal anesthesia decreases plasma norepinephrine concentrations and may improve uterine artery blood flow and fetal oxygen supply.
         (3) Induction of general anesthesia also compromises maternal airway reflexes. If the patient proves difficult to intubate, both maternal and fetal hypoxemia may follow.
   b. Maternal hypotension brought on by spinal blockade can worsen fetal condition. In *laboring* women, most studies report a low frequency of maternal hypotension associated with spinal anesthesia.
   c. Clinical studies report little difference in neonatal outcome after emergency cesarean section with regional or general anesthesia.[1]

PHYSIOLOGIC EFFECTS OF SPINAL ANESTHESIA
Central Nervous System

1. Intrathecal local anesthetics block both efferent and afferent nerve conduction.
2. The site and degree of this effect remain unclear.
   a. Efferent blockade
      i. Motor
         (1) Weakness is common with even small doses of intrathecal local anesthetics.
         (2) Even dense abdominal surgical anesthesia may not completely block motor function in the lower extremities.
         (3) Intensity of motor block is related to dose and type of local anesthetic used.
         (4) The addition of epinephrine increases the intensity of motor block.
      ii. Sympathetic impulses
         (1) Small, thinly myelinated, preganglionic sympathetic nerve fibers are more susceptible to local anesthetic blockade than are larger, more heavily myelinated sensory fibers.
         (2) In the cephalad regions of blockade, low concentrations of local anesthetic may block sympathetic but not sensory impulses.
         (3) The exact extent of this "zone of differential blockade" is uncertain.
            (a) Blockade of the ability to perceive cold extends two to three segments above the level of sensory blockade.
            (b) Skin temperature rises six or more segments above the level of sensory block.
            (c) Other methods suggest that spinal anesthesia produces incomplete sympathetic blockade.
               (i) Sweat glands are regulated by the sympathetic nervous system. Their activity can be assessed by measuring changes in skin conductance. These studies suggest that sympathetic nerve activity persists below the level of sensory block.
               (ii) The hemodynamic and catecholamine responses to a cold pressor test (plunging a hand in a bucket of ice-cold water for 2 minutes) also can serve as an index of sympathetic nervous system function.
                  1. Upper thoracic sensory block does not change the heart-rate response to the cold pressor test and

blunts, but does not eliminate, the blood pressure and cardiac index changes.
2. Plasma epinephrine and norepinephrine concentrations increase in some, but not all, patients.
(d) Incomplete blockade of the sympathetic nervous system could explain the occurrence of tourniquet and visceral pain despite the presence of adequate levels of sensory block.
b. Afferent sensory blockade
   i. As with the sympathetic nervous system, somatosensory activity may persist despite the presence of surgical anesthesia.
      (1) Intrathecal bupivacaine prolongs the latency and decreases the amplitude of, but does not eliminate, somatosensory evoked potentials elicited below the level of block.
      (2) Direct spinal cord stimulation can be perceived in the presence of profound peripheral anesthesia.
   ii. These results suggest that the primary site of spinal anesthesia-induced conduction blockade lies within the dorsal root ganglia and spinal rootlets, not in the spinal cord itself.

Cardiovascular System: Hypotension

Spinal anesthesia profoundly alters maternal hemodynamics. Hypotension, the most clinically significant hemodynamic effect of spinal anesthesia, can occur rapidly. If untreated, hypotension can be severe and harm both mother and infant.

Incidence and Severity
1. Varies with definition, frequency of measurement, method of measurement (manual versus automatic cuff), and prophylactic therapy (if any).
2. Significant hypotension complicates 50% to 60% of spinal anesthetics in nonlaboring parturients.
3. Hypotension develops less often in laboring women.
4. In supine parturients, not receiving intravenous fluids, maternal blood pressure decreases by an average of 44%.

Etiology
1. Sympathetic blockade (Fig. 16.1).
   a. Increases venous capacitance.
   b. Decreases arteriolar tone.
   c. Decreases cardiac output.
   d. Mesenteric venodilation from sympathetic blockade of the splanchnic circulation is the most important cause of this increased venous capacitance.
   e. All these effects are more pronounced if the mother lies supine without left uterine displacement.

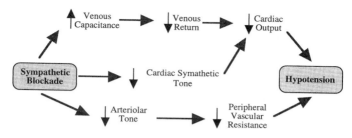

Fig. 16.1.   Mechanism of hypotension during spinal anesthesia.

2.   Cardiac sympathectomy
   a.   Hypotension is more common in patients with sensory blockade above T5 and hence significant blockade of cardiac sympathetic nerves.
   b.   Clinically, some degree of cardioaccelerator fiber blockade develops whenever the level of sensory block extends above T6 to T8.
      i.   In this setting, compensatory tachycardia does not routinely accompany decreases in blood pressure.
      ii.   More commonly, heart rate decreases as blood pressure decreases.

Fetal Effects of Spinal Anesthesia

UTERINE/PLACENTAL BLOOD FLOW
1.   In the absence of significant hypotension, spinal anesthesia lacks significant effect on intravillous blood flow.
2.   Despite the high incidence of maternal hypotension, spinal anesthesia does not produce any consistent changes in uterine artery pulsatility index (a measure of resistance to uterine blood flow).

FETAL BLOOD FLOW
1.   Maternal spinal anesthesia has minimal effects on fetal blood flow.
2.   Fetal aortic or umbilical blood flow and myocardial contractility do not change.
3.   Peripheral, and possibly placental, resistance may decrease.

FETAL/NEONATAL EFFECTS OF MATERIAL HYPOTENSION
1.   The effect of maternal hypotension on the fetus/neonate varies with its severity and duration.
2.   Maternal position, volume status, and drug therapy also may alter the consequences of hypotension.
3.   Severe, prolonged hypotension can lead to fetal bradycardia (Table 16.1).
4.   The fetal effects of transient maternal hypotension are less clear.
   a.   Studies examining neonatal outcome after maternal infusion of dextros containing intravenous fluids often

Table 16.1. Relation between the severity and duration of maternal hypotension after induction of spinal anesthesia and the incidence of fetal bradycardia

Minimal Maternal Systolic BP after Spinal Anesthesia (mm Hg)	No. of Patients	Incidence of Fetal Bradycardia (%)
>100	9	0
90–99	1	0
80–89	0	0
70–79	3	0
60–69	5	20
50–59	8	38
<50	3	67
Duration of Maternal Systolic BP <80 mm Hg (min)		
0–1.9	8	0
2.0–3.9	8	0
4.0–5.9	3	33
>6	9	44

BP, blood pressure.
Source: Data from Ebner H, Barcohana J, Bartoshuk AK. Influence of postspinal hypotension on the fetal electrocardiogram. *Am J Obstet Gynecol* 1960;80:569.

report slightly lower umbilical pH values in infants whose mothers developed transient hypotension versus those whose mothers remained normotensive.

  b. Studies using non–dextrose-containing fluids often find no deleterious effects of transient maternal hypotension.

5. Thus, although severe maternal hypotension may have significant fetal implications, transient decreases in maternal blood pressure are well tolerated. Infants of diabetic mothers may be more sensitive to the maternal hemodynamic effects of spinal anesthesia.

Factors Influencing the Severity of Maternal Hypotension

1. Labor and left uterine displacement probably have the most significant effects on the incidence of hypotension.
2. Anesthesiologists use a variety of strategies to lower the incidence and impact of maternal hypotension.

LABOR

1. Laboring patients are less inclined to develop hypotension than are nonlaboring women.
2. There are several possible explanations for this phenomenon.
  a. Laboring women usually receive intravenous fluids while hospitalized. Thus, these patients may simply be

better hydrated than are those seen for elective cesarean delivery.
- b. Descent of the fetal head into the pelvis lessens aortocaval compression.
    - i. This may improve the subsequent efficacy of left uterine displacement.
    - ii. In addition, left uterine displacement allows the blood (300 mL) squeezed from the uterus with each contraction to reach the maternal central circulation and help support blood pressure.

PATIENT POSITIONING

1. Uterine displacement
    - a. The hemodynamic effects of spinal anesthesia in the parturient are greatly aggravated by aortocaval compression.
    - b. Maintaining adequate left uterine displacement is probably the single most important step in minimizing the maternal and fetal impact of spinal anesthesia–induced hypotension.
2. Head-down tilt
    - a. Trendelenburg positioning is a traditional treatment for spinal anesthesia–induced hypotension.
    - b. Studies in both pregnant and nonpregnant patients show that 10 to 15 degrees of head-down tilt has little or no effect on the blood pressure response to spinal anesthesia.

VOLUME

1. Crystalloid
    - a. Hydration with 1 L of 5% dextrose in Ringer's lactate (D_5RL) (plus an intramuscular injection of 0.4 mg atropine) caused a slight increase in central venous pressure (CVP) but eliminated hypotension after induction of spinal anesthesia in one study.
    - b. Unfortunately, most subsequent studies suggested that prehydration has only limited ability to prevent maternal hypotension.
        - i. Despite infusion of up to 2 L crystalloid solution before induction of spinal anesthesia, over 50% of nonlaboring women will experience at least transient hypotension.
        - ii. Rapid redistribution of crystalloid out of the intravascular space may limit the efficacy of prehydration, although more rapid infusion may produce marked increases in CVP without any effect on the frequency of hypotension.[2]
        - iii. Volume loading not only increases maternal CVP but also increases release of atrial natriuretic peptide (ANP). Vasodilation and diuresis mediated by ANP may help explain the limited ability of prehydration to maintain maternal blood pressure during spinal anesthesia for cesarean section.
    - c. Whereas prehydration does not prevent maternal hypotension, it may blunt the fetal repercussions of

the maternal hemodynamic response to spinal anesthesia.

  i. In one study, increasing the volume of prehydration (from 500 to 999 mL to 1, 000 to 1,500 mL) did not alter incidence or severity of hypotension but did decrease the incidence of umbilical acidemia (uterine vein pH less than 7.20).[3]
  ii. In the less-hydrated group, the lower the maternal pressure, the lower the uterine vein pH and the greater the umbilical vein base deficit. In contrast, maternal hypotension did not correlate with umbilical acid–base status in the better hydrated group.
2. Colloid: As with crystalloids, colloid infusion appears to decrease but not eliminate maternal hypotension during spinal anesthesia for cesarean section.

LEG COMPRESSION

1. May limit hypotension, not by decreasing lower extremity venous capacitance, but by increasing peripheral resistance through compression of postcapillary vessels
2. Leg compression is effective only when relatively high pressures (more than 40 mm Hg) are applied by using either inflatable splints or Esmarch bandages.
3. Thromboembolic stockings, which produce a maximal pressure of 18 mm Hg, lack any effect on the frequency of severity of maternal hypotension.

VASOPRESSORS

1. Ephedrine is the vasopressor of choice in obstetrics. It has been used both to treat and to prevent maternal hypotension.
2. Timing and route of ephedrine administration
   a. Intramuscular ephedrine
      i. Prophylactic injection does not reliably prevent maternal hypotension.
      ii. Occasionally, intramuscular ephedrine induces maternal hypertension.
   b. Intravenous ephedrine
      i. Prophylactic injection (at first decline in maternal blood pressure)
         (1) May limit severity of maternal hypotension and frequency of nausea.
         (2) The effect on fetal acid–base status is unclear.
      ii. Ephedrine infusions may be more effective than intermittent bolus injections. A variable rate infusion (beginning at 5 mg per minute) may be more effective at maintaining maternal blood pressure.
3. Phenylephrine is an appropriate alternative to ephedrine. Consider its use in patients with tachycardia or in those who do not respond to ephedrine.

Summary

1. Spinal anesthesia has profound effects on the maternal cardiovascular system.
2. Expect significant hypotension.

3. Limit the severity and consequences of hypotension by assuring adequate left uterine displacement, infusing dextrose-free intravenous fluids, and using intravenous ephedrine to treat significant decreases in maternal blood pressure.

Respiratory Function
1. Levels of sensory blockade above T6
   a. Little change in forced vital capacity
   b. These levels significantly decrease expiratory flow rate (forced expiratory volume in 1 second and peak expiratory flow rate).
   c. Expiratory flow rates decrease even further with surgery and delivery of the infant.
   d. Epidural anesthesia for cesarean section has similar effects.
2. Pulmonary function remains depressed into the postoperative period.
3. Spinal anesthesia alone does not impair maternal oxygenation or ventilation; however, the interaction between anesthesia, surgery, and maternal respiratory disease may significantly impair the ability of some women to cough and mobilize their airway secretions.

SOME TECHNICAL ISSUES
Patient Preparation
Venous Access
1. Patients having a cesarean section should have a well-functioning, large-bore (at least 18-gauge) intravenous catheter.
2. Remember, cesarean section is a major intraabdominal operation with the potential for significant and rapid blood loss. Women undergoing even routine, elective cesarean delivery lose, on average, 1,000 mL of blood.

Aspiration Prophylaxis
1. These women should receive some type of acid aspiration prophylaxis.
2. I give them 30 mL of sodium citrate by mouth on the way to the operating room.

Prehydration
1. Attitudes toward prehydration have changed significantly in the past few years (see earlier). I no longer infuse large volumes of crystalloid within a few minutes of induction. Instead, I infuse fluids under gravity during transport to the operating room and while preparing to induce anesthesia.
2. The choice of crystalloid to be infused can have significant impact on neonatal outcome.
   a. Acute maternal infusion of as little as 10 g glucose causes significant maternal and, consequently, fetal hyperglycemia.
      i. The fetus secretes insulin in response to this hyperglycemia.
      ii. After delivery, with insulin (but not glucose) still present, fetal hypoglycemia can occur.

   b. Normal saline (0.9% NaCl), although free of glucose, con-
       tains a large amount of unbuffered chloride ion. Acute
       infusion of large volumes of 0.9% NaCl induces a mater-
       nal hyperchloremic metabolic acidosis and increases the
       risk of neonatal acidosis.
   c. Other available crystalloid solutions contain lactate and
       acetate as buffers (lactated Ringer's Plasmalyte). Theo-
       retically, these compounds could upset maternal and
       fetal carbohydrate metabolism, increasing the risk of
       neonatal hypoglycemia, but clinically, these problems
       have not been seen.

Maternal Position

1. Neither the sitting nor the lateral decubitus position offers
    any clear advantage during induction of spinal anesthesia.
    Onset of sensory block is slightly faster in the lateral posi-
    tion, but the final level is unaffected.
2. When inducing blockade in the lateral decubitus position,
    the side on which the patient lies does matter.
    a. If the patient assumes the left lateral position for induc-
        tion and then lies supine with left tilt for uterine dis-
        placement, blockade on the right side may not extend
        high enough for surgery.
    b. Inducing anesthesia with the patient in the right lateral
        position and then placing her supine with left tilt for uter-
        ine displacement helps to assure good bilateral blockade.
    c. A similar phenomenon occurs when using isobaric bupi-
        vacaine. Here, however, the greater extent of blockade
        develops on the nondependent side (0.5% bupivacaine is
        slightly hypobaric). Should this problem arise, rolling the
        patient from side to side evens the spread of analgesia.

How High a Level?

1. A level of sensory blockade above T10 will block the somatic
    sensations of cesarean section.
2. Eliminating visceral pain from peritoneal stimulation and
    uterine manipulation requires more extensive anesthesia.
3. Patients will tolerate the procedure with a T6 to T8 level of
    sensory blockade, but they will more likely need supple-
    mental systemic analgesics than will those with a higher
    level of block.
4. The level of *anesthesia* (loss of ability to perceive touch) may
    be more important than the level of analgesia (loss of sharp-
    ness to pinprick).
    a. In parturients, analgesia extends as much as nine seg-
        ments higher than anesthesia.
    b. Only when the level of *anesthesia* is above T5 will
        women be reliably pain-free during cesarean section.[4]
5. I strive for a level of sensory blockade between T4 and T1.
    a. I prefer having the block spread a little too high than
        not high enough.
    b. Occasionally, the level of sensory blockade creeps up
        into the cervical dermatomes.
        i. Place an extra pillow under the woman's head to
            limit further cephalad spread.

ii. Assess motor function by checking hand-grip strength and respiratory function (ask her to speak and breathe deeply).

iii. If the block extends so high that the patient cannot phonate or maintain her oxygen saturation above 95%, apply cricoid pressure and secure the airway to protect against possible aspiration.

iv. Fortunately, this complication occurs only rarely.

Drugs

Which Drug?

1. Tetracaine
    a. Often fails to provide good maternal sensory blockade.
    b. Twenty-five percent to 80% of parturients will require supplemental analgesia.
    c. Motor blockade persists long after the sensory block has regressed.

2. Hyperbaric lidocaine
    a. A rapid but unpredictable sensory anesthesia
    b. Short duration
        i. Rarely provides more than 60 minutes of surgical anesthesia
        ii. Patients often have significant pain on arrival in the recovery room.
    c. Recent reports of transient neurologic symptoms after lidocaine spinal anesthesia in nonpregnant patients have led many anesthesiologists (including me) to abandon its use.

3. Hyperbaric bupivacaine
    a. Probably the most widely, currently used local anesthetic for spinal anesthesia for cesarean section
    b. Produces better sensory block with less motor blockade than tetracaine.
    c. Has a longer duration than lidocaine.
    d. Hyperbaric 0.75% bupivacaine, in doses of 12 to 15 mg, provides good sensory blockade to at least the T6 dermatome.
        i. Sensory change begins within 4 to 6 minutes and peaks between 15 and 20 minutes.
        ii. It provides good maternal comfort for 60 to 120 minutes of intraabdominal surgery.

How Much Drug?

1. Neither height, weight, age, nor vertebral column length predict the intrathecal spread of hyperbaric local anesthetics in parturients (Fig. 16.2).

2. Recent data suggest that the extent of sensory blockade is determined by the volume of lumbosacral CSF.[5]

3. The physical properties of injected local anesthetic and the anatomic shape of the spinal column explain the behavior of hyperbaric spinal anesthesia
    a. Hyperbaric local anesthetics pool in dependent regions of the spinal column, and the distribution of local anesthetic within the CSF correlates with the spread of sensory blockade.

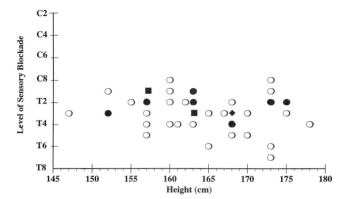

Fig. 16.2. Sensory blockade after subarachnoid injection of 12 mg hyperbaric bupivacaine in 50 term parturients. Sensory blockade develops independent of patient height. *Open circle,* **one patient;** *solid circle,* **two patients;** *square,* **three patients;** *diamond,* **four patients. (Source: Redrawn from Norris MC. Height, weight and the spread of spinal anesthesia for cesarean section.** *Anesth Analg* **1988;67:555, with permission.)**

    b. When the patient lies supine, the thoracolumbar spine slopes 8 to 12 degrees in the cephalad direction.

    c. Hyperbaric solutions pool in the lowest part of the thoracic curvature (T5 to T6).

    d. They produce sensory blockade into the upper thoracic dermatomes regardless of the distance between the site of injection and the base of the thoracic curve.

4. There is a weak, but statistically significant correlation between the extent and duration of sensory blockade produced by isobaric local anesthetics and patient height.[6] One model suggests that a 10-cm increase in height would be associated with a 1.1-dermatome decrease in the level sensory block.

5. Within the commonly used range of hyperbaric drug doses (7.5 to 12.0 mg of hyperbaric bupivacaine or 7 to 15 mg of hyperbaric tetracaine), similar levels of sensory blockade develop, despite varying doses of drug injected.

    a. Larger doses of drug produce more dense but not more extensive sensory blockade.

    b. When the dose of local anesthetic increases further (15 mg of bupivacaine or 18 mg of tetracaine), it exceeds the capacity of the upper thoracic curvature, and more extensive dermatomal spread follows (Fig. 16.3).

Improving the Quality of Block

1. The most reliable way to improve the quality of spinal anesthesia is to inject an adequate amount of drug. For cesarean section use:

    a. Hyperbaric bupivacaine 15 mg.

    b. Hyperbaric tetracaine 18 mg.

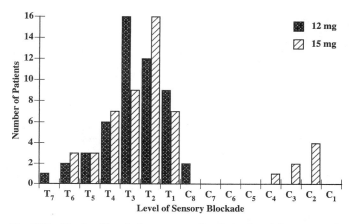

Fig. 16.3.   Maximal level of sensory analgesia to pinprick, measured 15 minutes after subarachnoid injection of 12 or 15 mg hyperbaric bupivacaine in term parturients. The mode shifts from T3 to T2 with the larger dose of drug. (Source: Data from Norris MC. Patient variables and the subarachnoid spread of hyperbaric bupivacaine in the term parturient. *Anesthesiology* 1990;72:478; and Norris MC. Height, weight and the spread of spinal anesthesia for cesarean section. *Anesth Analg* 1988;67:555.)

2. Other adjuvants may improve intraoperative analgesia.
    a. Fentanyl
        i. Dose: 6.25 to 50.0 μg. Doses greater than 25 μg are associated with significant pruritus and somnolence.
        ii. Fentanyl improves intraoperative and postoperative analgesia.
        iii. Its effect is more significant with smaller (i.e., less than or equal to 12 mg bupivacaine) doses of intrathecal local anesthetic.
    b. Epinephrine 200 μg will improve the quality of intraoperative analgesia produced by small doses of intrathecal bupivacaine. Epinephrine also increases the intensity of motor block and slightly prolongs the regression of sensory block
    c. Intrathecal morphine 200 μg both improves the quality of intraoperative blockade and provides prolonged postoperative analgesia. The combination of epinephrine and morphine is more effective than either drug alone. Not surprisingly, however, intrathecal morphine increases the incidence of nausea, vomiting, and itching.

Conclusion
1. Any of the three local anesthetics mentioned can, if given in high enough doses, provide good maternal comfort during cesarean section.

2. Because it provides excellent sensory blockade and reasonable duration motor block, I prefer hyperbaric bupivacaine for most cesarean sections.
    a. I routinely use 15 mg of 0.75% bupivacaine with 8.25% dextrose (Table 16.2).

Table 16.2.   Spinal anesthesia for cesarean section: suggested technique

Preparation	Large-bore peripheral IV
Premedication	30 mL sodium citrate within 15 min of induction
Prehydration	1.0 L balanced saline solution (i.e., Plasmalyte) within 15–30 min of induction
	Infuse under gravity.
	Do not delay induction for fluid infusion.
Positioning	Sitting or right lateral decubitus
Induction	Identify the subarachnoid space.
	Small-gauge pencil-point needle (≤24 gauge)
	L2–L3 interspace or lower
	Midline or paramedian approach (paramedian approach often easier when patient is in the lateral decubitus position)
	Inject local anesthetic.
	15 mg 0.75% bupivacaine with 8.25% dextrose
	Add morphine if desired for postoperative analgesia.
Maintenance	Position patient supine with 10–15 degrees of left uterine tilt
	Administer ≤50% oxygen by face mask.
	Monitor maternal blood pressure every 1–2 min for 20 min, then every 3–5 min.
	Continue fluids until maternal blood pressure stabilizes.
Hypotension	Well hydrated
	5–10 mg ephedrine when BP <90 mm Hg or mother symptomatic
	Poorly hydrated
	10 mg ephedrine when BP begins to decrease

BP, blood pressure.

b.   Those who wish to use smaller doses of local anesthetic should consider adding opioid or epinephrine to improve the quality of sensory blockade.

COMBINED SPINAL–EPIDURAL ANESTHESIA

1.   One limitation of spinal anesthesia is its finite duration.
   a.   Hyperbaric bupivacaine 15 mg readily provides 90 to 120 minutes of good operating conditions.
   b.   Occasionally, however, cesarean section lasts longer.
2.   A combined spinal–epidural anesthetic
   a.   Has rapid onset of spinal anesthesia and the flexibility of epidural catheterization.
   b.   Is also a good technique in patients with poor anatomic landmarks. In these women (especially the morbidly obese parturient), I find it easier first to find the epidural space with an 18-gauge needle and then to use the needle-through-needle technique to enter the subarachnoid space.
3.   There are a few technical issues to consider before using a combined spinal–epidural anesthetic for cesarean section.

Patient Position

1.   With the needle-through-needle technique, the success rate for dural puncture is slightly higher if the patient is sitting, not lying on her side.
2.   Sitting position
   a.   Hyperbaric drug will pool caudally while the epidural catheter is being inserted and secured.
      i.   The level of sensory block may not be high enough for surgery.
      ii.   This problem is most significant when smaller (10-mg) doses of hyperbaric drug are used.
   b.   Limit this risk by injecting a larger dose of bupivacaine and minimizing the time spent inserting and fixing the epidural catheter.
   c.   If the level of sensory block is rising too slowly, place the operating table in a 5- to 10-degree head-down tilt, as needed.
   d.   If the level is still inadequate, dose the epidural catheter (see later).
3.   Lateral position
   a.   The level of spinal anesthesia may ascend too high during insertion and fixation of the epidural catheter. (In most parturients, the hips are wider than the shoulders. When the patient is lying on a horizontal surface, the vertebral column slopes toward her head.)
   b.   Position the patient with pillows under her head and shoulders to produce an uphill slope of the cervical and thoracic spine. Even if final patient positioning is delayed, hyperbaric drug will not ascend to the cervical nerve roots.

Epidural Anesthesia in the Presence of Spinal Blockade

1.   There are two things to consider when preparing to inject epidural local anesthetics in the presence of spinal anesthesia:
   a.   First: detecting a subarachnoid catheter.

      b. Second: the impact of dural puncture and spinal anesthesia on the spread of epidurally injected drugs.

2. Subarachnoid injection of additional local anesthetic may produce dangerously high sensory blockade.

    a. One way to detect subarachnoid catheter placement is to wait until the spinal sensory level has regressed several segments before injecting a small (i.e., 5 mg of bupivacaine) subarachnoid test dose. Although this approach has its merits, waiting until the spinal begins to recede may increase the risk that the patient will feel pain before effective epidural anesthesia can be established.

    b. Instead, cautiously dose the epidural catheter about 1 hour after the induction of spinal anesthesia.

       i. Initially inject a small dose of epidural local anesthetic bupivacaine (1 mL 0.5%) and watch carefully for any sign of rising blockade (i.e., numbness or weakness of the upper extremities, or, if the patient is heavily sedated, look for a decrease in blood pressure or heart rate, or a change in respiratory pattern).

      ii. Wait 5 minutes between successive injections of drug.

      iii. Using small doses and waiting 5 minutes between injections minimizes the risks of unrecognized intrathecal or intravenous injection.

3. When dosing an epidural catheter in the presence of spinal anesthesia, small amounts of epidural local anesthetic can significantly raise the level of sensory blockade.

    a. Pressure within the epidural space caused by fluid injection is transmitted to the subarachnoid space and can displace intrathecal local anesthetic and raise the level of sensory blockade. Epidural injection of both saline and local anesthetic can extend the preexisting spinal block by this mechanism.

    b. The dural hole left by the spinal needle allows increased subarachnoid passage of epidurally injected drug.

    c. Clinically, extensive sensory block is likely to be a problem only after unrecognized intrathecal injection of local anesthetic.

4. Choose the concentration and volume of drug injected according to the anticipated remaining duration of surgery.

    a. If the operation will be finished in 15 to 30 minutes, and the patient still has at least a T4 level of sensory blockade, 10 mL 0.25% bupivacaine will help provide immediate postoperative analgesia.

    b. If surgery will be extensive or prolonged (i.e., a cesarean hysterectomy), "replace" the regressing spinal anesthetic with an epidural injection of 15 to 20 mL 0.5% bupivacaine.

SPINAL ANESTHESIA AFTER FAILED EPIDURAL BLOCK

1. Occasionally, epidural injection of local anesthetic fails to produce adequate surgical anesthesia. Case reports suggest that intrathecal injection of 9 to 15 mg hyperbaric bupiva-

caine in this setting may place the patient at greater risk of extensive sensory block and respiratory compromise. These reports raise some interesting questions:
   a. Does performing a spinal anesthetic after a previous epidural increase the risk of dangerously high block?
   b. What are the mechanisms of this excessive spinal block?
   c. Is spinal anesthesia contraindicated after a failed epidural?
   d. Can changes in spinal anesthetic technique reduce the risk of high block?
2. Does failed epidural anesthesia increase the risk of high spinal block?
   a. One retrospective series found an 11% incidence (three of 27) of sensory block above C8 when spinal anesthesia was induced after a failed epidural, compared with 0.2% (one of 643) when spinal block was used as the initial anesthetic.[7] However, sensory change can often be detected above C8 after intrathecal injection of hyperbaric bupivacaine 15 mg, but respiratory compromise requiring intubation is extremely rare.
   b. Others report complications in small case series ($n = 12$ or 30) of spinal anesthesia after failed epidural block.[8]
3. Possible mechanisms
   a. Fluid within the epidural space may compress the thecal sac, forcing intrathecally injected drugs to higher levels.
   b. The fresh dural hole may allow rapid diffusion of previously injected epidural local anesthetic.
   c. Both of these possibilities require local anesthetic to remain in the epidural space. In young patients, injected volume readily escapes the epidural space through the intervertebral foramina and is unlikely to play a role in the spread of a subsequent intrathecal injection.
   d. Alternatively, after epidural injection, local anesthetic diffuses into the subarachnoid space in amounts too small to block nerve conduction. After subsequent intrathecal injection, the epidurally injected drug combines with the spinal drug to extend the upper level of sensory blockade.
4. Several approaches may limit the risk of high sensory block after failed epidural anesthesia.
   a. While the first impulse may be to use a small dose of intrathecal local anesthetic, this approach risks inadequate intensity and duration of anesthesia.
5. Suggested technique
   a. Unless concerned about technical difficulty (i.e., a patient with poorly palpable spinous processes), induce anesthesia in the right lateral position to minimize the risk of postural hypotension.
   b. Base the dose of local anesthetic on the extent of the existing epidural block. Usually use 10 to 15 mg hyperbaric bupivacaine.
   c. After drug injection, carefully position the patient supine with left uterine displacement and place an extra pillow under her head.

   d. Monitor the patient's respiration and upper extremity motor function carefully.

   e. Despite these precautions, an occasional parturient will develop an excessively high level of sensory blockade. If so, apply cricoid pressure and rapidly induce general anesthesia with a small dose of thiopental and use succinylcholine to facilitate intubation.

  6. This situation serves most of all as a reminder to monitor patients receiving labor epidural analgesia carefully and immediately replace any catheter that does not function as expected.

REFERENCES

1. Marx GF, Luykx WM, Cohen S. Fetal-neonatal status following caesarean section for fetal distress. *Br J Anaesth* 1984;56:1009.

2. Rout CC, Akoojee SS, Rocke DA, Gouws E. Rapid administration of crystalloid preload does not decrease the incidence of hypotension after spinal anaesthesia for elective caesarean section. *Br J Anaesth* 1992;68:394.

3. Caritis SN, Abouleish E, Edelstone DI, Mueller-Heubach E. Fetal acid-base state following spinal of epidural anesthesia for cesarean section. *Obstet Gynecol* 1980;56:610.

4. Russell IF. Levels of anaesthesia and intraoperative pain at caesarean section under regional block. *Int J Obstet Anesth* 1995; 4:71.

5. Carpenter RL, Hogan QH, Liu SS, Crane B, Moore J. Lumbosacral cerebrospinal fluid volume is the primary determinant of sensory block extent and duration during spinal anesthesia. *Anesthesiology* 1998;89:24.

6. Schnider TW, Minto CF, Bruckert H, Mandema JW. Population pharmacokinetic modeling and covariate detection for central neural blockade. *Anesthesiology* 1996;85:502.

7. Furst SR, Reisner LS. Risk of high spinal anesthesia following failed epidural block for cesarean delivery. *J Clin Anesth* 1995;7:71.

8. Stoneham M, Souter A. Spinal anesthesia for caesarean section in women with incomplete extradural analgesia. *Br J Anaesth* 1996;77:301.

Anesthesia and Cardiac Disease

Maternal cardiac disease complicates 1% to 2% of pregnancies and is a significant cause of maternal mortality. The Report on Confidential Enquiries into Maternal Deaths in the United Kingdom 1991–1993 recorded 41 deaths (including four late deaths) due to cardiac disease, approximately twice the number recorded in each of the previous two triennia.[1] This increase was due mostly to more acquired heart disease (27 cases), including nine cases of ruptured thoracic aortic aneurysm. Migration from developing countries is maintaining the number of cases of rheumatic heart disease. In developed countries, the prevalence of ischemic heart disease in women in the reproductive age group appears to be increasing. Both factors may increase the importance of heart disease as a cause of maternal mortality. Areas of substandard care highlighted by the UK report included delay in referral to senior and specialist help, inadequate cooperation between specialists involved in patient care, and a perceived reluctance to perform chest radiographs in pregnancy.

GENERAL CONSIDERATIONS

1. Because of the increased risks associated with labor and delivery and operative delivery in these patients, it is essential that the obstetric anesthesiologist be involved as early as possible in their care.
2. A plan of analgesic and anesthetic management should be made in consultation with all specialist care providers, clearly documented, and repeatedly reviewed during the antenatal course. The obstetric anesthesiologist faces two principal concerns:
   a. Can epidural analgesia be safely used for labor and delivery?
   b. What is the safest method of providing anesthesia for cesarean section? (This debate usually devolves to a choice between epidural and general anesthesia.)

Regional Anesthesia

1. Women with most cardiac lesions withstand the hemodynamic effects of a carefully conducted epidural block better than a labor and delivery without the benefit of effective analgesia.
2. Patients with valvular stenosis or right-to-left intracardiac shunts may not tolerate the high sympathetic block associated with epidural anesthesia for cesarean delivery. Even women with regurgitant valvular lesions that normally improve with epidural analgesia may not withstand a poorly conducted block.
3. Whatever the circumstances, induce epidural blockade by using incremental doses of drug. Monitor closely the hemodynamic response to block.
4. Epidural or spinal opiates can provide excellent analgesia for the first stage of labor and avoid the deleterious effects of sympathetic blockade; however, neuraxial opioids alone

rarely provide adequate analgesia for the second stage of labor. They also do not ensure sufficient pain relief for operative delivery.

Systemic Analgesia for Labor

1. Maternal anticoagulation precludes major conduction analgesia.
2. The standard regimen of intermittent intramuscular meperidine provides neither adequate analgesia nor cardiovascular stability.
   a. Continuous intravenous infusion or patient-controlled analgesia (PCA) with meperidine or fentanyl is a reasonable alternative.
   b. The neonate may require intravenous naloxone at delivery.

General Anesthesia

1. The hemodynamic response to induction and intubation can produce significant cardiac compromise.
   a. Use rapidly acting intravenous agents to induce a profound level of anesthesia before attempting laryngoscopy and intubation.
   b. Use mostly opioids in severely ill patients (i.e., 10 µg per kilogram fentanyl followed by 50 to 100 mg thiopental [or a small dose of etomidate] and then a rapidly acting muscle relaxant).
   c. Alert the person caring for the infant to the likelihood of opioid-induced respiratory depression.
2. Maintenance
   a. Use the inhalational agent most appropriate to the patient's cardiac lesion for maintenance of anesthesia.
   b. Remember, nitrous oxide increases pulmonary vascular resistance.
   c. After delivery, supplemental opiates safely deepen maternal anesthesia.
   d. Rocuronium is an appropriate nondepolarizing muscle relaxant.

Monitoring

1. Use all available noninvasive cardiovascular monitors.
2. Consider central venous pressure (CVP) monitoring for patients with significant symptoms.
3. Reserve systemic and pulmonary artery catheters for the most severe cases.
4. Continue monitoring after delivery, if necessary, in a critical care unit.
   a. The greatest risk of circulatory overload arises during the first 48 hours after delivery as the contracted uterus displaces blood into the systemic circulation.
   b. If using epidural anesthesia, continue injecting local anesthetics so that the receding sympathetic block does not compound the increase in blood volume.

Vasoactive Drugs

1. Use vasopressors and oxytocic agents cautiously.

    a. Consider using a pure constrictor, like phenylephrine, in patients with stenotic valvular lesions.

    b. Patients with regurgitant valvular lesions or poor left ventricular function should respond better to an agent with inotropic activity, such as ephedrine.

    c. If an oxytocic agent is necessary, then use synthetic oxytocin.

       i. Avoid bolus doses, because significant, albeit transient, systemic hypotension can occur.

      ii. Ergot alkaloids cause a sustained increase in systemic vascular resistance.

2. β-Blockers are increasingly used in pregnancy, particularly in the management of mitral stenosis.

    a. Can prevent pulmonary edema

    b. Decrease the need for closed mitral valvotomy during pregnancy

    c. Do not contraindicate incremental epidural anesthesia

       i. Be careful with the high block required for cesarean delivery.

      ii. Significant bradycardia is possible, and the heart's ability to respond to decreased afterload is impaired.

Antibiotic Prophylaxis

1. Antibiotic prophylaxis against bacterial endocarditis is widely given to patients with valvular cardiac disease; however, the American Heart Association recommends this therapy only in a few, specific settings.[2]

2. Endocarditis prophylaxis is *not* recommended for:

    a. Cesarean section.

    b. Other gynecologic procedures in uninfected tissue.

       i. Urethral catheterization

      ii. Dilation and curettage

     iii. Therapeutic abortion

     iv. Sterilization procedures

      v. Insertion or removal of intrauterine devices

3. Endocarditis prophylaxis is optional for vaginal delivery in high risk patients (Tables 17.1 and 17.2).

VALVULAR HEART DISEASE

Mitral Stenosis

1. The most common isolated valvular lesion seen in pregnancy

2. The dominant lesion in most cases of mixed mitral valve disease

3. Hemodynamically, mitral stenosis is a fixed obstruction to left ventricular filling.

4. Maternal mortality during pregnancy is 1%, but the risk may increase to 14% to 17% if patients develop atrial fibrillation.

    a. Life-threatening pulmonary edema can develop with remarkable speed in women with previously asymptomatic mitral stenosis.

    b. Seen in immigrants from emerging nations who may be unaware that they have heart disease.

Table 17.1.   Cardiac conditions associated with endocarditis

High risk

    Prosthetic cardiac valves, including bioprosthetic and homograft valves

    Previous bacterial endocarditis

    Complex cyanotic congenital heart disease (e.g., single ventricle, transposition of the great vessels, tetralogy of Fallot)

    Surgically constructed systemic pulmonary shunts or conduits

Moderate risk

    Most other congenital cardiac malformations (other than the following negligible risk conditions: isolated secundum atrial septal defect, repaired atrial or ventricular septal defect, repaired patent ductus arteriosus without residua, and mitral valve prolapse without regurgitation)

    Acquired valvular dysfunction (e.g., rheumatic heart disease)

    Hypertrophic cardiomyopathy

    Mitral valve prolapse with regurgitation or thickened valvular leaflets

Source: After Dajani AS, Taubert KA, Wilson W, et al. Prevention of bacterial endocarditis. Recommendations by the American Heart Association. *JAMA* 1997;277:1794.

Table 17.2.   Prophylactic antibiotic regimens for genitourinary procedures

Situation	Agents	Regimen
High-risk patients	Ampicillin plus gentamicin	Ampicillin 2.0 g IV or IM plus gentamicin 1.5 mg/kg (not to exceed 120 mg) within 30 min of starting procedure; 6 h later, ampicillin 1.0 g IM or IV or amoxicillin 1.0 g PO
High-risk patients allergic to ampicillin/ amoxicillin	Vancomycin plus gentamicin	Vancomycin 1.0 g IV over 1–2 h plus gentamicin 1.5 mg/kg (not to exceed 120 mg); complete injection/infusion within 30 min of starting procedure. (No second dose of vancomycin or gentamicin recommended.)

Source: After Dajani AS, Taubert KA, Wilson W, et al. Prevention of bacterial endocarditis. Recommendations by the American Heart Association. *JAMA* 1997;277:1794.

5. Balloon dilatation has proved successful after failed medical therapy if the valve is pliable with no or minimal regurgitation.
   a. Patients may be able to discontinue medication and deliver vaginally after balloon valvuloplasty.
   b. Risks to the fetus can be minimized by shielding the abdomen and pelvis from radiation. The use of transesophageal echocardiography shortens fluoroscopic time.

Evaluation

1. Determine the New York Heart Association (NYHA) functional classification (see Chapter 2).
2. Exclude remediable exacerbating features such as anemia, infection, and tachycardia.
3. Review the patient's medications.
4. Look for signs and symptoms of severe disease (i.e., an opening snap within 80 ms of the second heart sound and features of pulmonary hypertension).
5. The electrocardiogram (ECG) may show atrial fibrillation or, if sinus rhythm, a broad, notched P wave in lead II (P mitrale). Evidence of right ventricular hypertrophy on ECG suggests pulmonary hypertension.
6. Radiographic findings include a straight left-heart border, left atrial enlargement, and Kerley's B lines. Upper lobe blood diversion is a common finding in pregnancy and is not a helpful sign.
7. Echocardiography will exclude other valvular lesions and allow assessment of left ventricular function (invariably good in isolated mitral stenosis, but decreased in a few patients with mixed valvular lesions).
8. Direct measurement or Doppler flow studies across the valve can provide objective assessment of mitral valve area.

Anesthesia and Analgesia

1. Avoid maternal tachycardia.
   a. The pressure gradient across the valve is inversely proportional to the square of the diastolic filling time.
   b. A small increase in heart rate (decreased diastolic filling time) will cause a marked increase in left atrial pressure.
   c. β-Blockers can control heart rate.
2. Use epidural block for labor analgesia unless it is specifically contraindicated.
   a. Sympathetic blockade helps attenuate changes in venous volume associated with uterine contractions.
   b. Do not give extra fluid before induction. Instead, infuse fluid as indicated by central volume status.
   c. In symptomatic patients, a central venous catheter may help assess volume status. Strongly consider a pulmonary artery catheter in NYHA functional classes III and IV.
3. If epidural analgesia is contraindicated
   a. NYHA functional classes I and II manage well with intermittent parenteral analgesia, provided maternal heart rate is kept under control. Meperidine is not the ideal agent because it may cause a tachycardia.

b. For NYHA grades III and IV, intermittent analgesia is insufficient. In these cases, try a continuous or patient-controlled intravenous opioid infusion.

4. Cesarean section
   a. NYHA class I and II patients tolerate the higher epidural block required for operative delivery. Monitor cardiac preload and adjust it as necessary.
   b. Even NYHA grades III and IV may fare better with epidural anesthesia.
      i. Although these patients do not tolerate any sudden *reduction* in cardiac afterload, they are often on the brink of pulmonary edema, with very high pulmonary arterial and venous pressures. Any sudden *increase* in afterload or heart rate (such as after intubation) may precipitate pulmonary edema.
      ii. The venodilation produced by slow incremental epidural anesthesia should improve maternal hemodynamics.
      iii. In this setting, pulmonary artery pressure must be monitored. Maintain adequate left ventricular preload during the onset of sympathetic blockade. Avoid fluid overload.
   c. General anesthesia
      i. Obtund the adrenergic response to intubation with β-blockers, opioids, or both.
      ii. Etomidate is the most suitable intravenous induction agent.
      iii. Rocuronium may be a more suitable (combining cardiovascular stability with rapid onset) agent than succinylcholine.
      iv. Maintain anesthesia with halothane or enflurane in air and oxygen. Isoflurane reduces systemic vascular resistance. Nitrous oxide can increase pulmonary artery pressure. After delivery, give a long-acting opioid.

5. These patients are at the greatest risk of pulmonary edema immediately postpartum.
   a. Blood volume expands as the uterus contracts and the vasodilator effects of regional blockade wear off.
   b. Because of the high incidence of early postpartum pulmonary edema, consider giving furosemide 20 to 40 mg intravenously with delivery of the placenta. Then, closely monitor the patient's volume status for the next 24 to 48 hours.

Mitral Regurgitation

1. Usually improves during pregnancy
   a. Decreased systemic vascular resistance
   b. Increased blood volume
2. Encourage forward blood flow. Epidural analgesia/anesthesia with fluid preloading:
   a. Reduce systemic vascular resistance.
   b. Maintain left ventricular filling pressure.
   c. Avoid bradycardia.
3. Atrial fibrillation, requiring anticoagulant therapy, is common.

4. If general anesthesia is required, limit the pressor response to intubation. Avoid myocardial depression. A vasodilator infusion may be a useful adjunct. In severe cases, an inotrope may be necessary.

Mitral Valve Prolapse

1. The vast majority of patients with this common congenital lesion are asymptomatic and have trivial regurgitation.
2. Decreased left ventricular volume increases the degree of prolapse. Avoid volume depletion and tachycardia.
3. Patients with significant or symptomatic regurgitation should be managed as for mitral regurgitation.

Mixed Mitral Valve Disease

1. Manage these patients according to the dominant lesion, as assessed by echocardiography.
2. The combination of both significant stenosis and regurgitation may impair left ventricular function, in which case the patient will not tolerate β-blockade. Here, keep the heart rate between 80 and 100 beats per minute with digoxin.
3. Epidural labor analgesia and invasive monitoring are appropriate.

Aortic Stenosis

Evaluation

1. Uncommon in pregnancy.
2. Patients with aortic stenosis poorly tolerate:
   a. Decreased afterload.
      i. Stenosis limits the ability to increase stroke volume in response to decreased systemic vascular resistance.
      ii. Diastolic pressure (and time) determine oxygen delivery to the thickened left ventricle.
   b. Shortened diastolic filling time: Tachycardia may lead to ischemia and cardiac failure.
   c. Bradycardia: decreased cardiac output, cardiac failure.
3. Unlike mitral stenosis, absence of symptoms does not necessarily suggest mild disease. However, women who are asymptomatic before pregnancy, have a normal ECG, and good left ventricular function, should have no trouble.
4. Echocardiographic evaluation can assess the pressure gradient across the valve, valve area, and ventricular performance.
   a. Pressure gradients (as assessed by Doppler) can be misleading, as they depend on flow velocity.
   b. Doppler output flow velocity should increase during pregnancy.
      i. The severity of mild-to-moderate disease is usually overestimated during pregnancy.
      ii. On the other hand, a low gradient does not necessarily imply mild disease and may reflect severely impaired left ventricular function.
      iii. A decrease in Doppler flow velocity or the development of tachycardia, dyspnea, or angina signals danger. If these occur, hospital admission, bed rest, and β-blocker therapy are needed. β-Block-

ade helps provide diastolic time for coronary flow and left ventricular filling.

5. If possible, the pregnancy should be sustained until the fetus is viable and delivered before dealing with the mother's valve.

   a. If required earlier, balloon valvulotomy may buy time but creates substantial regurgitation.

   b. The valve area and systolic ejection time also should be considered (valve area less than 1 cm^2 implies severe disease; values less than 0.6 cm^2 are critical).

Anesthesia and Analgesia

1. In mild cases, epidural blockade can be used for both vaginal and abdominal delivery. Continuous-infusion techniques minimize hemodynamic changes.

2. For severe cases, local anesthetic–induced sympathectomy may decrease afterload and precipitate maternal decompensation.

   a. Combined spinal–epidural analgesia can avoid the need to give large bolus injections of local anesthetic.

      i. Induce analgesia with intrathecal opioids (i.e., sufentanil 5 μg or fentanyl 25 μg).

      ii. Immediately start an epidural infusion of a diluted local anesthetic/opioid solution to maintain analgesia once the intrathecal opioid effect wanes.

      iii. Remember, epinephrine-induced tachycardia may be harmful.

   b. Severe aortic stenosis is often accompanied by aortic insufficiency, which improves with decreased afterload.

3. These patients can receive either general or regional (epidural) anesthesia for cesarean section.

   a. For general anesthesia, carefully control the hemodynamic response to intubation (see Mitral Stenosis above).

   b. Induce regional anesthesia slowly. Monitor blood pressure frequently or continuously. Treat hypotension with phenylephrine if the heart rate also is low.

4. Monitoring

   a. Noninvasive monitoring is sufficient in mild cases.

   b. For severe cases, especially if the patient needs a cesarean section, use direct arterial pressure monitoring and a pulmonary artery catheter to guide anesthetic and perioperative fluid management.

Aortic Regurgitation

1. Any reduction in heart rate or increase in systemic vascular resistance can cause acute volume overload in a chronically distended left ventricle.

2. The sympathetic block associated with epidural anesthesia reduces systemic vascular resistance and improves cardiac output.

3. If general anesthesia has to be used, consider a continuous vasodilator infusion. Avoid myocardial depression, and attempt to suppress the intubation response.

4. Pulmonary artery catheters are not particularly useful because an increase in left atrial pressure occurs late in the disease process.

Hypertrophic Obstructive Cardiomyopathy (Idiopathic Hypertrophic Subaortic Stenosis)

1. This uncommon condition occurs in young people and may complicate pregnancy.
2. Although it is hemodynamically and symptomatically similar to valvular aortic stenosis, the management is sufficiently different to warrant separate consideration.
   a. Like aortic stenosis, decreases in systemic vascular resistance are poorly tolerated.
   b. However, increased myocardial contractility and the Valsalva maneuver significantly increase the subvalvular obstruction.
   c. Pay close attention to maternal volume status.
   d. Use fluids to avoid decreases in left ventricular volume. Injudicious fluid therapy, however, may precipitate pulmonary edema.
   e. Tachycardia, which increases the obstruction, increases the risk of decompensation.
   f. If hypotension develops, use a vasoconstrictor without inotropic activity (phenylephrine).
   g. Continuous intraarterial blood pressure monitoring may help detect sudden changes in left ventricular outflow obstruction.
3. These patients may benefit from carefully conducted epidural analgesia for labor and delivery.
   a. Epidural block can prevent the effects of stress and pain on the outflow obstruction.
   b. Sudden sympathectomy, however, can prove hazardous.
4. The extensive sympathetic block associated with epidural anesthesia for cesarean section is more problematic.
   a. Many experts prefer general anesthesia for abdominal delivery.
      i. Use opioids to blunt the tachycardia and increased cardiac output associated with laryngoscopy and intubation.
      ii. Halothane is the most appropriate inhalational agent for maintenance of anesthesia.
      iii. If the left ventricle fails, treat hypotension and tachycardia by using a vasopressor and propranolol.
      iv. Inotropic therapy worsens the obstruction and is contraindicated.
   b. Others report that carefully conducted epidural anesthesia also can produce excellent maternal and fetal outcomes.[3]
      i. These women had central venous catheters. Volume was infused to maintain CVP at normal or slightly above normal (≥ 8 cm water)
      ii. Increments of epidural local anesthetics were given slowly, with continued monitoring and intravenous fluid infusion.

Peripartum Cardiomyopathy

1. New left ventricular dilatation and congestive cardiac failure during the third trimester of pregnancy or in the first 6 months postpartum without obvious cause or prior evidence of cardiac disease
2. It complicates 1 in 3,000 to 30,000 deliveries.
3. Some patients are taking anticoagulants because of the possibility of mural thrombosis.
4. If not contraindicated, epidural analgesia or anesthesia is strongly indicated for vaginal or cesarean delivery.
   a. Decreased systemic vascular resistance improves cardiac output.
   b. Epidural anesthesia avoids the myocardial depressant effects of general anesthesia.
   c. These women need little or no additional volume before induction of regional block.
   d. As epidural analgesia usually improves maternal cardiac function, reserve invasive monitoring for symptomatic patients and those requiring abdominal delivery.
5. General anesthesia
   a. Avoid increases in afterload and negative inotropic agents.
   b. Use invasive monitors.
   c. Isoflurane or sevoflurane would be the inhalational agents of choice.
   d. Consider the use of a vasodilator infusion, and have inotropic support available.
6. The availability of cardiac transplantation has improved the outlook for those with persistent dysfunction.

ARRHYTHMIAS

1. Any disturbance of cardiac rhythm should be treated promptly.
2. Supraventricular arrhythmias are particularly problematic in patients with rheumatic heart disease and occur commonly in mitral valve disease.
   a. Atrial fibrillation occurring during pregnancy may increase the maternal mortality rate to as high as 19%.
   b. Patients with chronic atrial fibrillation should be taking digoxin or propranolol to control ventricular rate. They also may be using anticoagulants to prevent thromboembolic complications.
   c. Sudden onset of atrial fibrillation or supraventricular tachycardia with severe cardiac compromise should be treated by direct-current cardioversion.
      i. Often this is best done in the operating room under general anesthesia.
      ii. Energy discharges of approximately 1 watt per second per kilogram usually suffice.
      iii. Although transient fetal arrhythmias may occur, cardioversion during pregnancy does not adversely affect mother or child.

PREVIOUS VALVE REPLACEMENT

1. Increasing numbers of these patients are being seen.
2. Usually, patients with a properly working valve prosthesis are hemodynamically normal.

   a. Pulmonary hypertension and atrial fibrillation may persist after mitral valve replacement.
   b. Stenosis of tissue valves and perivalvular regurgitation should be excluded, and ventricular function should be assessed before anesthesia.

Anticoagulant Therapy

1. The use of anticoagulants is the most common problem in patients with mechanical prostheses.
2. This therapy may contraindicate epidural anesthesia.
3. Antiplatelet agents alone are ineffective anticoagulants, but they are occasionally used as an adjunct to subcutaneous heparin.
4. Heparin
   a. Should be stopped the evening before planned delivery.
   b. Restart 3 to 24 hours after delivery.
   c. A 12-hour delay after the last heparin dose usually ensures normal coagulation.
   d. Check partial thromboplastin time and platelet count before beginning a major conduction anesthetic.
   e. Patients receiving low-molecular-weight heparin (LMWH) may be at greater risk of bleeding complications. LMWH should be stopped 24 hours before planned delivery and not restarted until 24 hours postpartum.[4]
   f. Remove the epidural catheter as soon as it is no longer needed and at least 2 hours before restarting the anticoagulant therapy. Epidural hematoma has been described after catheter removal in a patient receiving anticoagulant therapy.
5. Patients in labor while receiving anticoagulant therapy
   a. Protamine can reverse the effects of heparin (but not with LMWH).
   b. Patients taking warfarin should receive fresh-frozen plasma to prevent hemorrhagic complications.
      i. The baby will remain anticoagulated and often is delivered by urgent cesarean section to avoid the trauma of vaginal delivery.
      ii. This operation should be done with the patient under general anesthesia if time does not permit confirmation of anticoagulant reversal in the mother and induction of regional block.
      iii. Manage maternal blood loss as it occurs; there are limited options for treating a thrombosed valve or thromboembolism.

PREVIOUS HEART TRANSPLANTATION

1. There have been a number of successful pregnancies after heart or heart–lung transplantation.
2. Potential problems
   a. Immunosuppression may need to be adjusted during pregnancy because of increased drug clearance.
   b. The denervated heart
      i. Resting heart rate is increased because of absent vagal tone.
      ii. Indirectly acting agents (i.e., ephedrine) will have no effect on heart rate.

      iii. Upregulation of β-adrenergic receptors may increase sensitivity to directly acting agents.

      iv. The heart rate effects of anesthetics are sympathetically mediated and will not occur in these patients. Direct myocardial depressant effects will dominate.

3. Pregnancies tend to be complicated, with a high incidence of premature labor and pregnancy-associated hypertension.

4. Epidural analgesia is not contraindicated, but preload must be maintained.

PRIMARY PULMONARY HYPERTENSION

1. Peripartum maternal mortality may exceed 60%.
2. These patients should be advised not to become pregnant.
3. Management includes early admission and hospitalization beginning around 28 weeks of gestation. A team approach is essential.

Evaluation

1. Assessment includes a history, clinical examination, ECG, echocardiography, and chest radiograph.
2. Definitive assessment of right ventricular dysfunction must be made by pulmonary artery catheter.
   a. Poor prognostic signs
      i. A cardiac index less than 4.0 L per minute per square meter.
      ii. Right atrial pressure greater than 10 mm Hg.
      iii. Pulmonary vascular resistance greater than 1,000 dynes per second per cm^{-5}.
3. Some of the increased pulmonary vascular resistance may be pharmacologically reversible.
   a. Prostacyclin (10 ng per kilogram per hour), diltiazem (20 mg per hour), or isoproterenol (0.4 mg per hour) may decrease pulmonary vascular resistance and pulmonary artery pressure and increase cardiac output.
   b. A marked reduction in pulmonary vascular resistance is not the most common response, and the efficacy of pulmonary vasodilation appears to decrease as the pregnancy progresses.
4. After the initial hemodynamic assessment, the ECG provides an ongoing estimate of systolic pulmonary artery pressure and atrial and ventricular size.
   a. Increasing right ventricular failure requires bed rest, digitalis, and diuretics.
   b. Avoid hypoxia by the continuous administration of oxygen.
   c. Prophylactic low-dose heparin, 10,000 U twice a day, should be administered in the face of low cardiac output and bed rest.

Labor and Delivery

1. Vaginal delivery is preferable to cesarean section because the latter appears to lead to a poorer maternal outcome.
2. Regardless of the mode of delivery, these women require intensive monitoring.

a. Systemic and pulmonary artery catheters and continuous estimation of oxygen delivery by oximetry are essential. Associated tricuspid incompetence may make it difficult to insert a pulmonary artery catheter.

b. Anticipate the potential for severe bradycardia. Have atropine, isoproterenol, and transvenous pacing facilities available.

c. Pay meticulous attention to blood loss to avoid hypovolemia.

   i. Any decrease in venous return aggravates the reduced right ventricular output.

   ii. A decrease in right ventricular output, in turn, leads to hypoxia, which further increases pulmonary vascular resistance, creating a vicious cycle.

      (1) Unless broken, this cycle leads to progressive ventricular failure, hypoxemia, and acidosis in both mother and fetus.

      (2) Death ultimately follows.

Labor Analgesia

1. Induce epidural analgesia with small incremental boluses of 0.25% bupivacaine.
2. Maintain analgesia with a continuous infusion.
3. Judicious doses of epidural opioids should improve analgesia without risking respiratory depression.
4. Use more concentrated local anesthetics for second-stage anesthesia.

Cesarean Delivery

1. Risks

   a. Epidural anesthesia: extensive sympathetic blockade, hypotension, and worsening pulmonary hypertension. Successful use of this technique has been reported.

   b. General anesthesia: a marked increase in pulmonary vascular resistance associated with laryngoscopy and tracheal intubation

      i. A suggested technique begins with etomidate and fentanyl 10 µg per kilogram for induction, vecuronium for muscle relaxation, and early intubation.

      ii. Isoflurane is the volatile agent of choice because it is associated with the least myocardial depression.

      iii. Avoid hypoxia, hypercarbia, high intrathoracic pressures, and acidosis.

      iv. Maintain maternal hypocapnia.

      v. Consider continuing invasive monitoring and mechanical ventilation postoperatively.

2. Drugs to be *avoided* include ergometrine, oxytocin, prostaglandin $F_{2\alpha}$, ketamine, and nitrous oxide.

3. If needed, use pulmonary vasodilators (sodium nitroprusside, nitroglycerin, prostaglandin E, isoproterenol).

   a. Monitor for systemic hypotension, arterial hypoxemia, fall in cardiac output, and fetal and uterine side effects.

   b. Use oxygen delivery as the therapeutic endpoint.

4. Inotropic support (dopamine, up to 10 µg per kilogram per minute, or dobutamine) may be required to improve right ventricular function.

5. Increasing preload with volume loading is usually unsuccessful and may precipitate right ventricular ischemia.

MYOCARDIAL INFARCTION

1. Rare during pregnancy: estimated incidence of 1 in 10,000
   a. The greatest frequency is in the third trimester in women older than 35 years.
   b. Maternal mortality approximates 37% to 50%. Mortality is increased if the infarct occurs in the third trimester, if the patient is younger than 35 years, if she delivers within 2 weeks of her infarct, or if she has a cesarean section.

2. Newer therapies include intracoronary thrombolysis with tissue plasminogen activator (TPA) and primary percutaneous transluminal coronary angioplasty (PTCA).

3. Normal electrocardiographic findings in pregnancy include reversible ST-, T-, and Q-wave changes. These aberrations can be differentiated from those indicating heart disease by echocardiographic assessment of ventricular wall motion.

4. Predelivery assessment should include Holter monitoring and exercise testing, if appropriate. In addition, two-dimensional echocardiography and radionuclide ventriculography can assess left ventricular function.

5. Mode of delivery
   a. Vaginal delivery with epidural analgesia
      i. Eliminates stress, reduces blood loss, provides hemodynamic stability, and allows early ambulation.
      ii. The course of labor and delivery are unpredictable.
   b. Cesarean delivery under epidural anesthesia
      i. Eliminates the capriciousness of vaginal delivery.
      ii. May be associated with greater blood loss and increased cardiopulmonary and metabolic demands.
   c. Hypotension
      i. Treat with phenylephrine
      ii. Ephedrine increases myocardial work owing to β-stimulation.
      iii. Metaraminol is a potent coronary vasoconstrictor.

6. Patients with poor ventricular function may require a pulmonary artery catheter to monitor cardiac function. Nitroglycerin (0.5 mg per kilogram per minute) may help provide coronary artery vasodilation. Maintain diastolic pressure to allow subendocardial perfusion.

CONGENITAL HEART DISEASE

1. Congenital heart disease is now more common in pregnancy because of the prolonged survival of children with these lesions.

2. Most patients who are asymptomatic or barely symptomatic before pregnancy will be fine.

    a. The impact of congenital heart disease on pregnancy depends primarily on the ability to increase stroke volume or to tolerate a reflex increase in heart rate.

    b. Remember, the presence of congenital heart disease does not preclude superimposed preeclampsia or peripartum cardiomyopathy.

3. Initial diagnosis of a congenital lesion may sometimes occur at the antenatal clinic when a murmur, produced by the increased cardiac output, is heard. Most commonly, echocardiography will reveal an atrial septal defect, although restrictive ventricular septal defects, patent ductus arteriosus, pulmonary stenosis, and acyanotic Ebstein's anomaly may be found.

4. In general, if the patient wants children, pregnancy should not be delayed unless corrective surgery is planned. The heart disease can only get worse and the risks increase.

5. Optimal management requires a team effort with active involvement of the anesthesiologist.

6. The risk of pregnancy and the likelihood of a successful outcome must be determined individually. The literature does not provide categorical answers. Common sense and applied hemodynamic principles are most useful.

Left-to-Right Shunt

Atrial Septal Defect

1. Serious clinical manifestations do not usually occur until the fourth or fifth decade.

2. Pregnant patients with an atrial septal defect but without evidence of pulmonary hypertension or right ventricular failure require little additional management.

3. Use epidural analgesia for labor, vaginal delivery, and cesarean section. This technique avoids increases in systemic vascular resistance, which could increase left-to-right shunting.

4. If a general anesthetic is required, avoid exacerbating preexisting pulmonary hypertension.

5. Patients with atrial septal defect are prone to supraventricular arrhythmias, which are poorly tolerated.

    a. Acute supraventricular tachycardia in association with either hypotension or right ventricular failure should be managed with direct-current cardioversion or intravenous β-blockers.

    b. In less acute situations, patients should be digitalized.

    c. Usually, patients with uncorrected atrial septal defect do not develop supraventricular arrhythmias until they are past childbearing age.

6. In patients with uncorrected defects, blood loss can force left-to-right shunting, to the sudden detriment of left ventricular and coronary flow.

Ventricular Septal Defect

1. Asymptomatic patients with a small ventricular septal defect and no evidence of pulmonary hypertension tolerate pregnancy well and require no intervention.

2. Examine those with a large ventricular septal defect to exclude respiratory infection, pulmonary hypertension, bacterial endocarditis, and ventricular failure.
3. Anesthetic management.
    a. Continuous lumbar epidural analgesia prevents marked increases in systemic vascular resistance due to pain.
        i.   Optimal for labor and vaginal delivery.
        ii. Also preferred for operative delivery.
    b. These patients do not tolerate increases in heart rate associated with endotracheal intubation (tachycardia increases left-to-right shunt and decreases cardiac output). If using general anesthesia, include enough opioid to reliably block the hemodynamic response to endotracheal intubation.
    c. Marked increases in systemic vascular resistance may require low-dose vasodilator therapy with either sodium nitroprusside or phentolamine.
    d. To counteract the development of a right-to-left shunt and hypoxemia, treat significant decreases in systemic vascular resistance with small doses of vasopressor.
    e. Either of two mechanisms may incite peripheral cyanosis:
        i.   An increase in the left-to-right shunt (due to increased systemic vascular resistance) may cause pulmonary edema. Volume overload, however, is an uncommon cause of pulmonary edema in the adult. More likely, the increased right ventricular workload leads to right ventricular failure and, ultimately, biventricular failure and pulmonary edema with a low cardiac output.
        ii. Alternatively, an increase in pulmonary vascular resistance or a decrease in systemic vascular resistance may reverse interventricular flow and produce right-to-left shunt.
        iii. Diagnosis and treatment.
            (1) Cyanosis accompanied by low cardiac output (poor peripheral perfusion, decreased urine output, increased CVP) should be treated with 100% oxygen, inotropic support, and vasodilation.
            (2) Hypotension and cyanosis with signs of increased cardiac output (warm peripheries, full pulse) suggest right-to-left shunting and should be managed with 100% oxygen, lightening of depth of anesthesia, and small doses of a vasopressor until the blood pressure increases and the shunt reverts.

Patent Ductus Arteriosus

This lesion is serious only if the patent ductus arteriosus is large and surgically uncorrected. Look for signs and symptoms of left or right ventricular failure, pulmonary hypertension, and shunt reversal. Treat asymptomatic patients with no evidence of ventricular dysfunction as normal. Use continuous epidural analgesia for labor and vaginal and operative delivery, but take care to avoid excessive reduction of systemic vascular resistance.

When using general anesthesia, avoid changes in systemic vascular resistance and myocardial depressants.

Corrected Lesions
1. Successful pregnancy is possible after the Fontan operation.
   a. Increasing systemic venous pressure during pregnancy causes discomfort due to hepatic congestion and edema of the lower extremities.
   b. Atrial thrombosis is a major threat, and some patients may need continuous anticoagulant therapy.
2. Ventricular function needs careful assessment after the Mustard and Senning operation for transposition, as eventually the right ventricle, which handles the systemic circulation, will fail.
   a. Successful pregnancy has been reported.
   b. The development of atrial arrhythmias, particularly flutter, can be a major problem.

Right-to-Left Shunt
Tetralogy of Fallot
1. Mortality
   a. High for mother and fetus with uncorrected lesions.
   b. After correction, fetal mortality remains increased.
2. Anesthetic management of uncorrected women.
   a. Avoid decreased systemic vascular resistance (increases right-to-left shunt).
   b. Avoid decreased blood volume, venous return, and myocardial depression (decrease cardiac output).
   c. Labor analgesia
      i. Epidural and intrathecal local anesthetics may decrease venous return and systemic vascular resistance.
         (1) Manage with increased uterine displacement and intravenous fluids.
         (2) Be careful with vasopressors that can increase pulmonary vascular resistance (and right-to-left shunt) (i.e., phenylephrine).
      ii. However, epidural or intrathecal opioids may be useful for first-stage analgesia.
      iii. Intravenous opioids by continuous infusion or PCA may be useful.
   d. Cesarean section: general anesthesia
      i. Maintain a slightly increased CVP.
      ii. An opioid-based technique avoids the myocardial depression caused by volatile agents.
      iii. Patients with infundibular obstruction may decompensate in response to a decrease in right ventricular filling, a faster heart rate, or depressed myocardial contractility, which decrease cardiac output or increase right-to-left shunt.
         (1) Sign: increased peripheral cyanosis
         (2) Treatment: Give 100% oxygen and fluids, deepen the anesthetic, and eliminate any tachycardia with β-blockade.

Eisenmenger Syndrome

1. Pulmonary hypertension threatens a pregnant woman's life whether associated with a central shunt in the Eisenmenger syndrome or when solitary, as after previous closure of a nonrestrictive ventricular septal defect or arterial duct. The right-to-left shunt may be at the atrial, ventricular, or aortopulmonary level.

2. Laparoscopic sterilization under general anesthesia should be advised for all young women with Eisenmenger syndrome.
   a. Patients first seen when pregnant should be told the risks, and therapeutic abortion advised.
   b. Those who decide to continue their pregnancy should be admitted to the hospital as soon as the resting oxygen saturation decreases, definitely before the end of the second trimester.
   c. Treatment includes bed rest, which minimizes right-to-left shunting and maximizes fetal growth, prophylactic heparin, nasal oxygen, continuous pulse oximetry, and careful fetal monitoring.

3. Maternal and fetal outcome depend on the severity of the pulmonary hypertension.
   a. Maternal mortality ranges between 12% and 33%.
   b. Sudden death is not usual.
      i. Postmortem examination reveals no cause.
      ii. Systemic vasodilation, bradycardia, and increasing right-to-left shunt usually precede cardiac arrest.

4. Management
   a. Avoid increases in pulmonary vascular resistance (see section on primary pulmonary hypertension).
      i. Oxygen may reduce peripheral or pulmonary vascular resistance.
      ii. Assess peripheral oxygen saturation both before and after oxygen therapy.
   b. Avoid decreases in systemic vascular resistance, because it will markedly increase right-to-left shunt.
      i. Sympathetic blockade with local anesthetics is contraindicated.
      ii. First-stage analgesia can be provided by neuraxial opioids.
      iii. Pudendal block can provide second-stage analgesia.
      iv. Because of the high incidence of thromboembolism, some patients may require a low-dose (45 IU per hour) intravenous infusion of heparin throughout labor, precluding use of an epidural catheter.
   c. General anesthesia should be used for cesarean section. Maintain generous hydration, avoid systemic vasodilatation, and promptly replace blood loss.
   d. Monitoring should include ECG, S_aO_2, and CVP.
      i. Use fluids to maintain CVP.
      ii. Give supplementary oxygen.
      iii. The high risk of arrhythmias, thrombi, paradoxical emboli, pulmonary artery rupture, patent ductus arteriosus occlusion, and misleading data contraindicate the use of a pulmonary artery catheter.

iv. A decrease in oxygen saturation equates with an increase in right-to-left shunt.
   (1) In the presence of a patent ductus arteriosus, right hand and foot saturations can be used simultaneously to monitor the degree of shunt.
      (a) Blood flow to the right arm is predominantly preductal and represents right heart output.
      (b) Blood flow to the foot is postductal and represents left heart output.
e. Increases in heart rate and stroke volume raise right ventricular oxygen consumption. Right ventricular failure should be treated with inotropic support.

Potentially Fragile Aortas
1. Marfan or Ehlers–Danlos syndromes.
   a. Increased risk of aortic dissection or rupture during pregnancy.
   b. β-Blockade should continue throughout pregnancy.
2. Women with Marfan syndrome, whose aortic root is already dilated, or who have a family history of aortic rupture should be advised to delay pregnancy until after aortic root replacement.

Coarctation of the Aorta
1. A rare congenital vascular defect occurring in approximately 1 in 2,000 to 3,000 women
   a. Two percent of these cases involve the abdominal aorta.
   b. Maternal mortality approaches 4%, with death usually due to aortic rupture or dissection.
   c. Hypertension is a common associated feature, usually requiring β-blockade for control.
   d. Evaluation.
      i. Magnetic resonance imaging is a safe and reliable means of confirming a clinically suspected coarctation during pregnancy.
      ii. Echocardiography can exclude bicuspid aortic valve and other cardiac lesions.
   e. Maternal and fetal mortality and morbidity are not increased after surgical correction.
2. Asymptomatic patients require no additional care.
3. In uncorrected patients, avoid decreases in systemic vascular resistance, heart rate, and left ventricular filling, although survival to term pregnancy implies well-developed collateral flow.
4. Epidural anesthesia has not been recommended in the past because of the potential for bleeding into the epidural space from enlarged collaterals.
   a. Hard clinical evidence to support this stance is lacking.
   b. Neuraxial opioids can provide adequate analgesia and allow rapid detection of any compromise from an expanding hematoma.
   c. Alternatives include intravenous opioid infusion or inhalation analgesia.

5. General anesthesia is probably the better choice for cesarean section.
    a. Maintain heart rate, myocardial contractility, and vascular resistance.
    b. Manage maternal bradycardia by removing the precipitating cause and giving atropine or isoproterenol.

Congenital Aortic Stenosis

1. Anesthetic and hemodynamic considerations are similar to those for acquired aortic stenosis.
2. In the developed world, the majority of cases of aortic stenosis are congenital in origin.
3. Investigations should look for other associated lesions.

Congenital Pulmonary Stenosis

1. Asymptomatic patients with little right ventricular dysfunction require no additional intervention.
2. In other women, avoid changes in right ventricular filling pressure, decreased heart rate, decreased systemic vascular resistance, and myocardial depressants.
3. Use epidural local anesthetics cautiously.
    a. Neuraxial or systemic opioids, inhalation agents, and pudendal blocks are alternatives for labor and vaginal delivery.
    b. If using epidural local anesthetics, carefully monitor CVP and maintain systemic vascular resistance with ephedrine.
4. General anesthesia is recommended for cesarean section.
    a. Sustain vascular resistance, heart rate, and myocardial contractility.
    b. Withdraw volatile agents, and give inotropic support for any evidence of right ventricular failure.

REFERENCES

1. *Report on confidential enquiries into maternal deaths in the United Kingdom 1991–1993.* London: HMSO, 1996.
2. Dajani AS, Taubert KA, Wilson W, et al. Prevention of bacterial endocarditis. Recommendations by the American Heart Association. *JAMA* 1997;277:1794.
3. Autore C, Brauneis S, Apponi F, Commisso C, Pinto G, Fedele F. Epidural anesthesia for cesarean section in patients with hypertrophic cardiomyopathy: a report of three cases. *Anesthesiology* 1999;90:1205.
4. Horlocker TT, Wedel DJ. Neuraxial block and low-molecular-weight heparin: balancing perioperative analgesia and thromboprophylaxis. *Reg Anesth Pain Med* 1998;23:S164.

Anesthesia and Hematologic Disease

Hematologic problems facing the obstetric anesthesiologist are most commonly those of anemia and coagulation defects.

1. Chronic anemia
   a. Understand the physiologic consequences of decreased oxygen delivery and the effects of any underlying disease.
   b. As the risks of transfusion are increasingly recognized, blood must only be for specific indications, not solely in response to laboratory values.
2. Problems of coagulation usually involve the amount or function of platelets and clotting factors. The greatest, and yet unresolved, problem is the relation between platelet count and the safe use of regional anesthesia.

PATHOLOGIC ANEMIA IN PREGNANCY

1. Anemia, defined as a hemoglobin (Hb) concentration less than 11.0 g per deciliter, is due to an absolute reduction in red cell mass rather than a dilutional effect, and is very common in pregnancy.
2. Mild anemia poses little risk to mother and fetus. Fetal oxygen consumption is reduced only in severe anemia or in the presence of placental problems.

Indications and Risks of Blood Transfusion

1. There is no set minimum Hb concentration for labor, vaginal delivery, or cesarean section. In most practices, red cell transfusion is overused and could be markedly decreased if the Red Cross–recommended minimum Hb of 7 g per deciliter were used to assess transfusion requirements.
2. Ultimately, the decision to transfuse red blood cells (RBCs) should be based on the clinical condition of the patient, not on an arbitrary Hb level.
   a. A higher Hb may be required in hypermetabolic states, such as sepsis, or poor oxygen-delivery states, such as heart failure or myocardial ischemia.
   b. Tissue repair is not adversely affected until an Hb of 5 g per deciliter or less.
   c. Patients without cardiorespiratory symptoms do not need transfusion if their Hb concentration is greater than 7 g per deciliter.
3. Transfusion of blood and blood products carries a small but definite risk of disease transmission (Table 18.1).

Anesthetic Concerns in the Anemic Patient

1. Maintain plasma volume
2. Transfuse in the presence of hemodynamic instability or ongoing blood loss.
3. Monitor both end-tidal carbon dioxide (to prevent respiratory alkalosis) and temperature (to avoid hypothermia).

Table 18.1.   Current risk of transfusion-transmitted infections (per unit infused)

Disease	Risk
Hepatitis A	Rare
Hepatitis B	1/66,000–1/200,000
Hepatitis C	1/120,000
Hepatitis G	Unknown
HIV-1	1/563,000–1/825,000
Bacterial contamination	
Platelets	1/2,400
RBC	?–1/1,000,000
Malaria	1/4,000,000
Cytomegalovirus	Variable

Source: After Menitove JE. Transfusion-transmitted infections: update. *Semin Hematol* 1996;33:290, with permission.

4. Postoperative management of the severely anemic patient includes oxygen and prevention of shivering.
    a. Shivering can increase oxygen consumption by 35% to 40%.
    b. Normal oxygen demand can be met by an Hb of 5 to 7 g per deciliter (equivalent to a hematocrit of 21%) when intravascular volume is adequate.
    c. Despite a lower hematocrit (23%), nontransfused patients have similar lengths of hospital stay and incidences of postoperative infection and wound complications compared with transfused patients with higher hematocrits (28%).
    d. It is acceptable to discharge asymptomatic patients to home with an Hb of 7 g per deciliter and adequate oral therapy.

Erythropoietin (EPO)
1. Maternal EPO increases substantially during normal pregnancy, and at term, plasma concentration is two to four times higher than in nonpregnant and nonanemic controls.
    a. In the fetus, EPO also is the major regulator of erythropoiesis.
    b. Regulation of erythropoiesis takes place independently in the two circulations because the placenta forms a barrier to both endogenous and recombinant EPO.
2. Recombinant human EPO (rHuEPO)
    a. Has been used to treat the anemia associated with renal failure in pregnancy.
    b. Also has been used, with concurrent intravenous iron, to treat iron-deficiency anemia during pregnancy.
    c. Treatment may be associated with serious side effects.
        i.   Seizures in a small percentage of patients
        ii. A tendency to thrombotic events associated with increased fibrinogen and improved platelet function
        iii. Development or worsening of hypertension

    d. Still, EPO therapy for the treatment of long-term anemia or to avoid recurrent transfusions is probably a viable alternative in pregnant patients.

Autologous Blood Donation
1. Safe during pregnancy
2. No serious fetal effects were noted during autologous blood donation in 272 parturients.
3. Indications might include the management of placenta previa or accreta or elective cesarean hysterectomy.
4. However, the high cost of autologous donation and the low rate of transfusion in cesarean section patients (1.1%) makes it hard to justify this alternative.

Iron-deficiency Anemia in Pregnancy
1. The most common cause of anemia in pregnancy
2. It is characterized by hypochromic and microcytic red cells with a blunted reticulocyte response.
3. Treatment
    a. Usually with oral iron
    b. Early treatment may reduce the need for transfusion.
    c. Rarely, with severe deficiency, intramuscular or intravenous iron may be necessary. Intravenous iron may cause anaphylaxis.

Megaloblastic Anemia Due to Folate Deficiency in Pregnancy
1. Folate deficiency
    a. The most common cause of macrocytic anemia in pregnancy
    b. It may be associated with premature births, and severe and prolonged deficiency may lead to neural tube defects and development of cleft palate in the fetus.
    c. It is diagnosed by a peripheral smear, which usually shows large hypersegmented polymorphonuclear leukocytes.
    d. Folate is usually supplemented routinely during pregnancy, but the dose may need to be increased in the setting of exaggerated consumption, such as in sickle cell disease.
2. Severe vitamin B12 deficiency is very rare during pregnancy, as it leads to sterility, and the needs of pregnancy are easily met by the large body stores of this vitamin.

Sickle Cell Anemia
1. An inherited disorder with a structurally abnormal β-globin chain of the Hb molecule.
2. Sickle hemoglobinopathies can be classified into major or minor disorders (Table 18.2).
    a. The most common sickle cell disorder is the heterozygous form of hemoglobin S (HbAS), which occurs in 1 in 12 adult African Americans.
    b. The most common major sickle hemoglobinopathy is the homozygous form, hemoglobin S (HbSS), with an incidence of 1 in 625 African Americans.

Table 18.2.   Classification of sickle hemoglobinopathies

Minor disorders
    Sickle cell trait (HbAS)
    Hemoglobin C trait (HbAC)
    Hemoglobin C disease (HbCC)
    Hemoglobin SE disease (HbSE)
    Hemoglobin SD disease (HbSD)
    Hemoglobin S-Memphis (HbS-Memphis)
Major disorders
    Sickle cell anemia (HbSS)
    Hemoglobin SC disease (HbSC)
    Hemoglobin S β-thalassemia (HBS β-Thal)

Source: After Rust OA, Perry KG Jr. Pregnancy complicated by sickle hemo-globinopathy. *Clin Obstet Gynecol* 1995;38:472, with permission.

3. The additional physiologic demands of pregnancy increase the frequency of complications of sickle cell disease.
4. Sickle cell disease is associated with increases in both maternal and perinatal mortality.

Sickle Cell Crisis
1. Almost all the signs and symptoms of sickle cell anemia are the result of hemolysis, vaso-occlusive crisis, and increased susceptibility to infection.
2. The sudden onset of these clinical manifestations is known as sickle cell crisis, which is most often caused by vaso-occlusive disease.
    a. Symptoms of vaso-occlusive crisis include recurring attacks of pain involving the skeleton, chest, and abdomen and occur as a result of sickling in the microcirculation.
    b. Antenatal crises have been reported in 35% of affected parturients, with an increased incidence later in pregnancy.
    c. Treatment involves fast and adequate pain relief, fluid replacement, and antibiotics if infection is suspected.
    d. Intravenous fluids correct dehydration and reduce viscosity.
    e. Use systemic opioids, if necessary, to treat pain.
        i.   Analgesia can be maintained by continuous infusions or patient-controlled analgesia (PCA).
        ii. Epidural analgesia can be used for labor pain in a patient in crisis.
    f. Partial-exchange transfusions are an important therapeutic maneuver.
    g. Simple additive transfusions are not indicated in patients whose Hb has not decreased by at least 2 g per deciliter below the stable state and is more than 5 g per deciliter.

Preoperative Preparation
1. A conservative approach to preanesthetic preparation of these patients is appropriate.
2. Prophylactic transfusion does not improve outcome.

Anesthetic Care
1. Rigorously avoid hypoxemia, cold, acidosis, and dehydration.
   a. Provide a warm operating suite (or labor room), warming blanket, and humidified inspired gases, and avoid hypoventilation.
   b. Measure arterial blood gases for evidence of metabolic acidosis.
2. Choice of anesthetic technique is less important than avoidance of precipitating factors and careful attention to detail.
   a. Epidural blockade, with careful attention to proper prehydration and gradual onset of sensory blockade, may be better than spinal anesthesia, which may result in sudden hypotension and the subsequent need for vasopressors.
   b. Wrap the legs in elasticized bandages to reduce stasis in the lower extremities.
   c. Use lateral tilt and avoid aortocaval compression, because massive sickling can occur in the lower limbs, even in those with sickle cell trait. Monitor lower limb oxygen saturation with a pulse oximeter on the foot to assess the adequacy of uterine displacement.
   d. Treat hypotension initially with fluids and then ephedrine.
3. Complications can continue to arise postoperatively.
   a. Pay persistent attention to a warm environment, fluid intake, oxygen, and analgesia.
   b. Epidural opioid analgesia, with careful monitoring for respiratory depression, is ideal.
   c. Encourage early mobilization and vigorous chest physiotherapy.

Thalassemia
1. A family of inherited disorders that result in decreased synthesis of β-globulin or α-globulin, leading to reduced Hb concentration.
2. The thalassemia syndromes are named by the type of chain that is inadequately represented.
   a. Two major groups: α- and β-thalassemias
   b. Affect the synthesis of HbA, which is made up of two α and two β chains.
   c. The globin chains in thalassemia are structurally normal.
   d. It is the quantity that is reduced.
3. β-Thalassemias are most common.
   a. Categorized as minor, intermedia, or major (Cooley's anemia)
      i. Patients with β-thalassemia intermedia may have increased hemolysis. If hemolysis induces significant anemia, these women may need preoperative transfusion.
      ii. Patients with thalassemia major will have severe anemia and will require frequent transfusions.
      iii. Strategies to ensure maximal effectiveness of transfusion include availability of safe blood, leukocyte-depleted RBC transfusion, and intensive iron chelation with subcutaneous desferrioxamine.

4.   Anesthetic considerations
  a.   Thalassemia minor and intermedia do not present many peripartum anesthetic problems.
  b.   Women with thalassemia major rarely become pregnant.
    i.   If they do, they may require up to 6 L of washed packed cells antenatally to maintain an adequate Hb.
    ii.   Women with hemosiderosis (from hemolysis and multiple transfusions) may have significant hepatic damage and lack clotting factors.
    iii.   Splenomegaly may lead to increased hemolysis and thrombocytopenia.
    iv.   Cardiac hemosiderosis leads to left ventricular mechanical dysfunction and, eventually, arrhythmias. Evaluate cardiac function with an electrocardiogram and echocardiography.
    v.   Examine the airway closely. Maxillary overgrowth secondary to extramedullary erythropoiesis can make visualization of the glottis difficult.
    vi.   During labor:
      (1)   Correct severe anemia early.
      (2)   Monitor volume status carefully. Women with severe left ventricular dysfunction will need a pulmonary artery catheter.
      (3)   Continuous-infusion epidural analgesia is appropriate for pain relief.
        (a)   Induce blockade slowly.
        (b)   Treat hypotension with phenylephrine 20 to 40 µg intravenously. This drug corrects hypotension more readily than does ephedrine without increasing the heart rate.
    vii.   Cesarean section
      (1)   Use epidural anesthesia.
      (2)   Provide postoperative analgesia with epidural opioids.
      (3)   Avoid spinal anesthesia in women with significant myocardial compromise.

Aplastic Anemia

1.   Patients with profound pancytopenia in pregnancy have a high mortality (33%) and a poor prognosis.
2.   Others, with less stem-cell depression, recover between pregnancies.
3.   Steroids often are used. Treatment with antilymphocyte globulin also has been reported.
4.   At term:
  a.   Transfuse the symptomatic, severely anemic parturient.
  b.   If the platelet count is adequate, major conduction anesthesia is safe.
  c.   Avoid unnecessary urinary and central venous catheters because of the risk of infection.

Fanconi's Anemia

1.   Pregnancy is rare and usually happens only in women with mild disease.

2. These patients have an increased incidence of hypertensive disorders.
3. The use of regional analgesia is based on the platelet count.
   a. Platelet transfusion is usually required at delivery.
   b. Significant bleeding, very low platelet counts, and the need for blood and platelet transfusion may complicate the postoperative course.

COAGULATION DISORDERS
Vascular Purpuras
Systemic Lupus Erythematosus (SLE)

1. About a third of patients with SLE have thrombocytopenia, although fewer than 5% have a platelet count less than 30,000 per cubic millimeter.
2. Occasionally, a more severe and abrupt-onset thrombocytopenia may be seen with platelet-associated immunoglobulin G (PA-IgG).
3. Treatment of thrombocytopenia is difficult, and the response to corticosteroids may be poor, although aspirin occasionally increases the platelet count.

Henoch–Schönlein Purpura

1. This usually benign vasculitis occurs in children and young adults.
2. Despite the purpura, prothrombin time (PT), activated partial thromboplastin time (aPTT), platelets, and bleeding time are often normal.
3. Regional anesthesia is not contraindicated.

Platelet Disorders
Spurious (Laboratory-induced) Thrombocytopenia

1. Any unexpected low platelet count should be checked manually. Platelet clumping, which may not be detected by automated counters, can occur under certain laboratory conditions.
2. Spurious thrombocytopenia has been reported in 0.85% to 1.9% of processed samples.

Incidental Thrombocytopenia

1. Routine platelet count is not indicated before regional anesthesia in healthy patients.
2. Still, a few (approximately 0.5%) healthy term parturients will have platelet counts below 100,000 per cubic millimeter.
3. These women can safely receive regional anesthesia and analgesia.

Autoimmune or Idiopathic Thrombocytopenic Purpura (ITP)

1. The most common autoimmune disease in childbearing women
2. Antibodies, usually IgG, are directed against the platelet membrane. But, PA-IgG is not always present and may not correlate with the clinical disease.
3. Multiple episodes of relapse and remission are common.

4. ITP cannot be distinguished from gestational thrombo-cytopenia with certainty because both diagnoses are based on low platelets without an apparent cause.
5. Although symptoms may worsen, pregnancy does not increase the risk of severe exacerbation of ITP.
6. Treatment during pregnancy
   a. Women with more than 50,000 per cubic millimeter platelets need no treatment.
   b. During the first and second trimesters, women with platelet counts between 30 and 50,000 per cubic milli-meter also need no treatment.
   c. Patients with clinical bleeding are first treated with oral corticosteroids, and between 70% and 90% of patients will respond within 3 weeks.
   d. High-dose intravenous immunoglobulin
      i. Initial treatment for third-trimester women with fewer than 10,000 per cubic millimeter platelets
      ii. Initial treatment for bleeding patients with pla-telet counts between 10 and 30,000 per cubic milli-meter.
      iii. Splenectomy
          (1) Usually reserved for women for whom med-ical treatment fails
          (2) Is rarely indicated
          (3) May be safely performed during the second trimester
      iv. Platelet transfusion
          (1) Limited benefit because of rapid consump-tion by circulating antibodies
          (2) Should be reserved for life-threatening hem-orrhage
7. Maternal antibodies may cross the placenta and affect the fetus.
   a. Infants with low platelet counts are theoretically at an increased risk of intracranial hemorrhage if delivered vaginally.
   b. Maternal platelet count, steroid therapy, or previous splenectomy are of limited use in predicting neonatal thrombocytopenia.
   c. The only reliable predictor of risk is a fetal platelet count.
      i. Before labor, this can be ascertained from a per-cutaneous umbilical blood sample, although this test confers some risk to the fetus.
      ii. A scalp sample during labor requires adequate cervical dilatation, and accuracy may be affected by dilution with amniotic fluid or by clotting of the sample.
      iii. However, there is no convincing evidence that mode of delivery affects the rate of intracranial hemorrhage, and it has been recommended that patients with ITP be managed according to obstet-ric indications.[1]
8. Maternal mortality is exceptionally rare, and postpartum hemorrhage is the most common complication.

a. The incidence of postpartum hemorrhage
  i. Correlates with the severity of thrombocytopenia.
  ii. Is more often associated with cervical or vaginal lacerations or episiotomies than with uterine atony.
b. A maternal platelet count greater than 50,000 per cubic millimeter should prevent excessive maternal bleeding at vaginal delivery or cesarean section.
9. Anesthetic management
  a. Consider regional anesthesia, in particular, spinal block, in asymptomatic women.
    i. Because of the increase in marrow turnover in ITP, platelets tend to be younger and larger and therefore more efficient.
    ii. Platelet transfusion to cover regional techniques is not recommended because the lifespan of the transfused platelets is indeterminable and may be very short because of circulating antibodies.
  b. Beware of potential bleeding during general anesthesia, especially intubation. Postoperatively, patients should be carefully monitored for any bleeding or respiratory obstruction secondary to airway trauma after intubation.

Thrombotic Thrombocytopenic Purpura (TTP)

1. A rare, severe disease characterized by thrombocytopenia, microangiopathic hemolytic anemia, transient neurologic abnormalities, fever, and renal failure
2. Diffuse intravascular thrombosis occludes capillaries and arterioles.
3. Pregnancy outcome is poor. Damage to maternal organs and placenta indirectly injures the fetus.
4. It may be confused with severe preeclampsia or abruption.
5. Treatment
  a. In the acute phase, plasma infusion or plasma-exchange therapy results in improvement in 90% of cases and may enhance maternal and fetal survival.
  b. Steroids, aspirin, and dipyridamole also are used.

Postpartum Hemolytic Uremic Syndrome

1. Resembles TTP, but it is characterized by acute renal failure associated with microangiopathic hemolytic anemia
2. Maternal mortality and long-term morbidity are high, and preterm delivery and intrauterine fetal deaths are frequent complications.
3. Treatment is as for TTP, but dialysis is often required.

Drug-induced Platelet Disorders

THROMBOCYTOPENIA

1. Many drugs can induce thrombocytopenia.
2. The most common pathway is through the formation of an immune complex, a mechanism that often involves IgG, which can cross the placenta and affect the fetus (see ITP).
3. Generalized bone-marrow depression (e.g., chloramphenicol) or a selective effect involving only the megakaryocytes (e.g., thiazides, tolbutamide) also may occur.

THROMBOPATHY

1. Many commonly used drugs can inhibit platelet lifespan and function.
   a. Dipyridamole inhibits primary aggregation.
   b. Penicillin, in high doses, but more commonly ticarcillin and carbenicillin, epsilon aminocaproic acid in high doses, and ethanol can interfere with platelet function.
   c. Heparin-associated thrombocytopenia occurs in 5% of patients receiving heparin therapy. This problem usually arises after 6 to 12 days.
   d. Diazepam, chlordiazepoxide, propranolol, and phentolamine also may decrease platelet function.
   e. Phenothiazines may alter platelet numbers and function.
   f. After stopping the offending drug, platelets should recover within 1 to 2 weeks.
2. Aspirin and other nonsteroidal antiinflammatory drugs (NSAIDs) impair platelet aggregation by inhibiting the formation of platelet thromboxane after binding with cyclooxygenase.
   a. A single dose of aspirin prolongs the bleeding time for 48 to 72 hours, and the duration of effect on platelet aggregation may be longer.
   b. Aspirin and NSAIDs are not associated with an increase in minor hemorrhagic complications in patients receiving spinal or epidural anesthesia.
   c. Anesthetic factors associated with a higher incidence of minor hemorrhagic complications include:
      i. Continuous spinal or epidural techniques as compared with single-injection epidural anesthesia.
      ii. Increasing needle gauge.
      iii. Increasing number of needle passes.[2]
   d. In parturients, aspirin 60 mg daily did not increase the risk of adverse events associated with epidural analgesia.[3]
   e. There are three reported cases of spinal hematoma after epidural anesthesia in patients taking NSAIDs, suggesting that this event is extremely rare.[4]

PREECLAMPSIA AND ECLAMPSIA

1. The most common cause of thrombocytopenia in pregnancy
   a. Platelet count is less than 150,000 per cubic millimeter in 34% of parturients with preeclampsia.
   b. Platelet count is less than 100,000 per cubic millimeter in 7.5%.
   c. Thrombocytopenia is probably due to platelet consumption. There also may be a defect in platelet function despite adequate platelet numbers.
2. Other abnormalities of coagulation occur only in conjunction with reduced platelet count. Therefore, platelet counts are useful screening tests, and other coagulation tests should be reserved for use only in the presence of thrombocytopenia.
3. The lowest platelet count compatible with safe regional anesthesia in the presence of normal clotting tests is unknown and controversial.

   a. Platelet counts between 60,000 and 100,000 per cubic millimeter have been suggested, but these recommendations are not evidence-based.

   b. Uneventful epidural analgesia has been described in 30 parturients with platelet counts between 69,000 and 98,000 per cubic millimeter.

THROMBOELASTOGRAPHY (TEG)

1. TEG may provide useful information about overall hemostasis before regional anesthesia.
2. The MA (maximum amplitude) of the TEG tracing is a measure of maximum clot strength and depends on fibrinogen concentration and the number and function of platelets.
3. MA correlates with platelet count in patients with severe preeclampsia and eclampsia, especially in women with platelet counts less than 100,000 per cubic millimeter.
4. In one study, the lower limit of MA in normal pregnancy (53 mm) correlated with a platelet count of 54,000 per cubic millimeter (95% CI, 40 to 75,000 per cubic millimeter). The authors suggested that a platelet count of 75,000 per cubic millimeter should be adequate for neuraxial blocks in preeclamptic patients.[5]

BLEEDING TIME

1. There is no evidence that:
   a. The bleeding time is a specific *in vivo* indicator of platelet function.
   b. The bleeding time can predict the risk of hemorrhage.
   c. The degree of bleeding from the skin accurately reflects the risk of bleeding elsewhere in the body.[6]
2. The bleeding time provides no useful information about the risk of bleeding within the spinal canal.

HELLP SYNDROME

1. Between 4% and 12% of women with severe preeclampsia may have hemolysis, increased liver enzymes, and low platelets (HELLP syndrome).
2. These patients are at very high risk of cesarean section.
3. Common complications include postpartum hemorrhage, excessive bleeding, disseminated intravascular coagulation (DIC), and wound hematoma.
4. Platelet counts continue to decrease after delivery.
5. Check the platelet count before both inserting and removing an epidural catheter, as the risk of epidural hematoma is probably as great at time of removal as that at insertion.

PRIMARY THROMBOCYTHEMIA

1. This disease is a rare myeloproliferative disorder with increased platelet counts and increased marrow megakaryocytes.
2. Symptoms may relate to either thrombosis or hemorrhage.
3. Treatment may include aspirin, low-dose subcutaneous heparin, plateletpheresis, and, rarely, antiproliferative drugs, such as busulfan.
4. Regional anesthetics are usually contraindicated.

Clotting Disorders

Lupus Anticoagulant (LA)

1. An antibody of the IgG, or occasionally IgM, class.
2. Its presence prolongs the aPTT and very rarely the PT.
3. Paradoxically, these patients are at risk of thrombosis, not bleeding.
4. Treatment is often with aspirin, prednisone, and heparin.
5. An isolated increase of the aPTT secondary to the presence of LA and not associated with thrombocytopenia is not a contraindication to regional anesthesia.
    a. First exclude other causes of prolonged aPTT.
    b. Laboratory evaluation may be time consuming and require more than one confirmatory test.
    c. Although the TEG readily diagnoses hypercoagulability, it does not consistently detect LA abnormalities.

von Willebrand Disease (vWD)

1. The most common inherited disorder of hemostasis in women
2. Incidence approaches 1%.
    a. The incidence of severe disease is much lower, about 1 in 10,000.
    b. It is similar to the frequency of classic hemophilia.
3. von Willebrand factor (vWF)
    a. Circulates in plasma as a complex with factor VIII.
    b. Is responsible for platelet adhesion to exposed collagen after vessel injury.
    c. Any abnormality or quantitative decrease of vWF may be associated with a factor VIII decrease.
4. Type 1 vWD
    a. The most common form of the disease
    b. Occurs in about 75% of patients
    c. Is characterized by a reduction in all forms of vWF
5. Type 2A vWD
    a. Ten percent of patients with vWD
    b. Absence of the large and intermediate-size multimers
    c. Absence of ristocetin-induced platelet agglutination
    d. Bleeding episodes are more common and severe than are those in type 1.
6. Type 2B vWD
    a. Seven percent of patients with vWD
    b. Only large multimers are absent.
    c. Ristocetin agglutination is increased.
7. Type 3 vWD
    a. Least common (1%)
    b. Clinically, the most severe
    c. The entire vWF molecule is undetectable in plasma, platelets, or endothelial cells, and as a result, factor VIII also is absent.
8. Evaluation
    a. The most sensitive test for vWD is ristocetin cofactor activity, which measures the ability of vWF to bind to the platelet membrane.
    b. The bleeding time is still used, even though its prolongation does not invariably predict bleeding tendency.

    c. Increased ristocetin-induced platelet agglutination identifies type 2B disease.

    d. The aPTT is prolonged only with marked reductions in factor VIII (type 3 vWD).

9. Desmopressin, which releases vWF from endothelial cells, may be useful in the bleeding patient.

    a. In type 1 disease, desmopressin produces a median 3.1- to 8.8-fold increase of factor VIII, with return to baseline within 4 to 6 hours.

    b. In the different subtypes of type 2, responsiveness to desmopressin is variable.

    c. Type 3 patients usually have no response.

10. In the past, some antihemophilic factor (AHF) preparations have lacked ristocetin cofactor activity. However, purified viral-inactivated plasma-derived products (AHF-vWF) are as effective as cryoprecipitate. They are preferred to cryoprecipitate, which involves the infective risks of blood transfusion.

11. The vWF and factor VIII increase during normal pregnancy. Most women with vWD have a variable increase in vWF and factor VIII during pregnancy, which depends in part on the severity of the disease.

12. Preoperative evaluation

    a. Determine the type of disease.

    b. Measure Hb, PT, aPPT, bleeding time, and, if possible, factor VIII, vWF, and ristocetin cofactor activity.

    c. Response to desmopressin is variable, and a test infusion a few weeks before surgery or delivery will provide important information.

    d. The most important determinant of abnormal hemorrhage at delivery is low factor VIII.

       i. With type 1 disease, factor VIII concentrations greater than 50% appear sufficient for vaginal delivery.

       ii. Bleeding may occur postpartum, as factor VIII and vWF concentrations decrease after delivery.

13. Anesthetic management

    a. Is guided by the preoperative test results.

    b. Regional anesthesia is considered safe in mild disease (type 1).

    c. With type 2 disease, blood products are usually required, even though factor VIII concentration increases in pregnancy. Successful epidural analgesia has been reported in these patients after transfusion of factor VIII concentrate.[7]

Hemophilia A (Classic Hemophilia)

1. Decreased factor VIII activity
2. vWF concentration and activity are not affected.
3. X-linked recessive disorder

    a. Women are usually the only carriers.

    b. One-tenth may experience excessive bleeding. Bleeding may occur if the patient develops lyonization (suppression of normal gene expression), is homozygous, or has a spontaneous gene mutation.

4. Diagnosis is made by history, prolonged aPTT, normal PT, and low factor VIII activity.

5. Pregnancy
   a. Factor VIII activity increases.
   b. Hemostasis after vaginal delivery requires factor VIII concentrations greater than 40% for at least 3 to 4 days.
   c. After cesarean section, levels greater than 50% for 4 to 5 days are needed.
   d. Factor VIII concentrate (AHF) is the treatment of choice to increase levels of factor VIII, with cryoprecipitate or fresh-frozen plasma reserved for emergencies.
   e. The half-life of factor VIII is about 8 hours.
   f. Factor VIII concentration may decrease dramatically within hours of delivery and should be monitored closely.
      i. If bleeding occurs, desmopressin may increase factor VIII activity.
      ii. Serious bleeding should be treated with AHF.
6. Regional anesthesia
   a. Safety depends on the severity of the factor VIII decrease.
   b. There is no contraindication in carriers with normal aPTT.
   c. Avoid regional anesthesia in patients with reduced factor VIII activity and prolonged aPTT.
   d. Check aPTT before removing any epidural catheter.

Hemophilia B (Christmas Disease)
1. Low factor IX and prolonged aPTT but normal factor VIII activity
2. Management is similar to that for hemophilia A.
   a. During normal pregnancy, factor IX activity does not increase as much as factor VIII.
   b. Female carriers of hemophilia B, who have low factor IX activity, are more likely to require specific factor replacement to raise their factor IX activity to safe levels for vaginal delivery (40%) or cesarean section (50%).

Factor XI Deficiency
1. Occurs only occasionally in pregnancy
2. It is usually a mild defect, although serious deficiencies may occur.
3. Treat with virally inactivated factor XI. Use fresh-frozen plasma if factor XI is not available.

Fibrinogen
1. Congenital abnormalities of fibrinogen include afibrinogenemia, dysfibrinogenemia, and hypofibrinogenemia.
2. Dysfibrinogenemia is less severe, many patients are asymptomatic, and in one series, only seven of 83 patients had mild-to-moderate bleeding.
3. If bleeding is a problem, cryoprecipitate or fresh-frozen plasma may be required.
4. The PT and aPTT may be normal, but thrombin and reptilase times will be prolonged.

Antithrombin III Deficiency
1. Antithrombin III (ATIII) is the major inhibitor of thrombin Xa and other serine proteases.

2. Deficiency is associated with a high risk of venous thrombosis (40% to 70%) and pulmonary embolism. These risks are markedly increased in pregnancy.
3. Measuring low plasma ATIII activity makes the diagnosis.
4. Treatment may require large doses of heparin. (Heparin exerts its anticoagulant effect by binding and activating ATIII.) Try to prolong the aPTT by 5 to 10 seconds.

ANTICOAGULANTS IN PREGNANCY

1. Anticoagulation may be necessary for the prevention or treatment of thromboembolic disease.
2. Warfarin
   a. Contraindicated in the first trimester in pregnancy because of embryopathy
   b. Often avoided in the second and third trimesters because of risks of chondrodysplasia punctata and fetal cerebral hemorrhage. However, the frequency of these fetal risks may have been overstated in the past, and warfarin may still have a place during pregnancy.[8]
3. Heparin
   a. Does not cross the placenta because of its relatively large molecular weight.
   b. Heparin-induced thrombocytopenia is a rare complication.
      i. Frequency: 2.4% for therapeutic heparin and 0.3% for prophylactic heparin
      ii. Check a platelet count 5 to 14 days after starting therapy.
   c. Pharmacokinetics: As pregnancy progresses, patients require increasing doses of heparin.
   d. Monitoring heparin therapy with aPTT
      i. Suggested target aPTT varies between 1.5 and 2.5 times normal.
      ii. The risk of bleeding complications with higher aPTT must be balanced against the risk of thrombosis at lower levels.
4. Anesthetic considerations
   a. Regional techniques are contraindicated in patients who are anticoagulated with either heparin or oral anticoagulants.
   b. Spinal hematoma has been reported after spinal and epidural block.
   c. Affected patients were often receiving some form of heparin therapy.
   d. Hematoma also can follow removal of an epidural catheter in anticoagulated patients.
   e. There is some evidence that regional anesthesia can be safely performed in the presence of abnormal coagulation.
   f. Repeated caudal injection of morphine and bupivacaine for the control of chronic pain has been reported in anticoagulated patients.[9]
   g. Others also have reported uneventful epidural block in partially anticoagulated patients.[10]
   h. Anticoagulation with heparin after lumbar puncture may increase the risk of spinal hematoma.

   i.   This risk may be most significant if heparin is started within 1 hour of the lumbar puncture, if the procedure was traumatic, or if there was concurrent treatment with aspirin.

   ii. Consider these factors before starting heparin therapy after a central neuraxial block.

5. Low-molecular-weight heparin (LMWH)
   a. Prevents venous thrombosis in pregnancy.
   b. Use in obstetrics is increasing.
   c. Twice-daily dosing appears to incur a high risk of epidural hematoma after neuraxial block.
   d. Consensus recommendations include the following:
      i.   Monitoring factor Xa level is *not* predictive of the risk of bleeding and is not recommended.
      ii. Regional anesthesia should be postponed until at least 24 hours after the last dose of LMWH.
      iii. After delivery:
           (1) Twenty-four hours should elapse before the first dose of LMWH.
           (2) An indwelling epidural catheter should be removed at least 2 hours before the first dose of LMWH.[11]

6. Thrombosis prophylaxis
   a. Subcutaneous heparin prophylaxis probably does not increase the risk of epidural hematoma.
   b. The response to subcutaneous heparin is very unpredictable.
      i.   Fifty percent of nonpregnant patients who receive 5,000 U of unfractionated heparin subcutaneously will have therapeutic heparin blood concentrations for up to 4 hours.
      ii. Many patients who are receiving heparin prophylaxis would benefit from epidural anesthesia or analgesia.
      iii. Some experts recommend delaying regional block for 4 to 6 hours after the last dose of unfractionated heparin.
      iv. If the block needs to be done sooner, measure the aPTT.
      v.   Remove the epidural catheter just before heparin is restarted after delivery.

REGIONAL ANESTHESIA IN THE PRESENCE OF COAGULOPATHY OR PLATELET DYSFUNCTION

1. Regional anesthesia is contraindicated in the presence of marked thrombocytopenia or coagulopathy as manifested by abnormal coagulation tests. Most published reports of spinal hematoma after epidural injection have been in patients with bleeding diatheses.

2. A more common situation is a pressing indication for spinal or epidural analgesia or anesthesia in a patient with borderline coagulation status.
   a. The indication for regional block must be balanced against the risks involved with an alternative choice.
   b. Excessive concern about the risk of bleeding may dissuade anesthesiologists from offering spinal or epidural

block. As a result, patients may be denied the benefits of these techniques for uncertain reasons.

3. The risk of vessel damage during insertion of an epidural catheter in the parturient is higher than the approximately 10% incidence reported in surgical patients.

   a. When 16- or 18-gauge Tuohy needles are used, 18% of parturients have detectable bleeding.

   b. Attempts to minimize the risk of bleeding include:

      i. Using a spinal instead of an epidural block: The lowest incidence of minor bleeding at the time of insertion is associated with the smallest needles.

      ii. Avoiding the use of a catheter: Either spinal or epidural single-injection techniques are associated with less risk of minor hemorrhage than are spinal or epidural catheters. Insertion of an epidural catheter is important in the genesis of an epidural hematoma.

      iii. Limiting the length of catheter inserted: Greater insertion is associated with a greater risk of vessel puncture.

      iv. The left lateral position

         (1) Is associated with less epidural vein distention.

         (2) May theoretically offer some advantages.

         (3) In obese women, it is easier to identify the epidural or subarachnoid space in the sitting position, which may be more important. The number of passes or difficulty identifying the epidural space is a risk factor for minor hemorrhage.

      v. Midline approach: Theoretically, this choice should be safer, as the epidural veins are located laterally in the space. However, no difference in the incidence of minor venous bleeding was shown between paramedian and midline approaches.

4. Anesthetic technique

   a. In early labor, opioids alone can be used by spinal or epidural routes.

   b. Later in labor, use only dilute local anesthetic–opioid mixtures.

   c. Assess motor function regularly.

   d. Postoperative care

      i. Monitor patients closely for symptoms or signs of cord compression.

      ii. A well-educated nursing staff is essential.

      iii. Pain management

         (1) Avoid local anesthetics.

         (2) Use only neuraxial opioids.

      iv. Remove the epidural catheter only when laboratory tests confirm normal hemostasis.

REFERENCES

1. Cook RL, Miller RC, Katz VL, et al. Immune thrombocytopenic purpura in pregnancy: a reappraisal of management. *Obstet Gynecol* 1991;78:578.

2. Horlocker TT, Wedel DJ, Schroeder DR, et al. Preoperative antiplatelet therapy does not increase the risk of spinal hematoma associated with regional anesthesia. *Anesth Analg* 1995; 80:303.
3. CLASP Collaborative Group. CLASP: a randomised trial of low-dose aspirin for the prevention and treatment of pre-eclampsia among 9364 pregnant women. *Lancet* 1994;343:619.
4. Wulf H. Epidural anaesthesia and spinal haematoma. *Can J Anaesth* 1996;43:1260.
5. Orlikowski CEP, Rocke DA, Murray WB, et al. Thrombelastography changes in pre-eclampsia and eclampsia. *Br J Anaesth* 1996;77:157.
6. Rodgers RPC, Levin J. A critical reappraisal of the bleeding time. *Semin Thromb Hemost* 1990;16:1.
7. Jones BP, Bell EA, Maroof M. Epidural labor analgesia in a parturient with von Willebrand's disease type IIA and severe pre-eclampsia. *Anesthesiology* 1999;90:1219.
8. Oakley CM. Anticoagulation and pregnancy. *Eur Heart J* 1995; 16:1317.
9. Waldman SD, Feldstein GS, Waldman HJ, et al. Caudal administration of morphine sulfate in anticoagulated and thrombocytopenic patients. *Anesth Analg* 1987;66:267.
10. Molnar LI, Rø JS. Epidural analgesia and anticoagulant therapy. *Anaesthesia* 1984;39:602.
11. Horlocker TT, Wedel DJ. Neuraxial block and low-molecular-weight heparin: balancing perioperative analgesia and thromboprophylaxis. *Reg Anesth Pain Med* 1998;23:S164.

Anesthesia and Coexisting Maternal Disease: Diabetes Mellitus, Obesity, Pulmonary, and Neurologic Disease

ANESTHETIC MANAGEMENT OF THE DIABETIC PARTURIENT

1. Abnormal maternal glucose homeostasis
2. Potentially impaired uteroplacental perfusion
3. High likelihood of cesarean delivery

Preoperative Evaluation

1. Assess the severity of maternal diabetes. Review maternal insulin requirements during pregnancy.
2. Look for renal, cardiac, neurologic, or vascular disease, or preeclampsia.
3. Examine the airway carefully. Diabetic patients with "stiff-joint" syndrome may have reduced neck and jaw mobility, which predisposes them to difficult intubation.
4. Review fetal well-being, fetal maturity, and estimated fetal weight.

Glucose Control

1. Maintaining normal maternal glucose is very important throughout gestation and peripartum.
   a. Patients in labor can be managed with slow infusions of insulin (1 U per 10 mL normal saline) and glucose (such as 125 mL per hour of D_5LR or D_5 normal saline; Table 19.1).
   b. Monitor blood glucose closely and adjust glucose and insulin infusions accordingly.
   c. Try to keep maternal glucose below 90 to 110 mg per deciliter.
      i. Avoid maternal hyperglycemia.
      ii. Do not use glucose-containing solutions for intravenous hydration before induction of regional anesthesia.
2. Maternal hyperglycemia (and consequent fetal hyperglycemia and hyperinsulinemia) contributes to fetal hypercarbia and acidemia.
   a. The placenta metabolizes maternal glucose to lactate, contributing to neonatal acidosis. Hydrogen ions then displace oxygen from hemoglobin, limiting fetal oxygen-carrying capacity and decreasing blood oxygen content (Haldane effect).
   b. Glucose in the maternal circulation crosses the placenta via facilitated diffusion and produces fetal hyperglycemia. In response, fetal insulin secretion increases, which may increase fetal glucose uptake and reduce

Table 19.1.   Suggested insulin and glucose infusion rates based on finger-stick glucose measurements

Glucose (mg/100 mL)	Insulin dose (U/h)	Intravenous fluids (125 mL/h)
<100	0	D$_5$LR
100–140	1.0	D$_5$LR
141–180	1.5	Normal saline
181–220	2.0	Normal saline
>220	2.5	Normal saline

Source: After American College of Obstetricians and Gynecologists. Diabetes and pregnancy. Technical Bulletin 200. Washington, DC: American College of Obstetricians and Gynecologists, 1994.

fetal oxygen content, presumably by increasing fetal oxygen consumption.
3. Maternal hyperglycemia at delivery also can cause neonatal hypoglycemia.
    a. Increased maternal glucose causes high umbilical venous glucose.
    b. This hyperglycemia stimulates fetal hyperinsulinemia.
    c. After delivery, hyperinsulinemia leads to neonatal hypoglycemia. (The neonate cannot readily mobilize glucose stores to maintain a normal serum glucose concentration.)
4. Diabetes further worsens fetal condition by hindering placental function and uteroplacental perfusion.
    a. Enlarged villi reduce the surface area over which gas exchange can occur.
    b. Maternal vascular disease impairs placental perfusion and delivery of oxygen and substrates to the fetus.
    c. These changes result in intrauterine growth retardation and a fetus at risk for hypoxemia and acidosis during the stress of labor.
5. Often the fetus of a diabetic mother has macrosomia.
    a. Large fetal size increases the likelihood of cephalopelvic disproportion and need for cesarean delivery.
    b. Vaginal delivery of a macrosomic fetus may require forceps or result in shoulder dystocia.
    c. The large uterus of a diabetic parturient may not contract well after delivery, resulting in uterine atony and postpartum hemorrhage.

Analgesia for Labor and Delivery
1. Systemic opioids and sedatives can provide analgesia during early labor.
    a. The neonate of the diabetic patient may be particularly sensitive to depression from sedatives.
    b. Prematurity further increases the susceptibility to central nervous depression from opioids and sedatives.

2. Regional analgesia
   a. In nondiabetic laboring parturients, epidural analgesia reduces circulating maternal plasma catecholamines and 11-hydroxycorticosteroids.
   b. This effect has two potential benefits for diabetic patients:
      i. Epinephrine and cortisol stimulate hyperglycemia and may contribute to difficulties with maternal glucose control.
      ii. Reducing circulating maternal catecholamines should improve placental perfusion.
   c. Before induction
      i. Establish normal intravascular volume status with a glucose-free solution.
      ii. Remember the potential for impaired uteroplacental perfusion.
      iii. Pay close attention to fetal monitoring and proper maternal positioning.
      iv. Avoid aortocaval compression.
   d. Juvenile-onset diabetic parturients may have lower epidural local anesthetic dose requirements.
   e. Spinal injection of opioids or local anesthetics can rapidly provide analgesia labor and vaginal delivery.
      i. A saddle block is appropriate should forceps delivery be necessary in a patient without a functioning epidural catheter.
      ii. Be prepared to proceed to cesarean delivery should the attempted forceps delivery fail.

Anesthesia for Cesarean Delivery

Patient Preparation

1. Do not use glucose-containing fluids for prehydration or volume replacement.
2. Insulin and glucose therapy after the nothing-by-mouth (NPO) period before elective cesarean delivery depends on the severity of the patient's disease. On admission, measure maternal glucose by finger-stick. Start an intravenous infusion of insulin (1 U per 10 mL normal saline) and glucose (such as 125 mL per hour of D_5LR or D_5 normal saline) as indicated (see Table 19.1). Thereafter, measure blood glucose frequently.
3. After delivery, insulin requirements decrease.
   a. Patients receiving insulin before delivery may develop hypoglycemia.
   b. Carefully monitor maternal glucose and adjust glucose or insulin therapy as indicated.

Anesthetic Technique

1. Good maternal and fetal outcome follows both regional and general anesthesia, provided the earlier issues are considered.
2. During general anesthesia, neonatal depression (defined as Apgar scores less than 7 at 1 minute) occurs more commonly in the infants of diabetic mothers. The increased likelihood of immaturity and prematurity in neonates of diabetic mothers may explain this higher risk of depression.

3. Spinal anesthesia is appropriate for cesarean delivery, provided that hypotension is avoided. Avoiding maternal hyperglycemia and treating hypotension aggressively (ephedrine 10 to 20 mg IV when systolic blood pressure decreases 10 mm Hg) ensure comparable neonatal outcome in normal and diabetic pregnancies receiving spinal anesthesia for cesarean delivery.
4. Epidural anesthesia
   a. As with spinal anesthesia, maternal hypotension may cause neonatal acidosis, particularly if the maternal diabetes is severe.
   b. Use care when giving large doses of epidural local anesthetics to a potentially acidotic fetus of a diabetic parturient. Local anesthetic ion-trapping, resulting in accumulation of the anesthetic in the neonate, is a theoretical concern.
5. The neonate
   a. Hypoglycemia (blood glucose less than 35 mg per deciliter in term infants) can occur.
   b. Clinical signs include poor tone, poor color, apnea, respiratory distress, lethargy, hypothermia, and seizures.

ANESTHETIC MANAGEMENT OF THE OBESE PARTURIENT

1. Obesity complicates 6% to 10% of pregnancies and is more common in older patients of greater parity.
2. Obese parturients develop preeclampsia, hypertension, and diabetes more commonly than do nonobese parturients.
3. Obese women also may have hypertriglyceridemia and coronary artery disease.
4. Obesity is a risk factor for a long, difficult labor and cesarean delivery.
5. Associated fetal problems include macrosomia, shoulder dystocia, and birth trauma.
6. Physiology of obesity
   a. Pulmonary function
      i. Decreased lung and chest-wall compliance due to chest-wall and abdominal fat
      ii. Increased work of breathing
      iii. Increased minute ventilation
      iv. Remember, pregnancy itself decreases functional residual capacity (FRC) and increases minute ventilation and oxygen consumption.
      v. Pulmonary function studies in obese nonpregnant patients show a restrictive ventilatory defect.
      vi. Obesity decreases the ventilatory response to hypercarbia.
      vii. The pulmonary changes of pregnancy can produce airway closure, ventilation–perfusion defects, and hypoxemia.
   b. Cardiovascular system
      i. Both pregnancy and obesity increase cardiac work.
      ii. This combination may produce symptoms of myocardial failure during pregnancy.
      iii. Obstructive sleep apnea can cause pulmonary hypertension and right heart failure.
      iv. Hypertensive disorders also are common.

Analgesia for Labor and Delivery

1. Use systemic medications with caution.
   a. Sedatives can contribute to hypoventilation and hypoxemia.
   b. The effective dose of opioids for labor analgesia in the obese patient may be unpredictable.
      i. Give opioids in small increments, titrating to the desired effect.
      ii. Should somnolence occur, use a pulse oximeter to assess oxygenation and the need for supplemental oxygen.
2. Regional analgesia can be very helpful in obese parturients.
   a. Adequate analgesia will diminish ventilatory requirements during labor.
   b. Regional analgesia can help maintain good oxygenation by preventing the cycle of hyperventilation with painful contractions and hypoventilation in the rest period between contractions.
   c. A continuous epidural block provides a means of anesthetizing the patient should cesarean or operative vaginal delivery become necessary.

Monitoring

1. Monitoring of both mother and fetus while establishing regional anesthesia can prove difficult in obese parturients.
2. The fetal heart rate may be difficult to trace with an external monitor, and having the patient sit for epidural placement can exacerbate this problem.
3. Accurately measuring maternal blood pressure is another challenge.
   a. An appropriately sized blood pressure cuff should be 20% to 30% as wide as the arm circumference.
   b. A thigh cuff on the upper arm or a large blood pressure cuff on the forearm may be necessary.
   c. Pulse oximetry can be very helpful in guiding the need for supplemental oxygen.

Epidural Technique

1. Identifying the epidural space, inserting a catheter, and successfully providing labor analgesia can prove a daunting task in obese parturients.
   a. Landmarks can be impossible to feel.
   b. The sitting position may be both technically easier for the anesthetist and more comfortable for the patient.
      i. Sitting allows identification of the patient's midline by drawing a line between the often easily palpated C7 spinous process and the gluteal fold.
      ii. Marks at the waist from undergarments or the fetal heart rate monitor belt can approximate the level of the L3–L4 or L4–L5 interspaces.
   c. The spinous processes above and below the interspace used can be identified, after local infiltration, by probing with a long 26-gauge spinal needle.
   d. An extralong epidural needle may be (rarely) needed to reach the epidural space.

2. Induction of labor analgesia
    a. Intrathecal opioids (with or without local anesthetic)
        i. Rapid onset
        ii. High certainty of proper placement (by observing cerebrospinal fluid [CSF] flow).
    b. Epidural injection of opioid and local anesthetic allows immediate testing of catheter location.
3. Maintaining labor analgesia
    a. Dilute local anesthetic–opioid solutions.
        i. Confirm proper catheter location (by demonstration of a bilateral block).
        ii. Minimize motor block (to allow the patient to move and assist with transfer, if needed).
    b. Concerns
        i. Both the gravid uterus and the obese abdomen contribute to aortocaval compression.
        ii. Dose the catheter slowly to avoid sudden hypotension and fetal compromise.
        iii. Epidural local anesthetics may spread farther in obese parturients, increasing the level of sensory blockade achieved with a given dose of drug.
4. Problems
    a. Not uncommonly, the epidural catheter needs replacement or repositioning to achieve and maintain continuous pain relief. In on series, 42% of morbidly obese (more than 300 lb) parturients needed multiple epidural catheters compared with 6% of normal-weight parturients.[1]
    b. Placing an epidural catheter early in labor allows time to assure proper function. In addition, the patient may be more cooperative than in more painful active labor.
    c. Accidental dural puncture
        i. Consider threading a catheter into the intrathecal space and conducting a continuous spinal anesthetic.
        ii. Either opioids or a combination of opioids and local anesthetics can be used for labor analgesia.
        iii. Consider a continuous intrathecal infusion of a dilute local anesthetic-opioid mixture at 2 mL per hour.

Anesthesia for Cesarean Section

1. The operating table may be narrow or unstable.
    a. Extra arm boards along the side can increase the width of the table.
    b. Some tables are not meant for patients over 300 lb.
2. Patient positioning.
    a. The supine position may exacerbate dyspnea, airway closure, and inadequate alveolar ventilation.
    b. A modified "lawn chair" position with both head and legs slightly elevated (knees flexed) may help maintain FRC and preserve venous return and patient comfort.
    c. Positioning the patient in a proper "sniffing" position also should improve patient comfort and airway access (Fig. 19.1).

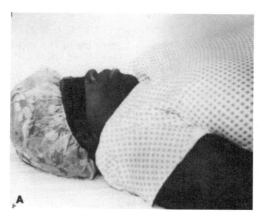

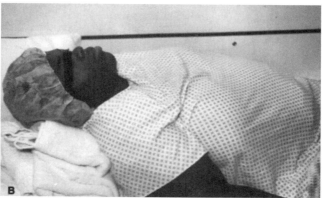

Fig. 19.1. A: An obese pregnant woman in the supine position. The inability to extend the head on the atlantooccipital joint prevents alignment of oral, pharyngeal, and laryngeal axes and limits access to the airway with the laryngoscope. **B:** Proper positioning includes elevation of the shoulders, flexion of the cervical spine, and extension of the head on the atlantooccipital joint (the "sniffing" position). The sniffing position helps align the oral, pharyngeal, and laryngeal axes and improves access to the airway. (Photographs courtesy of Dr. B. Leighton, Philadelphia, with permission.)

Surgical Technique

1. A Pfannenstiel incision may produce less postoperative pain and allow earlier ambulation.
2. However, the abdominal fat pad needs to be displaced cephalad to provide good surgical exposure. Doing so may compromise the patient's pulmonary status and contribute to caval compression and diminished venous return.
3. Carefully evaluate the hemodynamic and pulmonary affects of the patient's position.

Monitoring

1. Use a properly sized blood pressure cuff.
2. If noninvasive blood pressure monitoring is unreliable, consider an arterial catheter for measuring blood pressure and maternal blood gas tensions.
3. Parturients with severe hypertension or cardiac disease may require central hemodynamic monitoring.
4. Pulse oximetry is necessary to assess maternal oxygenation.
5. During general anesthesia, the ability to immediately measure end-tidal carbon dioxide is crucial.
6. Monitor the fetus during positioning and induction of anesthesia when at all possible.

Anesthetic Technique

EPIDURAL ANESTHESIA

1. Regional anesthesia, especially epidural block, has significant advantages over general anesthesia in obese patients, provided the patient can be positioned comfortably.
2. Advantages of epidural anesthesia
   a. The level of sensory blockade can be extended slowly and in a relatively controlled fashion. The slower onset of sympathetic block improves hemodynamic stability by allowing time to alter maternal position and volume status in response to changes in blood pressure.
   b. An epidural catheter can provide anesthesia for as long as needed.
   c. The catheter also can be used for postoperative analgesia.
3. Because local anesthetic requirements may be lower in obese patients, inject drug in small (5-mL) increments until an adequate level of blockade is achieved.

SPINAL ANESTHESIA

1. Advantages
   a. Distinct endpoint for needle placement (CSF)
   b. Rapid onset
   c. Profound anesthesia
2. Disadvantages
   a. Technical problems
      i. Small-gauge needles can deflect when passing through tissues.
      ii. Standard needles may not reach the subarachnoid space.
   b. Rapid onset (high-risk hypotension)
   c. Possibly unpredictable block height
      i. Weight does not influence the spread of blockade in patients weighing less than 94 kg.
      ii. Impact of greater weights on spread of blockade is unknown.
      iii. Excessive spread of block could be problematic.
   d. Inadequate duration of single-injection technique. (Cesarean sections in morbidly obese women are more likely to take over 1 hour compared with control patients.)

3. Alternative approaches
   a. Continuous spinal anesthesia
      i. Currently best done with 17- or 18-gauge Tuohy needle and a large-gauge polyamide catheter
      ii. Insert only 3 cm of catheter into the subarachnoid space.
      iii. Provide anesthesia with 0.5- to 1.0-mL boluses of local anesthetic.
   b. Combined spinal–epidural anesthesia
      i. Advantages
         (1) Often easier to identify epidural space than subarachnoid space
         (2) Can use a reduced dose of intrathecal local anesthetic and then extend or prolong block with epidural drugs
      ii. Disadvantages
         (1) It is difficult to test for intrathecal catheter location in the presence of extensive spinal anesthesia.
         (2) Extralong needles may be needed.

GENERAL ANESTHESIA

1. Inability to secure an airway is a leading cause of maternal mortality.
2. Obesity is an important risk factor for difficult intubation.
   a. If airway examination suggests a potentially difficult intubation, inform the obstetric staff that a rapid induction of general anesthesia could jeopardize maternal safety.
   b. If general anesthesia is necessary, allow time for either awake fiberoptic intubation or awake direct laryngoscopy.
   c. Factors that contribute to airway difficulties in the obese parturient
      i. A short neck with limited mobility may make it difficult to insert the laryngoscope into the mouth. A short-handled laryngoscope is helpful in this situation.
      ii. Redundant tissue in the airway may be difficult to displace with any laryngoscope blade. Use of the Bullard laryngoscope with an intubating stylet was reported to be useful in this situation.
   d. Airway management of the obese parturient: *maternal positioning*!
      i. Have the patient in the "sniffing" position, which includes flexion of the cervical spine with extension of the head on the atlantooccipital joint.
      ii. Support the patient's shoulders on blankets and further support the base of her skull with additional towels (see Fig. 19.1).
         (1) Helps the breasts to fall forward, increasing the space between the neck and the chest
         (2) Allows proper alignment of the oral, pharyngeal, and laryngeal axes
      iii. Confirm proper endotracheal placement with capnography.

e. Unpredicted difficult intubation
   i. Always be prepared to manage a difficult airway.
      (1) Have multiple laryngoscopes and endotracheal tubes immediately available.
      (2) Other supplies: laryngeal mask airway (LMA), fiberoptic bronchoscope, equipment for cricothyroid puncture and transtracheal jet ventilation
   ii. Set your priorities in advance. Know ahead of time the steps you will take if intubation proves difficult or impossible.
   iii. Failed intubation drill
      (1) Call for help.
      (2) One "best" attempt at intubation. (Multiple laryngoscopies will cause pharyngeal trauma and convert a "can't intubate, can ventilate" situation into a "can't intubate, can't ventilate situation.")
      (3) Move on to alternative methods to secure the airway (LMA, esophageal obturator, transtracheal ventilation).

3. Gastric acid aspiration
   a. Obese patients have even larger gastric volumes and lower gastric pH values than control parturients.
   b. Difficulties with intubation and the potential for multiple manipulations of the airway pose additional risks.
   c. Pharmacologic prophylaxis may decrease this risk. Consider clear antacids within 30 minutes of the planned surgery, H2-blockers, and metoclopramide.

4. Preoxygenation
   a. Obese parturients are at high risk for developing hypoxemia during the induction of anesthesia.
      i. Reduced FRC
      ii. Increased oxygen consumption (greater in obese versus nonobese parturients)
      iii. Increased risk of difficult ventilation or intubation
   b. In nonobese parturients, either 3 to 5 minutes of tidal breathing or four deep breaths of 100% oxygen provide adequate preoxygenation before the induction of anesthesia.
      i. Both techniques also provide effective preoxygenation in obese nonpregnant patients.
      ii. With both techniques, use high fresh gas flows (8 to 10 L per minute) to prevent rebreathing of exhaled nitrogen, and ensure a tight mask fit to avoid entrainment of room air.

5. Ventilation
   a. High F_iO_2
   b. Large tidal volumes or positive end-expiratory pressure (PEEP) will help maintain maternal oxygenation. If using PEEP, watch for adverse effects on cardiac output and blood pressure.

6. Pharmacokinetics
   a. Obese nonpregnant patients metabolize halothane more than do nonobese patients.

    b. Obese patients may have prolonged recovery times after steroid muscle relaxant (pancuronium, rocuronium, vecuronium). Obesity may alter the hepatic clearance of these drugs.

7. After completion of surgery, carefully evaluate the adequacy of ventilation, oxygenation, and airway reflexes before extubating the trachea. Assist ventilation in the early postoperative period as needed.

Postoperative Care

1. Pulmonary function abnormalities persist after cesarean delivery in obese patients.
   a. In obese nonpregnant patients undergoing abdominal surgery, oxygenation remains poor up to postoperative day 4.
   b. Possible etiologies for this hypoxemia include pain and inadequate ventilation, excessive sedation from analgesics, and diaphragmatic dysfunction.
   c. Good postoperative analgesia should promote early ambulation and good pulmonary toilet.
   d. Spinal or epidural opioids are helpful by providing good analgesia without excessive maternal sedation. In obese nonpregnant patients, epidural opioids for postoperative pain relief after abdominal surgery improves early postoperative pulmonary function.

2. Cardiac function
   a. Demands are highest immediately postpartum because of delivery of the placenta, the loss of the low-resistance placental bed, and autotransfusion of blood from the contracted uterus.
   b. Volume overload is possible during this time in patients with borderline cardiac function.
   c. Resolution of regional anesthesia-induced sympathetic blockade will contribute to this volume load, as will mobilization of interstitial edema in the preeclamptic patient.

3. Venous stasis and thrombosis
   a. Thromboembolic disease is a leading cause of death in obese parturients.
   b. Early ambulation, compression stockings, and subcutaneous heparin may help prevent venous thrombosis.

ANESTHETIC MANAGEMENT OF THE PARTURIENT WITH PULMONARY DISEASE

Asthma

Preoperative Evaluation

1. Assess the severity of asthma during pregnancy, symptoms (shortness of breath, cough, wheezing, chest tightness), medications (inhaled β-agonists, cromolyn sodium, corticosteroids, systemic corticosteroids, oral theophylline), and events that precipitate asthma (stress, exercise, allergens, infections).

2. Examine the patient for evidence of bronchospasm. Spirometry and, if necessary, arterial blood gases provide more information. When interpreting arterial blood gases, remember that a normal p_aCO_2 during pregnancy ranges from 32 to 34 mm Hg.

3. Try to optimize maternal pulmonary status before induction of labor or cesarean delivery. Maternal hypoxia and hypocapnia will impair fetal oxygenation.
4. Intrapartum bronchospasm
   a. Occurs in only 10% of parturients with asthma.
   b. Treatment
      i. Supplemental oxygen
      ii. Ensure adequate hydration.
      iii. Look for precipitating factors (i.e., upper respiratory infection, exposure to allergens)
      iv. Give inhaled β_2-adrenergic agonists (metoproterenol or albuterol).
      v. Parenteral corticosteroid therapy may be necessary if inhaled β-agonists do not relieve bronchospasm. Patients who have taken oral steroids to manage asthma during the previous year should receive steroid coverage during labor and delivery with intravenous hydrocortisone 100 mg every 6 hours. Note that patients receiving corticosteroids may have concomitant diabetes.

Anesthesia for Labor and Delivery

1. Systemic medications can provide analgesia and sedation in the early phases of labor.
2. In more active and painful labor, epidural analgesia has distinct advantages.
   a. In patients without analgesia, the pain of active labor increases minute ventilation and oxygen consumption.
   b. In the asthmatic patient, this hyperventilation and hypocarbia can precipitate bronchospasm.
3. For patients who do not receive epidural analgesia for labor, spinal anesthesia may be used for spontaneous or assisted vaginal delivery.

Anesthesia for Cesarean Section

EPIDURAL ANESTHESIA

1. Regional anesthesia offers significant advantages in asthmatic patients.
   a. Avoiding general anesthesia and endotracheal intubation may decrease the incidence of bronchospasm.
   b. In an awake patient, continuous verbal contact will elicit signs of respiratory difficulty.
   c. In the Closed Claims analysis of adverse respiratory events, there are eight cases of obstetric patients who experienced bronchospasm resulting in patient injury and lawsuit. Seven of the cases involved general anesthesia (two were patients who required conversion from regional to general anesthesia because of failed block and high block).[2]
2. Respiratory effects of epidural anesthesia
   a. While motor block accompanying the high levels of epidural anesthesia necessary for abdominal delivery can impair pulmonary function, arterial blood gas values are unchanged in asthmatic parturients.

b. High levels of epidural anesthesia can, however, reduce peak expiratory flow rates and may interfere with the ability to cough.
   i. Reassure the patient should the loss of sensation in the chest wall contribute to a feeling of shortness of breath.
   ii. If coughing is impaired, avoid sedatives that may further suppress coughing, and watch for problems with oral secretions or regurgitation.
3. Epinephrine (1:200,000) in epidural local anesthetics may aid in bronchodilation. However, no documentation exists that this small amount of absorbed epinephrine produces significant bronchodilation. This technique, however, is probably not harmful.

SPINAL ANESTHESIA

1. Most data suggest that extensive sensory and sympathetic blockades lack effect on respiratory function in these patients.
2. As with epidural anesthesia, reductions in peak expiratory flow rates occur during spinal anesthesia for cesarean delivery.

GENERAL ANESTHESIA

1. Rapid sequence induction and intubation can precipitate bronchospasm. Provide as deep a plane of anesthesia as possible to help prevent bronchospasm during intubation.
   a. Ketamine
      i. Good choice for induction of anesthesia in asthmatic parturients
      ii. Even in low doses (less than 0.5 mg per kilogram), it causes bronchodilation in nonpregnant patients with pulmonary disorders.
      iii. Bronchodilation begins within 1.5 minutes, and lasts 6 to 8 minutes.
      iv. Minimal neonatal depression occurs if the induction dose remains less than 1.5 mg per kilogram.
      v. Sympathetic stimulation increases maternal blood pressure and heart rate, limiting its use in hypertensive parturients.
   b. Propofol
      i. Dose: 2.0 to 2.5 mg per kilogram.
      ii. Produces less maternal hypertension but similar neonatal outcome as thiopental 4 to 5 mg per kilogram.
      iii. Reduces the incidence of bronchospasm and incites smaller increases in airway resistance after intubation compared with thiobarbiturates and etomidate.[3]
   c. Other techniques to prevent intubation-related bronchospasm
      i. Intravenous lidocaine
      ii. Small doses of opioid (such as fentanyl)
      iii. Because coughing and straining can trigger bronchospasm, avoid manipulation of the airway until full skeletal muscle relaxation has been achieved.

2. Intraoperative bronchospasm
    a. Give high concentrations of oxygen.
    b. Inhaled bronchodilators can be given via the endotracheal tube.
    c. Volatile anesthetics are potent bronchodilators and should be used to maintain anesthesia.
        i.   Halothane and isoflurane provide equivalent bronchodilation at high doses.
        ii. Animal data suggest that halothane is a better bronchodilator at lower doses (0.6 and 1.1 minimum alveolar concentration [MAC]).[4]
        iii. High concentrations of these anesthetics also may contribute to uterine atony and increase blood loss.
3. Extubation
    a. Awake extubation will minimize the chance of pulmonary aspiration of gastric contents.
    b. The endotracheal tube may prompt bronchospasm as the level of anesthesia wanes.
    c. Inhaled bronchodilators and small doses of intravenous fentanyl or lidocaine before emergence can help minimize airway reactivity during extubation.

UTERINE ATONY

1. Inhaled β-agonists and potent anesthetics are uterine relaxants.
2. Some uterotonics can be bronchconstrictors.
    a. Prostaglandin: $PGF_{2\alpha}$ is a potent bronchoconstrictor. Avoid the synthetic analogue of this prostaglandin, 15-methyl $PGF_{2\alpha}$, carboprost-tromethamine (Hemabate).
    b. Bronchospasm has been reported after the administration of ergot preparations ($n = 3$). (Two patients received the medication intravenously, and all three patients had a history of asthma.) The role of the ergot derivatives in these cases is a bit unclear.
    c. Use vigorous uterine massage and intravenous infusions of oxytocin as first treatment of uterine atony in the asthmatic patient.

CIGARETTE USE

1. Cigarette smoking during pregnancy has been associated with intrauterine growth retardation, spontaneous abortion, premature rupture of membranes, preterm birth, placenta previa, abruptio placentae, congenital anomalies, and sudden infant death syndrome.
2. Carbon monoxide
    a. Competes with oxygen for binding sites on hemoglobin in both the mother and the fetus.
    b. Increased carbon monoxide decreases fetal oxygen content.
        i.   Chronic hypoxemia alters both fetal and placental development.
        ii. The fetus redirects perfusion to priority organs (brain, heart, and adrenal glands) at the expense of overall growth.

       iii. The placenta increases in size, surface area, and vascularity to optimize fetal oxygenation. These changes predispose the mother to hemorrhagic complications.

3. Regional anesthetic techniques are appropriate for labor and vaginal or cesarean delivery.
   a. During induction, take care to avoid reductions in utero-placental blood flow with adequate maternal prehydration, left uterine displacement, and careful monitoring of blood pressure.
   b. Monitor the fetus to assess any potential anesthetic effects on fetal well-being.
   c. Regional anesthesia avoids airway manipulation and suppression of mucociliary clearance.
   d. The motor blockade that accompanies the high sensory level of blockade necessary for cesarean delivery may interfere with the ability of some parturients to cough intra- and immediately postoperatively.
4. General anesthesia for cesarean delivery has significant disadvantages for parturients who smoke.
   a. Airway reactivity increases in patients who smoke regularly.
   b. The induction of general anesthesia may provoke bronchospasm.
   c. General anesthesia inhibits mucociliary clearance and macrophage function in patients who smoke cigarettes. This action may increase the risk of postoperative pulmonary problems.
5. Postoperative care
   a. Cigarette smokers produce more airway secretions than do nonsmokers.
   b. Encourage aggressive postoperative pulmonary toilet with incentive spirometry and deep breathing and coughing.
   c. Avoid drugs that cause cough suppression (systemic opioids and sedatives) as much as possible.
   d. Postoperative analgesia with neuraxial opioids may minimize cough suppression and help maintain optimal pulmonary function.
6. Abstinence
   a. Postoperative respiratory complications decrease after 4 to 6 weeks.
   b. Carboxyhemoglobin concentrations decrease and oxygen delivery increases after as little as 48 hours.
   c. A few days of abstinence will improve mucociliary transport.

ANESTHETIC MANAGEMENT OF THE PARTURIENT WITH NEUROLOGIC DISEASE

Anesthetic care of the parturient with preexisting neurologic disease must be individualized. It should take into consideration the natural history of the patient's disease and the likelihood that a specific anesthetic technique or drug will alter the course of that disease. Some anesthesiologists hesitate, for example, to do a regional anesthetic in a patient with a neuropathy. If the patient's condition worsens after the anesthetic, they fear their anesthetic will be blamed for the problem. Others believe it is unfair to consider all patients with neurologic disease ineligible for the potential benefits of regional anesthesia for labor, delivery, or cesarean section. Consider each case individually. Consult with the patient, her neurologist, and her obstetrician to design a reasonable and safe anesthetic plan. Understand the pathophysiology of the neurologic problem, and consider the potential affects of anesthesia on the disease. Come to an agreement with the patient regarding anesthetic management before labor begins.

Seizure Disorder

1. Evaluation
   a. Be aware of the etiology of seizures in a given parturient (i.e., eclampsia, intracranial tumor or vascular abnormality, subarachnoid hemorrhage, metabolic disturbances, drug or alcohol withdrawal, trauma, and idiopathic).
   b. Review the patient's medications. Check their blood concentration and give supplemental drug if needed.
2. Labor epidural analgesia can significantly benefit these patients.
   a. Hypocarbia, which develops when labor pain causes maternal hyperventilation, lowers seizure threshold.
   b. Epidural analgesia limits this maternal hyperventilation in response to pain.
   c. Similarly, regional anesthesia is quite suitable for anesthesia for cesarean delivery.
3. Two anesthetics, enflurane and ketamine, can cause seizures.
   a. Enflurane
      i. High concentrations (2.5% to 3.0%) in the presence of hypocarbia lower the seizure threshold and cause convulsions.
      ii. At lower doses and with normocarbia, there is little risk of exacerbating a preexisting epileptic focus.
      iii. The presence of a seizure disorder probably does not contraindicate the use of enflurane in low doses during cesarean delivery.
   b. Ketamine
      i. Incites electroencephalogram (EEG) seizure activity when given to patients with preexisting seizure disorders.
      ii. It seems reasonable to avoid ketamine as an induction agent in parturients with epilepsy.
      iii. Also, avoid repeated doses of meperidine for labor or postoperative analgesia, as accumulation of the metabolite normeperidine has been reported to cause seizures.
4. Some seizure medications may alter anesthetic requirements.
   a. Phenytoin and carbamazepine antagonize nondepolarizing muscle relaxants.
   b. Phenobarbital increases hepatic metabolism of anesthetics by inducing hepatic enzyme function.

Multiple Sclerosis

1. A disease of the central nervous system characterized by nerve demyelination with intermittent exacerbations and improvements in symptoms
2. Hyperpyrexia, infection, electrolyte imbalance, emotional and physical stress, and fatigue can worsen symptoms or trigger relapses.
3. Parturients with multiple sclerosis who relapse tend to do so in the 3 months after delivery rather than during pregnancy.
4. Regional anesthesia
   a. Theoretical risks
      i. Local anesthetics may be neurotoxic when injected close to demyelinated nerves.
      ii. They could contribute to or be associated with exacerbations of the disease.
   b. Available data
      i. Currently available prospective longitudinal studies of pregnancy and multiple sclerosis have not included data about anesthesia for delivery.
      ii. Individual case reports and a case series document safe use of epidural block for labor analgesia and cesarean delivery.[5]
         (1) There is an association between the use of high concentrations of epidural local anesthetics and the incidence of postpartum relapse of multiple sclerosis. While this association is troubling, the number of patients reported was small.
         (2) Other factors (i.e., long, difficult labor; fetal malpresentation; difficult delivery) may increase both the need for high concentrations of local anesthetics and the risk of relapse of multiple sclerosis.
   c. Only sporadic case reports describe the use of spinal anesthesia in these women.
   d. Regardless of the type of neuraxial anesthesia selected, discuss the possibility of relapse with the patient preoperatively.
5. General anesthesia
   a. No technique has been associated with consistent alterations in relapse rate.
   b. There is one case report of hyperkalemia after succinylcholine administration, but the absence of other reports suggests a low incidence of this problem in these patients.
   c. Routine general anesthetic techniques are probably appropriate.

Myasthenia Gravis

1. Characterized by a lack of responsiveness of the postsynaptic acetylcholine receptor, probably due to antibodies to the receptor
2. Symptoms include weakness and easy fatigability associated with repetitive use of voluntary muscles.

3. Symptoms usually improve with anticholinesterase therapy, although other treatments including corticosteroids, immunosuppressives, and plasmapheresis may be required.
4. Pregnancy has a variable effect on the course of the disease. Not uncommonly, postpartum exacerbations arise.
5. Preoperative evaluation
   a. Know the muscles involved (respiratory, bulbar), current symptoms, ventilatory status, and anticholinesterase therapy.
   b. Continue anticholinesterase medications throughout the peripartum period to preserve muscle strength during the work of labor and delivery.

Labor Analgesia

1. Systemic medications may be used to provide labor analgesia to myasthenic patients, but give only small doses to avoid ventilatory depression.
2. Epidural analgesia will reduce the ventilatory work associated with painful labor without interfering with the muscles of respiration.

Anesthesia for Cesarean Section

1. Parturients with myasthenia gravis present a more difficult anesthetic challenge should they require cesarean delivery.
2. Anesthetic choice depends on the patient's ventilatory status and muscle strength.
3. Regional anesthesia
   a. Excessively high levels of spinal anesthesia can further impair ventilatory function.
   b. An epidural anesthetic may prove advantageous.
      i. The anesthetic level can be carefully titrated.
      ii. The level of motor blockade is lower and less profound than that seen with a comparable sensory level of spinal anesthesia.
   c. With any regional anesthetic technique, be prepared to intubate and support ventilation should muscle weakness and ventilatory failure develop.
   d. One can use neuraxial opioids for postoperative pain relief, minimizing the need for systemic opioids and sedative medications.
   e. Anticholinesterase medications may impede the metabolism of ester local anesthetics (i.e., 2-chloroprocaine). Use only amide local anesthetics in women taking these drugs.
4. General anesthesia
   a. May be appropriate for parturients with such significant respiratory compromise that they may not tolerate the stress of surgery under regional anesthesia.
   b. Consider the patient's unpredictable response to muscle relaxants.
      i. Succinylcholine
         (1) Both resistance and early onset of phase II block have been reported.
         (2) Long-term anticholinesterase therapy may decrease plasma cholinesterase activity and prolong the duration.

    ii. Nondepolarizing drugs
        (1) Because of the decreased number of func-
             tional acetylcholine receptors, myasthenic
             patients are very sensitive to nondepolariz-
             ing muscle relaxants.
        (2) In nonpregnant patients, adequate condi-
             tions for tracheal intubation can be obtained
             with sedative agents or volatile anesthetics
             alone.
        (3) The short-acting muscle relaxant miva-
             curium will have a substantially prolonged
             action in patients receiving long-term anti-
             cholinesterase therapy because of decreased
             plasma cholinesterase.
        (4) Rocuronium may be another alternative to
             rapid-sequence intubation, but expect a pro-
             longed duration.
  c. Suggested technique
      i. Awake intubation with topical anesthesia, or a
          rapid-sequence induction of anesthesia by using
          1.5 mg per kilogram succinylcholine or 0.6 mg per
          kilogram rocuronium.
     ii. Closely monitor neuromuscular function.
    iii. Before extubation, look for clinical evidence of full
          recovery of neuromuscular function (a negative
          inspiratory force of −40 cm water and a sustained
          head lift of greater than 5 seconds).
     iv. Prepare for the possibility of postoperative mechan-
          ical ventilation, especially in high-risk patients:
        (1) Duration of myasthenia gravis for longer
             than 6 years.
        (2) A history of chronic respiratory disease
             other than myasthenia gravis.
        (3) A dose of pyridostigmine greater than 750 mg
             per day.
        (4) A preoperative vital capacity less than 2.9 L.

Paraplegia and Quadriplegia

1. Paraplegic and quadriplegic patients are at risk for a vari-
    ety of medical complications, including anemia, urinary
    tract infections, decubitus ulcers, thromboembolic phe-
    nomena, respiratory compromise, and autonomic hyper-
    reflexia.
2. Preoperative evaluation of these patients must include assess-
    ment of the level of spinal cord injury, symptoms of autonomic
    hyperreflexia, ventilatory function, and hemoglobin.

Autonomic Hyperreflexia

1. Automomic hyperreflexia is seen in 85% of patients with
    spinal cord lesions at or above T6, although it has been
    described in parturients with lesions below T6.
2. Symptoms include flushing and sweating above the level of
    injury, severe hypertension, bradycardia, headache, and
    anxiety.

3. Mechanism
   a. Reflex sympathetic discharge, not modified or inhibited by supraspinal centers, follows distention or contraction of a viscus below the level of spinal cord injury.
   b. The vasculature in the region below the level of injury is very sensitive to catecholamines and responds with pronounced vasoconstriction.
   c. The resulting severe hypertension, via afferents from the carotid and aortic arch baroreceptors, stimulates vagally mediated bradycardia.
4. Triggers related to pregnancy
   a. Uterine contractions
      i. Paroxysmal hypertension may be the only sign of labor in patients with complete spinal cord transection.
      ii. Previously asymptomatic patients may first experience this problem during labor.
   b. Skin incision, perineal manipulation, suprapubic pressure, and distention of the bladder or rectum
   c. The more caudal the spinal segment receiving the afferent stimulation, the more potent the stimulus, and the greater the autonomic response.
      i. Maximum reaction occurs with stimuli to the anogenital area innervated by S2 to S4 nerve roots.
      ii. Autonomic hyperreflexia may first be seen in the late first stage or early second stage of labor with stretching of the perineum.
   d. Also may be triggered postpartum by abdominal or perineal pain caused by cesarean or vaginal delivery
5. If undiagnosed or untreated, extreme hypertension can lead to convulsions or cerebral hemorrhage. Measure blood pressure and heart rate frequently in at-risk patients. Consider invasive blood pressure monitoring with a radial artery catheter. Intravenous vasodilators should be immediately available to treat severe hypertension.

Labor Analgesia
1. Epidural analgesia can block autonomic hyperreflexia during labor. Consider placing the epidural catheter before elective induction of labor in patients with known histories of autonomic hyperreflexia.
2. Practical problems
   a. Catheter placement may be difficult because of the presence of scoliosis, spinal instrumentation, or reflex muscle spasms.
   b. In a patient with complete spinal cord transection, unintentional intrathecal injection of local anesthetic may be difficult to detect.
   c. Testing for intravascular injection should be done according to usual practice. There is no evidence that epinephrine-containing test doses are contraindicated in this population.
3. Choice of anesthetic
   a. Epidural fentanyl or morphine alone does not block autonomic hyperreflexia.

b. Epidural meperidine, probably via its local anesthetic effect, is effective.

c. As the level and adequacy of neural blockade cannot be assessed with the usual techniques in these patients, epidural local anesthetic should be given in concentrations suitable to completely block the pain of labor in normal patients. Boluses of 0.25% bupivacaine and infusions of 0.125% bupivacaine with and without fentanyl have been reported to block autonomic hyperreflexia successfully during labor.

d. Continuous epidural infusion may offer advantages over bolus administration to avoid the emergence of autonomic hyperreflexia symptoms between doses.

4. Consider leaving the epidural catheter in place for 24 to 48 hours after delivery, as autonomic hyperreflexia triggered by postpartum pain may occur.

Anesthesia for Cesarean Section

1. Epidural anesthesia also should work nicely for cesarean delivery.

2. Thoroughly evaluate ventilatory function and the ability to lie flat in patients with high spinal cord injury before induction.

3. If general anesthesia is necessary in the paraplegic parturient, beware of the potential for difficult intubation in patients with cervical injuries. Awake intubation may be indicated.

4. Succinylcholine
   a. Can cause hyperkalemia.
   b. Has been reported up to 1 year after injury.
   c. Rocuronium 0.6 to 1.0 mg per kilogram is a reasonable alternative.

5. Once the airway is secured, maintain an adequate depth of general anesthesia to prevent autonomic hyperreflexia during surgery.

6. As autonomic hyperreflexia also can occur postoperatively, adequate analgesia is important. Epidural (and presumably spinal) morphine appears to help limit postoperative sympathetic discharge due to pain.

Intracranial Vascular Lesions

1. Subarachnoid hemorrhage complicates 1 of every 10,000 pregnancies, a rate five times that of nonpregnant women of the same age.

2. Most intracranial bleeding follows rupture of either a berry (sacular) aneurysm or an arteriovenous malformation.

3. In a review of 154 patients, the average gestational age at the time of rupture for both aneurysms and arteriovenous malformations was 30 weeks. There was no correlation between type of lesion and incidence of rupture during parturition.[6]

4. Events that may increase the risk of bleeding include coughing, straining, emotional stress, lifting, or any sudden cardiovascular stress.

Preoperative Evaluation
1. What is the intracranial pathology?
2. What surgical intervention, if any, has been performed?
3. Has the lesion bled in the past?
4. Does the patient currently have symptoms attributable to intracranial blood (meningismus, headache) or increased ICP (headache, nausea, vomiting, altered sensorium)?
5. What is the obstetric plan (labor versus cesarean delivery)?
6. For patients whose lesions have been obliterated surgically, obstetric and anesthetic management proceed as usual.
7. For patients with uncorrected lesions, mode of delivery may depend on the timing of the subarachnoid hemorrhage during the gestation and the degree of maternal morbidity from the hemorrhage.[6]

Labor Analgesia
1. CSF pressure
   a. Increases markedly during painful uterine contractions and maternal pushing efforts.
   b. Decreases quickly when the Valsalva is released.
      i. Blood pressure increases simultaneously because of improved venous return.
      ii. This combination increases transmural stress on intracranial vessels.
2. Avoiding pain and bearing down is a priority in the laboring patient with an intracranial vascular lesion.
3. Continuous lumbar epidural or caudal anesthesia
   a. Can limit the hypertensive response to the pain of uterine contractions.
   b. Prevent "bearing down" during the late stage of labor.
   c. Provide anesthesia for forceps delivery.
4. Anesthetic management differs after acute intracerebral hemorrhage if the patient has increased ICP.
   a. As in the patient with an intact lesion, avoid events that can increase ICP.
   b. In these women, however, epidural anesthesia may not be the best way to accomplish this end.
      i. Cerebellar herniation may follow accidental dural puncture.
      ii. Injecting fluid into the epidural space also may increase CSF pressure. In patients with abnormal intracranial compliance after head trauma, lumbar epidural injection of 5 to 10 mL of bupivacaine or saline transiently increase ICP.
      iii. Proceed cautiously when injecting an epidural catheter in someone who may have reduced intracranial compliance. Inject the anesthetic in small increments, and observe the patient carefully for signs of increased ICP or decreasing blood pressure.
5. Systemic medications or lumbar sympathetic blocks may be used in patients in whom neuraxial anesthesia is thought to be contraindicated because of high ICP.
   a. Use opioids sparingly to avoid hypoventilation, hypercarbia, and cerebral venodilation.

b. Nitrous oxide and oxygen analgesia may help during labor and avoid the ventilatory depressant effects of systemic medications.

c. Minimize the hemodynamic effects of uterine contractions (hypertension, tachycardia) in these patients with appropriate antihypertensive therapy.

d. Pudendal block can provide pain relief during delivery.

Anesthesia for Cesarean Section

1. Goals
    a. Minimize hemodynamic disturbances.
    b. Prevent ICP increases.
2. Epidural anesthesia
    a. Pay strict attention to hemodynamic stability.
    b. Invasive arterial blood pressure monitoring may be useful.
    c. Consider prophylactic antiemetics (metoclopramide) to limit nausea and vomiting.
3. Certain situations (coma, high ICP, emergency surgery, simultaneous aneurysm clipping) may necessitate general anesthesia for cesarean delivery.
    a. In addition to invasive arterial pressure monitoring, central venous pressure monitoring may be useful in these situations to guide therapy directed at blood pressure control and maintenance of normal intravascular volume.
    b. Hemodynamic response to laryngoscopy and intubation
        i. Hypertension can rupture an aneurysm or arteriovenous malformation and will contribute to increases in ICP.
        ii. Provide deep anesthesia before airway manipulation.
            (1) Use fentanyl or other rapidly acting opioid.
            (2) Give a generous induction dose of thiopental (5 to 6 mg per kilogram).
            (3) Intravenous lidocaine and voluntary hyperventilation before the induction of anesthesia also will help blunt changes in ICP.
            (4) Wait for onset of complete muscle relaxation before attempting laryngoscopy.
        iii. Treat any increases in blood pressure aggressively. Infusions of nitroprusside or trimethaphan are helpful. Nitroprusside should be used only with direct arterial pressure monitoring to avoid precipitous hypotension.
        iv. When the risk of hemodynamic perturbations from a rapid-sequence induction is greater than the likelihood of aspiration, a slower induction of anesthesia may be indicated. The parturient with acutely increased ICP or recent bleed from an aneurysm would probably be in this category.
            (1) After preoxygenation, apply cricoid pressure and slowly induce anesthesia with barbiturate, opioid, and a nondepolarizing muscle relaxant.

   (2) Manually hyperventilate the patient via bag
         and mask.
   (3) Control blood pressure with antihyperten-
         sive medications or additional anesthetic.
   (4) Secure the airway only after the onset of
         complete paralysis.
   (5) Neonatal depression is predictable with this
         technique. Communicate with the pediatri-
         cian and be prepared to resuscitate the new-
         born as needed.
 4. After delivery, do not use ergot derivatives to treat uterine
     atony; they cause hypertension via α-receptor stimulation.
     Oxytocin has been used after delivery in these patients with-
     out a problem.

SUMMARY

 1. Proper anesthetic management of the parturient with med-
     ical problems requires knowledge of:
     a. The patient's disease.
     b. The impact of her pregnancy on her disease.
     c. The impact of her disease on the pregnancy and fetus.
     d. The impact of an anesthetic on both the patient and the
         fetus.
 2. Consult the patient's internist, endocrinologist, pulmonolo-
     gist, or neurologist to learn the extent and management of
     the medical problem.
 3. Discuss the delivery plan with the patient's obstetrician.
 4. Consider the side effects of the available anesthetic tech-
     niques and what specific agents are best used or avoided.
 5. Finally, spend time discussing these concerns with the
     patient. This is not always possible in the labor and delivery
     suite, where management plans change frequently. Talking
     to these patients in advance of delivery will allow time to
     gather information from the patient's primary physicians,
     discuss anesthetic options with the patient, and formulate
     an anesthetic plan.

REFERENCES

 1. Hood DD, Dewan DM. Anesthetic and obstetric outcome in mor-
     bidly obese parturients. *Anesthesiology* 1993;79:1210.
 2. Cheney FW, Posner KL, Caplan RA. Adverse respiratory events
     infrequently leading to malpractice suits. *Anesthesiology* 1991;75:
     932.
 3. Eames WO, Rooke GA, Wu RS, Bishop MJ. Comparison of the
     effects of etomidate, propofol, and thiopental on respiratory resis-
     tance after tracheal intubation. *Anesthesiology* 1996;84:1307.
 4. Brown RH, Zerhouni EA, Hirshman CA. Comparison of low con-
     centrations of halothane and isoflurane as bronchodilators. *Anes-
     thesiology* 1993;78:1097.
 5. Bader AM, Hunt CO, Datta S, Naulty JS, Ostheimer GW. Anes-
     thesia for the obstetric patient with multiple sclerosis. *J Clin
     Anesth* 1988;1:21.
 6. Dias MS, Sekhar LN. Intracranial hemorrhage from aneurysms
     and arteriovenous malformations during pregnancy and the puer-
     perium. *Neurosurgery* 1990;27:855.

Anesthesia and Maternal Substance Abuse

Substance abuse is a major public health problem in our society. Drug use crosses geographic and socioeconomic boundaries; patients under the influence of these substances are being seen not only in inner cities but also in small communities and private hospitals. Substance abuse during pregnancy is no longer a rare event. Many women of childbearing age are currently abusing at least one illicit substance.

Perinatal substance abuse has been linked to numerous maternal and neonatal complications and may alter the anticipated response to commonly administered anesthetics. The situations that may arise in this patient population have been attributed to many factors:

1. The direct and indirect effects of illicit drugs and contaminants.
2. Failure of many of drug-abusing patients to receive antenatal care.
3. Poor diet.
4. The presence of untreated coexisting diseases.

Of all the causative factors, prenatal care has the greatest impact on outcome.

Multiple drug use is common. Women who use cocaine are likely to use other drugs. Although all patients should be questioned regarding the use of illicit drugs, self-reporting underestimates actual use. Risk factors for substance abuse include lack of prenatal care, preterm labor, and cigarette smoking.

COCAINE

1. The prevalence of cocaine abuse in pregnant women dramatically increased during the past decade.
    a. Pregnant patients from many geographic, socioeconomic, and cultural groups abuse this drug.
    b. Although the exact extent of perinatal cocaine use is unknown, the epidemic of drug use has far-reaching effects.
2. Cocaine (benzoylmethylecgonine) is a naturally occurring alkaloid derived from the *Erythroxylon coca* plant, which is indigenous to Peru, Bolivia, and Ecuador.
    a. The drug is readily absorbed through mucous membranes and metabolized rapidly by the liver and plasma cholinesterases to water-soluble products that are excreted in the urine.
    b. Cocaine is highly lipid soluble and has a low molecular weight and ionization, thus allowing easy transplacental diffusion.
    c. The alkalinized form of cocaine can be smoked and is known as "crack."

d. The pharmacologic effects of cocaine are mediated via the norepinephrine, dopamine, and serotonin neurotransmitter systems. Because of inhibition of neuronal reuptake, extracellular norepinephrine accumulates, producing hypertension, tachycardia, and vasoconstriction.

Maternal Risks

Cardiovascular Effects

1. The effects of maternal cocaine use are incremental and cumulative, although erratic use, too, can produce severe complications.
2. Some cardiovascular effects of cocaine include:
   a. Hypertension.
   b. Cardiac dysrhythmias.
      i. Common: sinus tachycardia atrial extrasystoles, atrial tachycardia, and ventricular extrasystoles
      ii. Possible: ventricular tachycardia, ventricular fibrillation, and asystole
   c. Electrocardiographic changes.
      i. Prolongation of the PR, QRS, and QT intervals; increased QRS voltage
      ii. ST-T wave changes, and pathologic Q waves
   d. Myocardial ischemia.
      i. Coronary vasospasm produces transient ST elevation, similar to that seen in patients with Prinzmetal's angina.
      ii. Chronic cocaine use may cause an acceleration of atherosclerosis and lead to ventricular hypertrophy.
   e. Myocardial infarction.
      i. Incidence is unknown.
      ii. Myocardial infarction an occur after cocaine use in young, healthy women.
      iii. The time from cocaine use to infarction is variable, ranging from minutes to hours.
      iv. Both Q-wave and non-Q-wave infarcts occur.
      v. Infarcts are due to coronary artery spasm, thrombus, or a combination.
   f. Left ventricular (LV) dysfunction and failure.
      i. Direct negative inotropic effect
      ii. LV dysfunction is temporally related to cocaine use.
      iii. Users can develop severe global LV hypokinesis and greatly reduced ejection fractions.
      iv. Pulmonary edema and cardiomyopathy are reported.
3. Mechanisms
   a. Direct drug effects
   b. Indirect effects of catecholamine release
4. Pregnancy may increase the sensitivity to the cardiovascular effects of cocaine.
   a. In animals, pregnancy alters the metabolism of cocaine.
   b. The cardiac effects of pregnancy may make the parturient more susceptible to cocaine-induced abnormalities.

5. Recognition of the cocaine user
    a. Most deny drug use when interviewed by physicians.
    b. Physical examination may be misleading due to difficulty in differentiating between preeclampsia and cocaine use.
    c. In urban hospitals, approximately 60% of parturients without prenatal care seen in the labor suite tested positive for cocaine.

Fetal Risks
1. Neonatal and fetal complications of maternal cocaine abuse are numerous and include:
    a. Intrauterine fetal death.
    b. Congenital abnormalities.
    c. Cerebral infarction.
    d. Central nervous system (CNS) irritability.
    e. Increased incidence of fetal desaturation.
    f. Fetal myocardial ischemia.
2. The risk of these complications remains high even after accounting for confounding variables such as age, race, alcohol abuse, and smoking.
3. Mechanisms
    a. Vasoconstriction of uterine and umbilical vessels
    b. Altered placental prostaglandin production, favoring thromboxane, which may cause vasoconstriction and decreased uteroplacental blood flow
    c. Direct effect on several biochemical processes within the placenta: The function of the placental serotonin transporter may be severely impaired by cocaine use.
4. The American College of Obstetricians and Gynecologists (ACOG) has made several suggestions in response to the growing problem of cocaine use during pregnancy[1]:
    a. A drug history should be taken on all patients.
    b. A woman acknowledging cocaine use should be counseled and offered support mechanisms to aid in her abstinence.
    c. Periodic urine testing should be considered to encourage abstinence.
    d. Testing the mother and neonate may be useful in some clinical situations, such as unexplained fetal growth retardation, prematurity, or abruptio placenta.

Detecting Cocaine Abuse
1. Current laboratory screening methods for cocaine metabolites include gas chromatography, mass spectrometry, and radioimmunoassay. With some of these tests, there is a significant lag between sending the sample and reporting of results.
2. Instant latex agglutination tests for cocaine metabolites in maternal urine can provide an accurate result within several minutes.
3. Hair and meconium testing may prove useful in the detection of cocaine use in pregnancy.

Legal Implications
1. Legal controversies surrounding maternal rights and the status of the fetus are complex and vary among states.

2. Confusion regarding antenatal toxicology testing arose
    after a 1993 lawsuit against the Medical University of
    South Carolina.[2]
    a. This lawsuit was brought by three women who were
        incarcerated after positive urine toxicologic tests and
        refusal to attend substance abuse and prenatal care clin-
        ics. The suit claimed that the University had violated the
        patients' rights to privacy and liberty and their rights to
        refuse medical treatment and to procreate.
    b. This case demonstrates the importance of assessing the
        ethical and legal standing of drug-testing policies.
        i.   Toxicologic testing of parturients, *per se,* should not
             be abandoned when it is considered clinically im-
             portant for the safe treatment of mother or fetus.
        ii. However, safeguards to avoid bias and to protect
             patients' rights must be considered.

Anesthetic Considerations
1. Because cocaine-abusing patients have a higher incidence of
    cesarean section for "fetal jeopardy," anesthesiologists may
    meet these women in an emergency setting.
2. Potential problems
    a. Severe hypertension from generalized vasoconstriction
    b. Severe hypotension because of cocaine-related hemor-
        rhage
3. Choice of anesthetic
    a. General endotracheal anesthesia
        i.   Hemodynamically compromised parturient
        ii. Abruptio placenta after cocaine use has been well
             described
        iii. Placenta previa also may be related to cocaine use
             and can be another cause of bleeding.
    b. Regional anesthesia
        i.   Epidural or spinal anesthesia have been used suc-
             cessfully.
        ii. Hemodynamic perturbations and ephedrine resis-
             tance can occur.

General Anesthesia
1. Stimulation, as with laryngoscopy during induction of gen-
    eral anesthesia, can produce severe hypertension in the
    cocaine-abusing patient. To limit this risk, blood pressure
    should be pharmacologically controlled before induction and
    intubation.
    a. β-Blockade with propranolol
        i.   Is contraindicated in the cocaine-abusing patient.
        ii. May cause unopposed α-adrenergic stimulation
             and worsen the hypertension.
        iii. Also may enhance cocaine-induced coronary vaso-
             constriction.
    b. Hydralazine
        i.   May produce profound maternal tachycardia.
        ii. Does not restore uterine blood flow.
    c. Labetalol
        i.   Safe use reported

ii. Better hemodynamic effects than hydralazine in animal studies

2. Anesthetics
   a. Avoid halothane due to the risk of cardiac arrhythmias.
   b. Isoflurane has been used without incident. Cocaine toxicity during isoflurane anesthesia may be associated with increased systemic vascular resistance and cardiac arrhythmias.
   c. Ketamine
      i. May potentiate the cardiac effects of cocaine by further increasing catecholamine concentrations.
      ii. May precipitate myocardial depression and hypotension if the patient is unable to mount a further catecholamine release.

3. Succinylcholine
   a. Prolonged blockade, presumably due to a depletion of cholinesterases involved in cocaine metabolism, has been reported.
   b. Succinylcholine can be safely used in standard doses. If cholinesterase deficiency occurs, the ensuing neuromuscular block should not last as long as the surgery.
   c. Use a nerve stimulator to ensure that the effect of the succinylcholine has terminated before giving nondepolarizing muscle relaxants to these patients.

Regional Anesthesia

1. Profound hypotension may follow sympathetic blockade.
2. The cocaine-abusing patient may not respond as expected to ephedrine.
   a. Apparently, these women cannot develop a tachycardia in response to this indirect-acting agent.
   b. Should these patients develop ephedrine-resistant hypotension, they do respond to small doses of phenylephrine.

Postoperative Care

1. Vigilant postoperative monitoring is essential.
2. Signs and symptoms of cocaine toxicity may arise hours after the drug exposure.
3. Cocaine users may have silent myocardial ischemia with episodes of ST elevation during the first weeks of withdrawal.

AMPHETAMINES

1. Sympathomimetic agents
2. Profound CNS stimulation
3. They are abused individually or with others, such as cocaine.
4. Acute ingestion produces signs and symptoms that mimic cocaine abuse and also may be mistaken for preeclampsia.
5. Amphetamines and pregnancy
   a. Patients often receive little or no prenatal care.
   b. Amphetamines may cause uteroplacental vasoconstriction and precipitate worrisome fetal conditions.
   c. They are associated with intrauterine growth retardation, intrauterine fetal death, and abruptio placenta.

6. Anesthetic considerations
   a. Acute ingestion can increase the dose requirement (minimum alveolar concentration [MAC]) for general anesthetics.
   b. Chronic use decreases MAC.
   c. Amphetamines produce an accumulation of norepinephrine. Avoid halothane and other potentially arrhythmogenic agents.
   d. Reports have described cardiac arrest in amphetamine-abusing patients undergoing cesarean section under regional and general anesthesia.

OPIOIDS

1. Approximately 250,000 women in the United States are intravenous drug abusers, with 90% of childbearing age.
2. Perinatal abuse of opioids is associated with the human immunodeficiency virus and acquired immunodeficiency syndrome, hepatitis, endocarditis, and pulmonary, renal, and cardiac disease.
3. Acute withdrawal syndrome may occur, producing tremors, anxiety, muscle pains, nausea, vomiting, anorexia, gastrointestinal pain, tachycardia, hypertension, and mydriasis.
   a. These signs and symptoms peak 48 to 72 hours after the last drug exposure.
   b. Opioid antagonists or agonist-antagonists can precipitate acute withdrawal. Avoid them in known or suspected addicts.
4. Overdose
   a. Coma, miosis, or respiratory depression
   b. Risk of regurgitation and aspiration. If in doubt about the patient's ability to protect her airway, secure it with a cuffed endotracheal tube.

Methadone

1. Used for the treatment of pregnant opioid addicts.
2. Fetal-neonatal effects
   a. A high incidence of nonreactive nonstress tests.
   b. May alter fetal CNS neurotransmitters and change fetal behavior.
   c. Infants born to mothers taking methadone weigh more than infants of heroin users.
   d. Newborn withdrawal, neurobehavioral depression, and death are risks.
   e. Regardless of side effects, methadone maintenance poses far fewer hazards, both to mother and fetus, than continued use of intravenous heroin.
3. Pregnancy and methadone
   a. Metabolism may be altered in late gestation.
   b. Once daily dosing may be inadequate in pregnant patients.
   c. Giving a twice-daily dose may reduce fetal stress.
   d. Regardless of drug or regimen, to avoid maternal withdrawal, daily opioid administration must continue during labor and postpartum.

Intentional Acute Withdrawal

1. Not recommended
2. Occasionally undertaken during pregnancy
   a. Reasons
      i. Patient refusal to take methadone
      ii. Lack of methadone maintenance program in the patient's vicinity
      iii. Patient request
      iv. Patient is so disruptive to the treatment setting that other patients are jeopardized.
      v. It has long been suggested that women should be withdrawn only in the second trimester of pregnancy.
         (1) First-trimester withdrawal may result in spontaneous abortion.
         (2) Third-trimester withdrawal may cause premature labor.
         (3) There is little evidence to support these claims.

Anesthetic Considerations

1. Regional anesthetic techniques offer many advantages.
2. Spinal and epidural analgesia can provide pain relief without opioids.
   a. The opioid-abusing patient may be intolerant to pain because of decreased endogenous opioid peptides.
   b. A regional anesthetic can provide pain relief without opioids, which many rehabilitated addicts fear will precipitate readdiction.

ETHANOL

1. There are an estimated 15 million alcoholics in the United States; approximately one-fourth of them are women.
2. Alcohol abuse has been associated with numerous maternal abnormalities, including cardiomyopathy, decreased albumin concentration, coagulopathy, liver disease, ascites, and electrolyte abnormalities.
3. Alcohol is a known teratogen, and alcohol use during pregnancy is associated with the fetal alcohol syndrome.
   a. Craniofacial, cardiac, renal, and musculocutaneous abnormalities
   b. Children with complete fetal alcohol syndrome are usually born to mothers who consume large amounts of alcohol throughout pregnancy.
   c. However, because a safe level of alcohol intake in pregnancy has not been established, total abstinence is considered the safest course.
4. Anesthetic considerations
   a. Regional anesthesia
      i. Safe in the absence of coagulopathy or neuropathy, both of which have been associated with end-stage disease
      ii. Occasional failures because of psychotic or combative behavior

b.   General anesthesia
   i.   Aspiration: Alcohol both increases gastric acid secretion and decreases protective reflexes.
   ii.   Severe hypoalbuminemia and cardiac manifestations of alcohol abuse may increase sensitivity to the effects of myocardial depressants.
   iii.   Tolerance and an expanded plasma volume will increase the dose requirement for induction agents.

REFERENCES
1. ACOG. Committee opinion: Committee on Obstetrics: maternal and fetal medicine: number 114. *Int J Gynecol Obstet* 1998; 41:102.
2. Jos PH, Marshall MF, Perlmutter M. The Charleston policy on cocaine use during pregnancy: a cautionary tale. *J Law Med Ethics* 1995;23:120.

Anesthesia and Preeclampsia/Eclampsia

Hypertensive disorders are the third leading cause of pregnancy-related mortality. Death is due primarily to cerebrovascular or other central nervous system (CNS) event. Pregnancy-induced hypertension (PIH), or preeclampsia, alters function in many organ systems. The physiologic changes of a pregnancy complicated by preeclampsia may differ markedly from those of a healthy gestation. Recognition of these differences allows modifications to provide optimal care for these high-risk parturients.

Although mild preeclampsia may have few anesthetic implications, severe disease requires special consideration. Preoperative evaluation requires additional and more frequent laboratory evaluation. Patients may need invasive hemodynamic monitoring. Control of blood pressure assumes a high priority.

In obstetric anesthesia, several plans must be developed for each patient. A patient seen for a trial of labor and vaginal delivery may eventually require cesarean section. Although some indications for cesarean delivery can be managed semi-electively, others may be true emergencies. The anesthetic plan must cover all of these possibilities. Be flexible. Plan ahead. Communicate actively with the obstetrician.

PREOPERATIVE ASSESSMENT
Hemoglobin and Hematocrit

1. Provides an initial estimation of volume status
   a. The "physiologic anemia of pregnancy" rarely permits a hematocrit greater than 36% at sea level.
   b. Attribute higher values to intravascular volume contraction.
2. Ten percent of patients with severe preeclampsia develop a microangiopathic hemolytic anemia associated with thrombocytopenia and increased liver enzymes (HELLP syndrome).
3. Even in milder forms of preeclampsia, endothelial cell damage and vasospasm cause destruction of red cells.
   a. Increased heme catabolism increases production of carboxyhemoglobin and causes a leftward shift of the oxyhemoglobin dissociation curve.
   b. Normally, pregnancy shifts half-saturation pressure (p50) rightward to approximately 30 mm Hg. In preeclampsia, p50 is 24.4 mm Hg, to the left of even the nonpregnant value.
   c. This leftward shift decreases the release of oxygen to the fetus at the placenta.
      i. Impaired oxygen delivery may have a profound effect on maternal and fetal outcome.
      ii. A maternal base deficit greater than −8.0 mEq per liter may predict fetal acidosis, fetal death, and maternal end-organ ischemic injury.[1]

Coagulation

Laboratory Evaluation

1. Disseminated intravascular coagulation is rare in the pre-eclamptic patient.
   a. It is most commonly associated with placental abruption or fetal death.
   b. Absent thrombocytopenia (less than 100,000 per cubic millimeter), it is extremely unlikely that a woman with severe preeclampsia will have an abnormal fibrinogen or prolonged prothrombin time (PT) or partial thromboplastin time (PTT).
2. Platelet count alone is an appropriate initial screen of coagulation status.
3. Reserve additional tests for women with abruption, hemorrhage, fetal death, or severe liver dysfunction.
4. The D-dimer assay
   a. Uses monoclonal anti-D-dimer antibody to detect degradation products of stable (cross-linked) fibrin.
   b. Specifically detects *in vivo* clot dissolution.
   c. Presence in preeclamptic women correlates consistently with increased fibrin-degradation products and platelet counts less than 100,000 per millimeter. This test may help define a subset of patients with severe disease.
      i. Compared with preeclamptic women negative for D-dimer, positive women have higher blood pressures, greater proteinuria, higher serum creatinine, and more abnormal liver function tests.
      ii. Positive women also have a higher incidence of cesarean section and premature delivery.
5. Thrombocytopenia
   a. The most common coagulopathy in preeclampsia
   b. It occurs in about 20% of cases.
   c. Platelet function also may be abnormal.
6. Despite the concerns about abnormal platelet function, there are no definitive reports of epidural hematoma in preeclamptic patients after epidural anesthesia.

Clinical Evaluation

1. Routine use of bleeding time to make clinical judgments is, at best, inconvenient. In addition, the test provides little useful information.
   a. No existing data support its use to predict adequacy of hemostasis.
   b. No data show that bleeding from the skin can predict bleeding elsewhere in the body.
   c. There is no evidence that the bleeding time will prolong sufficiently in advance of serious bleeding to allow intervention or a change in management.[2]
2. Currently, thromboelastography (TEG) suffers many of the same limitations of the bleeding time.
3. Instead of relying on laboratory tests, examine women with preeclampsia carefully for clinical signs of abnormal coagulation. Look for bleeding from gums, intravenous (IV) sites, and other sources.

Aspirin
1. Aspirin inhibits thromboxane synthesis and corrects the imbalance of thromboxane and prostacyclin production seen in preeclampsia. Low-dose aspirin in pregnancy may prevent preeclampsia in subgroups of women at increased risk of the disease.
2. Aspirin impairs platelet function. Fortunately, low-dose aspirin therapy does not increase the risk of bleeding-related complications during pregnancy. These women can safely receive regional anesthesia without additional laboratory evaluation.

Guidelines
1. A recent survey questioned academic and private anesthesiologists about coagulation and preeclampsia; most practitioners in both groups would:
   a. Place an epidural anesthetic in a parturient taking one aspirin a day.
   b. Require only a platelet count in mild preeclampsia.
   c. Also require a PT and PTT in severe preeclampsia.[3]
2. The TEG has not found widespread use in obstetric anesthesia. However, preeclamptic and eclamptic patients with a platelet count above 60,000 per cubic millimeter have normal TEG values.[4]
3. Recommendations
   a. Screening platelet count on all women with the diagnosis of preeclampsia
   b. If the initial value is greater than 150,000 per cubic millimeter, no further workup is required.
   c. If less than 150,000 per cubic millimeter, repeat the test to rule out a rapid downward trend.
   d. The safe lower limit for platelet count before epidural placement is unknown.
      i. Using 100,000 per cubic millimeter as an arbitrary cut-off has no supporting outcome data.
      ii. No laboratory test can substitute for careful patient evaluation and the clinician's judgment.
4. Thrombocytopenia or other coagulopathy in a patient with an *in situ* epidural catheter
   a. The literature offers no definite guidelines.
   b. It seems prudent to allow the platelet count to normalize before removing the catheter.
   c. The longer a catheter is left in place, the greater the chance that it will damage or migrate into a blood vessel.
   d. In patients with HELLP syndrome, the nadir of the platelet count often occurs 1 to 3 days after delivery. Recovery to a concentration greater than 100,000 per cubic millimeter may require 5 to 6 days.
   e. Alternatively, wait until platelet count begins to recover and make sure the patient has no clinical signs of bleeding.
   f. If the catheter is removed while the patient is thrombocytopenic, frequent neurologic examinations must be

performed to detect potential spinal cord compression from an epidural hematoma.

Renal Function

1. Intravascular volume depletion and renal artery vasospasm can decrease creatinine clearance and cause oliguria. Hypovolemia is the most common cause of oliguria in these women.
2. Maternal urine output is probably the best way to assess volume status in the absence of invasive hemodynamic monitoring.
3. When creatinine values exceed 1.0 mg per deciliter in the parturient, significant renal dysfunction is present, and the excretion of drugs such as magnesium sulfate will be compromised.

Liver Function

1. Laboratory examination may reveal increased liver enzymes due to vasospasm and ischemia.
2. Patients with preeclampsia may complain of right upper quadrant or epigastric pain due to stretching of the liver capsule. Subcapsular hemorrhage, hematoma, or liver rupture can occur.
3. When associated with HELLP syndrome, coagulopathy and hemolysis increase maternal morbidity.
4. Assure large-bore IV access and blood, fresh-frozen plasma, and platelet availability if hepatic involvement is suspected.

Nervous System

1. Complete a neurologic examination before any anesthetic intervention.
   a. Deficits due to cerebral edema, cerebral hemorrhage, or a postictal state already may exist.
   b. Headaches, visual disturbances, including cortical blindness, and seizures characterize CNS involvement.
2. The etiology of eclampsia is unknown.
   a. Histopathologic examination of the brain reveals numerous hemorrhages, capillary thrombi, and small infarcts.
   b. Computed tomography (CT) in the eclamptic patient with recurrent seizures may reveal structural lesions.
      i. Changes seen resemble those found in hypertensive encephalopathy in nonpregnant patients: cerebral edema, cerebral vein thrombosis, and low-density white matter.
3. The indications for CT or magnetic resonance imaging (MRI) in the eclamptic patient are controversial. Patients who have focal signs, decreasing level of consciousness, or recurrent seizures despite therapeutic concentrations of magnesium or phenytoin need further evaluation.

Evaluation of the Fetus

1. Intrauterine growth retardation, oligohydramnios, extreme prematurity, and uteroplacental insufficiency can contribute to fetal intolerance of labor.

2. Fetal evaluation includes documentation of fetal presentation, estimated weight, biophysical profile, nonstress testing, and possibly an oxytocin contraction test.
3. Hypertensive parturients are much more likely than normotensive women to develop ominous fetal heart rate patterns during labor.

MONITORING

1. Basic intrapartum monitoring of a parturient with preeclampsia should include:
   a. Automated noninvasive blood pressure.
   b. Accurate intake and output measurements (usually requiring a urinary bladder catheter).
   c. Hourly examination of deep-tendon reflexes.
   d. Fetal scalp electrode as soon as the cervix is adequately dilated.
   e. An intrauterine pressure catheter to monitor strength and frequency of contractions and timing of any decelerations.
2. I do not continuously monitor maternal electrocardiogram (ECG) unless I also am monitoring cardiac filling pressures.

Invasive Hemodynamic Monitoring

General Considerations

1. Most obstetric patients are young and healthy.
2. Many hospitals hesitate to provide labor and delivery units with the expertise and equipment needed to care for critically ill parturients.
3. Nursing issues
   a. Without nurses trained in critical care and comfortable with invasive monitoring, attempts to treat these patients aggressively in the labor unit will not succeed and could be dangerous.
   b. Placing a laboring patient in an intensive care unit (ICU) does not allow optimal monitoring of the fetus and disrupts the unit's normal routine.
   c. Ideally, the labor and delivery unit should have an ICU bed staffed by nurses comfortable with invasive monitoring and knowledgeable about critical care issues.
   d. As an alternative, the patient could be co-nursed by both an ICU and labor and delivery nurse.
   e. The anesthesiologist becomes an important and necessary source of information and support for the nursing service in this situation.

Arterial Catheter

1. Possible indications for intraarterial blood pressure monitoring:
   a. Sustained diastolic blood pressure greater than 90 mm Hg
   b. Use of potent vasodilators, such as nitroprusside or nitroglycerin
   c. Induction of regional or general anesthesia with the potential for rapid blood pressure changes

    d. Inability to obtain accurate blood pressure measurements by cuff in a morbidly obese patient

    e. The need for repeated sampling for arterial blood gas tensions or other laboratory studies (especially if venipuncture is difficult because of edema, obesity, or IV drug abuse

    f. The patient with a coagulopathy (avoids repeated venipuncture)

Pulmonary Artery Catheter

1. Presently accepted indications for use of a pulmonary artery (PA) catheter in the parturient with severe preeclampsia:

    a. Severe hypertension unresponsive to conventional antihypertensive therapy

    b. Pulmonary edema

    c. Persistent oliguria unresponsive to fluid challenge

2. Pulmonary artery catheters can be used safely in a labor and delivery suite and may offer useful clinical information. Advantages of this approach include:

    a. Consolidation of care when the pathophysiology is unique to pregnancy (such as severe preeclampsia).

    b. Fetal monitoring.

    c. The ability to provide immediate medical and surgical management.

Central Venous Pressure or Pulmonary Artery Catheter?

1. Central venous pressure (CVP) monitoring alone may provide misleading information.

    a. CVP cannot reliably predict pulmonary artery occlusion pressure (PAOP).

    b. When CVP and PAOP do correlate, the gradient varies too widely to have any predictive value.

    c. The relation between CVP and PAOP becomes discordant when systemic vascular resistance (SVR) increases, and acutely increases left ventricular afterload.

    d. CVP may be the more accurate index of true intravascular volume, especially when the value is low.

    e. PAOP reflects the risk of pulmonary edema and the amount of left ventricular dysfunction.

    f. Although CVP is rarely low in the presence of an increased PAOP, higher CVP values are difficult to interpret.

2. The PA catheter provides far more information than does volume status.

    a. CVP gives no indication of cardiac output.

    b. Noninvasive measures of cardiac output (impedance cardiography and Doppler velocimetry) provide little assessment of filling pressures.

    c. Colloid osmotic pressure (COP)

        i. Is lower in patients with preeclampsia than in normal parturients, perhaps due to proteinuria.

            (1) Imbalance of Starling forces across the pulmonary capillary membrane is a possible mechanism for pulmonary edema in severe preeclampsia.

(2) A PAOP/COP gradient of less than 4 mm Hg may allow excessive fluid flux out of the pulmonary vasculature.
(3) The COP reaches its nadir postpartum, whereas filling pressures often increase before the onset of postpartum diuresis.

ii. If COP measurements are used, they can be combined with PAOP measurements to guide fluid therapy and use of diuretics.

3. Risk
   a. Most of the risks of central monitoring (i.e., carotid or subclavian artery puncture, pneumothorax, dysrhythmias, hematoma, or infection) are related to obtaining central venous access and are common to both CVP and PA catheter placement.
   b. The additional risks of placing the PA catheter, such as pulmonary infarction and rupture of the PA, are very rare in this patient population.
   c. Because the risks of access are similar, the more comprehensive information obtained from the PA catheter provides a favorable risk–benefit ratio.
   d. If concerned about central venous access in a patient with abnormal coagulation studies, insert the CVP or PA catheter through the antecubital basilic or external jugular vein.

Hemodynamic Profile

1. No single hemodynamic profile describes all parturients with preeclampsia.
   a. Some women have a hyperdynamic state with increased cardiac output and low-to-normal filling pressures in the face of high SVR.
   b. Others have a depressed cardiac index with low filling pressures and high vascular resistance.
   c. Some women have elevated filling pressures and cardiac failure.
   d. Different profiles may predict different outcomes (Table 21.1).

2. Serial measurements suggest that women destined to develop preeclampsia have significantly higher cardiac outputs and lower SVR from early gestation compared with parturients who remain normotensive. Vasodilation of terminal arterioles may increase the risk of end-organ damage by exposing capillary beds, especially the renal glomeruli, to systemic pressures. The resultant endothelial damage incites platelet adherence, vasospasm, and the clinically overt disease we see in patients with severe preeclampsia. Thus, women with preeclampsia present a spectrum of hemodynamic patterns reflecting the variable extent of endothelial and end-organ damage.

PERIOPERATIVE MANAGEMENT OF SPECIAL PROBLEMS
Eclampsia

1. Convulsions occur in the antepartum or intrapartum periods in 63% of cases of eclampsia.

Table 21.1. Maternal and neonatal parameters based on maternal systemic vascular resistance before treatment in severe preeclampsia

| Parameter | Vascular Resistance (dyne/s/cm²) | | |
	Low <800	Normal 800–1,500	High >1,500
CI (L/min/m²)	6.0	5.0	2.0
LVSWI (g/m/m²)	83.3	50.5	20.5
Birth weight (g)	3,591	2,645	1,740
Incidence of emergency delivery (%)	0	50	66.7
Incidence of newborn pH <7.2 (%)	0	33.3	50

CI, cardiac index; LVSWI, left ventricular stroke work index.
Source: After Yang JM, Yang YC, Wang KG. Central and peripheral hemodynamics in severe preeclampsia. *Acta Obstet Gynecol Scand* 1996;75:120, with permission.

2. Management
   a. Airway support, oxygen by mask, left uterine displacement, and cricoid pressure
   b. Do not force an oral airway or tongue blade into the patient's mouth; this action may cause vomiting or break teeth. A simple jaw lift should suffice.
   c. Intubate if the seizure is prolonged, if regurgitation occurs, or if ventilation cannot be maintained.
   d. If necessary, treat the seizure with thiopental 75 mg instead of a long-acting sedative such as diazepam.
   e. Focal seizures, or seizures in the presence of a therapeutic magnesium concentration, should raise the suspicion of a structural lesion or intracerebral hemorrhage
3. Magnesium sulfate
   a. The anticonvulsant of choice in North America.
   b. Magnesium sulfate prevents recurrent seizures in women with eclampsia.
   c. It is commonly used to prevent seizures in women with preeclampsia.
   d. A nontherapeutic serum concentration may permit recurrent seizures.
   e. Infuse magnesium sulfate as a bolus dose of 4 to 6 g over a 20-minute period, and repeat once if seizures recur.
   f. Mechanism of action
      i. Unknown
      ii. Magnesium enhances production of prostacyclin by vascular endothelium, thereby promoting vasodilation and inhibiting platelet aggregation.
      iii. Magnesium dilates the smaller diameter intracranial vessels, possibly relieving cerebral ischemia.

iv. Magnesium blocks the excitatory amino acid
N-methyl-D-aspartate (NMDA) receptor. (Stimulation of the NMDA receptor can induce seizure
activity.)[5]
g. It is more effective than phenytoin (Dilantin) in hypertensive pregnant women.
h. Tocolytic effects can slow cervical dilation and increase
blood loss at delivery.
4. Eclampsia is rarely an indication for immediate delivery.
a. Give precedence to stabilization, monitoring, and neurologic evaluation of the mother to avoid unnecessary
maternal obstetric and anesthetic risks.
b. Once seizure activity stops, continue to give the mother
supplemental oxygen.
c. Fetal decelerations occur commonly during a seizure
because of maternal hypoxia and acidosis.
d. Unless placental abruption has occurred, fetal acidosis
will improve more quickly *in utero* than if delivery
occurs during or immediately after the seizure.

Oliguria

1. A common complication of severe preeclampsia
2. Although postpartum renal failure rarely occurs, most
physicians become anxious when urine output decreases
below 0.5 mL per kilogram per hour for several hours.
3. Because magnesium sulfate is cleared only by glomerular
filtration, oliguria also can increase the risk of magnesium
toxicity.
4. Management
a. Fluid challenge of 500 mL of crystalloid over a 20-minute period
b. Repeat once or twice.
c. If urine output remains unchanged or declines, consider
central venous or PA catheterization before further
fluid therapy.
5. Etiology may differ among women with preeclampsia.[6]
a. Most commonly, patients have low filling pressures,
hyperdynamic ventricular function, and a moderate
increase of vascular resistance, reflecting intravascular
volume depletion. These women respond to further volume infusion with an increase in PAOP, a decrease in
SVR, and no change in blood pressure.
b. Other women also have hyperdynamic ventricular function, but with higher filling pressures (9 to 18 mm Hg)
and normal SVR. In these women, renal artery vasospasm may be the cause of oliguria. In this group of
patients, urine production increases after vasodilator
therapy with hydralazine and cautious fluid administration.
c. Women who are oliguric and have elevated filling pressures also may benefit from low-dose dopamine (1 to
5 µg per kilogram per minute).[7]
d. Uncommonly, women will have depressed left ventricular function, increased PAOP, and a marked increase of

SVR. These patients need afterload reduction to relieve vasospasm and improve cardiac output.

Pulmonary Edema

1. A significant cause of maternal and perinatal morbidity and mortality
2. Most cases occur postpartum.
3. Medical, surgical, or obstetric complications that require large-volume crystalloid or colloid infusions (i.e., sepsis, abruption, disseminated intravascular coagulation, aspiration, or ruptured liver) increase the risk.
4. Older multigravidae and those with chronic hypertension are at greater risk.
5. Pulmonary edema normally occurs at a PAOP of 20 to 25 mm Hg, but if the patient also has a low COP, clinical symptoms may manifest earlier. Antepartum correction of COP with albumin leads to much higher filling pressures after delivery.
6. PA catheterization helps to determine the cause of pulmonary edema and to guide therapy (oxygen, diuresis, and possibly nitroglycerin).

ANTIHYPERTENSIVE THERAPY

1. The purpose of antihypertensive therapy is to prevent cerebral hemorrhage, pulmonary edema, and other maternal complications of acute hypertension, while preserving or improving uteroplacental circulation.
2. Strive to reduce maternal mean blood pressure to 105 to 110 mm Hg, but by no more than 30%.
   a. The fetus with uteroplacental insufficiency is an exquisitely sensitive monitor of perfusion.
   b. Fetal decelerations may limit the degree of blood pressure reduction.
   c. If hemodynamic monitoring is available, use these values to guide your choice of antihypertensive therapy. For example, the parturient with hyperdynamic left ventricular function and normal SVR may respond well to a negative inotrope (i.e., labetalol), whereas a vasodilating agent would best correct an increased vascular resistance in the presence of high filling pressures.
   d. A number of antihypertensive drugs can be used in obstetrics. Be aware of the safety and any potential harmful effects of the drugs chosen to control blood pressure (Table 21.2).
3. Magnesium sulfate is not an antihypertensive, although it attenuates the hyperreactive vascular responses in preeclampsia and has other beneficial effects. Most hemodynamic changes that accompany magnesium bolus and infusion are transient.

Direct-acting Vasodilators

Hydralazine

1. Hydralazine remains a popular drug for use in PIH.
2. It is a direct arteriolar smooth muscle dilator.
3. It improves renal and uterine blood flow.

Table 21.2. Reported adverse effects of antihypertensive therapy during pregnancy

Drug	Adverse Effect
Esmolol (Brevibloc)	Decreased in fetal arterial pO_2
	Equivalent maternal and fetal β-blockade
	Prolonged fetal β-blockade
	? Decreased fetal tolerance to asphyxia
Clonidine (Catapres)	Fetal hypoxemia
	Increased uterine tone
	Decreased uterine blood flow
Nifedipine (Adalat, Procardia)	Tocolysis
	Additive myocardial depression with magnesium
	Additive neuromuscular blockade with magnesium
	? Fetal hypoxemia with nicardipine infusion
ACE inhibitors (enalapril)	Neonatal hypotension
	Neonatal renal failure
	Teratogenicity

ACE, angiotensin-converting enzyme.

4. Onset is relatively slow (15 to 20 minutes).
   a. Time to peak effect varies considerably.
   b. Titration is difficult.
5. Effects last for hours.
6. It increases heart rate and cardiac index and decreases SVR.
7. Hydralazine can produce acute hypotension and fetal heart rate changes when given to a hypovolemic patient.

Nitroprusside
1. A potent arterial and venous dilator
   a. Cerebral vasodilation increases intracranial pressure, which may be detrimental in a postictal patient with an equivocal neurologic examination, or if a structural intracerebral lesion is suspected.
   b. Pulmonary vasodilation decreases hypoxic pulmonary vasoconstriction and could cause hypoxemia.
2. Advantages
   a. Fast onset, short duration, and rapid metabolism (plasma half-life of 12 seconds) make nitroprusside titratable as an infusion.
   b. Patients are rarely resistant.
   c. It preserves uterine blood flow.
3. Disadvantages
   a. Like all vasodilators, nitroprusside can cause severe hypotension when the patient is hypovolemic.

   b.   Heart rate will increase in response to the decrease in SVR.
   4.   The maximum acceptable dose of nitroprusside is 8.0 µg per kilogram per minute or 0.5 mg per kilogram per hour. If exceeding this amount, use another hypotensive agent.

Nitroglycerin
   1.   Produces venous and arterial dilation. Increased intracranial pressure (ICP) and decreased hypoxic pulmonary vasoconstriction are concerns.
   2.   Its short duration makes it easily titratable.
   3.   In animals, it partially restores uterine blood flow diminished by phenylephrine infusion.
   4.   In untreated preeclamptics, it reduces blood pressure, PAOP, and cardiac output. Volume expansion prevents the decrease in filling pressures and cardiac index.
      a.   After volume expansion, however, patients can develop a marked resistance to nitroglycerin's hypotensive effects.
      b.   The decrease in filling pressures may help correct the hemodynamic abnormalities associated with pulmonary edema.
   5.   Fetal heart rate variability also diminishes, possibly as a result of loss of cerebral autoregulation and increased ICP in the fetus.

Ganglionic Blocking Agents
   1.   Trimethaphan exerts its hypotensive effect by ganglionic blockade of sympathetic nerve impulses.
   2.   It can be used as an infusion or in bolus doses without causing reflex tachycardia.
   3.   Tachyphylaxis can develop during prolonged infusion.
   4.   Of the vasodilating agents, it has the largest molecular weight (597 dalton), which should limit its placental transfer.
   5.   Although it is not a direct cerebral vasodilator, ICP increases transiently during the induction of hypotension. The risk seems greatest when blood pressure decreases rapidly (less than 1 minute) to a mean below 60 mm Hg or in patients who already have critically increased ICP.
   6.   Pupillary dilation due to ganglionic blockade can be expected and should not cause concern.
   7.   Trimethaphan inhibits plasma cholinesterase and can prolong the duration of succinylcholine.

β-Receptor Blocking Agents
Labetalol
   1.   Very popular in obstetrics
   2.   Has nonselective β- and α_1-blocking properties in a ratio of about 7 : 1 when given intravenously.
      a.   It decreases SVR and blood pressure without changing heart rate or cardiac index.
      b.   Uteroplacental flow does not change, suggesting that labetalol reduces placental vascular resistance.
      c.   It does not produce significant adrenergic blockade in the fetus or newborn.

3. Peak effect after parenteral administration occurs within 10 minutes, but the dose–response is variable.
    a. Labetalol may fail to reduce blood pressure in 10% of patients.
    b. The required dose varies considerably, ranging from 20 to 300 mg.
    c. Women requiring the largest doses have the shortest duration of effect.

Esmolol

1. An ultra-short-acting β_1 selective blocking agent
    a. Elimination half-life of 9 minutes
    b. Metabolism is by hydrolysis by red blood cell esterases.
2. Animal studies have reported adverse fetal effects.
    a. Fetal arterial pO_2 decreases significantly.
    b. Isoproterenol challenge testing revealed fetal β-blockade that persisted for 30 minutes after completion of the esmolol infusion.
    c. It produces equivalent degrees of β-blockade in fetus and ewe.
3. There are no human studies of esmolol in pregnancy, but fetal bradycardia has been reported with its use.

Sympatholytic Agents

1. Gradually reduce blood pressure without reflex tachycardia
2. α-Methyldopa is a centrally acting α_2-receptor agonist with a long history of safe use in obstetrics. It provides a peripheral sympathectomy and has both parenteral and oral forms. Its main drawbacks are its long latency (6 hours) and only moderate efficacy. Additionally, it is contraindicated in patients with liver dysfunction, not uncommon in severe PIH.
3. Clonidine acts by the same mechanism as α-methyldopa, but it is not available in a parenteral form. Although it seems to be safe in long-term use in parturients with chronic hypertension, IV use in animals caused fetal hypoxemia, increased uterine tone, and decreased uterine blood flow. The patch formulation has been used for long-term postpartum control of blood pressure, but patients can develop rebound hypertension after removing the patch.

Calcium Channel Blocking Drugs

1. Verapamil
    a. Available in oral and IV forms
    b. No maternal tachycardia
    c. IV infusion decreases maternal blood pressure and increases cardiac index without altering uterine or umbilical or uteroplacental blood flow.
2. Nifedipine
    a. Can be given orally or sublingually.
    b. Is primarily a vasodilator and causes reflex maternal tachycardia.
    c. Nimodipine and nicardipine have similar actions.
3. Limitations
    a. These agents produce significant uterine relaxation, which can be problematic during labor induction and augmentation.

b. Interaction with magnesium, another calcium antagonist
   i. Could potentiate the neuromuscular effects of magnesium and increase the risk of cardiac or respiratory toxicity
   ii. Acute respiratory insufficiency has been reported when magnesium was given to patients receiving nifedipine for tocolysis or blood pressure control.

Angiotensin-Converting Enzyme Inhibitors
1. The use of these agents in pregnancy is associated with neonatal hypotension, neonatal renal failure, and teratogenicity.
2. Avoid these drugs.

ANALGESIA FOR LABOR AND VAGINAL DELIVERY
Epidural Analgesia
Advantages
1. Excellent pain relief
2. Reduction of maternal circulating catecholamine concentrations
   a. These women are more sensitive to catecholamines than are healthy parturients.
   b. Catecholamines, secreted in response to pain and stress, can increase blood pressure and compromise uteroplacental blood flow.
   c. The serum concentration of epinephrine decreases significantly after induction of epidural anesthesia.
   d. Uteroplacental blood flow increases.
3. Flexibility
   a. Once in place, the epidural catheter can provide effective anesthesia for labor and vaginal delivery or cesarean section.
   b. Early placement can avoid inducing general anesthesia if an urgent cesarean section is required.
   c. Epidural opioids can provide excellent postoperative analgesia if needed.
   d. Finally, sympathectomy can be maintained postpartum, if desired, to buffer intravascular volume changes during fluid mobilization.

Hemodynamic Effects
1. Historically, a fear of precipitous maternal hypotension has limited the use of epidural labor analgesia in some centers.
2. An extensive body of data now shows that epidural block is safe and effective in this patient population.
3. The incidence of maternal hypotension, abnormal fetal heart rate tracings, low Apgar scores, and neonatal ICU admissions does not differ whether or not women with preeclampsia receive epidural anesthesia.
4. Epidural blockade provokes little hemodynamic change in women with severe preeclampsia.
   a. Neither PAOP, CVP, nor cardiac index changed after epidural local anesthetic injection in women hydrated to a PAOP of 8 to 12 mm Hg.

b. Prudent use of fluids guided by clinical judgment and invasive monitoring when indicated will minimize risk of precipitous hypotension when using regional anesthesia in the preeclamptic patient.

c. Obstetric or medical complications, not fluids given before epidural placement, predispose to pulmonary edema.

Some Technical Issues

EPINEPHRINE

1. Controversy surrounds the use of epinephrine-containing local anesthetic solutions in women with preeclampsia.

2. Normal parturients have attenuated responses to endogenous and exogenous catecholamines.
   a. They become resistant to the chronotropic effects of isoproterenol.
      i. Pregnancy reduces the response to this synthetic catecholamine by fivefold.
      ii. Women who develop preeclampsia do not make these adaptations.

3. Preeclamptic patients have an exaggerated hypertensive response to norepinephrine infusion.

4. Accidental intravascular injection or excessive systemic absorption of epinephrine might cause an exaggerated heart rate or blood pressure response in a woman with preeclampsia.

5. Epidural epinephrine also may impair uteroplacental blood flow.
   a. Placental blood flow decreases by 34% when healthy patients undergo cesarean section with 0.5% bupivacaine with 2.5 µg per milliliter epinephrine (1 : 400,000).
   b. In healthy primigravidae, umbilical arterial resistance decreases after induction of labor epidural analgesia with plain lidocaine.
   c. Patients receiving epidural lidocaine with epinephrine (40 µg) fall into two groups:
      i. Those with an initially normal umbilical arterial resistance respond with a decline in uterine artery resistance.
      ii. Those with a high initial resistance have a further increase and can develop fetal heart rate decelerations.[8]
   d. The risks of epinephrine might be even greater in preeclamptic patients with generalized arteriolar vasospasm. During cesarean section in hypertensive parturients, vascular resistance increases in the uteroplacental circulation, including the fetal renal and middle cerebral arteries after local anesthetic with epinephrine.
   e. Lower concentrations of epinephrine (1 : 400,000) still improve the quality of epidural lidocaine, but may have fewer hemodynamic consequences.

6. Because of the increased responsiveness to vasopressors in women with preeclampsia, maternal and fetal sequelae could be disastrous should unintentional IV injection or systemic

absorption of epinephrine occur. If you decide to include epinephrine in your local anesthetic solution, use the lowest concentration possible, and use small incremental doses and meticulous technique to avoid intravascular injection.

Patient Preparation
1. Check a recent coagulation profile, at least a platelet count.
   a. Look at sequential values to evaluate whether or not a downward trend exists.
   b. If the platelet count is 70,000 to 100,000 per cubic millimeter but stable, and there are no clinical signs of coagulopathy, then proceed with epidural anesthesia.
   c. If ultrasound examination suggests abruption or fetal death, or if the patient has liver dysfunction associated with the HELLP syndrome, check the PT and PTT and fibrinogen concentration.
2. Evaluate volume status.
   a. A hematocrit greater than 36% or a urine output less than 0.5 mL per kilogram per hour suggests significant volume contraction.
   b. Patients who are not severely volume contracted need little crystalloid before induction of epidural block.
   c. In seriously ill patients requiring invasive hemodynamic monitoring, increase the CVP to a positive value or the PAOP to 5 to 10 mm Hg.
   d. Whatever the preload, give the local anesthetic slowly. This precaution allows adequate time to respond if hypotension develops as the level of blockade rises.

Suggested Technique
1. These patients can safely receive epidural or combined spinal–epidural labor analgesia.
2. Epidural analgesia
   a. Insert the catheter.
   b. Position the patient comfortably, with good uterine displacement.
   c. Induction: 3- to 5-mL increments of 0.125% bupivacaine with fentanyl 2 µg per milliliter or sufentanil 0.5 to 1.0 µg per milliliter. A total of 10 to 20 mL should be sufficient.
   d. Maintenance: continuous infusion or patient-controlled epidural analgesia (PCEA) with 0.0625% to 0.125% bupivacaine with fentanyl 2 µg per milliliter or sufentanil 0.3 to 0.5 µg per milliliter at 10 to 15 mL per hour (more dilute solutions will require greater infusion rates).
3. Combined spinal–epidural analgesia
   a. Induction
      i. Pure opioids (more itching)
         (1) Sufentanil 5 µg
         (2) Fentanyl 20 to 25 µg
      ii. Opioids plus local anesthetic (more hemodynamic changes)
         (1) Bupivacaine 2.5 mg plus sufentanil 1 to 2 µg
         (2) Bupivacaine 2.5 mg plus fentanyl 5 to 10 µg

b. Maintenance: Begin this infusion or PCEA within 30 minutes of intrathecal drug injection.
4. Monitor blood pressure by arterial catheter or at least every 2 minutes by automated cuff for 20 minutes after the initial dose of either epidural or intrathecal drug.
   a. If mean arterial pressure decreases more than 30% from baseline or if nonreassuring fetal heart rate patterns develop, use further left uterine displacement, a fluid bolus, and IV ephedrine 2.5 to 5.0 mg.
   b. In severely ill patients, evaluate filling pressures and SVR repeatedly as the level of sympathetic blockade rises. Monitoring trends in these measurements will help to guide fluid and vasopressor therapy.

Other Choices
1. Patient-controlled analgesia with fentanyl, nalbuphine, or meperidine can provide better labor analgesia than intermittent bolus injection.
2. Suggested techniques
   a. Fentanyl
      i. Loading dose: 1 to 2 µg per kilogram
      ii. Bolus: 50 µg
      iii. Lockout: 10 minutes
   b. Meperidine
      i. Loading dose: 50 mg (±25 mg promethazine)
      ii. Bolus: 10 to 15 mg
      iii. Lockout: 10 minutes
   c. Both of these techniques are associated with an increased use of naloxone during initial neonatal resuscitation.

ANESTHESIA FOR CESAREAN DELIVERY
Epidural Anesthesia
Advantages
STRESS RESPONSE
1. Epidural blockade markedly blunts the hormonal and hemodynamic responses to surgery.
   a. Extensive epidural blockade correlates with lower maternal plasma cortisol, glucose, insulin, and adrenocorticotropic hormone (ACTH) concentrations in women undergoing elective cesarean section.
   b. Epinephrine and norepinephrine concentrations increase markedly during general anesthesia, whereas these compounds decrease in patients given an epidural anesthetic.
2. Severely preeclamptic patients undergoing cesarean section have similar responses. Plasma concentrations of epinephrine, norepinephrine, ACTH, and β-endorphin increase with general anesthesia, but remain unchanged in preeclamptic parturients having an epidural anesthetic.

HEMODYNAMIC CHANGES
1. Dramatic hypertension is less likely to occur during epidural anesthesia than during general anesthesia.

2. Hypotension also may be more likely.
3. With careful attention to technique, either regional or general anesthesia can be safe for these women.[9]

UTEROPLACENTAL BLOOD FLOW

1. The effects of epidural anesthesia for cesarean section on uteroplacental blood flow in women with preeclampsia are unclear. Both pronounced increases and decreases in placental blood flow occur.
2. Induction of general anesthesia with 4 mg per kilogram thiopental and succinylcholine consistently decreases intervillous blood flow.

MISCELLANEOUS ADVANTAGES

1. Epidural anesthesia allows the mother to remain awake and may decrease the risk of aspiration.
2. When the patient is awake, neurologic status can be monitored.
3. Epidural blockade avoids the increases in ICP associated with a rapid-sequence induction of general anesthesia.
4. Regional anesthesia also exposes the premature neonate to less drug than does general anesthesia.

Some Technical Issues

1. Evaluate coagulation before proceeding with a regional anesthetic.
2. Consider the risks of IV and epidural injection of epinephrine.
3. Fluid management can be challenging.
   a. These women may require large volumes of crystalloid to maintain hemodynamic stability.
   b. There will be rapid volume shifts of 1,000 mL or more at the time of delivery.
4. Establish large-bore IV access.
   a. Hemodynamic changes during induction of epidural anesthesia may require treatment with rapid fluid infusion.
   b. Magnesium therapy may cause some degree of tocolysis and can contribute to uterine atony and blood loss.
   c. Patients with HELLP syndrome or liver injury may require blood products.
5. Choice of local anesthetic
   a. 2-Chloroprocaine
      i. Most rapid onset
      ii. Timely intervention to correct hypotension may be more difficult.
      iii. Slow titration is difficult with 2-chloroprocaine. Dosing at intervals of more than a few minutes will often fail to increase the anesthetic level.
      iv. Redosing will have to be done about every 30 minutes, so you may be faced with giving a bolus of drug just after delivery, when the incidence of hypotension is already high.
   b. Lidocaine
      i. Lidocaine is metabolized less efficiently in the preeclamptic patient, but this should not be of concern with a single dose for cesarean section.

ii. It requires the addition of epinephrine (at least
1 : 400,000) to provide adequate surgical anesthesia.
c. 0.5% Bupivacaine
i. Best for slow titration of anesthetic level
ii. Because bupivacaine provides less dense motor
and sensory blockade, the mother may require
supplemental analgesia.
(1) Adding fentanyl 100 μg to the local anesthetic solution will improve intraoperative
analgesia.
(2) Injecting the epidural catheter several times
during labor before extending the block for
cesarean section will significantly improve
the quality of blockade.
iii. Ropivacaine may have similar characteristics and
benefits but less potential for cardiotoxicity.

Suggested Technique

1. Assess coagulation status.
2. Assess volume status and determine need for invasive hemodynamic monitoring.
3. Administer aspiration prophylaxis (30 mL 0.3 M sodium citrate PO).
4. Insert additional 16-gauge IV catheter, separate from medication infusions. Hydrate with 20 mL per kilogram or until
CVP is positive or PAOP is 5 to 10 mm Hg. (If not invasive
monitoring, use urine output to guide volume therapy.)
5. Identify the epidural space and insert a catheter.
6. Aspirate the catheter for blood or cerebrospinal fluid.
7. Inject 2 to 3 mL 0.5% bupivacaine to detect subarachnoid
catheter location. Wait 3 to 5 minutes.
8. Inject an additional 0.5% bupivacaine in 3- to 5-mL increments to a total dose of 15 mL.
9. Assess hemodynamic changes in between each increment of
drug, and give additional IV fluids or vasopressor as needed.
Use ephedrine 2.5 to 5.0 mg unless maternal heart rate is
greater than 100 beats per minute; then use phenylephrine
50 to 100 μg.
10. When hemodynamics are stable and the patient has bilateral sensory analgesia to at least the T10 dermatome, proceed to the operating room.
11. Position the patient supine with left uterine displacement;
reestablish monitoring.
12. Inject an additional 0.5% bupivacaine, plus fentanyl 100 μg,
as needed, to raise the level of sensory blockade to at least
T4. (Most women will require a total of 20 to 25 mL local
anesthetic. Women who have been receiving a dilute local
anesthetic–opioid solution for labor analgesia may need less
drug at cesarean section.)
13. Continue to treat hypotension as dictated by hemodynamic
changes (i.e., volume versus pressor versus inotropic support). The significant hypotension that commonly occurs at
delivery in these women is most often due to blood loss and
hypovolemia.

14. If desired, inject preservative-free morphine 2 mg through the epidural catheter after the umbilical cord is clamped for postoperative analgesia.
15. For more urgent procedures in women with a functioning epidural catheter, use 2% lidocaine or 3% 2-chloroprocaine to provide more rapid sensory blockade. Infuse additional fluids simultaneously to maintain stable blood pressure. During labor, be certain that the epidural catheter is working effectively should cesarean delivery be needed. Good communication with the obstetric service should provide adequate warning of an impending operative procedure.

Spinal Anesthesia

1. Although controversial, a growing body of data suggests that spinal anesthesia is a reasonable choice for women with severe preeclampsia.
2. Both prospective and retrospective studies suggest that the hemodynamic changes associated with spinal and epidural anesthesia are similar in these women.[9,10]
3. Profound hypotension can occur with either technique.

General Anesthesia

Airway

1. The generalized edema seen in preeclampsia may produce glottic swelling, which can make endotracheal intubation extremely difficult.
2. Be prepared for a difficult airway. Marked facial edema, hoarseness, difficulty swallowing, or respiratory distress should warn of potential problems.
3. Glottic edema cannot be adequately assessed on routine airway examination. Have a small (i.e., 5.5-mm) endotracheal tube available.

AWAKE INTUBATION

1. The vascularity of the pregnant airway and our reluctance to premedicate parturients heavily just before delivery can make awake nasal or oral intubation traumatic for all involved.
2. A simple, comfortable method of anesthetizing the airway for nasotracheal intubation:
    a. Nebulize 4 mL 4% lidocaine and 1 mL 1% phenylephrine by face mask.
    b. Ephedrine nasal drops will improve nasal breathing.
    c. A small dose of IV fentanyl may help prevent coughing.
    d. Dilate the nares gently with a lubricated nasal airway.
    e. Introduce an appropriate-size endotracheal tube over the fiberoptic bronchoscope.
3. An approach to awake oral fiberoptic intubation:
    a. Use glycopyrrolate 0.4 mg IV to decrease oral secretions
    b. Slowly drip 1% lidocaine along the tongue and into the back of the throat.
    c. Keep the mouth open with a bite block.
    d. Advance the fiberoptic bronchoscope in the midline until you see the vocal cords.

Blood Pressure

1. Dramatic and dangerous hypertension can complicate intubation and cause pulmonary edema or cerebral hemorrhage.
2. Nitroglycerin
    a. Can reduce blood pressure before induction and limit the hypertensive response to intubation.
    b. Is less effective in the volume-expanded patient.
3. Labetalol
    a. Up to 1 mg per kilogram
    b. No reflex tachycardia
    c. Labetalol blunts hemodynamic response to laryngoscopy and intubation.
    d. It is occasionally ineffective.
4. Sublingual nifedipine also attenuates the hypertensive response to laryngoscopy and intubation, but it does not prevent maternal tachycardia.
5. Opioids
    a. Fentanyl 100 µg: safe, but does not reliably blunt maternal hemodynamics.
    b. Alfentanil (10 µg/kg) given just before induction effectively controls the pressor response to intubation without adversely affecting Apgar scores.
    c. Although there are no data yet, remifentanil might provide similar hemodynamic control at induction.

Maintenance

1. The choice of an inhalation agent for maintenance of the parturient with severe preeclampsia is not critical.
    a. Neither renal toxicity with enflurane nor liver dysfunction with halothane have been reported in preeclamptic parturients.
    b. Isoflurane, sevoflurane, or desflurane also is safe.
2. Remember that p50 shifts to the left in preeclampsia. Mechanical hyperventilation will shift the oxyhemoglobin-dissociation curve even farther to the left. Mechanical ventilation also decreases venous return and cardiac output. Both events decrease oxygen delivery to an already compromised fetus.

Magnesium and Muscle Relaxants

1. Therapeutic serum magnesium concentrations significantly potentiate nondepolarizing muscle relaxants.
2. Magnesium impairs neuromuscular transmission at multiple sites.
    a. Decreases presynaptic release of acetylcholine.
    b. Reduces sensitivity of the postjunctional muscle endplate.
    c. Depresses excitability of the muscle fiber membrane.
3. Clinically, magnesium increases the density and duration of nondepolarizing neuromuscular blockade.
4. The interaction of magnesium with depolarizing relaxants is more complicated.
    a. Magnesium has no effect on the onset or duration of a single dose of succinylcholine.
    b. Repeated doses or continuous infusions of succinylcholine produce competitive neuromuscular blockade (phase 2 block), which is enhanced by magnesium.

10. Carefully monitor neuromuscular function with a nerve stimulator when giving any muscle relaxant to a woman with preeclampsia who has received magnesium.

Suggested Technique
1. Administer aspiration prophylaxis.
2. Determine a need for invasive hemodynamic monitoring.
3. Insert an additional 16-gauge IV catheter, separate from medication infusions.
4. Evaluate the airway. Have smaller endotracheal tubes (5.5, 6.0 mm) available in the operating room.
5. In the operating room, place the patient in the left-tilt position and begin preoxygenation with 100% oxygen.
6. Use increasing doses of labetalol (5, 10, 20 mg) to lower blood pressure to a mean of approximately 105 to 110 mm Hg (diastolic blood pressure: approximately 90 to 95 mm Hg).
    a. If 1 mg per kilogram labetalol fails to provide adequate blood pressure control, carefully titrate nitroprusside.
    b. Stop either drug if a nonreassuring fetal heart rate pattern develops.
7. Rapid sequence induction with cricoid pressure
    a. Fentanyl 100 µg
    b. Thiopental 5 mg per kilogram
    c. Succinylcholine 1.5 mg per kilogram
8. Maintenance
    a. Before delivery
        i. Fifty percent nitrous in oxygen and 0.75% isoflurane
        ii. If fetal compromise, consider using 100% oxygen and 1.0% to 1.5% isoflurane.
        iii. Avoid hyperventilation.
    b. After delivery
        i. Increase nitrous oxide to 60% to 70% as tolerated.
        ii. Titrate morphine 0.2 to 0.3 mg per kilogram or fentanyl 3 to 5 µg per kilogram intravenously.
        iii. Decrease isoflurane.
    c. Muscle relaxation
        i. Use a nerve stimulator.
        ii. Titrate cisatracurium in 10-mg increments to maintain 80% to 90% blockade.
9. Treat hypotension at delivery based on hemodynamic changes (i.e., volume versus pressor versus inotropic support).
10. Infuse oxytocin immediately after delivery. Avoid ergot alkaloids, which can cause hypertension.
11. Emergence
    a. Reverse neuromuscular blockade.
    b. Discontinue nitrous oxide.
    c. Treat emergence hypertension with agents used at induction.
    d. Extubate when the patient is awake and can maintain a 5-second head lift.

POSTPARTUM CONSIDERATIONS
1. Care of the preeclamptic patient does not end with emergence and extubation.

2. Monitoring should continue for at least 24 hours after delivery, or until diuresis begins.
    a. Mobilization of fluid should begin by 24 hours.
    b. If a spontaneous diuresis does not occur, cardiac filling pressures will increase.
    c. If invasive monitoring is in place, follow CVP and PAOP closely. If they begin to rise without diuresis, small doses of diuretics or low-dose dopamine may help.
3. In HELLP syndrome, thrombocytopenia may not reach its nadir until 2 to 3 days after delivery.
    a. An upward trend in platelet count should be apparent by postpartum day 3.
    b. Resolution to a count above 100,000 per cubic millimeter may require 5 to 6 days.
4. Fourteen percent to 27% of eclamptic seizures occur after delivery. Women with HELLP syndrome are at especially high risk of postpartum eclampsia.
5. Patients will need to be changed from short-term (parenteral) to long-term (oral) blood pressure medications.
    a. Most patients will need treatment of their hypertension for up to 6 weeks after delivery.
    b. The efficacy of oral therapy should be documented before discharge.

REFERENCES

1. Wheeler TC, Graves CR, Troiano NH, Reed GW. Base deficit and oxygen transport in severe preeclampsia. *Obstet Gynecol* 1996; 87:375.
2. Rodgers RPC, Levin J. A critical reappraisal of the bleeding time. *Semin Thromb Hemost* 1990;16:1.
3. Beilin Y, Bodian CA, Haddad EM, Leibowitz AB. Practice patterns of anesthesiologists regarding situations in obstetric anesthesia where clinical management is controversial. *Anesth Analg* 1996;83:735.
4. Orlikowski CEP, Rocke DA, Murray WB, et al. Thromboelastography changes in pre-eclampsia and eclampsia. *Br J Anaesth* 1996; 77:157.
5. Cotton DB, Hallak M, Janusz C, Irtenkauf SM, Berman RF. Central anticonvulsant effects of magnesium on N-methyl-D-aspartate-induced seizures. *Am J Obstet Gynecol* 1993;168:974.
6. Clark SL, Greenspoon JS, Aldahl D, Phelan JP. Severe preeclampsia with persistent oliguria: management of hemodynamic subsets. *Am J Obstet Gynecol* 1986;154:490.
7. Kirshon B, Lee W, Mauer MB, Cotton DB. Effects of low-dose dopamine therapy in the oliguric patient with preeclampsia. *Am J Obstet Gynecol* 1988;159:604.
8. Marx GF, Elstein ID, Schuss M, Anyaegbunam A, Fleischer A. Effects of epidural block with lignocaine and lignocaine-adrenaline on umbilical artery velocity wave ratios. *Br J Obstet Gynaecol* 1990;97:517.
9. Wallace DH, Leveno KJ, Cunningham FG, Giesecke AH, Shearer VE, Sidawi JE. Randomized comparison of general and regional anesthesia for cesarean delivery in pregnancies complicated by severe preeclampsia. *Obstet Gynecol* 1995;86:193.
10. Hood DD, Curry R. Spinal versus epidural anesthesia for cesarean section in severely preeclamptic patients. *Anesthesiology* 1999;90:1276.

Vaginal Birth after Cesarean Section

The use of cesarean delivery in the United States more than quadrupled from 5.5% in 1970 to 25% in 1988. The almost 900,000 cesarean sections per year exceeded the combined yearly total of tonsillectomies, appendectomies, and mastectomies. The practice of automatic repeat cesarean section was primarily responsible for this increase. Part of a nationwide attempt to reduce the cesarean section rate included informing physicians that, in the absence of a contraindication to vaginal delivery, patients with a prior cesarean scar should be encouraged to attempt vaginal delivery by undergoing a trial of labor (TOL).

BACKGROUND

1. Before the late nineteenth century, too few mothers survived the cesarean delivery to even worry about subsequent pregnancies.
2. As maternal mortality from cesarean section decreased and patients became pregnant again, the question arose as to how to manage these subsequent deliveries.
   a. As early as 1903, the dangers of rupture of the previous uterine scar were recognized.
   b. At that time, rupture of a fundal uterine incision carried a 50% to 75% maternal mortality and was invariably fatal to the fetus.
   c. Thus, the dictum "once a cesarean, always a cesarean" was well received.
3. In 1921, because catastrophic rupture of the classic uterine incision occurred in 4% of patients, Kerr revived the use of the transverse lower uterine segment incision. This incision rapidly gained in popularity and comprised 90% of uterine incisions in 1976.
4. In subsequent pregnancies, a low transverse incision behaves differently than a classical (fundal) one.
   a. The classical scar is more than four times as likely to rupture.
   b. It also is more likely to rupture before labor.
   c. Rupture of the classical incision carries a higher fetal and maternal mortality.
5. In the 1950s and 1960s, there were sporadic reports of safe and successful TOL.
6. In 1995, the American College of Obstetricians and Gynecologists (ACOG) published clinical practice guidelines under the heading of "ACOG Practice Patterns,"[1] which were based on an extensive review and evaluation of the available literature on vaginal birth after cesarean section (VBAC).
7. For TOL and VBAC, ACOG made the following recommendations:
   a. Success rates of TOL
      i. Success rates for VBAC range from 60% to 80%.

b. Risks and benefits
    i. The benefits of a TOL outweigh the risks.
c. Candidates for VBAC
    i. In the absence of contraindications, a woman with one previous low-segment transverse uterine incision is a candidate for VBAC and should be counseled and encouraged to undergo TOL.
    ii. A woman who has two or more previous low-segment transverse uterine incisions, who has no contraindications, and who desires TOL should not be discouraged from doing so.
d. Contraindications
    i. A previous classic uterine incision is a contraindication for TOL.
    ii. Epidural analgesia is not a contraindication for TOL.
    iii. Oxytocin use for induction or augmentation of labor is not contraindicated.
    iv. Suspicion of macrosomia in a nondiabetic should not disqualify the patient from attempting VBAC.
    v. Available data are insufficient to determine the risks and benefits of TOL for patients with multiple gestation or breech presentation, or for use of prostaglandin gel.
e. Management of VBAC
    i. VBAC should not be limited to large subspecialty hospitals. Well-equipped basic and specialist hospitals with the capacity to respond to intrapartum emergencies can be appropriate settings for TOL.[1]

WHY DOES THE ANESTHESIOLOGIST NEED TO KNOW ABOUT VAGINAL BIRTH AFTER CESAREAN SECTION?

Risks

1. In a labor suite, the anesthesiologist is often the first physician called on to evaluate a patient's complaint of pain. In patients undergoing TOL, atypical pain may herald an obstetric complication rather than failure of the epidural catheter.
2. Fetal heart rate changes can follow the induction of neuraxial labor analgesia.
    a. These changes must be distinguished from those suggestive of uterine rupture.
    b. Early detection of impending uterine rupture requires a high index of suspicion.
        i. During TOL, a fetal bradycardia to 90 beats per minute or less, lasting longer than 1 minute, is often the first warning of uterine rupture.
        ii. When rupture occurs, the infant must be delivered immediately.
3. Attempting VBAC is low risk, but clearly not risk-free.
    a. Uterine rupture can complicate 0.5% to 0.8% of cases.
    b. Prompt intervention usually results in good maternal outcome.

     c. Hysterectomy due to irreparable uterine rupture may be required in 1 of 2,000 TOLs.

     d. Despite electronic fetal monitoring and careful observation, rupture-related birth asphyxia with neurologic sequelae may occur in 1 of 5,000 TOLs.

4. Patients and obstetricians also may express concerns about the effects of labor epidural analgesia on the progress of labor and the need for cesarean delivery.

     a. The obstetric anesthesiologist should be cognizant of these issues and able to participate in reasoned discussions with patients and other health care providers.

     b. Patients contemplating VBAC who have questions or concerns about earlier anesthetic experiences should seek early consultation to relieve anxiety and apprehension.

Outcome

1. Collected studies from 1950 to 1985 show that 60% to 80% of patients with a single previous cesarean section can deliver vaginally.

2. Patients with two or more prior cesarean sections can achieve up to a 69% VBAC rate.

3. Attempted VBAC will have a high rate of success regardless of the indication for the original operation.

4. Adopting a liberal VBAC program can significantly lower the cesarean section rate.

BENEFITS OF VAGINAL BIRTH AFTER CESAREAN
Maternal

1. Women are five to ten times more likely to die after cesarean than vaginal birth. Patients delivering abdominally are more likely to die of sepsis, pulmonary embolism, hemorrhage, and complications from anesthesia.

2. Febrile morbidity is 10.8 times more common following cesarean section than vaginal delivery.

     a. Women who fail VBAC have a good chance of developing infection.

     b. Because about 70% of VBAC patients succeed in delivering vaginally, the total febrile morbidity of VBAC patients is lower than that of patients delivering by elective repeat cesarean section.

3. VBAC avoids operative complications, such as injury to vital organs, blood transfusions, anesthetic complications, postoperative adhesions, and wound infections.

4. Patients delivering vaginally experience less discomfort and require less analgesia and nursing care. They recover more quickly, care for their infants, and return to work sooner. The hospital stay is 2 to 3 days shorter. The psychological benefits of shared labor and delivery experience for the patient and her spouse are immeasurable. Fetal–maternal bonding is more readily established.

5. Shunning elective repeat cesarean section saves from $2,000 to $3,000 per delivery; avoiding 200,000 elective repeat procedures would save approximately $600,000,000.

Fetal

1. Elective cesarean section increases the risk of iatrogenic prematurity and neonatal respiratory morbidity.
2. In the term newborn, the absence of labor before abdominal delivery can result in the syndrome of transient tachypnea or "neonatal wet lung." Final fetal lung adaptation to extrauterine respiration may require a few hours of labor. Transient tachypnea may require admission to the intensive care nursery. Occasionally, this syndrome leads to pulmonary hypertension.
3. Accidental scalpel lacerations can occur when the lower uterine segment thins and the surgeon is relatively inexperienced.
4. Subsequent pregnancies in patients with previous cesarean section present high risk to the fetus, owing to the likelihood of abnormal placentation or possible catastrophic uterine rupture.

RISK OF VAGINAL BIRTH AFTER CESAREAN
Uterine Rupture

1. There are two types of uterine rupture:
   a. Complete or true rupture
      i. Involves the entire thickness of the uterine wall, usually with extrusion of uterine contents.
      ii. Symptoms occur suddenly and explosively.
      iii. There usually is pain, hemorrhage, shock, and significant fetal and maternal morbidity and mortality.
      iv. A classical uterine scar usually splits this way. The unscarred uterus also may suffer true rupture following trauma.
      v. This type of rupture is rarely seen in low transverse uterine scars.
   b. Incomplete uterine rupture
      i. Does not involve the entire thickness of the uterine wall; there usually is overlying peritoneum, which prevents extraperitoneal extrusion.
      ii. Because there is frequently no associated bleeding or extrusion of uterine contents, symptoms may be absent, atypical, or nonspecific.
      iii. Except when diagnosis is markedly delayed, fetal and maternal morbidity or mortality is rare.
      iv. This is the usual type of uterine rupture seen in the low transverse uterine scar.
      v. Synonyms include *occult, silent, window,* or *dehiscence.*
2. The risk of uterine rupture depends largely on the location of the uterine scar.
   a. The greatest risk follows a classical incision, which is a vertical cut in the thicker, more contractile upper uterine segment.
   b. Most uterine incisions (90%) are transverse in the passive, less contractile lower uterine segment.

       i. This portion of the uterus is thinner, less vascular, and only becomes fully formed during labor.

      ii. It is gradually stretched during labor, which may explain why a scar here is more prone to dehisce rather than completely rupture.

  c. Low vertical, J- and T-shaped uterine incisions are more likely to rupture than is the uncomplicated low transverse scar.

3. Most ruptures of the intact uterus follow accidents, traumatic obstetric maneuvers (i.e., version and extraction, forceps delivery), obstructed labor, or oxytocin use in the grand multipara. Following rupture of the intact uterus, maternal mortality is 14% and fetal mortality is 76%. In contrast, fetal mortality falls to 35% and maternal death rarely occurs with rupture of previous cesarean scars.

4. The most common cause of uterine rupture is reportedly the separation of a prior cesarean section scar. Although uterine rupture and dehiscence of the transverse scar do occur during TOL, this complication does not present a greater risk of maternal or fetal mortality than does elective repeat cesarean section.

5. Risk factors associated with uterine rupture
   a. Excessive oxytocin, dysfunctional labor (primarily active-phase arrest disorders, failure of dilation and descent), and history of two or more cesarean sections
   b. Epidural anesthesia, macrosomia, history of previous vaginal delivery after cesarean section, unknown uterine scar, and prior cesarean section for cephalopelvic disproportion (CPD) are not associated with uterine rupture.[2]

6. Complications associated with uterine rupture
   a. Maternal death
   b. Fetal asphyxia and death
   c. Maternal hemorrhage requiring blood transfusion
   d. Hysterectomy or major artery ligation

Diagnosis of Uterine Rupture

1. Because of its rarity and protean manifestations, uterine rupture is not easy to diagnose early.

2. The clinician must maintain a high index of suspicion in any patient with a uterine scar. The few premonitory signs may be indistinguishable from the normal aches, pains, and "bloody show" of labor. The classic symptoms of uterine rupture arise in fewer than 25% of cases (Table 22.1).

3. Abdominal pain is an inconsistent finding that is neither sensitive nor specific.
   a. If present, pain usually is described as severe suprapubic shearing or tearing.
   b. Some physicians fear that epidural labor analgesia may mask the pain of uterine rupture.
      i. There is a growing consensus that this apprehension is not valid.
      ii. However, "breakthrough pain" must be carefully evaluated in these women. The anesthesiologist may be the first physician to diagnose uterine rupture, provided that unusual pain is recognized as

Table 22.1. Signs and symptoms of uterine rupture of the gravid uterus (scarred or unscarred)

Signs and Symptoms of Uterine Rupture	Incidence (%)
Pain	0 to 50–80
Fetal distress	50–75
Vaginal bleeding	17–67
Recession of presenting part	25–50
Shock	0–50
Readily palpable fetal parts	17
Peritoneal signs	17

a symptom of obstetric complication rather than a failure of an epidural block.

4. The clinical manifestations of uterine rupture depend on:
   a. Location of the rupture.
   b. Completeness of the tear.
   c. Degree of hemorrhage.
   d. Presence of communication with the peritoneal cavity.
      i. Complete ruptures that communicate with the peritoneal cavity can extrude blood and other irritants intraabdominally.
      ii. Subsequent irritation of the diaphragm can cause referred shoulder pain.
5. Complete ruptures may be sudden and explosive, associated with severe pain and shock.
6. Incomplete ruptures may develop more gradually.
   a. The pain may be less intense, with abdominal tenderness instead of cardiovascular collapse.
   b. If blood distends the broad ligament, the pain may be felt down the leg.
   c. If the bleeding is retroperitoneal, the patient may complain of back pain and there may be no peritoneal signs.
7. Fetal distress
   a. Signals uterine rupture in 20% to 60% of monitored patients.
   b. There may be fetal bradycardia or severe variable decelerations.
   c. Intrauterine pressure monitoring
      i. May show progressive increases in baseline intrauterine pressure.
      ii. Or a sudden loss of uterine tone may accompany fetal heart rate changes.

Treatment of Uterine Rupture
1. Early diagnosis is the key to minimizing maternal and fetal morbidity and mortality.
2. Resuscitation of the mother must start simultaneously with preparations for immediate surgical intervention.
3. Shock does not contraindicate surgery when intraperitoneal hemorrhage is suspected.

4. Fetal outcome depends largely on the timeliness of the operation. As soon as the diagnosis of uterine rupture is suspected, it is important to proceed with cesarean section immediately. In one series, no infants had significant perinatal morbidity when delivered within 17 minutes of the onset of prolonged bradycardia.[3]

Failed Vaginal Birth after Cesarean
1. Patients who fail a TOL have a higher likelihood of febrile morbidity following repeat cesarean section compared with women who have an elective operation. This risk is greater than that seen in patients undergoing primary cesarean section during labor.
2. Indications for repeat cesarean section in these patients include arrest disorders or failure to progress (72%) and fetal distress (15%).

Fetal Risk
1. Whether the VBAC patient is at greater risk for late fetal demise than is her unscarred counterpart is unknown.
2. Although the low transverse scar is more likely to dehisce than to rupture, delayed diagnosis of complete rupture is associated with poor perinatal outcome.

Medicolegal Risks
1. Medicolegal problems can arise if there is an adverse result from TOL.
   a. It is important to involve the patient actively in the decision process.
   b. She must be aware that there are risks associated with both VBAC and repeat cesarean section.
   c. The mere presence of a prior scar puts her at a higher risk for uterine rupture.
2. Obstetricians and courts have questioned the ACOG guideline suggesting that only 30 minutes pass from decision to delivery. In one case, the court considered this ACOG "30-minute rule" to mean the maximum time, and it ruled that delivery within 30 minutes may not be adequate in certain situations.[3]
3. Although thousands of patients have undergone VBAC with generally good outcomes, most published experience took place in hospitals where obstetricians, anesthesiologists, and operating room personnel were immediately available and could perform cesarean sections within 10 to 15 minutes. In many obstetric suites, this response time from the onset of ominous fetal heart tracing to delivery may be impossible.

OBSTETRIC CONSIDERATIONS FOR VAGINAL BIRTH AFTER CESAREAN SECTION
Patient Selection
1. Women with one previous cesarean scar, in the absence of contraindication to vaginal delivery, should be counseled and encouraged to undergo TOL.

2. Those with more than one uterine scar who wish to attempt VBAC and in whom no contraindication to vaginal birth exists should not be discouraged.
3. A previous low vertical scar and an estimated fetal weight greater than 4,000 g are not contraindications to TOL.

Use of Oxytocin for Induction or Augmentation of Labor

1. Some fear that use of oxytocin increases the risk of uterine rupture during TOL.
2. There seems no reason to believe that a given uterine pressure achieved by oxytocin administration is any more dangerous to the uterine scar than is the same pressure produced during natural labor.
3. A uterus strong enough to withstand spontaneous labor should be able to withstand a properly induced labor as well.
4. In properly selected cases, with careful surveillance and precisely controlled administration, the use of oxytocin for induction or augmentation of labor in a patient with a prior low-segment cesarean section appears safe.

Multiple Prior Cesarean Section Scars

1. The success rate of VBAC in women after multiple previous cesarean deliveries varies between 45% and 81%.
2. The number of previous scars does not affect the dehiscence rate.

Previous Low-Segment Vertical Incision

1. The reported incidence of rupture of the low vertical scar is 1.3% compared with 2.2% for the classic and 0.7% for the low transverse scar.
2. Most available data suggest that VBAC is safe in patients with one or more low vertical scars.

Unknown Type of Uterine Scar

1. VBAC in women with an unknown uterine scar is a highly controversial issue.
2. In some practices, it may be difficult to consistently document the type of uterine scar.
3. In these settings, the risk of uterine rupture appears comparable between women with low transverse scars and unknown scars.
4. Some obstetricians will allow patients with an unknown uterine scar to attempt labor, provided intensive maternal and fetal monitoring are carried out and facilities are available to perform emergency operation.[4]

Previous Cesarean Section for Failure to Progress

1. Patients with a history of cesarean section for failure to progress or CPD should not be automatically excluded from considering a TOL.
2. Arrest of labor after reaching complete cervical dilation before the original cesarean delivery may increase the risk of failed TOL. In one study, only 13% of these women had a successful VBAC compared with 64% whose original cesarean section was for any other indication.[5]

Macrosomic Fetus

1. Some recommend cesarean delivery for macrosomic (more than 4,000 g) infants to avoid traumatic birth injuries, including shoulder dystocia.
2. There is even greater concern about delivering these babies in the presence of uterine scar.
3. Still, in most circumstances, women with a suspected macrosomic fetus can be safely offered a TOL.

Postterm Pregnancy

1. Seven percent to 12% of pregnancies are postterm (more than 42 weeks' gestation).
2. The fetal dangers associated with prolonged pregnancy include oligohydramnios and possible cord accidents, macrosomia and birth trauma, meconium passage and aspiration, placental insufficiency, perinatal hypoxia, and death.
3. Elective repeat cesarean section, usually scheduled shortly after completion of 38 weeks, theoretically should avoid these problems.
4. Women with postterm pregnancies can safely and successfully complete a TOL.

ANESTHETIC CONSIDERATIONS

When planning the anesthetic for these women, consider a variety of issues.

What Is the Incidence of Emergent Cesarean Section in Patients Attempting Vaginal Birth after Cesarean?

1. The incidence of uterine rupture during TOL is less than 0.5%.
2. These patients are also at risk for the other common causes of emergency cesarean section (i.e., abruptio placentae, cord prolapse, fetal intolerance to labor).

What Is the Risk of Epidural Labor Analgesia in Vaginal Birth after Cesarean Patients?

1. A previous cesarean section is not a contraindication to the use of epidural labor analgesia.
2. Some worry that labor epidural analgesia delays diagnosis of uterine rupture.
   a. Effective analgesia may mask pain associated with rupture.
   b. Maternal hypotension and compensatory tachycardia caused by hemorrhage from uterine rupture may be mistaken for sympathetic blockade.
   c. The cessation of uterine contractions after fetal extrusion may be misinterpreted as the temporary decrease in uterine activity sometimes seen after induction of epidural analgesia.
3. Epidural analgesia dose not alter the presentation of uterine rupture.
   a. Nonreassuring fetal heart rate changes are the most common presenting sign.
   b. Abdominal pain alone is reported by fewer than 25% of women suffering uterine rupture.

4. The diagnosis of uterine rupture may be simplified in the presence of epidural analgesia.
   a. View with suspicion any pain that "breaks through" a functioning epidural block.
   b. At low anesthetic concentrations used to relieve labor pain, axons are exposed to just slightly more than minimal blocking concentration of drug.
   c. More intense stimuli, such as uterine rupture, abruptio placentae, or acute bladder distention, can provoke an impulse that may be conducted through the "blocked" segment of the axon.
   d. Similarly, peritoneal irritation from blood or amniotic fluid underneath the diaphragm can cause referred pain in the shoulder.
5. Suggested technique
   a. Establish effective analgesia and bilateral sensory change.
   b. Maintain analgesia with an infusion of a dilute local anesthetic–opioid solution (patient-controlled epidural analgesia with such a solution also is acceptable).
   c. Monitor the anesthetic level frequently.
   d. The level of sensory blockade usually can be rapidly extended if immediate operative intervention is required. Three percent 2-chloroprocaine or 2% lidocaine are equally useful for this purpose.

CONCLUSION

The literature about VBAC must be viewed in proper perspective. Most studies are nonrandomized and retrospective. They usually were conducted in teaching institutions with continuous obstetric and anesthesia coverage. The frequently quoted incidence of uterine rupture of 0.7% to 2.2% is many times higher than the overall rate of rupture of both scarred and unscarred uteri. It is a mistake to think that VBAC patients are so low risk that they can be managed as if they did not have a uterine scar. The mere presence of a uterine scar places a woman at greater risk for uterine rupture than her unscarred counterpart. Low-segment incision scars are safer than scars after classic incision. The slower progress of the tear in a low-segment scar allows the clinician more time to make the diagnosis and act before catastrophe occurs. However, the signs and symptoms of rupture are less definite and may be atypical. Rupture of the low-segment scar may occur with serious consequences for the fetus and mother if the diagnosis is not made early and managed promptly.

REFERENCES

1. American College of Obstetricians and Gynecologists. Vaginal delivery after previous cesarean birth. ACOG Practice Patterns, August 1995.
2. Leung AS, Farmer RM, Leung EK, Madearis AL, Paul RH. Risk factors associated with uterine rupture during trial of labor after cesarean delivery: a case-control study. *Am J Obstet Gynecol* 1993;168:1358.

3. Flamm BL. Once a cesarean, always a controversy. *Obstet Gynecol* 1997;90:312.
4. Pruett KM, Kirson B, Cotton DB. Unknown uterine scar and trial of labor. *Am J Obstet Gynecol* 1988;159:807.
5. Hoskins IA, Gomez JL. Correlation between maximum cervical dilatation at cesarean delivery and subsequent vaginal birth after cesarean delivery. *Obstet Gynecol* 1997;89:591.

Intraamniotic Infection

Infection within the uterus, a common cause of morbidity during pregnancy, can complicate anesthetic management. This condition has been termed *chorioamnionitis, amniotic fluid infection,* and *intrapartum fever;* however, the term *intraamniotic infection* (IAI) alludes to both the site and symptoms of the disease. IAI occurs in as many as 10% of parturients. Diagnosis is usually based on the combination of a fever 37.8°C or higher (100°F or higher) plus two or more of the following:

1. Maternal tachycardia (greater than 100 beats per minute).
2. Fetal tachycardia (greater than 160 beats per minute).
3. Maternal leukocytosis (white blood cell count greater than or equal to 15,000).
4. Uterine tenderness.
5. Foul-smelling amniotic fluid.

The diagnosis may be based primarily on a maternal temperature exceeding 38°C with no other apparent source of infection.

FEVER AND THE ACUTE-PHASE RESPONSE

1. The parturient must be febrile to have clinically significant IAI.
   a. This elevation in body temperature is merely one facet of the cascade of events, termed the *acute-phase response,* that occurs after exposure to pathogenic organisms.
   b. Initially, endothelial cells and cells of the immune system are activated to produce cytokines, such as interleukin-1 and tumor necrosis factor.
   c. These compounds, in turn, affect the functioning of almost every organ system and lead to the production of other acute-phase reactants, including C-reactive protein, serum amyloid A protein, α_1 acid glycoprotein, and fibrinogen.
   d. Together, these compounds bolster the host's defenses and enable the body to rid itself of the infectious threat.
2. Fever is caused by the effects of endogenous (from the acute-phase response) and exogenous (bacterial) pyrogens on temperature-regulating centers, such as the hypothalamus and its lamina terminalis.
3. The change in body temperature triggers both behavioral and autonomic responses.
   a. For example, a warm person is inclined to seek a cooler environment, change to cooler clothing, and adjust the temperature of the room.
   b. Activation of the autonomic nervous system leads to increased sweating and peripheral vasodilatation to increase evaporative heat loss.

TEMPERATURE REGULATION IN THE PARTURIENT AND FETUS

1. During pregnancy, heat is produced and dissipated by many factors (Table 23.1).

**Table 23.1. Competing forces in temperature regulation
in the parturient**

	Heat Gain	Heat Loss
Without conduction anesthesia	↑ Basal metabolic rate	Hyperventilation
	Uterine contractions	Perspiration
	Vascular and lymphatic engorgement	
After conduction anesthesia	Vasoconstriction above block	Vasodilatation within block
	↓ Hyperventilation	↓ Muscle activity
	↓ Sweating with sympathetic block	Transfer of heat from core to periphery
		Central effects of medications in the epidural and spinal spaces

2. By the fifteenth week of gestation, basal metabolic rate has
   started to increase. Oxygen uptake and heart rate continue
   to increase until after delivery. Eventually, these sources of
   heat are coupled with heat from muscular exertion during
   labor. Uterine contractions are a constant and important
   source of heat at term. Lymphatic and vascular engorgement also may contribute to a rise in the mother's temperature, although this effect should last less than 24 hours.
3. The active metabolism of the developing fetus produces
   large quantities of heat. The fetus has two available methods to eliminate heat. The uteroplacental circulation can
   rapidly regulate fetal temperature. In addition, the amniotic
   fluid provides a reservoir for heat that crosses fetal skin.
   The human fetus generally remains 0.4°C warmer than its
   mother.

Effects of Labor
1. The pain of labor causes the parturient to hyperventilate.
2. Hyperventilation, with the accompanying perspiration, leads
   to heat loss.

Effects of Analgesia
1. Neuraxial analgesia upsets the balance between heat-produc-
   ing and -eliminating mechanisms.
   a. Once contraction pain is relieved, labored breathing
      subsides.
   b. Local anesthetic–induced sympathectomy produces
      vasodilatation within the blocked area.

   c. Heat transfers from the core to the periphery.

   d. Both sympathectomy and analgesia decrease sweating.

2. Less well understood are the central effects of spinal and epidural anesthesia. Unblocked areas have altered responses to heating and cooling.

   a. Shivering and vasoconstriction occur 1°C lower than in nonanesthetized individuals.

   b. Sweating does not begin until a higher temperature is reached.

3. As all of these forces come into play, maternal body temperature fluctuates widely.

   a. Without regional anesthesia, heat-dissipating mechanisms predominate, and maternal temperature slowly decreases until delivery.

   b. Relief of labor pains leads to a stabilization of the core temperature.

   c. Occasionally, the parturients' temperature rises slowly throughout labor.

4. Labor epidural analgesia and maternal temperature

   a. Maternal temperature often increases slightly after 4 to 6 hours of continuous epidural analgesia.

   b. Usually, maternal temperature remains below 37.5°C.

   c. However, epidural analgesia during labor is an independent predictor of maternal fever (temperature greater than 38°C).[1]

      i. Controversy surrounds the fetal–neonatal implications of epidural analgesia and maternal fever.

      ii. Some authors report more neonatal sepsis evaluations in babies whose mothers receive epidural labor analgesia, even in the absence of maternal fever.[2]

      iii. Others report increased sepsis evaluations only in relationship to maternal fever.[1]

      iv. These discrepancies probably represent different local triggers for neonatal sepsis evaluation.

      v. Most often, maternal fever is associated with signs of placental inflammation, whether or not the patient receives labor epidural analgesia.[3]

Effects of Maternal Fever

1. The elevation of body temperature that occurs during the acute-phase response assists in the fight against the invading organism.

   a. Heart rate and cardiac output increase while peripheral resistance decreases, helping immune system cells and proteins reach their targets.

   b. Higher temperatures at target sites improve the performance of these protective factors.

   c. The more efficient circulation also delivers oxygen and nutrients to satisfy increased demand.

2. Changes in the mother's body temperature alter fetal metabolism.

   a. With mild elevations in maternal temperature (1°C), fetal temperature also rises to maintain the fetal–maternal gradient.

      i.   Fetal heart rate increases.
     ii.   The fetus copes well. Mean blood pressure, arterial pH, pO_2 and pCO_2 remain unchanged.

b. With marked increases in maternal body temperature (1.5°C to 2.0°C), compensatory mechanisms show signs of failure.

      i.   The fetus finds it increasingly difficult to dispose of its heat, and the fetal–maternal gradient widens.
     ii.   Uterine activity increases.
    iii.   Uterine and umbilical blood flows decrease.
    iv.   Fetal cardiac output declines, and fetal blood pressure may fall.
     v.   When fetal heart rate cannot increase further, dysrhythmias begin to appear.
    vi.   The fetus may become hypoxemic, but often the fetal p_aO_2 is maintained.
   vii.   As the fetal p_aCO_2 rises, pH declines.
  viii.   The worsening fetal hypoxemia and acidosis can lead to fetal injury or even death.

INTRAAMNIOTIC INFECTION

Etiology

1. The organisms that give rise to IAI can gain entry to the uterus in various ways.

   a. Most commonly, pathogenic bacteria ascend from the lower genital tract.

      i.   Parturients with bacterial vaginosis are more likely to develop IAI.
     ii.   Frequent vaginal examinations and internal fetal monitors are other ways that bacteria are introduced through the cervix.

2. When barriers to invasion by pathogens are removed, such as when the amniotic membranes are ruptured, infection of the uterus is much more likely.

   a. Premature rupture of membranes exposes the woman to the risk of infection for a longer time. IAI occurs in over 20% of parturients whose membranes have been ruptured for more than 24 hours. For each hour of ruptured membranes or internal monitoring, the probability of IAI increases by approximately 2%.

   b. Conversely, IAI may predispose to premature rupture of membranes. The inflammatory response and the neutrophils that it attracts can lead to the release of proteolytic enzymes that may weaken the amniotic membrane.

3. IAI can occur with intact membranes. Other routes for infection to reach the uterus include hematogenous spread from a distant site, retrograde seeding from the peritoneal cavity through the fallopian tubes, and iatrogenic introduction of organisms during invasive procedures.

Intraamniotic Infection and Preterm Labor

1. Efforts have been made to link the inflammatory response associated with IAI with preterm labor.
2. Inflammation stimulates the production of prostaglandins, which mediate cervical ripening and induce labor.

3. Some species of bacteria, such as *Clostridium,* produce phospholipase, which can cleave arachidonic acid and increase the amount of prostaglandins present in the infected area. Bacterial endotoxins produced by gram-negative bacteria also can directly stimulate prostaglandin production. These bacteria, in concert with the inflammatory response they initiate, can impair placental membrane integrity and predispose it to premature rupture.

Diagnosis

1. Clinical IAI is diagnosed on the basis of multiple nonspecific signs and symptoms (Table 23.2).
2. An elevated temperature usually must be present for the diagnosis to be entertained.
3. The degree of leukocytosis required to diagnose IAI is unclear. Noninfected women can have a white blood cell count well above 15,000 per milliliter, especially postpartum. Other factors, such as exogenous steroids, also elevate the white blood cell count.
4. Laboratory tests have played a limited role in the diagnosis of IAI because of their disappointing predictive values. Serum concentration of C-reactive protein, an acute-phase reactant, can be measured, and samples of amniotic fluid can be gram-stained and cultured. Amniotic fluid also can be assayed for leukocyte esterase, glucose, cytokines, ceramide lactoside, short-chain organic acids, and fetal fibronectin.

Maternal Complications

1. Pregnancies complicated by IAI often are associated with dysfunctional labor. However, a cause-and-effect relationship is unclear. A low-grade infection in the uterus may be detrimental to uterine contractility and yet not be extensive enough to cause overt symptoms.
2. The dystocia seen in IAI leads to a higher than usual percentage of patients requiring oxytocin augmentation.
   a. The amount of oxytocin required to increase uterine contractility and induce cervical change may be increased.
   b. These patients often fail to make adequate progress. In pregnancies complicated by IAI, this failure to progress,

Table 23.2.   Criteria used in the diagnosis of intraamniotic infection

Criteria	Frequency (%)
Fever (>37.8°C)	100
Maternal tachycardia (>100 beats/min)	20–80
Leukocytosis (>15,000 cells/mm³)	36–90
Fetal tachycardia (>160 beats/min)	40–70
Foul amniotic fluid	4–22
Uterine tenderness	4–25
Fetal distress	<5

combined with the increased incidence of nonreassuring fetal heart patterns, increases the cesarean section rate by two-to threefold (26% to 53%).

3. Infectious processes that begin before delivery increase the risk of postpartum infection.

Maternal Septicemia

1. The bacteria involved with IAI can enter the bloodstream and produce symptoms of septicemia in 8% to 12% of patients.

2. The appearance of symptoms of sepsis in the parturient with IAI marks a significant turning point in the clinical course. The condition of both mother and fetus may deteriorate more rapidly, and delivery of the fetus becomes more urgent.

3. Unfortunately, the diagnosis of sepsis often is not obvious, especially in the early stages, and requires a high index of suspicion.

4. Untreated septic patients can develop pronounced and life-threatening signs of shock. These women require fluid resuscitation and cardiovascular support with inotropes and vasopressors. Close monitoring in an intensive care setting is appropriate, because other conditions, such as disseminated intravascular coagulation, pneumonia, and lung abscess, may develop.

Fetal Complications

1. Infecting organisms can reach the fetus by hematogenous spread or through the amniotic fluid.
   a. Fetal bacteremia may follow infection and inflammation of the placenta and umbilical cord.
   b. The fetus may swallow or aspirate pathogens in the amniotic fluid.

2. Fetal well-being may be jeopardized within a short time of membrane rupture.
   a. More than 10% of neonates born more than 24 hours after rupture of membranes may be bacteremic.
   b. Infants born prematurely after infection-induced preterm labor are exposed to the risks of survival with immature organ systems.
   c. At birth, fetuses who survive prolonged exposure to intrauterine infection are at increased risk for infection of almost every major organ system.

Obstetric Management

1. Early administration of antimicrobials decreases the incidence of neonatal sepsis and shortens the length of the neonates' hospital stay.

2. Giving antibiotics to women whose membranes have ruptured prematurely not only reduces maternal and fetal morbidity, but can safely prolong pregnancy.

ANESTHETIC CONSIDERATIONS

Before inducing regional anesthesia in a febrile parturient, the risk-benefit ratio of either proceeding with or withholding the anesthetic must be considered. Regional anesthesia provides needed labor pain relief. At the same time, the procedure could expose the patient to infectious risks that may not arise for weeks or even months. Withholding treatment is not without risk. Should the patient need a cesarean section, difficulty with the intubation caused by infection-induced airway edema could prove to be life threatening. The two main infectious complications associated with neuraxial analgesia are spinal epidural abscess and meningitis. Both occur rarely, but can have devastating effects if not diagnosed and treated promptly and effectively.

Abscess

Risk

1. The incidence of spinal–epidural abscess is surprisingly low: 0.2 to 1.2 times per 10,000 hospital admissions.
2. It is probably even rarer among obstetric patients, as only ten cases have been reported in the literature. Two of these cases occurred in the absence of anesthesia. However, an accurate estimate of the frequency of this complication cannot be made based on the appearance of case reports.

Source of Infection

1. Infecting organisms may reach the epidural space by several routes.
   a. During needle or catheter insertion, microbes can be transferred from anesthetist to the patient. Poor aseptic technique can be involved, or organisms from the nasopharynx of the anesthesia provider can reach the epidural needle.
   b. Anesthetic medications can become contaminated, especially if drawn from multidose vials. Luckily, contamination of local anesthetics is rare.
2. The source of the infection may be within the patient's own body.
   a. During a regional technique, organisms can be brought from more superficial areas of the back to the vicinity of the spinal canal.
   b. If a catheter is left in place, a path is available for the infection to continue its spread.
   c. The catheter can act as a nidus for infection. Hematogenous spread from a distant site is a danger in bacteremic patients. Disruption of small vessels in the epidural space occurs in 8% of epidural placements. Blood from these vessels can introduce pathogenic organisms into the epidural space.

Symptoms

1. Days to months can pass before symptoms of spinal–epidural abscess appear. Then, a typical progression classically occurs.
   a. First there are complaints of fever and backache.
      i. Most patients complain of deep back pain, and the majority are febrile.
      ii. Leukocytosis and an elevated erythrocyte sedimentation rate are common.
   b. Complaints due to radiculopathy follow shortly.

   c. Sensory deficits and muscle and sphincter weakness eventually are found and progress finally to paralysis.
  2. The rate of neurologic deterioration varies from hours to weeks.

Diagnosis
  1. Definitive diagnosis of spinal–epidural abscess involves radiologic imaging.
  2. Computed tomography (CT) scanning will show most of the important structures.
  3. Myelography can help visualize the soft tissue. However, it adds to the infectious risk of the diagnostic process, but some abscess lesions cannot be diagnosed with CT imaging alone.
  4. Magnetic resonance imaging (MRI) is as sensitive as CT scanning and can identify associated conditions, such as disc herniation or cord infarct. It also is more helpful in demarcating the extent of the lesion. Unfortunately, MRI may not distinguish between frank pus, granulation tissue, and hematoma. It also may not differentiate between epidural and subdural lesions. These deficiencies may be corrected by enhancing the signal intensity with gadolinium.

Treatment
  1. Management usually involves surgical exploration and drainage, followed by antibiotic therapy for at least 2 to 4 weeks.
  2. Medical therapy alone has been used successfully in some cases, but it increases the risk of further neurologic deterioration.
  3. Outcome depends on the degree of neurologic impairment at the time of diagnosis and the length of time it has been present before surgery.

Meningitis
  1. Infection of the subarachnoid space is rare following regional anesthesia. However, meningitis after the dural barrier has been breached by a spinal needle is well documented.
  2. Isolated cases of meningitis in obstetric patients have been reported after spinal, or epidural, combined spinal–epidural, and continuous spinal anesthesia.
  3. The causes of septic meningitis—contamination of equipment of anesthetics, nonsterile techniques, or bacteremia or infection at the site of injection—are similar to those of abscess formation. In addition, detergent residues on needles or syringes and coring of tissues by the spinal needle can produce aseptic meningitis.
  4. The onset of symptoms can vary from days to weeks. Once the characteristic fever, headache, and stiff neck appear, the infection must be treated aggressively with antibiotic therapy to prevent further deterioration.

Risk of Dural Puncture
  1. Whether introducing a needle into the subarachnoid space of bacteremic patients increases the risk for developing meningitis has been debated for decades.

2. Interestingly, the diagnosis of meningitis is made routinely by lumbar puncture (LP) in patients suspected of having the condition. However, some have long warned that this diagnostic maneuver may initiate the disease.
3. However, studies of diagnostic LP in both bacteremic and nonbacteremic individuals have found no increased risk of meningitis associated with dural puncture.

RISK OF REGIONAL ANESTHESIA
IN INTRAAMNIOTIC INFECTION

1. Only three retrospective studies have examined the risk of epidural or spinal anesthesia in patients with clinical IAI.
2. The first reviewed records of 115 parturients with IAI symptoms. Only 39, all of whom had first received antibiotics, were symptomatic at the time of anesthetic induction. There were no infectious anesthetic complications.[4]
3. A larger study found no infectious complications related to 279 regional anesthetics in women with clinically diagnosed IAI. This study included three women who may have been bacteremic at the time of anesthetic induction. None had received antibiotics.[5]
4. In the largest study, there were no infectious complications among 531 patients who received a regional anesthetic and whose placentas were positive for chorioamnionitis on pathologic examination after delivery. One-fourth of the patients with fever and three-fourths of those with leukocytosis just before anesthetic induction did not receive previous antibiotic therapy. Also, the epidural catheter was left in place for at least 24 hours after delivery in dozens of women who were febrile and who had elevated white blood counts without complications.[6]
5. Unfortunately, all of these studies may be skewed by the fact that sicker patients may not have been offered the option of regional anesthesia. These studies may have only established the safety of regional techniques if the infectious symptoms have not advanced past a certain point.

Recommendations

1. Parturients at risk for IAI but who are currently asymptomatic can be given a regional anesthetic without hesitation. No prior administration of antibiotics is needed.
2. Parturients who are febrile but show no other signs or symptoms of infection also may receive a regional anesthetic. If no antibiotic is administered before the anesthetic induction, these women most likely will follow an uneventful course. However, lacking prospective and conclusive proof of the safety of regional block in women with untreated IAI, the prudent course may be to give at least one dose of antibiotic before the anesthetic.
3. Febrile parturients with foul-smelling amniotic fluid or other signs and symptoms of IAI should be treated. In the absence of conclusive evidence to the contrary, antibiotics should be given before regional anesthesia.

4. Parturients who are overtly septic need antipyretic analgesics and antibiotic therapy before regional anesthesia can be considered. Here, the risk of spreading the infection while placing the regional block may be too high unless the patient shows signs of responding to the antimicrobial medication. However, even in these women, the risk of spinal or epidural infection after neuraxial analgesia may be less than the risks of alternative therapies.

5. If an epidural catheter has been placed before signs of sepsis were noted, the catheter need not be removed. An epidural catheter in a properly treated patient would not be expected to serve as a nidus for infection. As always, vigilance is the key to safe practice, and a discharge at the insertion site (but not erythema alone) should dictate immediate removal of the catheter.

SUMMARY

1. Intraamniotic infection complicates up to 10% of pregnancies and is associated with significant maternal and fetal morbidity. Most infections ascend from vaginal flora, but bacteria also can arrive from the bloodstream.

2. Mild infection is well tolerated by mother and fetus, but more serious cases can lead to maternal and fetal acidosis and fetal compromise.

3. Diagnosis of IAI must be made from multiple insensitive and nonspecific signs and symptoms.

4. Regional anesthesia can upset heat balance and cause a mild elevation in core temperature in parturients.

5. Risks of regional anesthesia include spinal epidural abscess and meningitis. These complications occur infrequently and must be balanced against the benefits of the procedure.

REFERENCES

1. Philip J, Alexander JM, Sharma SK, Leveno KJ, McIntire DD, Wiley J. Epidural analgesia during labor and maternal fever. *Anesthesiology* 1999;90:1271.

2. Lieberman E, Lang JM, Frigoletto F, Richardson DK, Ringer SA, Cohen A. Epidural analgesia, intrapartum fever, and neonatal sepsis evaluation. *Pediatrics* 1997;99:415.

3. Dashe JS, Rogers BB, McIntire DD, Leveno KJ. Epidural analgesia and intrapartum fever: placental findings. *Obstet Gynecol* 1999; 93:341.

4. Ramanathan J, Vaddadi A, Mercer BM, Sibai B, Angel JJ. Epidural anesthesia in women with chorioamnionitis. *Anesth Rev* 1992;19:35.

5. Bader AM, Gilbertson L, Kirz L, Datta S. Regional anesthesia in women with chorioamnionitis. *Reg Anesth* 1992;17:84.

6. Goodman EJ, DeHorta E, Taguiam JM. Safety of spinal and epidural anesthesia in parturients with chorioamnionitis. *Reg Anesth* 1996;21:436.

Peripartum Hemorrhage and Maternal Resuscitation

Peripartum hemorrhage remains a leading cause of maternal morbidity and mortality (10 to 2,000 per 100,000 live births). In emerging nations, peripartum hemorrhage is among the leading causes of death in women of childbearing age. Excessive bleeding occurs in 5% to 8% of pregnancies.

INITIAL EVALUATION

1. Preanesthetic evaluation of any obstetric patient involves a directed history and physical examination. Look for medical illnesses, prior surgeries, and obstetric complications that can increase the risk of maternal hemorrhage (Table 24.1). On physical examination, look for signs and symptoms of abnormal coagulation or hypovolemia (Table 24.2). Patients at high risk for peripartum hemorrhage may need additional laboratory evaluation (Table 24.3).

2. If a parturient presents with vaginal bleeding, assess the nature and quantity of blood loss. It can be difficult to quantitate the exact amount of hemorrhage. During pregnancy, hemodynamic changes may not be apparent until significant bleeding has occurred. Measurement of orthostatic changes in blood pressure and heart rate can give an indication of volume status (Table 24.4).

3. General considerations for the parturient predisposed to hemorrhage include preparation for surgical delivery of the fetus, volume resuscitation, and transfusion of blood and blood products as indicated by clinical status.

   a. The potential for rapid fluid administration requires at least one, preferably two, large-bore intravenous catheters.

   b. An indwelling urinary catheter and, in some cases, central access and an intraarterial catheter may be indicated.

   c. In at-risk patients, send a blood sample for type and screen.

   d. If transfusion is likely, have 2 to 4 U of packed red blood cells readily available.

   e. Equipment for rapid transfusion and fluid warming should be prepared.

   f. In addition to the anesthesiologist and obstetrician, key personnel, such as operating room staff and blood bank and laboratory technicians, should be alerted to the situation.

ANTEPARTUM HEMORRHAGE

1. Vaginal bleeding in early pregnancy may be due to:
   a. Ectopic pregnancy.
   b. Spontaneous abortion.
   c. Trophoblastic disorders.

Table 24.1.   Maternal conditions that can increase the risk of peripartum hemorrhage

Bleeding disorders
  von Willebrand
  Coagulation abnormalities
Anemia, history of uterine myoma, polyps
Pregnancy-related disorders
  Pregnancy-induced thrombocytopenia
  Preeclampsia
  HELLP syndrome
  Chorioamnionitis
  Abnormal fetal presentation
  Placenta previa
Previous uterine surgery
  Low transverse cesarean section
  Myomectomy
Grand multiparity
Multiple gestation, macrosomia
Maternal trauma
Medications
  NSAIDs
  Warfarin
  Heparin
Illicit drug use (cocaine)

HELLP, hemolysis, elevated liver enzymes, and low platelet count; NSAIDs, nonsteroidal antiinflammatory drugs.

Table 24.2.   Physical findings suggesting increased risk of maternal hemorrhage

Signs of abnormal coagulation
  Bruises
  Petechiae
  Bleeding gingiva
  Bleeding from IV sites
  Hematoma at IM injection sites
Signs of hypovolemia or anemia
  Skin turgor
  Pale conjunctiva
  Syncope
  Mental status changes
  Nausea
  Abdominal pain unrelated to contractions
  Vital signs changes
    Hypotension
    Tachycardia
    Orthostatic hypotension

IV, intravenous; IM, intramuscular.

Table 24.3. Laboratory evaluation of the parturient at risk of hemorrhage

Hemoglobin/hematocrit
Prothrombin time
Partial thromboplastin time
Fibrinogen
Platelet count

      d. Local vaginal and cervical lesions.
      e. Malignancy.
      f. Coagulation disorder.
  2. The most common causes of bleeding during midpregnancy include:
      a. Abnormalities of placental implantation (i.e., placenta previa)
      b. Placental abruption.
      c. Preterm labor.

Placenta Previa
  1. Positioning of the placenta over or very near the cervical os
      a. Risks disruption during cervical dilation.
      b. Blocks the passage of the fetus through the birth canal.
  2. It can be total (20% to 43% of cases), partial (31%), or marginal. Premature placental separation can contribute to the bleeding seen with a partial placenta previa.

Incidence
  1. Placenta previa is the leading cause of third-trimester maternal hemorrhage and is responsible for one-third of antepartum hemorrhages.
  2. It occurs in approximately 5 in 1,000 deliveries.
  3. Two major causes of maternal death in women with placenta previa are severe hemorrhage and complications of disseminated intravascular coagulation (DIC).
  4. Fetal mortality is 4% to 8%, most often due to complications of prematurity.

Risk Factors and Pathophysiology
  1. Both uterine and placental factors may increase the risk of placenta previa.
  2. Maternal age and parity: Women over 30 years of age are three times more likely to have placenta previa than are women less than 20 years. This finding may be related more to parity than age. Uterine vasculature is altered and endometrial blood flow is decreased to areas of previous placental implantation (i.e., previous pregnancies, abortions). To maintain adequate perfusion in a subsequent pregnancy, the placenta implants over a larger surface, increasing the risk that it will encroach on the cervical os.
  3. Cigarette smoking: Chronic mild hypoxemia due to exposure to nicotine and carbon monoxide from maternal cigarette smoking may cause compensatory placental hypertrophy. The larger placenta may be more likely to cover the cervical os.

Table 24.4.   Classification of hemorrhage in the 60-kilogram gravida at 30 weeks' gestation

Class	Volume Lost	Clinical Findings
Modest bleeding	≤15% of blood volume (≤900 mL)	Mild tachycardia Variable pallor Normal blood pressure Normal respirations Negative capillary blanching test Negative tilt test Normal urine output
Moderate bleeding	20%–25% of blood volume (1,200–1,500 mL)	Tachycardia (heart rate 110–130) Diastolic hypertension, decreased pulse pressure Moderate tachypnea Positive capillary blanching test Positive tilt test Urine output 25–40 mL/h
Severe bleeding	30%–35% of blood volume (1,800–2,100 mL)	Marked tachycardia (heart rate 120–160) Cold, clammy, pallid skin Hypotension Tachypnea (respirations 30–50/min) Oliguria
Massive bleeding	≥40% of blood volume (≥2,400 mL)	Profound shock No peripheral blood pressure discernible (systolic blood pressure <80 mm Hg) Peripheral pulses absent Marked tachycardia Circulatory collapse Oliguria or anuria

Source: After Baker RN. Evaluation and management of critically ill patients. In: Wynn RM, ed. *Obstetrics and gynecology annual: 1977,* vol. 6. New York: Appleton-Century-Crofts, 1977:295; and Beneditti TJ. Obstetric hemorrhage. In: Gabbe SG, Niebyl JR, Simpson JL, eds. *Obstetrics: normal and problem pregnancies,* 2nd ed. New York: Churchill Livingstone, 1991:573, with permission.

4. Previous uterine surgery: Low transverse uterine incision at cesarean delivery is the greatest single risk factor for placenta previa. Here, the placenta may be more likely to implant over the uterine scar, or the scarred area of the uterus may not grow normally during a subsequent gestation. (More than 90% of ultrasonographically diagnosed placenta previas will resolve by term. This phenomenon, often called "placental migration," does not represent separation and reattachment of the placenta at a more cephalad site. Instead, proportionally greater development of the fundus and body of the uterus during the second and third trimesters pulls the placenta away from the cervical os. A scarred lower uterine segment will not grow normally, which may impair "migration" of a low-lying placenta.)

Diagnosis
1. Placenta previa often is identified early in gestation by ultrasound.
   a. Placenta previa is seen in 6% to 45% of second-trimester ultrasounds.
   b. Ultrasound may miss 7% of cases of placenta previa.
2. Transvaginal ultrasound provides greater resolution and can accurately diagnose placenta previa without increasing the risk of hemorrhage.
3. Magnetic resonance imaging (MRI) provides superior picture quality compared with ultrasound. It is useful in differentiating a low-lying placenta from partial previa and determining the margins of a posterior placenta.

Obstetric Management
1. The management of a patient with placenta previa depends on several factors, including the gestational age and condition of the fetus, severity of hemorrhage, degree of placenta previa, and whether or not active labor is present.
2. Ideally, delivery is postponed until the fetus is mature. However, fetal or maternal compromise may necessitate urgent intervention.
3. Mild hemorrhage before fetal lung maturity
   a. Expectant management can improve fetal outcome.
   b. Tocolysis, weekly ultrasonography, and blood transfusions as indicated may allow extension of pregnancy to close to term.
   c. The benefits of further fetal maturation must be weighed against the risk of maternal hemorrhage.
4. Compared with other interventions, such as blood transfusions and improved prenatal care, cesarean section has ultimately proved to be the most significant factor in reducing both maternal and perinatal mortality in cases of placenta previa.

Placenta Accreta, Increta, and Percreta
1. When the placenta abnormally attaches to or invades the myometrium in areas where the decidua basalis is absent or deficient, normal placental separation is impaired.

2. *Placenta accreta* is the collective term for abnormal placental adherence. Further classification is based on the degree to which the chorionic villi penetrate the myometrium:
    a. Placenta accreta: Villi adhere to the surface of the myometrium.
    b. Placenta increta: Villi invade through the myometrial surface.
    c. Placenta percreta: Villi erode through the uterine wall.
3. The frequency of placenta accreta has increased in the past decade due to the rising number of cesarean deliveries. Placenta accreta is identified clinically in 1 of 2,600 deliveries and is confirmed by histopathologic examination in 1 of 4,000.
4. Risks factors
    a. The risk of placenta accreta rises significantly in parturients with a history of both placenta previa and cesarean delivery.
    b. Other factors associated with placenta accreta include multiparity, leiomyomas, endometritis, manual removal of placenta, adenomyosis, and Asherman syndrome (intrauterine adhesions and uterine synechiae).
5. Placenta percreta, although rare (0.03 per 1,000 deliveries), risks significant morbidity and severe hemorrhage. Placental invasion involving nearby organs, such as the bladder and bowel, can occur. Treatment involves surgical removal of areas of placental penetration.
6. Diagnosis
    a. Most often at the time of placental separation or during cesarean section
    b. Placental invasion in early pregnancy can be diagnosed by ultrasonography.
    c. Transvaginal color Doppler sonography can provide further evidence of the extent of placenta accreta. Both of these modalities are associated with false-positives due to technical limitations.
    d. MRI can provide a definitive diagnosis in addition to accurate localization of the placenta in relation to the cervix.
7. Adherent placenta is the most common indication for peripartum hysterectomy, which usually is performed at cesarean section.

Interventional Radiologic Approaches to Placenta Accreta
1. Interventional radiologic techniques are becoming instrumental in decreasing the morbidity and mortality in the parturient with massive hemorrhage.
    a. Selective embolization of pelvic vessels immediately after cesarean section can help control bleeding and, if successful, can eliminate the need for further surgery and, in some cases, preserve the uterus.
    b. Angiographic procedures also are performed preoperatively.
        i. Prophylactic embolectomy catheter placement may decrease the incidence of coagulopathy, transfusion requirements, and postpartum complications.

      ii. Balloon occlusion of the infrarenal aorta may prevent rapid blood loss during cesarean hysterectomy. After delivery, a previously placed balloon catheter can be inflated to control bleeding during surgical removal of the uterus with adherent placenta.

     iii. Percutaneous bilateral internal iliac artery balloon catheters, placed under fluoroscopic guidance before elective cesarean delivery, can be used in a similar manner.

Conservative Therapy

1. Nonsurgical management, or "conservative treatment," is advocated by some for special cases. This approach involves leaving the placenta intact after cesarean delivery and delaying hysterectomy. In some instances, the placenta completely resorbs. This option may be preferable when surgical excision may be technically difficult, such as a placenta percreta extending to the bowel and bladder.
2. In selected cases, "conservative management" with pharmacologic therapy can preserve fertility. Methotrexate has been used to promote involution of trophoblastic tissue that makes up the adherent placenta.

Placental Abruption (Abruptio Placenta)

1. Separation of a normally implanted placenta from the uterus before delivery of the infant.
2. Separation allows bleeding into the layer between the placenta and myometrium (decidua basalis).
3. The ensuing decidual hematoma isolates, compresses, and impairs the function of adjacent placental tissue.
4. Continued bleeding from the decidual spiral arteries enlarges the hematoma. Maternal hemorrhage is varyingly concealed within the uterine cavity or passed per vagina.
5. Although abruption can occur at any time, it is most common in the third trimester.

Incidence

1. Placental abruption occurs in 0.6% to 1.0% of pregnancies.
2. Placental abruption carries serious consequences for both mother and fetus. It is associated with 6% of maternal deaths during pregnancy. Stillbirth, preterm delivery, and fetal death occur with increased frequency. Perinatal mortality may be as high as 50%.

Symptoms

1. The amount of blood loss, percentage of functioning placenta, and development of coagulopathy affect the severity of clinical presentation.
2. Symptoms include:
    a. Painful vaginal bleeding.
    b. Uterine tenderness.
    c. Uterine hypertonus.
    d. Back pain.
    e. Preterm labor.

      f. Hypovolemia or shock.

      g. Fetal heart rate abnormalities or fetal demise.

3. Milder cases may go unnoticed.

4. Ultrasound may identify a retroplacental clot in the uterine cavity, yet the absence of clot does not exclude a severe abruption.

5. Blood loss usually is underestimated.

    a. The amount of blood passed vaginally may mislead.

    b. The uterus can hide significant blood loss without maternal evidence of hypotension or anemia. As much as 4,000 mL of blood may be concealed.

        i. Here, fetal heart rate abnormalities may be the only indication of hemorrhage.

       ii. The more concealed the bleeding, the greater is the risk of coagulopathy.

6. Continued blood loss with extravasation of blood, placental tissue, and amniotic fluid into the systemic circulation may cause systemic clotting abnormalities and consumptive coagulopathy.

    a. These problems complicate up to 50% of abruptions.

    b. The severity of coagulopathy correlates with both the duration and the amount of placental separation.

    c. Fetal death increases the risk of coagulopathy to 30%.

Risk Factors

1. Hypertension, either chronic or pregnancy induced, is the most common risk factor.

2. Prolonged premature rupture of membranes increases preterm deliveries. The risk of abruption increases when gestational age is less than 34 weeks and when membranes have been ruptured more than 24 hours.

3. Patients with a history of placental abruption are at increased risk of recurrence (5% to 17%) in a subsequent pregnancy.

4. Cigarette smoking and alcohol and cocaine use have been implicated.

5. Transabdominal trauma, such as occurs with motor vehicle accidents, may precipitate abruption.

6. Abruption also has been reported after percutaneous umbilical blood sampling.

Uterine Rupture

1. A rare, potentially catastrophic complication that occurs in approximately 0.05% to 0.09% of pregnancies

2. The risk increases with previous uterine surgery, such as cesarean section (particularly classical incisions) and myomectomy.

    a. Rupture of fundal scars from classical incisions may occur at any time and has been reported as early as 16 to 20 weeks.

    b. Rupture of lower segment scars is seen later in pregnancy.

    c. The highest maternal and fetal morbidities occur with rupture of an unscarred uterus.

3. True uterine rupture (total separation of the wall of the uterus) is very rare. Spontaneous rupture occurs in areas of previous uterine surgery and uterine abnormalities, such as placental implantation over previous scarring (placenta accreta).
4. Uterine scar dehiscence occurs with previous lower segment uterine incisions.
5. Signs and symptoms vary but may include:
    a. Increasing atypical abdominal pain.
    b. Vaginal bleeding.
    c. Uterine tenderness.
    d. Loss of contractions.
    e. Uterine hypertonus.
    f. Fetal heart rate abnormalities.
    g. Hypovolemia, shock, and loss of fetal heart tones are seen in more severe cases.
6. It is unlikely that the use of dilute local anesthetic–opioid mixtures for labor analgesia will mask the pain of uterine rupture. However, increased vigilance is appropriate.

Fetal Hemorrhage

1. A rare event and poses no threat to the mother
2. A small amount of blood loss can be catastrophic to the fetus.
    a. The fetus at term has a blood volume of 78 mL per kilogram, or approximately 300 mL.
    b. A loss of 30 to 40 mL may produce evidence of fetal stress.
    c. A loss of 100 mL is life threatening.
3. Fetal blood loss most often occurs into the maternal circulation.
4. Loss of up to 10 mL happens in 1 in 200 to 1 in 714 births.
5. Life-threatening hemorrhage (greater than 150 mL) complicates 1 of 800 births.
6. Causes of fetal hemorrhage include:
    a. Scalp sampling.
    b. Forceps delivery.
    c. Umbilical cord trauma.
    d. Medical conditions (von Willebrand disease, idiopathic thrombocytopenic purpura).
    e. Velamentous insertion of the umbilical cord.
        i.   Umbilical vessels travel to the fetus from the placenta within the thin membrane of the amniotic sac instead of the cushioning, protective Wharton jelly of the umbilical cord.
        ii. This is more common in multiple gestations.
    f. Vasa previa.
        i.   "Vessels going ahead," describes velamentous insertion of the umbilical cord in front of the presenting part of the fetus.
        ii. The diagnosis is made on palpation of pulsatile vessels in an unruptured sac during vaginal examination.
        iii. It is most often diagnosed accidentally with elective rupture of the membranes.
        iv. Tragically, perinatal mortality with rupture is 75% to 100%.

v.   Treatment involves immediate delivery, usually by emergent cesarean section.

vi.   Fetal salvage requires a high index of suspicion, with plans for infant volume resuscitation at delivery.

ANESTHETIC MANAGEMENT OF THE BLEEDING PARTURIENT

Cesarean Section

1. In the past decade, the number of cesarean sections has increased steadily.
2. The average blood loss during cesarean section is 900 to 1,100 mL.
3. The physiologic changes of pregnancy allow parturients to tolerate up to 1,000 mL of blood loss without a change in hematocrit, blood pressure, or cardiac output.
4. Factors associated with increased blood loss during cesarean delivery include:
   a. General anesthesia.
   b. Chorioamnionitis.
   c. Preeclampsia.
   d. Prolonged active phase of labor.
   e. Second-stage arrest.
   f. Hispanic ethnicity.
   g. Classic uterine incision.

Anesthesia for the Parturient at Risk for Hemorrhage

Assessment

1. The choice of anesthetic for cesarean section depends on several factors including, but not limited to, the urgency, amount of expected blood loss, and the volume and coagulation status of the parturient.
2. Examine each patient to determine current volume status, potential for intraoperative blood loss, and risk of cesarean hysterectomy.
3. Fetal status also will determine the urgency of the situation.
4. Close communication with the obstetrician aids in initial assessment.
5. Careful assessment of blood loss and current volume status is an important step in formulating an anesthetic plan.
   a. Patients who are significantly hypovolemic, who are still bleeding, or who have coagulation abnormalities are poor candidates for regional anesthesia.
   b. Stable, well-hydrated patients with little or no active bleeding can be good candidates for regional block.

Preparation

1. Check the availability of blood and blood products.
2. When anesthetizing women with placenta previa or suspected placenta accreta, have 2 to 4 U of packed red blood cells immediately available. Even stable parturients presenting for elective cesarean delivery because of placenta previa can have significant, rapid hemorrhage.
3. Insert two large-bore intravenous catheters to allow rapid fluid resuscitation.

4. Prepare rapid-transfusion and blood-warming devices. Warming blood and intravenous fluids will help maintain temperature stability.
5. Having extra personnel available to help may prove life saving.

Management
1. Regional anesthesia
   a. Hemodynamics
      i. Sympathectomy induced by regional block impairs the mother's ability to cope with sudden hypovolemia.
      ii. Although hemorrhage may lead to maternal hypotension, this problem usually is readily treated with intermittent boluses of ephedrine or phenylephrine.
      iii. If blood loss and hypotension persist, a continuous infusion of epinephrine or norepinephrine can be titrated to maintain maternal blood pressure. Use maternal symptoms (i.e., nausea, light-headedness) to guide therapy.
   b. If cesarean hysterectomy becomes necessary, the operation may outlast a single-injection spinal anesthetic. Plan ahead. If needed, induce general anesthesia in a calm, controlled manner. Do not wait until the block has regressed significantly and the patient is suffering severe pain. Continuous spinal, combined spinal–epidural, or continuous epidural block are appropriate alternatives if you suspect a prolonged procedure at the outset.
2. General anesthesia
   a. Possible indications
      i. Actively bleeding, hypovolemic parturients can develop profound hypotension with regional anesthesia.
      ii. Women with chronic abruption and significant coagulopathy should not receive regional block.
      iii. When the maternal or fetal condition mandates immediate delivery (i.e., within 5 to 10 minutes)
   b. Induction
      i. Initial choices depend on volume status.
         (1) A reduced dose of thiopental (3 mg per kilogram) or ketamine 0.5 to 1.0 mg per kilogram is safe in moderately hypovolemic women.
         (2) In the severely compromised parturient, muscle relaxant alone may be the only safe choice.
         (3) Ketamine
            (a) Causes central nervous system-mediated catecholamine release.
            (b) In most hypovolemic patients, this effect supports heart rate and blood pressure.
            (c) However, peripheral vasoconstriction may have reached its maximum in a severely volume depleted patient. In

this situation, ketamine cannot induce further vasoconstriction, and its cardiac depressant effects can result in hypotension and potential cardiac arrest.

ii. The remainder of a rapid-sequence induction, including application of cricoid pressure, succinylcholine 1.0 to 1.5 mg per kilogram intravenously, and endotracheal intubation, proceeds as usual.

iii. After securing the airway, maintain anesthesia with 50% nitrous oxide in oxygen and careful titration of volatile agent.

3. Central venous access may be helpful to guide volume status; however, blood loss, urine output, and maternal hemodynamics usually provide enough information. An intra-arterial catheter may be beneficial if multiple blood samples for hematocrit, coagulation studies, and acid-base analysis are needed.

POSTPARTUM HEMORRHAGE (PPH)

1. Responsible for over 75% of complications after delivery
2. Definition: blood loss in excess of 1,000 mL after vaginal or cesarean delivery

Retained Placenta

1. Retention of the placenta *in situ* beyond 30 minutes after delivery is abnormal and occurs in 1 in 300 deliveries. If all or part of the placenta remains within the uterus, it prevents contraction of the uterus, inciting atony and ongoing blood loss.
2. Retained placenta may be the first sign of placenta accreta.
3. Obstetric management consists of manual removal of the placenta with or without curettage.
   a. In a hemodynamically stable patient, analgesia for this procedure can be provided by paracervical block with intravenous sedation, extending a preexisting epidural anesthetic or spinal block.
   b. Inhalational analgesia with 50% nitrous oxide in oxygen and intravenous opioid also is an option.
   c. General anesthesia rarely is necessary. In addition, the amount of volatile agent needed for uterine relaxation (greater than or equal to 2 minimum aleveolar concentration [MAC]) can aggravate hypotension.
4. Occasionally, uterine relaxation will be needed to allow the placenta to pass a tightly contracted lower uterine segment.
   a. Intravenous nitroglycerin 50 to 100 μg provides uterine relaxation within 30 seconds without significant hemodynamic effect. Uterine muscle tone returns within 1 minute of injection.
   b. Using nitroglycerin may avoid the need for general anesthesia.
   c. Once the placental fragments have been removed, intravenous oxytocin usually is sufficient to induce uterine contraction.

Vaginal and Cervical Lacerations
1. Cervical lacerations from delivery are a significant cause of PPH.
2. A laceration, as opposed to uterine atony, should be suspected when bleeding persists despite good uterine tone.
3. For mild cases, anesthesia can be provided by the obstetrician: a paracervical block for cervical lacerations or a pudendal block for vaginal or perineal repair. Extending a previously placed epidural or instituting a spinal anesthetic to a T10 sensory level is an option in a hemodynamically stable patient.

Uterine Atony
1. Uterine atony is the most common cause of PPH and occurs in 2% to 5% of vaginal deliveries (Table 24.5).
2. Diagnosis: flaccid uterus and steady uterine bleeding
3. Initial therapy consists of uterine massage and oxytocin infusion. Prostaglandins can further aid in increasing uterine tone.
4. If these pharmacologic maneuvers are unsuccessful, surgical intervention may be necessary to prevent catastrophic hemorrhage.

Uterine Inversion
1. Uterine inversion occurs in about 1 in 3,600 vaginal deliveries. Although rare, it has been reported during cesarean delivery.
2. Fundal implantation of the placenta may be the underlying cause.
3. It usually arises when fundal pressure and traction on the umbilical cord are used to facilitate delivery of the placenta.
4. Severe hemorrhage and immediate hypotension, often out of proportion to blood loss, occur rapidly.

Table 24.5.   Conditions associated with uterine atony

Grand multiparity
Previous tocolysis
Uterine leiomyomas
Overdistended uterus
   Multiple gestation
   Macrosomia
   Polyhydramnios
Molar pregnancy
Uterine rupture
Dysfunctional labor
   Prolonged second stage
   Secondary arrest of labor
   Protracted active stage
Oxytocin
   Prolonged induction of labor
Retained placenta/products of conception

5. Treatment
   a. Forcing the everted fundus back through the cervical os
   b. Uterine relaxation usually is required. Relaxation can be achieved by β-agonist tocolytics, intravenous nitroglycerin, potent inhaled anesthetics, or magnesium sulfate.
   c. Nitroglycerin is an ideal agent, as it provides rapid onset of relaxation of short duration.
   d. If these measures fail, general anesthesia at greater than 2 MAC via an endotracheal tube provides uterine relaxation but can worsen maternal hypotension.
   e. An epidural catheter can be used for analgesia but does not provide uterine relaxation.
   f. If the uterus cannot be replaced manually, laparotomy may be required. Once the uterus is repositioned, give intravenous oxytocin to increase uterine tone and prevent further blood loss.

Distant or Secondary Postpartum Hemorrhage
1. Late PPH occurs after 24 hours but within 6 weeks of delivery.
2. Causes of hemorrhage beyond 48 hours after delivery include infection, retained placenta, dislodgment of a hematoma, and coagulopathy.

Amniotic Fluid Embolism
1. Incites approximately 10% of maternal deaths during pregnancy
2. Clinical presentation includes restlessness, sudden dyspnea, cyanosis, hypotension, coagulopathy, and seizures. Severe coagulopathy and subsequent massive PPH are related to the presence of placental and fetal material in the maternal circulation.
3. Treatment consists mainly of cardiorespiratory resuscitation, including transfusion of blood and blood products as needed.

Obstetric Management of Postpartum Hemorrhage
Pharmacologic Management
1. Oxytocin infusion (10 to 30 U per liter) will decrease blood loss after most uncomplicated vaginal or cesarean deliveries.
2. Methylergonovine (Methergine) 0.20 mg intramuscularly
   a. Produces intense uterine contraction and arterial constriction.
   b. The most worrisome side effect is severe hypertension.
3. 15-Methyl prostaglandin $F_{2\alpha}$ (Hemabate)
   a. Is very effective uterotonic.
   b. Side effects
      i. Are due to smooth muscle contraction.
      ii. Include an increase in pulmonary artery pressure and pulmonary vascular resistance, bronchoconstriction, and severe hypertension.
      iii. Use with caution in parturients with cardiorespiratory disease, especially asthma.

Surgical Management

1. Transvaginal and uterine packing with gauze can be a temporizing measure to control blood loss.
2. Surgical interventions before hysterectomy to control bleeding include ligation of pelvic vessels, including the uterine, ovarian, and hypogastric arteries.

Angiography

1. Selective embolization of pelvic vessels is very effective in the treatment of PPH.
   a. After catheterization of the femoral artery, an aortogram can locate bleeding pelvic vessels.
   b. After selective embolization of the involved vessels, a repeat angiogram confirms adequate hemostasis.
   c. Arterial catheters typically are left *in situ* for 24 to 48 hours in the event of continued hemorrhage.
2. Angiographic techniques are perhaps of greatest benefit to those patients in whom a significant risk of PPH is identified before actual hemorrhage occurs. Parturients with known placental abnormalities or bleeding disorders can have balloon catheters placed before delivery. These catheters subsequently can be used after delivery of the fetus to control bleeding before hypogastric artery ligation or hysterectomy.

Anesthetic Management of Maternal Hemorrhage

Transfusion

1. Ideally, typed and cross-matched blood should be transfused. If only the blood type is known, type-specific blood can be given in an emergency. When the blood type is unknown, type O-negative packed red blood cells should be used.
2. Evaluating blood loss
   a. Visual estimation of blood loss is inaccurate.
   b. Blood loss during primary PPH often is underestimated.
   c. Hemodynamic signs and serial hematocrits are more accurate methods of determining the need for transfusion.
3. The American Society of Anesthesiologists (ASA) has published "evidence-based" recommendations for transfusion of blood and blood products.[1]
   a. Red blood cells
      i. Transfusion rarely is necessary when the hemoglobin (Hb) concentration is greater than 10 g per deciliter.
      ii. In cases of acute blood loss, in which Hb is 6 g per deciliter or less, transfusion of red blood cells is usually indicated.
      iii. When Hb falls between 6 and 10 g per deciliter, the decision to transfuse should be based on several factors, including adequacy of oxygen-carrying capacity, hemodynamic signs, and potential for continuing blood loss.

  b. Platelets
      i. Prophylactic transfusion is not warranted when thrombocytopenia is due to platelet destruction, such as in idiopathic thrombocytopenic purpura.
      ii. Transfusion is not necessary when platelet count (PC) is greater than or equal to 100×10^9/L.
      iii. Transfusion is indicated when PC is less than or equal to 50×10^9/L.
      iv. For PC between 50 and 100×10^9/L, transfusion is determined by risk of bleeding.
      v. Transfusion is indicated if there is known platelet dysfunction and microvascular bleeding.
  c. Fresh-frozen plasma
      i. Amount: 10 to 15 mL per kilogram or for a minimum of 30% of plasma factor level
      ii. Correction of specific factor deficits when concentrates are not available
      iii. Correction of microvascular bleeding with elevated prothrombin time (PT) and partial thromboplastin time (PTT) (greater than 1.5 times normal)
      iv. In massive transfusion (more than one blood volume), when PT and PTT values cannot be obtained rapidly
      v. Should not be used for increasing plasma volume or albumin concentration
  d. Cryoprecipitate
      i. Nonbleeding patients with congenital fibrinogen deficiencies or von Willebrand disease that does not respond to desmopressin acetate
      ii. Patients with von Willebrand disease who are bleeding
      iii. Massive transfusion to correct microvascular bleeding in patients with fibrinogen levels less than 80 to 100 mg per deciliter or when fibrinogen levels cannot be measured rapidly

Autologous Blood Transfusion
  1. Several studies have found autologous blood donation by pregnant women to be safe and effective.
  2. Advantages
      a. Decreases the risk of infectious complications, transfusion reactions, and incompatibilities
      b. Predonation is particularly beneficial in cases of known adherent placenta, elective cesarean hysterectomy, placenta previa, and parturients with documented antigens.
      c. The threshold for transfusion of autologous blood may be lower.
  3. Disadvantages
      a. Costly
      b. Blood can be mislabeled.
      c. Does not completely prevent a need for homologous blood

Intraoperative Blood Salvage
  1. Blood collected from the operative field via suction can be collected, washed, and given back to the patient.

2. The use of banked blood can be dramatically decreased in cases of massive transfusion.
3. Concerns with the use of this procedure include intravascular transmission of amniotic fluid, air embolism, and infection.
4. Several reports have shown that standard processing techniques remove amniotic fluid and fetal tissue factor from salvaged blood.[2]
5. Reinfusion of salvaged blood lacks detectable effects on standard measures of coagulation function.[3]

Disseminated Intravascular Coagulation

1. PPH and massive transfusion may be complicated by coagulopathy.
2. Conditions associated with DIC include:
    a. Placental abruption.
    b. Amniotic fluid embolism.
    c. Prolonged fetal death *in utero.*
    d. Sepsis.
    e. Preeclampsia/eclampsia.
3. DIC results from activation of the clotting cascade. There is increased production of thrombin, activation of the fibrinolytic system, and fibrin deposition in the microcirculation. Clotting factors are consumed.
4. Laboratory testing reveals prolonged PTs and PTTs, low platelet counts and fibrinogen concentrations, and increased fibrin degradation products.
5. Immediate treatment includes supportive care and administration of blood and coagulation products as indicated by clinical status and laboratory tests. Elimination of the underlying cause is necessary for complete resolution.

REFERENCES

1. American Society of Anesthesiologists Task Force on Blood Component Therapy. Practice guidelines for blood component therapy. *Anesthesiology* 1996;84:732.
2. Catling SJ, Williams S, Fielding AM. Cell salvage in obstetrics: an evaluation of the ability of cell salvage combined with leucocyte depletion filtration to remove amniotic fluid from operative blood loss at caesarean section. *Int J Obstet Anesth* 1999;8:79.
3. Potter PS, Waters JH, Burger GA, Mraović B. Application of cell-salvage during cesarean section. *Anesthesiolgy* 1999;90:619.

Amniotic Fluid Embolism

Amniotic fluid embolism (AFE) is an incompletely understood syndrome, which can be catastrophic for both mother and fetus. Classically, AFE presents with a triad of hypoxia, hypotension, and coagulopathy. The onset and lethality of the physiologic derangements induced by AFE are remarkable. As many as 86% of cases are fatal; death occurs within half an hour in more than 50% of cases. Although rare, AFE ranks among the leading causes of maternal death.

EPIDEMIOLOGY OF AMNIOTIC FLUID EMBOLISM

1. Complicates 1 in 32,000 to 1 in 92,000 pregnancies
2. Carries a high risk of fatal outcome: causes 4.5% to 9.0% of peripartum maternal deaths
   a. In the United States, AFE ranks behind preeclampsia/eclampsia, obstetric hemorrhage, pulmonary thromboembolism, and obstetric infection as a cause of death.
   b. It causes nearly twice as many obstetric deaths as does anesthesia.
3. Our understanding of the factors that predispose to AFE is largely anecdotal.
   a. Advanced maternal age, multiparity, large fetal size, rapid labor, and oxytocin augmentation may increase the risk.
   b. Most cases occur in older parturients, with a mean age of 32 years.
   c. The incidence of AFE increases in multiparous patients; covariation of maternal age with increased parity may, at least partly, explain this association.
   d. Little evidence exists for macrosomia as a risk factor.
   e. Tumultuous labor or uterine stimulants are present in less than one-third of cases.
   f. Placental abruption occurs in up to 50% of cases; fetal death precedes clinical presentation in 40%.
4. Most often, AFE presents during labor (90% of cases). AFE also occurs during cesarean delivery, first- and second-trimester abortion, amniocentesis, and abdominal trauma. Some cases even present postpartum.

The American Registry

1. In 1988, an Amniotic Fluid Embolism National Registry was created.
2. A 1995 report detailed 46 cases that met the inclusion criteria.[1]
3. Its strict inclusion criteria and systematic evaluation have yielded significant insights.
   a. AFE presented most often during labor (Table 25.1).
   b. There was no correlation with ethnicity, age, oxytocin use, and rapidity or stage of labor.
   c. Maternal survival was 61%, although only 15% were neurologically intact. (Another report included 53 parturients who suffered AFE. Here, 84% of the mothers survived, most of whom (34/39) were neurologically intact.[2])

Table 25.1. Time of diagnosis of amniotic fluid embolism

Time	Percent of Cases
Labor	70
Cesarean delivery	19
Postpartum	11

Source: Data from Clark SL, Hankins GDV, Dudley DA, et al. Amniotic fluid embolism: analysis of the national registry. *Am J Obstet Gynecol* 1995;172:1158.

    d. Neurologically intact neonatal survival was 39% and appeared to be related to expeditious delivery.

    e. In several patients, clinical signs of AFE had a striking temporal relationship to artificial rupture of membranes or placement of an intrauterine pressure catheter.

    f. Of interest, 41% of parturients had a history of atopy, and 67% of fetuses were male. In concert with the high incidence of bronchospasm and hypotension in the presentation of AFE, the authors suggested that the syndrome would be more appropriately termed *anaphylactoid syndrome of pregnancy.*

    g. The major part of this clinical syndrome may be the result of mast cell degranulation and the release of histamine, tryptase, and other mediators. A study examining the presence and the pulmonary distribution of mast cell tryptase found similar results in women dying of AFE and those who died following anaphylactic shock.[3]

CLINICAL PRESENTATION

Presenting Symptoms

1. The clinical presentation of AFE syndrome often is dramatic.

2. Sometimes, nonspecific prodromal symptoms (nausea, vomiting, agitation, chills, apprehension, and restlessness) may precede overt evidence of AFE. The prevalence of these symptoms in the obstetric population renders them of limited use in predicting onset of AFE.

3. Rapid onset of severe cardiopulmonary compromise characterizes the initial phase of AFE syndrome.

    a. Usually, respiratory distress is the presenting symptom (Table 25.2), followed by severe hypotension and frequently, within minutes, cardiac arrest.

    b. Alternate initial presentations include cardiovascular collapse, uncontrolled hemorrhage, and seizures.

Table 25.2. Presenting symptoms in amniotic fluid embolism

Respiratory distress	57%
Hypotension	37%
Coagulopathy	13%
Seizures	10%

Due to frequent overlap of presenting symptoms, percentages sum to more than 100%.

      c. More atypical presentations of AFE have included abdominal pain, chest pain, ventricular tachycardia, and worrisome fetal heart rate patterns.

4. Mortality is very high during the initial phase. In one review, over half the women died within 30 minutes of onset of symptoms. A later hemorrhagic phase develops in 40% to 50% of patients.

Cardiopulmonary Effects

1. The chief cardiovascular manifestation of AFE is severe hypotension, usually out of proportion to any blood loss. Tachycardia typically accompanies the rapid drop in blood pressure. Clinical and invasive monitoring data frequently suggest left ventricular dysfunction.

2. Electrocardiographic findings are nondiagnostic.

3. Usually, clinical evidence of pulmonary edema, such as rales, frothy pink sputum, and jugular venous distention, develops rapidly.

      a. In up to 70% of patients, a chest radiograph reveals some degree of pulmonary edema.

      b. Although left ventricular filling pressures may increase, the degree of pulmonary edema often is out of proportion to this rise, suggesting involvement of both cardiogenic and noncardiogenic mechanisms.

      c. Adult respiratory distress syndrome frequently will develop in those who survive the acute event.

4. Arterial blood gas tensions in AFE typically reveal severe hypoxemia and metabolic acidosis with incomplete respiratory compensation.

Invasive Monitoring

1. Left ventricular failure is the only consistent finding in humans suffering from AFE.

      a. Case reports consistently describe significant left ventricular dysfunction based on clinical criteria, nuclear scanning, echocardiography, or calculation of left ventricular stroke work index.

      b. Diminished coronary artery blood flow may explain these observations.

2. In addition to left ventricular failure, some patients have low calculated systemic vascular resistance.

3. Unfortunately, the earliest data from any of these patients was obtained 70 minutes after the onset of clinical symptoms. Because mortality in excess of 65% occurs within 30 minutes of initial symptoms, invasive monitoring information from longer term survivors may not represent all cases of AFE, especially those with more sudden and catastrophic presentations.

Coagulopathy

1. Some degree of coagulopathy will develop in 40% to 70% of patients who survive the immediate effects of AFE.

2. Conditions ranging from subclinical coagulopathy with transient abnormalities in laboratory studies to fully developed disseminated intravascular coagulation with life-threatening hemorrhage may arise.

3. Laboratory values will reflect consumption of clotting factors with decreased fibrinogen and platelet count, elevated fibrin split products, and prolonged prothrombin and partial thromboplastin times.
4. Clinically, the patient will exhibit persistent vaginal or incisional bleeding and oozing from venipuncture sites.
5. The simultaneous development of uterine atony, possibly secondary to direct inhibition of myometrial contractility by amniotic fluid, often complicates the coagulopathy.
6. The underlying mechanism of AFE-associated disseminated intravascular coagulation is unclear. Tissue factor, trophoblastic material, and factor X activator may play a role.
7. Clinical signs of coagulopathy may precede other evidence of AFE. Rarely, coagulopathy has been reported as the sole manifestation of presumptive AFE.

Neurologic and Other Manifestations

1. Seizures, likely secondary to cerebral hypoxia, occur in 10% to 20% of AFE cases. Hypoxic brain injury has caused severe disability in survivors.
2. Acute renal failure due to prolonged hypoperfusion also may follow.
3. AFE appears to have no permanent cardiac or pulmonary sequelae; survivors generally return to baseline cardiopulmonary function.
4. Fetal distress is inevitable following onset of AFE symptoms. Maternal hypoxemia and hypotension drastically reduce transplacental oxygen delivery. The fetus rarely survives unless delivered immediately. Fetal distress also may precede the development of maternal symptoms, reflecting the extreme sensitivity of the fetus to even asymptomatic maternal hypoxemia.

Differential Diagnosis

1. Clinically, it is difficult to differentiate AFE from other serious peripartum complications.
2. Pulmonary thromboembolism, venous air embolism, systemic sepsis, myocardial infarction, decompensation of significant valvular disease, and peripartum cardiomyopathy can cause acute cardiovascular collapse in the parturient.
3. Both severe preeclampsia and placental abruption cause a coagulopathy that is clinically indistinguishable from that of AFE.
4. Other complications to be considered in the differential diagnosis of AFE include eclampsia, cerebral hemorrhage, aspiration of gastric contents, severe supine hypotensive syndrome, uterine rupture, and systemic toxicity of local anesthetic agents.

AMNIOTIC FLUID IN THE MATERNAL CIRCULATION
Amniotic Fluid Composition

1. Amniotic fluid volume increases rapidly during pregnancy, from approximately 50 mL at 12 weeks of gestation to a maximum of 1 L at term.

2. In the first half of pregnancy, amniotic fluid has essentially the same electrolyte composition as maternal plasma. Particulate matter is nearly absent.
3. As pregnancy progresses, fetal urine output makes the fluid hypotonic and increases its concentration of urea and creatinine. Varying amounts of particulate matter of fetal origin accumulate. This debris consists of desquamated fetal skin cells, lanugo and scalp hairs, vernix caseosa, mucin, and, occasionally, meconium.
4. Amniotic fluid also contains prostaglandins and other arachidonic acid metabolites, which may play an important role in the pathophysiology of AFE.

Entry into Maternal Circulation

1. Amniotic fluid entry into the maternal circulation requires communication between the amniotic sac and the maternal venous system.
   a. Endocervical veins are commonly lacerated during labor as the upper portion of the uterus becomes part of the lower uterine segment. Following membrane rupture, uterine contractions may force amniotic fluid into these vessels. Because cervical veins frequently tear during normal labor, with no apparent ill effects on the parturient, this mechanism most likely lacks a primary role in AFE syndrome.
   b. Placental abruption commonly occurs in cases of AFE. Possibly, premature separation of the placenta allows amniotic fluid entry through the placental implantation site.
   c. Disruption of the fetal membranes appears necessary for the development of AFE. The amniotic sac breaks before the onset of symptoms in most cases. When not apparent, concealed rupture has occurred, with intact membranes continuing to cover the cervical os.
2. Evidence exists for and against the routine entry of amniotic fluid into the maternal circulation.
3. Amniotic fluid debris is routinely found in maternal lungs after AFE. Lung specimens rarely contain amniotic fluid debris in parturients who die of other causes.
4. Unlike amniotic fluid, trophoblastic embolism is more common during pregnancy. Postmortem, evidence of trophoblastic tissue can be found in maternal lung in 40% of cases. Between 30% and 80% of parturients have trophoblastic cells in their peripheral circulation. However, these findings are clouded by the histologic difficulty in distinguishing trophoblastic cells from maternal megakaryocytes. Reliable differentiation may require sophisticated immunohistochemical analysis techniques.

Significance of Fetal Debris

1. Detection of fetal squamous cells in the maternal pulmonary circulation has been proposed as pathognomonic for AFE; however, reliable differentiation of fetal from adult squamous cells may not be possible.

    a. Examination of mixed venous blood from patients with indwelling pulmonary artery catheters commonly reveals squamous cells.

    b. In parturients, some cells may be of fetal origin, but most are contaminants during cannulation.

    c. Squamous cells, lanugo, and mucin can be found in pulmonary artery blood from parturients.

2. The lack of specificity of squamous cells in the maternal circulation has prompted a search for more sensitive markers of amniotic fluid in the maternal circulation. Zinc coproporphyrin and amniotic fluid–derived, mucin-type glycoprotein (sialyl Tn [STN], $NeuAc_{\alpha 2}$-6GalNAc) are recent candidates.

TREATMENT

1. Initial supportive therapy should be based on maternal and fetal symptoms (Fig. 25.1).

2. Use appropriate vasoactive drugs as guided by invasive monitoring.

Cardiopulmonary Resuscitation

1. With a potential first-hour mortality of 65%, considerable attention should be focused on the ABCs of cardiopulmonary resuscitation.

2. Hypoxemia is a nearly universal finding in early AFE. Many patients have survived the initial insult, yet ultimately die of complications of cerebral hypoxia. Early oxygen supplementation, preferably via an endotracheal tube, is imperative.

3. AFE patients frequently need blood pressure support to provide acceptable perfusion pressures for maternal vital organs and the fetus. Start with volume, ephedrine, and left uterine displacement.

4. Should full cardiac arrest occur, controversy surrounds the effectiveness of closed-chest cardiopulmonary resuscitation in parturients.

    a. It is unlikely that adequate placental and fetal oxygen delivery can be sustained during cardiopulmonary resuscitation.

        i. Diminished venous return in the supine position impairs cardiopulmonary resuscitation in the antepartum patient.

       ii. Lateral tilt introduces technical difficulty and mechanical disadvantage.

      iii. Even optimal cardiopulmonary resuscitation produces only 30% of normal cardiac output.

    b. Expeditious delivery may improve maternal and neonatal outcomes after cardiac arrest.

    c. Immediate and rapid preparation for cesarean delivery must start once maternal cardiac arrest occurs. Of course, aggressive resuscitation and continuous cardiopulmonary resuscitation should continue during this time.

5. Once initial stabilization and appropriate noninvasive monitoring (electrocardiogram, pulse oximetry, blood pressure monitor) have been accomplished, attention should focus on the differential diagnosis.

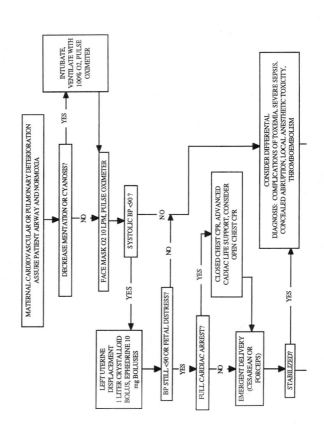

MATERNAL CARDIOVASCULAR OR PULMONARY DETERIORATION
ASSURE PATIENT AIRWAY AND NORMOXIA

DECREASE MENTATION OR CYANOSIS?

YES → INTUBATE, VENTILATE WITH 100% O2, PULSE OXIMETER

NO → FACE MASK O2 10 LPM, PULSE OXIMETER

SYSTOLIC BP <90 ?

YES → LEFT UTERINE DISPLACEMENT 1 LITER CRYSTALLOID BOLUS, EPHEDRINE 10 mg BOLUSES

NO → CONSIDER DIFFERENTIAL DIAGNOSIS: COMPLICATIONS OF TOXEMIA, SEVERE SEPSIS, CONCEALED ABRUPTION, LOCAL ANESTHETIC TOXICITY, THROMBOEMBOLISM

BP STILL <90 OR FETAL DISTRESS?

NO

YES → FULL CARDIAC ARREST?

YES → CLOSED CHEST CPR, ADVANCED CADIAC LIFE SUPPORT, CONSIDER OPEN CHEST CPR

NO → EMERGENT DELIVERY (CESAREAN OR FORCEPS)

STABILIZED?

YES

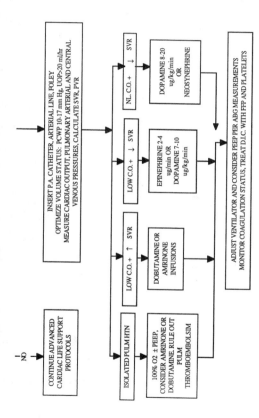

Fig. 25.1. A therapeutic algorithm for amniotic fluid embolism syndrome. BP, blood pressure; CPR, cardiopulmonary resuscitation; PA, pulmonary artery; HTN, hypertension; SVR, systemic vascular resistance; PVR, pulmonary vascular resistance; CO, cardiac output; PEEP, positive end-expiratory pressure; ABG, arterial blood gas; DIC disseminated intravascular coagulation; FFP, fresh-frozen plasma.

   a.   Clinical AFE syndrome is rare.
   b.   Conditions that easily mimic AFE include complications of preeclampsia (severe cerebral hemorrhage, hepatic rupture, eclamptic seizure with aspiration), overwhelming sepsis, concealed abruptio placenta, and intravenous or cerebrospinal fluid–mediated local anesthetic toxicity.
6.   If AFE appears likely and severe sepsis has been excluded, some clinicians advocate administering a very large bolus of steroids, possibly combined with H1 and H2 blockers.[1] This therapy is based on the similarities of AFE to anaphylaxis and the data linking inflammatory mediators to the clinical manifestations of AFE.

Invasive Monitoring

1.   Placement of arterial and pulmonary artery catheters is the next priority.
2.   Periodic arterial blood gas measurement will guide ventilator therapy.
3.   Intelligent use of a pulmonary artery catheter can be invaluable in choosing and titrating vasoactive drugs, as well as in optimizing volume status (see Fig. 25.1).

Blood Product Therapy

1.   Delayed coagulopathy (disseminated intravascular coagulation) develops in 40% of patients who survive the initial insult of AFE.
2.   Concomitant uterine atony also may occur.
3.   Frequent laboratory evaluation of coagulation profiles (fibrinogen, fibrin split products, prothrombin time, partial thromboplastin time, and platelet counts) provides a basis for therapy.
4.   Treat this usually self-limited coagulopathy with factor (fresh-frozen plasma) and platelet replacement.
5.   Treat uterine atony with methergonovine and avoidance of volatile anesthetics. Use prostaglandin $F_{2\alpha}$ only with extreme caution, as it may further complicate matters by inciting severe hypoxemia and hypotension.

CONCLUSION

1.   AFE syndrome remains a significant cause of maternal morbidity and mortality.
2.   Although the symptom complex involving maternal hypotension, hypoxemia, and coagulopathy clearly exists, the link to amniotic fluid remains unproved. Amniotic fluid commonly enters the maternal circulation, yet clinical AFE syndrome is rare. Amniotic fluid has a highly variable ability to activate complement and arachidonic acid pathways. Women vary tremendously in their susceptibility to complement activation and prostaglandin synthesis. Current knowledge suggests that clinical AFE syndrome results when a significant volume of amniotic fluid, high in complement-activating ability, enters the circulation of a woman predisposed to excessive complement and arachidonic acid metabolite response.

3. The diagnosis of AFE rests on excluding potential imitators, and therapy is essentially supportive. Early invasive monitoring helps optimize intravascular volume and use of appropriate vasoactive drugs.

REFERENCES

1. Clark SL, Hankins GDV, Dudley DA, et al. Amniotic fluid embolism: analysis of the national registry. *Am J Obstet Gynecol* 1995; 172:1158.
2. Gilbert WM, Danielsen B. Amniotic fluid embolism: Decreased mortality in a population-based study. *Obstet Gynecol* 1999; 93:973.
3. Fineschi V, Bambassi R, Gherardi M, Truillazzi E. The diagnosis of amniotic fluid embolism: an immunohistochemical study for the quantification of pulmonary mast cell tryptase. *Int J Legal Med* 1998;111:238.

Intraoperative Anesthetic Complications

Obstetric anesthesia is remarkably safe, but a number of minor and major complications can and do occur. This chapter attempts to describe some common and uncommon obstetric anesthesia complications that are diagnosed and treated intraoperatively. Complications that present or are treated postoperatively are discussed in Chapter 33. For each complication, consider the following:

1. Why is a given event harmful to mother or fetus?
2. Why is the parturient at greater risk of a given complication than is her nonpregnant counterpart?
3. Can the complication be prevented?
4. Can the effects of the complication be minimized or eliminated even if the complication occurs?
5. How can I best manage the consequences of a complication?

HYPOTENSION

1. Hypotension is the most common complication of obstetric regional anesthesia.
2. The incidence of hypotension during spinal anesthesia for cesarean section can be decreased by using left uterine displacement, intravenous (IV) fluids, and IV venoconstrictors.

Why Are Obstetric Anesthesiologists So Worried about Hypotension?

1. Severe hypotension can prove fatal for both mother and fetus.
2. "Spinal shock" was once a common cause of maternal mortality.
3. Infants delivered after severe hypotension lasting more than 4 minutes may be acidotic and have poor Apgar scores.
4. Mild hypotension produces few maternal symptoms but may be poorly tolerated by the fetus. Uterine blood flow falls in proportion to the decrease in maternal blood pressure (BP).

What Constitutes Treatment-requiring Hypotension in a Parturient?

1. Maternal and fetal conditions are unaffected if the systolic pressure remains above 100 mm Hg or falls less than 30% (whichever is greater).
2. The fetal effects of mild-to-moderate maternal hypotension depend on the duration of hypotension and maternal hydration. A healthy fetus tolerates hypotension for up to 4 minutes.
3. Generous maternal IV fluid administration blunts the fetal acidosis following maternal hypotension during spinal anesthesia for cesarean section.

Why Are Parturients So Susceptible to Hypotension?

Aortocaval Compression

1. Compression of the inferior vena cava and the aorta by the abdominal contents occurs rarely in nonpregnant patients but almost universally among parturients. The inferior vena cava

is an easily collapsed blood vessel that frequently gets caught betweem the gravid uterus and the maternal vertebral bodies.
2. The following increase the incidence and severity of aortocaval compression.
   a. Supine position
      i. Obstruction of the inferior vena cava produces supine hypotension (a decrease in systolic BP of 30 mm Hg or a systolic BP of 80 mm Hg) in 6% to 11% of term parturients.
      ii. Aortic compression can occur in 37% of supine term parturients.
   b. Hypovolemia
   c. Spinal or epidural anesthesia
      i. This induces a form of distributive hypovolemia.
      ii. Hypotension during spinal or epidural anesthesia occurs when the cardiac preload (not the afterload) decreases.

Uterine Contractions
1. The uterus compresses the more posteriorly placed vena cava only between contractions. Maternal hypotension occurs more frequently during caval obstruction (between contractions).
2. Aortic occlusion occurs almost exclusively during uterine contractions, regardless of maternal body position.

Early Labor, the Absence of Labor, or Nonengagement of the Fetal Head
1. Laboring women have a lower incidence of hypotension than do nonlaboring parturients during epidural or spinal anesthesia for cesarean section.
2. Aortic compression is more frequent if the cervix is dilated less than 5 cm or if the fetal head is not engaged in the pelvis.

Rapid Development of Sympathetic Nerve Block
1. Sympathetic nerve block develops more quickly in pregnant than in nonpregnant women during regional anesthesia.
2. Intrinsic homeostatic mechanisms then are less able to compensate for this sympatholysis as it develops.

What Is the Best Way to Prevent or Treat Hypotension?
Left Uterine Displacement
1. The full left or right lateral position completely relieves aortocaval compression.
2. Elevating the mother's right hip 10 to 15 cm improves femoral arterial BP and often completely relieves aortocaval compression. In some patients, tilting the uterus to the right is more effective than leftward tilt.
3. Left uterine displacement will decrease, but not eliminate, the risk of hypotension following the induction of neuraxial anesthesia.

Intravenous Hydration
1. Despite a 40% increase in blood volume, parturients appear hypovolemic when facing the twin assaults of a total sympathectomy and compressed abdominal blood vessels.

2. Rapid infusion of crystalloid solutions is well tolerated by healthy parturients, but fails to completely prevent hypotension (55% versus 71%).[1]
3. Colloid infusions also have only a modest effect on the frequency of hypotension (45% versus 85%).[2]
4. Clinical recommendations
    a. Labor analgesia (epidural injection of dilute local anesthetic–opioid mixtures or intrathecal injection of opioids with or without small doses of local anesthetic).
        i. Prehydration is unnecessary and may decrease the frequency and intensity of uterine contractions.
        ii. Continue infusing IV fluids at maintenance rates (125 mL per hour).
        iii. Have dextrose-free fluid available to treat any hypotension that may arise.
    b. Spinal or epidural anesthesia for cesarean section
        i. Infuse dextrose-free fluids under gravity while preparing and inducing anesthesia.
        ii. Give additional fluid to treat any hypotension that may arise.

Pressors

EPHEDRINE

1. Remains the pressor of choice in most obstetric situations
2. In hydrated parturients during cesarean section, prompt treatment of hypotension with IV ephedrine rapidly restores maternal BP and cardiac output. Timely therapy also ensures excellent neonatal outcome. Ephedrine also elevates maternal heart rate and cardiac inotropy.
3. Ephedrine crosses the placenta, increases fetal heart rate and beat-to-beat variability, and transiently affects the neonatal electroencephalogram.
4. Administration
    a. Although many methods have been described, no method of ephedrine administration reliably prevents maternal hypotension.
    b. Inject ephedrine 5 to 10 mg intravenously as needed to maintain a parturient's BP within her normal range. Maternal symptoms (nausea, vomiting, lightheadedness) and fetal heart rate changes can guide therapy.
5. Limitations
    a. Occasionally, ephedrine fails.
    b. Some women develop mostly a tachycardia from the drug's β-agonist actions.
    c. Switching to phenylephrine, an α_1-agonist, usually corrects the hypotension quickly.

PHENYLEPHRINE

In well-hydrated, laterally tilted parturients, phenylephrine 50 to 100 μg restores maternal BP and cardiac preload without compromising neonatal acid-base status, Apgar scores, or neurobehavioral scores.

MALPOSITIONED EPIDURAL NEEDLES AND CATHETERS
Unintended Dural Puncture
Diagnosis

1. The gold standard for clinical diagnosis of intrathecal needle or catheter position is the development of spinal anesthesia after the injection of an appropriate amount of local anesthetic.
2. In parturients, spinal anesthesia is diagnosed by the onset of sensory anesthesia at 2 to 3 minutes and motor nerve block at 3 to 5 minutes after injection of one of the following: lidocaine 30 to 45 mg, bupivacaine 5 to 15 mg, or 2-chloroprocaine 40 to 100 mg.
3. Recognizing a dural puncture is simple if clear fluid flows in a continuous stream from the epidural needle or catheter. Occasionally, one can aspirate a small (0.2 to 2.0 mL) amount of clear fluid after injecting saline or local anesthetic. On which side of the dura did the fluid originate?
   a. A urine dipstrip is a convenient, but not infallible, testing method (Table 26.1).
   b. Small amounts of fluid aspirated from epidural catheters before reinjection may have a physiologic pH and test positive for glucose despite the absence of a dural puncture.

Initial Management

1. Puncture of the dura occurs in 1.0% to 2.5% of attempted obstetric lumbar epidural anesthetics.
2. Usually the dura is punctured with the needle, and cerebrospinal fluid (CSF) is visible in the needle hub. Four courses of action then are possible:
   a. Pull the needle out and reidentify the epidural space.
      i. This risks a second dural puncture, but it allows insertion of an epidural catheter.
      ii. Many recommend choosing a different interspace for this second attempt. I do so only if the first approach proved problematic.
      iii. The incidence of unintended subdural or intrathecal cannulation is higher than if the previous dural puncture had not occurred. Inject epidural drugs slowly and test the patient for spinal anesthesia.
   b. Convert to a single-shot spinal anesthetic.
      i. This option is reasonable at cesarean section. Also, if inducing labor analgesia, inject a small

Table 26.1.   Urine test strip properties of fluids that might be aspirated from the epidural space

Fluid	pH	Glucose	Protein
Cerebrospinal fluid	7	0–1+	Trace–1+
Saline	5	0	0
Local anesthetic	5	0	2+ – 4+
Epidural aspirate, no dural puncture	7	0–2+	Trace

dose of preservative-free opioid with or without local anesthetic. Then, the patient will be more comfortable during any subsequent attempts to insert an epidural catheter.

   ii. Limitations

     (1) The tip of the epidural needle may be only partially subarachnoid. (Insert a long spinal needle through the epidural needle and inject through it.)

     (2) Injected solutions may flow back out of the needle along with additional CSF. (Keep the plunger depressed for a few moments after injection; then remove needle and syringe together.)

  c. Thread a catheter and manage as a continuous catheter spinal anesthetic.

    i. The Food and Drug Administration (FDA) has recalled spinal catheters smaller than 25 gauge, but larger catheters may be used.

    ii. If one follows this course, *do not inject lidocaine* in any form through the spinal catheter.

    iii. Limitations

     (1) Drug resistance (tachyphylaxis) can occur if repeated injections are needed during a prolonged labor or operative anesthetic. Continuous infusion of a dilute local anesthetic-opioid mixture at approximately 2 mL per hour may limit the frequency of this problem.

     (2) Maldistribution of injected drug can occur if the catheter is directed to the caudal end of the spinal canal. Changing baricity and patient position may be needed to produce an appropriate level of sensory blockade. Keep local anesthetic doses within the range used for single-injection spinal anesthesia.

  d. Pull the needle back until CSF no longer drips, and thread a catheter into the "epidural space."

    i. This approach is occasionally effective, but sometimes the catheter will still enter the subarachnoid space. At other times, it may miss both epidural and subarachnoid spaces.

3. Occasionally, the dura appears to have been punctured by the catheter: No fluid is seen in the epidural needle, but CSF is aspirated freely through the catheter. In this situation, leave the catheter *in situ* and initiate spinal catheter anesthesia, or remove the catheter entirely and replace it.

Management of Epidural Catheters Placed after Dural Puncture

Should One Decrease the Epidural Dose of Local Anesthetic?

1. Cases of high or total spinal anesthesia after epidural injection into an interspace adjacent to a dural puncture have been reported.

2. Dural puncture increases drug passage across the meninges and slightly increases the dermatomal spread of epidurally

injected bupivacaine. The magnitude of this effect is proportional to the size of the dural hole.
3. Titrate subsequently injected epidural drugs to effect, especially if injecting concentrated drugs for surgical anesthesia.

Can One Safely Administer 2-Chloroprocaine?
1. Although preservative-free 2-chloroprocaine is available (Nesacaine-MPF), other manufacturers still sell 2-chloroprocaine containing metabisulfite for epidural use.
2. Carefully identify the type of drug you are injecting.

Does a Dural Puncture Decrease the Incidence of Successful Epidural Block in a Subsequent Pregnancy?
No, although these patients may be at greater risk of a subsequent dural puncture.

Subdural Anesthesia
1. Unintended subdural, epiarachnoid anesthesia is clinically recognized during 0.1% to 0.8% of attempted epidural anesthetics. The true incidence may be much higher.
2. Subdural injection occurs more frequently during attempted subarachnoid needle placement; subdural injection complicates 10% to 13% of attempted myelograms.
3. The clinical picture can be confusing, for the characteristics of a subdural anesthetic are not halfway between those of spinal and epidural anesthetics. The chief clinical features of subdural anesthesia following injection of 2 to 10 mL of local anesthetic are:
   a. Delayed anesthetic onset.
      i. Most authors report a lag of 5 to 45 minutes between local anesthetic injection and the first signs of sensory block.
   b. Extensive sensory block, frequently extending to cervical levels.
      i. Although the sensory block is extensive, it frequently is patchy or asymmetric and may be one-sided.
   c. Loss of consciousness accompanying high sensory blocks.
      i. Unlike the epidural space, the subdural space does extend intracranially.
      ii. Hypotension
          (1) Maternal BP requires treatment, but the severity of hypotension is less than that accompanying total spinal anesthesia.
   d. Variable motor block.
   e. Respiratory depression.
      i. Respiration is usually compromised, although total apnea is uncommon.
      ii. Prolonged time to complete clinical recovery.
      iii. Most patients recover fully in 2 to 6 hours, but an 11-hour recovery has been reported.
4. Subdural anesthesia is rarely reported following injection of larger volumes of local anesthetic. Perhaps the fluid pressure from larger-volume injections ruptures the arachnoid membrane and produces a total spinal anesthetic.

Risk Factors

1. Factors that increase the risk of subdural anesthesia include:
   a. Previous back surgery.
   b. Immediately preceding dural puncture at the same or adjacent interspace.
   c. Rotating the Tuohy needle 180 degrees (with gentle needle advancement) following identification of the epidural space—*not* rotating the needle with gentle needle retraction.

Management

1. The initial subdural injection usually provides a more extensive block than is desired clinically.
2. Provide hemodynamic and respiratory support as needed.
3. Although few authors report a second, deliberate subdural injection, the nature of a subdural block (extensive sensory analgesia with little motor or sympathetic nerve block) makes it appropriate for labor.
4. Most anesthesiologists opt to replace the subdural with an epidural catheter.

High/Total Spinal or Subdural Anesthesia

1. Excessively extensive spinal anesthesia is seen most frequently in the following clinical circumstances:
   a. Unrecognized dural puncture by the epidural needle or catheter.
      i. This event complicates 0.2% of epidural anesthetics. Treat every bolus of epidural local anesthetic as a subarachnoid test dose.
   b. Spinal anesthesia for cesarean section initiated immediately following institution of a patchy epidural anesthetic (see Chapter 16).
   c. Attempted spinal or epidural anesthesia following accidental dural puncture.
      i. This may be either a spinal or a subdural anesthetic (see previous).
   d. Unexpectedly high block during a primary spinal anesthetic for cesarean section.
   e. High spinal block following administration of the initial local anesthetic "test dose" during the induction of epidural anesthesia.
      i. Spinal anesthesia requiring intubation and ventilation has occurred after injection of 50 mg of 2-chloroprocaine and 15 mg of bupivacaine.

Management

1. If the patient develops extensive sensory and motor block, profound hypotension, apnea, and loss of consciousness, do the following (quickly!):
   a. Place the patient supine with left uterine displacement.
   b. Apply cricoid pressure.
   c. Administer oxygen, by positive pressure mask ventilation, if possible.

d.   Intubate the trachea once appropriate supplies and a competent assistant are in the room and the patient is well oxygenated (if possible).
   i.   Inject succinylcholine 1 mg per kilogram intravenously to optimize visualization.
   ii.   Also give a small dose of thiopental if the BP permits.
   iii.   Once an airway is established, continue ventilation until the patient regains consciousness and can maintain a 5-second head lift or good hand grip.
e.   Administer fluids and pressors vigorously to maintain an adequate BP.
2.   Proper management of cervical (but not cerebral) levels of spinal blockade is not so obvious. At what point is a spinal too high? Most patients who appear anxious, complain vigorously of shortness of breath, and have a weaker than normal hand grip need only reassurance. Proceed to endotracheal intubation and general anesthesia when:
   a.   The patient is unable to maintain oxygen saturation greater than 95% despite breathing oxygen via a face mask.
   b.   The patient can whisper but can no longer phonate. Now, the patient may be neither ventilating adequately nor able to cough effectively to expel any foreign material that impinges on her vocal cords.
      i.   Apply cricoid pressure.
      ii.   Inject 1 to 3 mg per kilogram thiopental (based on BP) and 1.5 mg per kilogram succinylcholine.
      iii.   Ventilate with 100% oxygen until the patient is well oxygenated (if possible or necessary).
      iv.   Intubate and finish the case as a general anesthetic.

Unintended Intravenous Placement of Epidural Needle or Catheter

1.   During attempts to identify the epidural space, veins are cannulated in 5% to 15% of parturients versus 2.8% of nonpregnant patients.
2.   Can one lower the incidence of epidural venous cannulation?
   a.   Injecting 10 mL of saline or dilute local anesthetic before threading the epidural catheter halves the incidence of venous cannulation.
   b.   Injection of 3 mL of fluid does not decrease the incidence of blood vessel puncture.
3.   Can one detect all catheters located in epidural veins?
   a.   *No.*
      i.   Aspirate before each dose.
      ii.   Never inject a potentially dangerous bolus of drug.
         (1)   Never inject more than 25 mg bupivacaine at once.
         (2)   Limit all injections to 5 mL at a time.
   b.   Detecting IV catheters
      i.   Aspriation

          (1)   Simplest method

          (2)   Efficacy depends on the type of catheter.

              (a)   Aspiration fails to detect 33% to 67% of IV single-holed (open-tip) catheters.

              (b)   Aspiration will detect almost all IV multi-holed catheters.[3]

   ii.   Epinephrine 15 µg

          (1)   Widely used

          (2)   Limitations

              (a)   Parturients are less sensitive to the chronotropic effects of epinephrine than are nonpregnant women. Some never develop a tachycardia after IV epinephrine.

              (b)   Cyclical maternal heart rate changes occur during painful labor. In 12% to 45% of actively laboring women, maternal heart rate increases more than 30 beats per minute with each painful uterine contraction. Most "positive" epinephrine responses do not occur in women with IV catheters.[4]

  iii.   Doppler (air) method

          (1)   Precordial Doppler monitoring during injection of 1 to 2 mL of air through the epidural catheter detects most intravenously located epidural catheters.

          (2)   Independent of changes in maternal heart rate or chronotropic responsiveness; more appropriate than epinephrine for use in laboring women.

          (3)   Reminder: When using this test, rule out intrathecal catheter location first. (Intrathecal air will cause a headache).

   iv.   Type of catheter

          (1)   Effects the efficacy of the above tests.

          (2)   Single-holed catheters

              (a)   Aspiration is often falsely negative (i.e., not aspirating blood does not rule out IV catheter location).

              (b)   False-negatives are rare with epinephrine or air. False-positive responses are possible (i.e., a negative test rules out IV catheter location, but some positive tests occur in appropriately sited catheters).

          (3)   Multi-holed catheters

              (a)   Aspiration detects more than 95% of IV catheters.

              (b)   Both falsely negative and falsely positive responses can occur with epinephrine or air.

                  (i)   False-positives

                      1.   Air: A catheter may lie near, but not in, a disrupted blood vessel.

          2. Epinephrine: Pain-induced tachycardia may occur simultaneously with drug injection.

    (ii) False-negatives

          1. Multi-holed catheters also can be multicompartmental (i.e., one hole can lie in the epidural space and another in a blood vessel).

          2. The hole through which injectate exits the catheter depends on the speed of injection.

             a. Slow injection: Solution leaves through the most proximal hole.

             b. Fast injection: Solution exits uniformly from all holes.

4. Every dose is a "test dose." Aspirate carefully before each injection. Never give enough drug in a bolus to cause harm. Assume catheters that do not work properly are IV. Remove and replace them.
5. What should one do with an IV catheter?
   a. Remove and replace it.
   b. Withdraw the catheter unit until aspiration is negative, But,
      i. The catheter is often still IV.
      ii. The catheter is no longer in the epidural space.

BUPIVACAINE: A POTENT CARDIOELECTROPHYSIOLOGIC POISON

1. Bupivacaine is the most popular and also the most arrhythmogenic local anesthetic currently used in parturients.
2. IV injection of large doses of bupivacaine (greater than or equal to 35 mg) can cause maternal cardiac arrest and death.

Pathophysiology

1. Bupivacaine blocks fast sodium channels, slow calcium channels, and potassium channels.
2. Bupivacaine causes arrhythmias because it dissociates from myocardial sodium channels much more slowly than it binds to them, particularly at physiologic maternal heart rates.
   a. Bupivacaine is 16 times as potent as lidocaine in inducing cardiac arrhythmias.
   b. Both lidocaine and bupivacaine enter myocardial sodium channels quickly during the action potential. Lidocaine dissociates ten times faster during diastole.
   c. Bupivacaine accumulates in myocardial sodium channels and then impairs impulse conduction at all levels.
3. Intracerebral bupivacaine produces ventricular arrhythmias and hypertension by increasing autonomic nervous system outflow from the brainstem.

Arrhythmias

1. Wide QRS complex
2. AV nodal block of varying degree
3. Polymorphic ventricular tachycardia, which can progress to torsades de pointes
4. Bradycardia with electromechanical dissociation
5. Asystole

Confounding Factors

1. Bupivacaine administration by rapid IV bolus injection
   a. Bupivacaine is very lipid soluble and highly protein bound. At steady state, plasma free drug concentration is low. During rapid IV injection, toxic amounts of free drug can reach the heart and the brain before lipid uptake and protein binding occur. In addition, the percent of bound drug decreases with increasing serum concentrations of bupivacaine.
2. Hypoxia and acidosis
   a. Profound hypoxia and acidosis develop within 90 seconds of the start of bupivacaine-induced convulsions in both humans and anesthetized dogs.
3. Hyperkalemia or hyponatremia
4. Presence of other drugs that decrease electrical conduction in the heart
   a. This is a long list, including class I antiarrhythmics (quinidine, procainamide, lidocaine, disopyramide, etc.), calcium entry blockers, and β-blockers.

Available Antiarrhythmics

1. Bretylium
   a. In anesthetized dogs, bretylium 20 mg per kilogram proved beneficial. Bretylium corrected bupivacaine-induced alterations in cardiac output, stroke volume, heart rate, and systemic vascular resistance (SVR).
2. Isoproterenol
   a. In isolated rabbit hearts, isoproterenol 1 to 2 µg per milliliter corrects bupivacaine-induced prolongation of electrical conduction. Isoproterenol is an effective antiarrhythmic in other torsades de pointes conditions.
3. Magnesium
   a. Pretreating dogs with magnesium sulfate prevented widening of the QRS complex and QT interval but did not affect PR interval prolongation or the seizure dose of bupivacaine. Magnesium has not been used to treat bupivacaine-induced arrhythmias, although magnesium successfully treats torsades de pointes arrhythmias due to other causes.
4. Diazepam or midazolam
   a. Benzodiazepines terminate dysrhythmias caused by minute bupivacaine doses applied to the brainstem and thus may treat confounding γ-aminobutyric acid-mediated cerebral autonomic components of the arrhythmia.

Benzodiazepines can treat or prevent further seizure activity.

Treatment

1. Treatment frequently involves a prolonged and difficult cardiac resuscitation.
2. Because bupivacaine cardiac arrest occurs so rarely and volunteer studies have obviously not been done, the following treatment recommendations are based on animal studies, case reports, and treatments that work in related conditions.
   a. Ventilate and oxygenate immediately.
      i. Profound hypoxemia, hypercarbia, and acidosis occur more quickly in bupivacaine cardiotoxicity than in almost any other condition.
      ii. Resuscitation is more difficult in the face of hypoxia and acidosis.
      iii. Intubate the trachea quickly, but do not delay ventilation pending tracheal intubation.
   b. Perform closed-chest cardiac massage as needed.
   c. Prevent aortocaval compression.
      i. In anesthetized dogs, partial inferior vena cava compression lengthened the time to successful resuscitation and significantly increased the amounts of epinephrine and bicarbonate required.
      ii. Because preventing aortocaval compression while maintaining effective closed-chest cardiac massage may prove nearly impossible, one should strongly consider:
   d. An emergency cesarean section.
      i. In one case report, a mother could not be resuscitated until after the fetus was removed. Both the mother and the baby survived.
   e. Antiarrhythmics
      i. Ventricular tachycardia:
         (1) Bretylium 5 mg per kilogram intravenously every 30 seconds to a maximum dose of 30 mg per kilogram
      ii. Ventricular fibrillation:
         (1) Bretylium as above, plus epinephrine 1 mg intravenously, followed by direct current cardioversion
      iii. Bradycardia with electromechanical dissociation or asystole:
         (1) Epinephrine 0.75 mg and atropine 0.8 mg intravenously, followed by epinephrine 0.5 mg and atropine 0.4 mg intravenously every 45 seconds until the pulse and BP are stable.

FETAL HEART RATE CHANGES FOLLOWING REGIONAL ANALGESIA FOR LABOR

1. Fetal heart rate changes occur in about 15% of patients receiving either epidural bupivacaine, or intrathecal fentanyl or sufentanil labor analgesia.

2. After either epidural bupivacaine or intrathecal sufentanil labor analgesia, prolonged fetal bradycardia (heart rate less than 100 beats per minute for more than 2 minutes) is seen in 3% to 4% of patients with previously normal fetal heart rate patterns.
   a. The fetal bradycardias generally occur about 10 to 20 minutes after the patient is pain-free.
   b. Fetal bradycardia appears related to rapid progression of labor or excessive uterine activity.
      i. Maternal catecholamines (especially epinephrine) can inhibit uterine activity during painful labor.
      ii. Epinephrine, which has a serum half-life of about 3 minutes, disappears quickly after labor pain has been relieved.
      iii. This decrease may disinhibit factors that promote uterine activity (i.e., oxytocin). If uterine hypertonus develops, prolonged decelerations may follow.
3. Treatment
   a. Turn off the oxytocin infusion.
   b. Administer oxygen by face mask.
   c. Turn the patient on her side or into the knee–chest position.
   d. Palpate the abdomen for uterine contractions; recommend terbutaline or nitroglycerin if uterine tachysystole or hypertonus is present.
   e. Check BP; give IV fluids or ephedrine as needed.
   f. With IV fluids and tocolysis, few of these patients require emergent cesarean delivery. If an operative delivery seems indicated, recheck the fetal heart rate just before prepping the abdomen. In most cases, the fetal heart rate will have recovered during transit to the operating room.

RESPIRATORY ARREST AFTER INTRATHECAL SUFENTANIL OR FENTANYL

1. Severe respiratory depression or respiratory arrest rarely follows intrathecal administration of fentanyl or sufentanil.
2. Pathophysiology
   a. Intrathecal injection is a very effective way to deliver opioids to brainstem respiratory centers.
   b. Measurable respiratory depression occurs commonly after intrathecal fentanyl and sufentanil.
3. Presentation
   a. Often, these patients also received parenteral opioids.
   b. Somnolence is a common early sign.
   c. Patients become unresponsive with profound respiratory depression or complete apnea within 5 or 10 minutes of intrathecal injection.
4. Treatment
   a. Position the patient supine with left uterine displacement.
   b. Ventilate with 100% oxygen.
   c. Administer naloxone 0.4 to 0.8 mg IV (or endotracheal intubation).

MISCELLANEOUS
Broken Needles/Catheters
Needles
1. Open-ended needles are most prone to breakage at the junction of the hub and the shaft of the needle.
   a. Do not bury needles to the hub.
   b. Surgical exploration may be needed for needle retrieval if the hub and shaft separate.
2. Needles with recessed holes (such as the Sprotte needle) may bend (and, very rarely, break) at the thinnest point of the metal after a high-velocity impact with bone.
3. Broken needles should be removed because they can migrate and cause further tissue damage.

Epidural Catheters
1. The tip of an epidural catheter may shear if withdrawn through the epidural needle.
   a. Catheter shearing occurs more frequently with Teflon-coated polyvinyl chloride than with nylon or polyamide catheters.
   b. Such catheter tips may be left *in situ* if the patient is asymptomatic.
2. Catheters may knot on themselves if excessive amounts are threaded into the epidural space. Most such catheters have been removed intact with gentle, steady traction.

Headache of Immediate Onset
1. Immediate, severe headache can follow subarachnoid or subdural injection of air.
2. Patients usually recover spontaneously over 1 to 5 days.

Ulnar or Radial Nerve Injury
1. Automatic BP cuffs positioned over the elbow of thin parturients who are actively moving their arms may cause acute radial or ulnar nerve injury.
2. Injury may occur after less than 1 hour of automated cuff use.
3. Unlike nerve injuries under general anesthesia, which primarily are caused by ischemia of the vasa nervorum, these injuries probably are caused by mechanical intussusception of the myelin sheath.

Air Emboli
1. Air can enter the venous sinuses of the gravid uterus.
2. Precordial Doppler monitoring detects venous air embolism in 10% to 65% of cesarean section patients.
3. Awake patients experiencing air emboli may complain of chest pain or dyspnea.
4. Cyanosis, low oxygen saturation, or end-tidal carbon dioxide tension, hypotension, and cardiac dysrhythmias may occur when larger amounts of air are entrained.
5. Treatment of a (rare) clinically significant air embolism consists of flooding the operative field, discontinuing nitrous oxide administration, placing the patient in a steep head-down and

left-tilted position, and providing cardiac resuscitation as needed.

Electrocardiographic Changes during Cesarean Section

1. Electrocardiographic ST-segment changes occur in 25% to 64% of cesarean section patients.
2. The cause of this phenomenon is unknown, but it is not associated with regional wall motion abnormalities, decreased cardiac ejection fraction, abnormal postoperative 12-lead electrocardiograms, or elevated myocardial creatine kinase.

GENERAL ANESTHESIA

Failed Intubation

1. Occurs roughly ten times more often in parturients than in other surgical patients.
2. The incidence of failed intubation during general anesthesia for cesarean section ranges from 1 in 140 to 1 in 1,000 cases.
3. Intubation difficulties, with or without pulmonary aspiration, are the primary cause of anesthesia-related maternal mortality.

Why Is Tracheal Intubation of Obstetric Patients So Difficult?

1. Anatomic changes related to pregnancy
   a. Edema of the larynx, nasopharynx, and tongue. Airway edema, present to some degree in all parturients, contributes to difficult intubations in some preeclamptic patients and healthy patients following strenuous bearing-down efforts.
   b. Capillary engorgement. The mucosa of the airway is friable and bleeds easily.
   c. Pregnancy-induced anatomic changes can turn a difficult airway into an impossible airway.
2. Mammary hyperplasia and increased anteroposterior chest diameter. These anatomic changes decrease the distance from the chin to the chest and make it more difficult to insert the laryngoscope blade in the mouth.
3. Emergency operations. Most difficult or failed intubations occur during emergent, not elective, general anesthesia. The urgent or emergent clinical situation leads many to proceed without sufficient attention to airway assessment, patient positioning, or other anesthetic options.

Prevention

1. Decreasing the incidence of intubation failures requires careful preparation of personnel and equipment, much of which needs to occur long before the case is anticipated.
2. Carefully assess the airway in all obstetric patients. This assessment need not take much time. Honesty, not egotism, is essential in this endeavor.
3. Be prepared to suggest or insist on an anesthetic plan not involving rapid-sequence general anesthesia. This approach can be difficult when facing an agitated obstetrician concerned about fetal well-being; however, an excessively fetocentric view helps neither mother nor baby.

4. Anticipate difficult situations and plan ahead for regional anesthesia. Routine preoperative evaluation of laboring women and early induction of neuraxial analgesia can significantly decrease the frequency of emergency general anesthesia.
5. Optimize the position of the bed and the patient's head before inducing general anesthesia.
    a. Use pillows, blankets, or towels to raise the patient's head and shoulders and place her in the "sniffing position" (see Chapter 19, Fig. 19.1).
    b. This body position permits gravity to keep the breasts and chest out of the way of the laryngoscope handle and minimizes the amount of lift necessary to expose the larynx.
6. Equipment
    a. Never induce general anesthesia with inadequate or unchecked equipment or inadequate assistance.
    b. Have a variety of laryngoscope blades and endotracheal tube sizes immediately available.
    c. Use smaller endotracheal tubes than one would use in nonpregnant women (i.e., a cuffed 6.0- or 6.5-mm tube). Always keep a cuffed 5.5-mm tube available.
7. Develop a failed intubation protocol and review and practice it periodically (Fig. 26.1).
    a. All personnel administering general anesthesia to obstetric patients must know where the relevant emergency airway and ventilation equipment is stored.
    b. Practice the techniques involved during routine general anesthetics in nonpregnant patients at low risk of aspiration.
    c. Laryngeal mask airway
        i. Can be used to ventilate the patient if one cannot intubate and cannot ventilate the patient by mask. Remember, the laryngeal mask airway does not

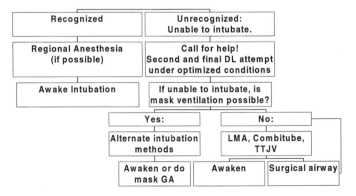

Fig. 26.1. Simplified version based on the American Society of Anesthesiologists Difficult Airway Algorithm. DL, direct laryngoscopy; LMA, laryngeal mask airway; TTJV, transtrachial jet ventilation; GA, general anesthesia.

protect against aspiration. Continue cricoid pressure until the aiway is secured or the patient is awake.
ii. Can be used as a conduit for endotracheal intubation.

Aspiration

1. Pulmonary aspiration has long been recognized as a clinical problem. One-third of obstetric anesthesia-related malpractice claims involve aspiration of gastric contents (versus 2% of the non-obstetric suits).[5]
2. Compared with nonpregnant women, parturients have
   a. Larger gastric volume.
   b. More frequent esophageal reflux.
   c. Elevated intragastric pressure.
   d. Low concentrations of plasma motilin (and thus low gastric motility) and high concentrations of plasma gastrin (and thus high gastric acid production).
3. Gastric emptying
   a. Slowed slightly by the pain of labor
   b. Unaffected by epidural local anesthetics
   c. Profoundly delayed by parenteral and somewhat delayed by epidural opioids
   d. Laboring women may have solid food in the stomach for up to 24 hours after a meal.

Pathophysiology

1. Tracheal instillation of 1 to 4 mL per kilogram of any liquid produces hypoxia, hypotension, and wheezing. The further clinical course depends on the nature of the liquid aspirated.
   a. Saline: Hypoxia and hypotension are mild and completely resolve in 30 minutes with no sequelae.
   b. Acid:
      i. Produces an immediate chemical pneumonitis, the severity of which depends on the liquid's pH and volume.
      ii. Instillation of liquid with a pH below a critical value (in humans, somewhere between 1.75 and 2.5) produces severe lung injury.
      iii. Acid aspiration produces moderate-to-severe hypoxemia and hypotension.
         (1) Transudation of plasma occurs rapidly, producing intravascular hypovolemia and pulmonary edema.
         (2) Adult respiratory distress syndrome then develops, with alveolar hyaline membrane formation.
         (3) If the patient survives the initial event, the lungs may heal without scarring. Patients with acid aspiration uncomplicated by bacterial pneumonia recover in 4 to 5 days.
   c. Food:
      i. Large chunks can obstruct airways.

ii.   Liquid food produces less hypoxemia, hypotension, and fluid transudation than acid but more hypercarbia and acidosis.
iii.   Food aspiration heals with granuloma formation.
d.   Bile-contaminated gastric juice is usually fatal in both patients and animals.

Diagnosis

1.   Frequently, the aspiration is observed. However, one should suspect aspiration with:
   a.   Hypoxia.
   b.   Pulmonary edema.
   c.   Bronchospasm.
   d.   Isolated laryngospasm.
   e.   Cough.
   f.   Apnea followed by tachypnea, tachycardia, or hypotension.
2.   Symptoms usually present within 2 hours.
3.   Roentgenograms show localized or diffuse patchy alveolar infiltrates or, in severe cases, opacification of large lung fields.
4.   Aspiration occurs most often in the right lower lobe (the straightest path from the trachea) or the most dependent lung area (frequently the right upper lobe in supine patients).
5.   The clinical course usually follows one of three paths:
   a.   Rapid deterioration and death (12%).
   b.   Rapid, sustained clinical improvement (62%).
   c.   Rapid improvement followed by decline due to bacterial pneumonia (26%).

Therapy

RECOMMENDED THERAPY

1.   Intubation and positive-pressure ventilation with positive end-expiratory pressure (PEEP). Because ventilation may need to be continued for several days, avoid excessively high oxygen concentrations to prevent additional damage from oxygen toxicity. Use just enough oxygen to maintain oxygen saturation above 90%.
2.   Careful intravascular fluid replacement. Plasma volume can decrease 35% within 2 hours of a massive acid aspiration. Institution of mechanical ventilation with PEEP can further depress cardiac output and arterial pressure. These patients frequently have obvious pulmonary edema yet are oliguric secondary to hypovolemia. Central venous or pulmonary artery pressure monitoring may be needed to guide therapy.
3.   Bronchoscopy ONLY if needed to clear food from the airway.
4.   Rigid maintenance of asepsis during tracheal tube care.

THERAPIES THAT ARE NOT RECOMMENDED

1.   Lavage: Bronchial transudation neutralizes bronchial fluid pH within 30 minutes of massive acid aspiration. Lavage spreads the noxious aspirate to previously uninvolved lung areas.
2.   Steroids: Once enthusiastically prescribed after aspiration, they are clinically ineffective.

3. Prophylactic antibiotics: These are also clinically ineffective and may increase late mortality by promoting the growth of resistant bacteria. Obtain bronchial fluid cultures regularly and use antibiotics to treat documented bacterial infection.

Prophylaxis
1. Pharmacologic agents frequently are used to decrease the volume and acidity of gastric contents.
2. Antacids: 30 mL 0.3 M sodium citrate (Bicitra) will raise gastric pH for 15 to 30 minutes. Do not use magnesium- and aluminum-containing antacids (i.e., Maalox) because aspiration of aluminum/magnesium hydroxide produces acute pulmonary pathology (as severe as that produced by acid instillation), which evolves into chronic granulomatous bronchopneumonitis and heals with extensive scar formation.
3. Agents to raise the gastric pH: ranitidine, cimetidine, or omeprazole.
4. Metoclopramide
    a. Increases gastric motility (an effect that is blocked by opioids or atropine).
    b. Increases lower esophageal sphincter pressure.

Prevention
1. Avoid mask general anesthesia in parturients.
2. When general anesthesia is necessary, use a rapid-sequence anesthetic induction with cricoid pressure and insert a cuffed endotracheal tube. Unfortunately, now that obstetric patients receiving general anesthesia are routinely intubated, deaths from failed intubation are replacing deaths from aspiration.
3. No completely effective measures exist to prevent aspiration or failed intubation in parturients. A major contributing factor is that awake intubations in parturients, as currently performed, usually are so uncomfortable and time consuming that the technique is rarely seriously considered. Can new awake intubation techniques improve this situation?

REFERENCES
1. Rout CC, Rocke DA, Levin J, Gouws E, Reddy D. A reevaluation of the role of crystalloid preload in the prevention of hypotension associated with spinal anesthesia for elective cesarean section. *Anesthesiology* 1993;79:262.
2. Riley ET, Cohen SE, Rubenstein AJ, Flanagan B. Prevention of hypotension after spinal anesthesia for cesarean section: six percent hetastarch versus lactated Ringer's solution. *Anesth Analg* 1995;81:838.
3. Norris MC, Fogel ST, Dalman H, Borrenpohl S, Hoppe W, Riley A. Labor epidural analgesia without an intravascular "test dose." *Anesthesiology* 1998;88:1495.
4. Norris MC, Ferrenbach D, Dalman H, et al. Does epinephrine improve the diagnostic accuracy of aspiration during labor epidural analgesia? *Anesth Analg* 1999;88:1073.
5. Chadwick HS, Posner K, Caplan RA, Ward RJ, Cheney FW. A comparison of obstetric and nonobstetric anesthesia malpractice claims. *Anesthesiology* 1991;74:242.

Anesthesia and the Compromised Fetus

Few situations in anesthesia are as anxiety provoking as sudden fetal compromise requiring emergent delivery. Yet, more often than not, a vigorous neonate is delivered after an emergency cesarean section, mocking the frantic efforts of those trying to rescue it from a hostile *in utero* environment. There are several reasons for this phenomenon:

1. Limited ability to directly assess fetal status.
2. Lack of clearly defined criteria to determine at what point "fetal distress" will result in permanent neurologic injury or death.
3. Once "fetal distress" is suspected, many feel that only immediate operative delivery meets the standard of care expected of a reasonably prudent physician.

DEFINITION

1. *Fetal distress* is an imprecise, poorly defined term, which is applied indiscriminately to a variety of intrapartum events and fetal conditions:
   a. Abnormal or "nonreassuring" fetal heart rate patterns.
   b. Intrauterine growth restriction.
   c. Oligohydramnios.
   d. Meconium-stained amniotic fluid.
   e. Newborns born with low Apgar scores or umbilical cord blood pH.
2. None of these conditions carries much, if any, prognostic significance. The majority of fetuses with these diagnoses are vigorous at birth and have no adverse long-term sequelae.
3. Perinatal asphyxia can cause neonatal injury.
   a. Asphyxia occurs when there is an interruption of fetal oxygen supply or respiratory gas exchange.
   b. Asphyxia leads to fetal hypoxemia and hypercarbia. Prolonged hypoxemia deprives fetal tissues of oxygen (hypoxia) and leads to anaerobic glycolysis, lactic acid production, and metabolic acidosis.
   c. However, all fetuses are born hypoxemic, with a mixed respiratory and metabolic acidosis, and are, in a sense, "asphyxiated." Only severe, prolonged asphyxia is thought to be of consequence.
4. The challenge, then, is to apply the term *fetal distress* only to "persistent fetal asphyxia that, if not corrected or circumvented, will result in permanent neurologic damage or death."[1]

PHYSIOLOGIC RESPONSE TO ASPHYXIA

1. Decreased fetal breathing and body movement in an effort to decrease oxygen consumption.

2. Redistribution of blood from splanchnic and peripheral vascular beds toward the brain, heart, adrenal glands, and placenta.
3. In response to asphyxia, fetal oxygen consumption decreases by 50%, mostly from metabolic changes in underperfused vascular beds. Anaerobic glycolysis in these areas gradually produces a metabolic acidosis.
4. Severe, prolonged hypoxemia impairs myocardial contractility, decreases cardiac output, and leads to intense vasoconstriction and hypoperfusion of all vascular beds. Both metabolic and respiratory acidosis ensue, with irreversible organ damage, hypotension, bradycardia, and, eventually, fetal death.

CAUSES OF FETAL DISTRESS

1. Most often, fetal deterioration follows a continuum as a chronically compromised or stressed fetus is further deprived of nutritional blood flow and becomes hypoxemic and distressed.
2. The exact cause of fetal distress is seldom known with certainty, but can be categorized as originating from the mother, her uterus, the placenta, the umbilical cord, or the fetus.
   a. Fetal perfusion and oxygen delivery depend primarily on uterine blood flow, which varies directly with maternal arterial perfusion pressure. Hypotension, from decreased maternal cardiac output due to aortocaval compression, sympathetic blockade, or hypovolemia, directly lowers placental perfusion. Chronic maternal vascular diseases, such as hypertension, diabetes, or systemic lupus erythematosus, produce uterine vascular insufficiency. Oxygen delivery to the fetus may be inadequate, with severe maternal anemia or hypoxemia despite the preservation of adequate uterine blood flow. Although uterine blood vessels are dilated maximally at term, α-adrenergic stimulation from endogenous or exogenous catecholamines will cause intense vasoconstriction.
   b. Uterine contractions transiently decrease intervillous blood flow in proportion to their duration, intensity, and frequency.
   c. Umbilical cord occlusion can dramatically reduce blood flow to the fetus. The risk of umbilical cord compression is enhanced by the presence of oligohydramnios and also can depend on maternal position. Other conditions that predispose to sudden umbilical cord occlusion from umbilical cord prolapse include multiple gestation after the birth of the first baby and nonvertex fetal presentations with rupture of membranes.
   d. Conditions that interfere with oxygen delivery within the fetal circulation, such as fetal anemia or arrhythmias, may result in acute fetal distress.

Diagnosis

1. The effects of moderate, transient hypoxemia are reversible and of little consequence.

**Table 27.1. Diagnostic modalities used
to detect fetal distress**

Antepartum
  Nonstress test
  Contraction stress test
  Biophysical profile
    Fetal breathing movement
    Gross body movement
    Fetal tone
    Amniotic fluid volume
    Fetal heart rate analysis
  Doppler ultrasound
    Umbilical blood flow velocity
Intrapartum
  Continuous electronic fetal heart rate monitor
  Intermittent auscultation of fetal heart rate
  Fetal pulse oximetry
  Fetal scalp capillary blood pH
Postpartum
  Apgar scores
  Umbilical cord blood gas analysis
  Neurobehavioral testing

2. It is more important to detect inadequate perfusion that, if not corrected, will cause irreversible fetal damage. Detection must be followed by timely intervention to either restore fetal oxygen delivery or remove the fetus from the hostile intrauterine environment.
3. Presently, there are no clinically useful diagnostic tests that allow us to specifically detect insufficient fetal oxygen delivery. Instead, we rely on modalities that indirectly measure fetal status (Table 27.1).

Antepartum

1. The biophysical profile
   a. Evaluates the five discrete biophysical variables listed in Table 27.1.
   b. The presence of a normal parameter is awarded two points, whereas the absence of that parameter is scored as zero.
      i. The compromised fetus will attempt to conserve oxygen by suspending diaphragmatic and limb movement.
      ii. Oligohydramnios may indicate poor fetal renal perfusion and is defined by an amniotic fluid index (AFI) less than or equal to 5.
      iii. The final component of the biophysical profile consists of a nonstress test using external fetal heart rate monitoring.
   c. A biophysical profile less than 6 is a sensitive, specific, and highly predictive indicator of acidotic umbilical cord blood.

2. Doppler ultrasound measurement of fetal umbilical artery blood flow velocity waveforms reflects placental vascular resistance. Umbilical artery Doppler velocimetry may help predict poor perinatal outcome and confirm the presence of fetal compromise during labor.

Intrapartum

FETAL HEART RATE

1. Electronic fetal heart rate analysis remains the principal intrapartum diagnostic modality used to detect fetal compromise.
2. Observation of the baseline heart rate, variability, and periodic changes in heart rate associated with uterine contractions provides an indirect assessment of fetal status.
3. Because these parameters are under the direct control of the central nervous system (CNS), a normal fetal heart rate tracing is thought to represent an intact axis between the CNS and cardiovascular system. Asphyxia interferes with this axis and produces characteristic changes in the fetal heart rate tracing as the fetus moves through a continuum of decompensation (Table 27.2).
   a. At first, a neurologically intact fetus will develop a tachycardia in an attempt to increase cardiac output and oxygen delivery in response to asphyxia.
   b. With progressive hypoxemia and acidosis, the fetus attempts to divert blood flow to the brain, heart, and adrenal glands through intense vasoconstriction to other vascular beds. A dramatic increase in systemic vascular resistance and reflex bradycardia or deceleration of the fetal heart rate ensues.
   c. Fetal heart rate decelerations are mediated by chemoreceptor and baroreceptor stimulation of the vagus nerve and can be categorized as early, variable, or late according to their timing in relation to the onset of a uterine contraction.

Table 27.2.   Fetal heart rate characteristics

	Baseline Heart Rate (beats/min)	Variability (beats/min)	Periodic Changes
Normal	120–160	3–25	Accelerations Early decelerations
Fetal stress	Tachycardia	>3–5	Variable decelerations Late decelerations (moderate to severe)
Fetal distress	Bradycardia	ABSENT, unresponsive to stimuli	Variable decelerations Late decelerations (moderate to severe)

      i. Early decelerations are a benign vagal response to fetal head compression and do not indicate asphyxia.

     ii. Variable decelerations represent umbilical cord compression and often occur whenever amniotic fluid volume is decreased. Repetitive or prolonged umbilical cord compression can lead to progressive fetal asphyxia and acidosis, manifested by persistent fetal bradycardia.

    iii. Late decelerations are associated with more serious fetal hypoxemia from uteroplacental insufficiency. They are characterized by smooth, uniform, U-shaped decelerations that produce a delayed, but mirror, image of the uterine contraction. The latency between the onset of the contraction and the beginning of the deceleration shortens as fetal hypoxemia worsens.

d. Beat-to-beat variability of the fetal heart rate

      i. The most important parameter in predicting fetal hypoxemia

     ii. It represents the constant push-pull effect of the sympathetic and parasympathetic nervous systems exerted on the fetal heart and indicates an intact axis between the central nervous and cardiovascular systems.

    iii. It may be diminished or absent with fetal sleep cycles, hypoglycemia, and maternally administered narcotics and sedatives. Loss of variability caused by these conditions usually is reversed by fetal scalp or vibroacoustic stimulation.

    iv. Persistent, irreversible loss of beat-to-beat variability, devoid of accelerations or decelerations in the fetal heart rate tracing, correlates well with umbilical artery acidemia at birth, and should alert the clinician to the development of true fetal distress requiring immediate delivery.

4. Electronic fetal heart rate monitoring (EFM), when used correctly, can increase the chance of detecting the rare event of fetal distress. It is clear, however, that EFM has several limitations (Table 27.3).

a. Specific fetal heart rate abnormalities do correlate with subsequent neurologic damage (cerebral palsy).

      i. Multiple late decelerations and decreased beat-to-beat variability are associated with an increased risk of cerebral palsy.[2]

     ii. However, children who develop cerebral palsy represent only 0.19% of the fetuses displaying such findings. Thus, 99.8% of fetuses with multiple late decelerations and decreased beat-to-beat variability do not develop cerebral palsy. Assuming 10% of electronically monitored labors show these fetal heart rate patterns, there will be 516 unnecessary interventions performed for each child "saved" from cerebral palsy.

Table 27.3.   Limitations of electronic fetal heart rate monitoring

1. Interpretation is subjective.
2. It uses only one physiologic variable (fetal heart rate) to assess fetal status.
3. False-positive diagnosis of fetal asphyxia is high.
4. False-positive tracings cause a high incidence of unnecessary operative interventions.
5. It indicates the same short- or long-term neurologic outcome as auscultation of fetal heart tones.

---

       b. Despite its introduction into clinical practice nearly 30 years ago, continuous EFM has done little to prevent intrapartum and neonatal death or to improve short- or long-term neurologic morbidity.

FETAL SCALP pH
1. The use of fetal scalp capillary blood sampling to confirm the diagnosis of fetal distress has been nearly abandoned in contemporary obstetric practice.
2. The fetal heart rate response to scalp blood sampling is probably a more useful indicator of fetal acidemia (pH less than 7.20). Significant fetal acidosis is unlikely if manual fetal scalp stimulation produces fetal heart rate acceleration or increased short-term variability.

MECONIUM
1. Its significance is poorly understood.
2. Meconium-stained amniotic fluid occurs in up to 44% of pregnancies and has never been consistently associated with abnormal fetal heart rate tracings, acidosis, or low Apgar scores.
3. Its presence should prompt the obstetrician to look for other signs of fetal compromise and to take special precautions at the time of delivery to prevent the potentially devastating consequences of meconium aspiration syndrome. Intrapartum amnioinfusion of saline can wash meconium from the amniotic cavity and decrease the incidence and severity of meconium aspiration.

Postpartum
1. The Apgar score
    a. Performed 1 and 5 minutes after birth
    b. A quick method of assessing the clinical status of the newborn
    c. Scores at 1 and 5 minutes correlate poorly with neurologic outcome.
    d. Persistently low scores (less than 3) at 10, 15, and 20 minutes identify infants at high risk of death or severe neurologic impairment.

e. Do not retrospectively attribute low Apgar scores to intrapartum asphyxia. The term *asphyxia* should be reserved for clinical situations in which all of the following are present:

   i. Profound metabolic or mixed acidemia (pH less than 7) on an umbilical cord arterial blood sample.

   ii. An Apgar score of 0 to 3 for longer than 5 minutes.

   iii. Neonatal neurologic manifestations (seizures, coma, hypotonia).

   iv. Multisystem organ dysfunction (cardiovascular, gastrointestinal, hematologic, pulmonary, or renal).[3]

2. Acidosis, identified by umbilical cord blood gas analysis, correlates poorly with neonatal status and subsequent neurologic development.

   a. Most neonates with an umbilical artery pH less than 7.20 are vigorous at birth and show no adverse short- or long-term sequelae.

   b. The frequency of poor neurologic outcome rises only with umbilical artery pH less than 7.[4]

FETAL RESUSCITATION

1. Obstetric management of the stressed fetus must strike a delicate balance.

   a. Aggressive surgical intervention leads to frequent cesarean section, instrumental delivery, and maternal morbidity.

   b. Surgery performed too late may produce a damaged infant.

2. There are several noninvasive maneuvers that may improve fetal condition and avert or postpone the need for surgical intervention. Because the etiology of fetal distress often is multifactorial and seldom known with certainty, these measures should be implemented simultaneously with the hope that one or a combination will improve the fetal status.

Alter Maternal Position

1. This improves fetal blood flow by relieving both aortocaval and umbilical cord compression.

2. Aortocaval compression

   a. Impairs uterine blood flow by direct compression of the aorta and decreased venous return.

   b. Remember, maternal brachial artery blood pressure may be normal in the presence of aortic compression and decreased uterine blood flow.

3. Trendelenburg or knee–chest positions may relieve umbilical cord compression by the fetal presenting part.

Administer Maternal Oxygen

1. Maternal hyperoxia can increase oxygen delivery to the fetus if uterine hypoperfusion, umbilical cord compression, or uterine hypertonus do not impede blood flow.

2. Supplemental oxygen delivered by high-flow face mask increases maternal and fetal transcutaneous pO_2 in both normal and "high-risk" parturients in labor.

3. Although the absolute rise in umbilical venous pO_2 seems insignificant (from 28 to 47 mm Hg), it results in a dramatic increase in fetal oxygen saturation (from 65% to 87%), reflecting the steep slope of the fetal oxyhemoglobin dissociation hemoglobin curve at these pO_2 values.

Improve Maternal Circulation

1. Maternal hypotension decreases uterine artery blood flow and intervillous perfusion.
2. It is poorly tolerated by the compromised fetus and should be treated rapidly with dextrose-free crystalloid infusion and a vasopressor.

Decrease Uterine Tone

1. Because the blood vessels that perfuse the placenta traverse the myometrium, uterine contractions decrease placental perfusion in proportion to their frequency, intensity, and duration.
2. Even transient reductions in blood flow may cause acute decompensation in a fetus with limited placental reserve.
3. When nonreassuring fetal signs occur, immediately stop exogenous oxytocin.
4. Next, consider improving placental perfusion by using medications that acutely decrease uterine tone.
   a. Terbutaline 0.25 mg injected intravenously or subcutaneously significantly improves fetal heart rate tracings, fetal acid-base status, and neonatal outcome and should be routine practice when uterine hypertonus is suspected. Terbutaline is well tolerated by most parturients but may produce mild tachycardia, hypotension from systemic vasodilation, and, in diabetics, problems with glucose homeostasis.
   b. Nitroglycerin also can provide acute uterine relaxation. Intravenous or sublingual administration can rapidly produce transient uterine relaxation with little impact on maternal hemodynamics.

Consider Amnioinfusion

1. Widely used for the treatment of persistent variable decelerations, which are most likely due to umbilical cord compression
   a. Normal saline is infused transcervically through an intrauterine pressure catheter either in a set amount (250 to 500 mL) or by titration until variable decelerations resolve. The addition of this fluid to the uterine cavity seems to cushion and protect the umbilical cord from compression due to maternal position or uterine contractions.
   b. Amnioinfusion decreases the frequency and severity of variable decelerations in labor, leads to lower instrumental and cesarean delivery rates, and improves umbilical artery and venous blood gas values.
   c. Reported complications include umbilical cord prolapse, uterine overdistention, dehiscence of a prior low-trans-

verse cesarean section scar, fetal bradycardia, and one
report of amniotic fluid embolism.

2. In addition to treating persistent variable decelerations,
   amnioinfusion is used to dilute meconium and decreases the
   frequency and severity of meconium aspiration syndrome in
   the neonate.

ANESTHETIC MANAGEMENT: GENERAL PRINCIPLES

Anticipation

1. Acute fetal distress seldom arises without warning.
2. Routine preoperative evaluation can predict most emergency cesarean deliveries
   a. Preoperative assessment allows identification of risk
      factors for abdominal delivery (Table 27.4).
   b. Parturients with any of these risks can be encouraged
      to have an epidural catheter placed early in labor.
   c. Using epidural anesthesia for cesarean section can pre-
      vent many of the serious maternal complications asso-
      ciated with general anesthesia.

Communication

1. The obstetrician should obtain an antepartum anesthesia
   consultation when any factors are present that may increase
   the risks of either regional or general anesthesia:
   a. Intrinsic or induced coagulopathy.
   b. Prior back surgery with instrumentation.
   c. Severe scoliosis.
   d. Airway abnormality or history of difficult intubation.
   e. Malignant hyperthermia susceptibility.
2. A preoperative consultation allows advance discussion about
   the risks and benefits of the anesthetic plan and can allay
   much anxiety.
3. Open communication among obstetric, nursing, and anesthesia personnel throughout labor is essential. At the first
   sign of fetal deterioration, the anesthesiologist should be

**Table 27.4. Characteristics of parturients who seem likely
to require abdominal delivery**

Failure to progress in labor
Cephalopelvic disproportion
Nonengaged fetal head
Persistent occiput posterior head
Breech presentation
Abnormal fetal heart rate tracing
Need for fetal scalp pH analysis
Multiple gestation
Suspected intrauterine growth retardation
Vaginal birth after cesarean section
Preeclampsia

notified to allow preparations for provision of anesthesia for delivery. The earlier the anesthesiologist is notified, the less likely the parturient will be subjected to the risks of a rushed general anesthetic.

ANESTHESIA FOR VAGINAL DELIVERY

1. When antepartum surveillance suggests that the fetus is not thriving in the intrauterine environment, prompt delivery may be indicated.
2. Despite the possibility of fetal compromise, obstetricians often attempt to achieve either a spontaneous or instrumental vaginal delivery.
3. Most often, labor will be induced. Labor is stressful even to a normal fetus, and the compromised one, with marginal physiologic reserve, may decompensate.
4. Lumbar epidural analgesia, induced early in labor, may prevent a rushed general anesthetic should fetal distress arise and may improve uteroplacental perfusion, probably by reducing maternal circulating catecholamines.

Analgesia

1. Goal: a functioning epidural catheter that can be used at cesarean section, if needed
2. Choices: Both epidural analgesia or combined spinal–epidural (CSE) analgesia can be appropriate. Establish effective labor analgesia. Maintain pain relief with a continuous infusion of a dilute local anesthetic–opioid mixture.
3. Risks
   a. Fetal heart rate changes
      i. Clinically significant fetal heart rate changes follow induction of labor analgesia in 2% to 20% of cases.
      ii. The frequency of clinically significant fetal heart rate changes is the same with either epidural or CSE anesthesia.
      iii. Most are due to uterine hypertonus or rapid progression of labor.
      iv. Emergency cesarean section is rarely required.
   b. Misplaced epidural catheters
      i. The precise location of catheters inserted with the CSE technique may not be determined for some time. (Intrathecal analgesia makes it difficult and unnecessary to "test" the epidural catheter.)
      ii. Epidural catheters also fail.
      iii. In experienced hands, both techniques are very reliable ways to place a catheter into the epidural space.[5]
   c. Catheter failure
      i. Even previously functioning epidural catheters will occasionally fail at cesarean section (5% to 8% of catheters).
      ii. Failure is more likely if the catheter has required multiple interventions during labor.[6]

Choice of Local Anesthetic

1. Subtle neonatal neurobehavioral changes have been reported in association with all local anesthetics. These effects are short lived and correlate better with the route of delivery than with the drug used.
2. Theoretically, 2-chloroprocaine should be the local anesthetic of choice in the presence of fetal compromise.
    a. It is hydrolyzed rapidly by maternal plasma cholinesterase to an inactive metabolite.
    b. Fetal acid-base status does not affect its placental transfer.
    c. The maternal and neonatal *in vitro* half-lives of 2-chloroprocaine are 21 and 43 seconds, respectively.
    d. However, 2-chloroprocaine possesses several undesirable characteristics that make its use for continuous lumbar epidural analgesia impractical:
        i.   A short duration.
        ii. Profound motor blockade.
        iii. Antagonism of neuraxial opioids.
3. In practice, dilute concentrations of bupivacaine or ropivacaine safely produce excellent maternal analgesia with minimal motor blockade.
4. Operative vaginal delivery
    a. Use the existing epidural catheter to provide dense perineal anesthesia and pelvic relaxation.
    b. Rapid onset and minimal fetal transfer make 3% 2-chloroprocaine an ideal local anesthetic in this setting.
    c. Give 10 to 15 mL of pH-adjusted solution and rapidly treat any maternal hypotension that may occur.

Epinephrine

1. Epinephrine-containing local anesthetics can exaggerate the hypotensive response to epidural anesthesia from β_2-mediated vasodilation.
2. Unintentional intravascular injection of epinephrine may produce uterine artery vasoconstriction from a direct α-agonist effect and can precipitate acute fetal distress.
3. Epidural injection of epinephrine-containing local anesthetics in patients with underlying uteroplacental insufficiency increases placental vascular resistance. These patients seem more sensitive to the α-agonist, rather than β-agonist, effect of epinephrine.

Epidural Opioids

1. Provide excellent labor analgesia in combination with dilute local anesthetics.
2. Systemic opioids can decrease fetal heart rate beat-to-beat variability.
3. Epidural injection of 50 to 75 µg of fentanyl lacks effect on fetal heart rate patterns. Epidural fentanyl does not cause neonatal depression, as measured by Apgar scores and respiratory rates, immediately after delivery.
4. Even with a potentially compromised fetus, fentanyl 2 to 3 µg per milliliter or sufentanil 0.3 to 0.5 µg per milliliter can

safely be added to dilute local anesthetic solutions for epidural labor analgesia.

ANESTHESIA FOR CESAREAN SECTION

1. To formulate a plan to provide anesthesia for cesarean delivery of a compromised fetus:
   a. Determine the urgency of the situation.
   b. Assess both maternal and fetal status.
2. In this situation, clear, unequivocal communication between obstetrician and anesthesiologist is essential.
3. Any nonscheduled cesarean section is categorized as "emergency." These emergencies then are subdivided further into stable, urgent, or "stat."
   a. A stable emergency cesarean section is performed in the absence of acute decompensation.
      i. Usually these patients are not in labor.
      ii. Any anesthetic is appropriate.
   b. Cesarean section becomes urgent when labor is in progress and either the fetus begins to manifest signs of distress, or there are maternal contraindications to vaginal delivery.
      i. These deliveries should probably take place within 30 minutes.
      ii. Appropriate anesthetics:
         (1) Epidural anesthesia (if the patient has a functioning epidural catheter)
         (2) Spinal anesthesia
         (3) General anesthesia
   c. "Stat" cesarean section is performed when either the mother or fetus faces life-threatening danger if delivery is not performed immediately.
      i. Examples include severe maternal hemorrhage, uterine rupture, or prolonged fetal bradycardia with loss of short-term variability.
      ii. Appropriate anesthetics:
         (1) General anesthesia
         (2) In some cases:
            (a) Epidural anesthesia (if the patient has a functioning epidural catheter)
            (b) Spinal anesthesia
4. When notified of the need for an emergency cesarean section, learn the indication for the operation and proceed accordingly. Open communication and a good working relationship between anesthesiologist and obstetrician are essential.

Regional Versus General Anesthesia

1. In the absence of severe maternal hemorrhage or coagulopathy, most agree that regional anesthesia is appropriate for stable or urgent emergency cesarean sections.
2. Considerable controversy surrounds the choice of anesthetic for a "stat" cesarean section.
   a. Maternal outcome: The risk of maternal death associated with general anesthesia is 16.7 times greater than that associated with regional anesthesia.[7]

b. Neonatal outcome: For emergency cesarean section, rapid extension of an existing epidural block or induction of spinal anesthesia is associated with neonatal outcomes comparable to those after rapid-sequence induction of general anesthesia. Infants whose mothers receive regional anesthesia may have better Apgar scores and less need for ventilatory assistance immediately following delivery.

Preoperative Preparation

1. Have at all times, in the operating room:
   a. An anesthesia machine with breathing circuit and face mask.
   b. Suction apparatus.
   c. Equipment for endotracheal intubation, including a short-handled laryngoscope with an assortment of blades; cuffed, styletted endotracheal tubes ranging in size from 5.5 to 7.0 mm; No. 3 and No. 4 laryngeal mask airways; and a device for emergency cricothyrotomy and transtracheal ventilation.
   d. Medications for induction and maintenance of general anesthesia.
2. The patient must have at least one functioning large-bore intravenous catheter.
3. For premedication, give 30 mL of a nonparticulate antacid on the way to the operating room.
4. Continue to give supplemental oxygen while preparing to induce anesthesia and until delivery.
5. Monitor fetal heart rate as continuously as possible until delivery. Often, the fetal heart rate abnormality will resolve or improve, and cesarean delivery can either be averted or performed in a calm and organized fashion. An electronic scalp electrode can be used to monitor fetal heart rate until delivery, at which time it can be disconnected under the surgical drapes or delivered through the uterine incision. Continuous assessment of fetal status can influence the speed at which surgical dissection is performed. It also can provide invaluable information should airway difficulties arise during induction of general anesthesia.

Epidural Anesthesia

1. Unless maternal hemorrhage is present, an existing epidural catheter is the technique of choice for emergency cesarean section.
2. The choice of local anesthetic depends on the urgency of the situation.
   a. Bupivacaine at 0.5% for stable and urgent cesarean sections, when the patient must be ready for incision within 30 minutes:
      i. Bupivacaine provides dense sensory anesthesia without epinephrine.
      ii. The gradual onset of bupivacaine helps maintain maternal hemodynamic stability.
      iii. Epidural opioids can be added for intraoperative anesthesia and to provide postoperative analgesia.

      b. Lidocaine (2%) with 1 : 200,000 epinephrine or 3% 2-chloroprocaine for "stat" cesarean section. Adding NaHCO$_3$ to either solution will speed onset.

2. Technique: Begin dosing the epidural catheter before the patient is transported to the operating room.

      a. Aspirate.

      b. Inject 15 mL in 3- to 5-mL increments while checking maternal vital signs.

      c. Watch for overt signs of intravascular injection.

      d. After transport to the operating room, inject an additional 5 to 10 mL of local anesthetic as needed.

      e. If the surgeons are ready to proceed before the patient is fully anesthetized, supplemental local anesthetic can be injected in the incision, or small doses (10 mg) of intravenous ketamine can be given to the parturient. Continuous reassurance that discomfort will be brief can improve patient cooperation.

Spinal Anesthesia

1. In patients without a functioning epidural catheter, spinal anesthesia can avoid the need for general anesthesia at emergency cesarean section.

2. Hypotension

      a. Hypotension is more common during spinal than epidural anesthesia, but labor markedly decreases its frequency and severity.

      b. Because intravenous fluids do not reliably prevent maternal hypotension, do not delay induction of anesthesia to prehydrate the patient.

      c. Treat with additional intravenous fluids and ephedrine or phenylephrine.

3. Spinal anesthesia for "stat" cesarean section

      a. Prepare the spinal tray in advance.

      b. Continuously monitor fetal heart rate.

      c. The most experienced anesthesiologist present should make this attempt.

      d. Know when to quit: If there is ongoing fetal distress and the block is not in place by the time the surgeons are ready, abandon the technique and prepare for general anesthesia.

General Anesthesia

1. Indications

      a. Maternal request

      b. Maternal coagulopathy

      c. Maternal hemodynamic instability

      d. Severe fetal heart rate abnormality in a patient lacking adequate regional anesthesia

Preoxygenation

Four maximal inspirations of 100% oxygen provide equivalent preoxygenation to that of 3 minutes of tidal breathing.

Induction Agents

1. The ideal induction agent in the presence of fetal distress has not been determined.

2. Thiopental 4 to 5 mg per kilogram
   a. Although it crosses the placenta rapidly, thiopental rarely is associated with significant neonatal depression due to at least three factors:
      i. Rapid redistribution in the maternal circulation.
      ii. Dilution in the fetal inferior vena cava.
      iii. Uptake by the fetal liver.
   b. There is no reason to either expedite or delay delivery after anesthetic induction to limit the depressant effects of thiopental.
3. Methohexital, despite its shorter half-life, offers no advantage over thiopental.
4. Ketamine 1 to 2 mg per kilogram
   a. Rapidly crosses the placenta, and peak fetal blood concentrations develop in 1 to 2 minutes.
   b. Maternal mean arterial blood pressure and uterine blood flow are well preserved because of ketamine's sympathomimetic effects. Therefore, ketamine is a good choice for the hypotensive mother.
   c. Add a benzodiazepine after delivery to decrease the risk of emergence delirium.
5. Etomidate 0.3 mg per kilogram produces fewer maternal hemodynamic changes than does thiopental.
6. Propofol has been evaluated as an induction agent for elective cesarean delivery and lacks adverse effects on umbilical blood gas values or neurobehavioral scores.

Maintenance of Anesthesia

1. Maximize fetal blood flow and oxygen delivery.
2. Maintain left uterine displacement.
3. Give intravenous fluids and vasopressors to ensure stable maternal hemodynamics.
4. Give 100% oxygen until delivery of the asphyxiated fetus to maximize fetal pO_2 and oxygen saturation.
5. Use enough volatile agent to provide sufficient depth of anesthesia to limit maternal catecholamine release (especially when nitrous oxide is omitted). There is no evidence to suggest that one inhalational agent is superior to another when fetal compromise is present. Brief exposure (less than 15 minutes) to moderate concentrations of inhalational agents does not significantly alter fetal compensatory responses to asphyxia.
6. Maintain normocarbia.
   a. A low maternal p_aCO_2 shifts the oxyhemoglobin dissociation curve to the left, impairing oxygen delivery to the fetus.
   b. Aggressive positive-pressure ventilation decreases venous return, impairing maternal cardiac output and uterine perfusion.
   c. Likewise, avoid maternal respiratory acidosis because it leads to fetal carbon dioxide retention and worsening acid-base status.

Local Anesthetic Infiltration

1. It can provide anesthesia for emergency cesarean delivery in the following rare circumstances:

      a. Failed or contraindicated regional anesthesia with an inaccessible airway.
      b. Failed intubation with ongoing fetal distress.
      c. Supplementation of an inadequate regional blockade.
      d. Unavailability of trained personnel to administer other types of anesthesia.

2. It involves the infiltration of sequential layers in the midline of the lower abdominal wall with a large volume of dilute local anesthetic (typically 200 to 300 mL of 0.5% lidocaine with epinephrine).

3. Advantages: requires little technical skill, has a rapid onset, preserves maternal airway reflexes, and produces minimal fetal effects.

4. Disadvantages: incomplete and often unsatisfactory anesthesia, potential local anesthetic toxicity.

REFERENCES

1. Parer JT, Livingston EG. What is fetal distress? *Am J Obstet Gynecol* 1990;162:1421.

2. Nelson KB, Dambrosia JM, Ting TY, Grether JK. Uncertain value of electronic fetal monitoring in predicting cerebral palsy. *N Engl J Med* 1996;334:613.

3. American College of Obstetricians and Gynecologists. ACOG committee opinion no. 174: use and abuse of the Apgar score. *Int J Gynecol Obstet* 1996;54:303.

4. Helwig JT, Parer JT, Kilpatrick SJ, Laros RK. Umbilical cord blood acid–base state: what is normal? *Am J Obstet Gynecol* 1996; 174:1807.

5. Norris MC. Are CSE catheters reliable? *Int J Obstet Anesth* 1999 (*in press*).

6. Riley ET, Papasin J. Converting labor epidural analgesia to surgical anesthesia: success rates and factors associated with failure. *Anesthesiology* 1999:A41.

7. Hawkins JL, Koonin LM, Palmer SK, Gibbs CP. Anesthesia-related deaths during obstetric delivery in the United States, 1979–1990. *Anesthesiology* 1997;86:277.

The Premature Fetus

1. Definitions
   a. *Preterm birth:* delivery before 37 weeks' completed gestation.
   b. *Low birth weight:* birth weight less than 2,500 g regardless of gestational age, and very low birth weight less than 1,500 g.
2. Importance
   a. In developed nations, 5% to 10% of births are preterm.
   b. Approximately 45% of the preterm births follow preterm labor with intact membranes, 30% are a consequence of premature rupture of membranes (PROM), and 25% are secondary to fetal or maternal concerns.
   c. Prematurity is, by far, the leading cause of perinatal morbidity and mortality, accounting for between 69% and 83% of neonatal deaths.
3. Outcome
   a. Nearly 100% of nonanomalous neonates born after 32 weeks' gestation survive.
   b. When birth takes place in a tertiary care center, survival rates are 90% after 29 to 30 weeks' gestation and near 50% for 26 weeks' gestation.
   c. Prolonging an otherwise uncomplicated pregnancy by as little as 1 week will significantly decrease neonatal morbidity.
      i. The risk of respiratory distress syndrome (RDS) declines progressively until 36 weeks.
      ii. The frequency of patent ductus arteriosus and necrotizing enterocolitis fall steadily until 32 weeks.
      iii. High-grade intraventricular hemorrhage (IVH) diminishes rapidly after 27 weeks and is almost absent after 32 weeks.
      iv. The most dramatic decrease in risk occurs between weeks 25 and 26, when survival increases from 15% to 55%.

OBSTETRIC CONSIDERATIONS IN PREMATURITY
Fetal Evaluation

1. *In utero* fetal evaluation is the key to the rational therapy of premature labor (PML).
2. Estimating gestational age
   a. Pregnancy dates based on the last menstrual period often are in error.
   b. If performed early, ultrasound can accurately time pregnancy within 1 week.
3. Determining fetal lung maturity
   a. Analyzing amniotic fluid for components of lung surfactant.
   b. Lecithin–sphingomyelin (L/S) ratio increases rapidly between weeks 33 and 35 and is usually greater than 2 at 35 weeks' gestation. In the nondiabetic parturient,

an L/S ratio greater than 2 is associated with minimal risk of RDS. A value less than 1.5 predicts a significant risk of RDS.

c. Other amniotic fluid determinations of lung maturity include both phosphatidylinositol and phosphatidylglycerol. The presence of phosphatidylglycerol in amniotic fluid virtually assures the absence of RDS.

Tocolytic Drugs

β-Agonists

1. The advent of β-agonist tocolytic drugs has not had a significant impact on the frequency of preterm birth in Western Europe or North America.

2. Despite these pessimistic findings, tocolysis remains a cornerstone in the treatment of PML.

3. β-Agonists have multiple maternal physiologic effects. Side effects, many of which have important anesthetic implications, are common.

CARDIAC EFFECTS

1. Tachycardia, with maternal heart rates above 100 beats per minute, often is associated with tremor, palpitations, and chest pain. Heart rate may exceed 140 beats per minute with concurrent administration of drugs such as epinephrine, ephedrine, anticholinergics, or intravenous bolus oxytocin.

2. Arrhythmias, including premature ventricular contractions, premature nodal contractions, and atrial fibrillation have been reported.

3. Angina pectoris and associated electrocardiographic changes
    a. Pain usually resolves when the β-agonist is stopped.
    b. Enzyme changes suggesting myocardial damage are extremely rare.
    c. Electrocardiographic changes suggestive of myocardial ischemia (including ST depression and T-wave inversion) occur in over 70% of asymptomatic parturients receiving β-agonists.

PULMONARY EDEMA

1. Reported incidence is as high as 5%. Cases have involved oral, subcutaneous, and continuous intravenous infusions. The risk does not correlate with the total dose of drug or the rate of infusion. It usually occurs 24 to 72 hours after initial intravenous administration.

2. The etiology of the pulmonary edema is unclear. Possibilities include:
    a. Fluid overload.
    b. Catecholamine-related myocardial necrosis.
    c. Cardiac failure secondary to tachycardia.
    d. Downregulation of cardiac β-receptors due to chronic β-agonist exposure.

3. Neither pulmonary artery catheterization nor echocardiography has demonstrated left ventricular failure in these women. Increased pulmonary vascular permeability and decreased colloid oncotic pressure could cause noncardiogenic pulmonary edema.

4. Risk factors
   a. Simultaneous administration of glucocorticoids does *not* add to the incidence of pulmonary edema.
   b. Fluid overload
   c. Coexisting disease (including intraamniotic infection)
   d. Multiple gestation
5. Treatment
   a. Stop the β-agonist.
   b. Avoid other tocolytic drugs.
   c. Restrict fluids.
   d. Give supplemental oxygen.
   e. Effect diuresis with furosemide.
   f. Rarely, intubation, positive-pressure ventilation, and the addition of positive end-expiratory pressure will be needed.

METABOLIC EFFECTS

1. Hypokalemia
   a. Potassium concentrations of less then 3 mEq per liter are common.
   b. These are due to an influx of potassium into cells because of hyperinsulinemia and direct β_2-adrenoreceptor stimulation.
   c. Maternal hyperventilation can exaggerate hypokalemia.
   d. As total body potassium remains normal, replacement seldom is necessary.
2. Hyperglycemia and lactic acidosis
   a. Caused by β_2-receptor stimulation
   b. In nondiabetic parturients, blood glucose concentrations of 140 to 160 mg per deciliter are common.
   c. Lactic acidosis can develop.
   d. Maternal hyperglycemia can predispose to reactive neonatal hypoglycemia.
3. Maternal fluid retention is common and may decrease hemoglobin and plasma oncotic pressure.
4. Other side effects of the β-agonist tocolytics include nausea, vomiting, insomnia, tremors, and headache.

ANESTHETIC IMPLICATIONS

1. β-Agonist tocolytics produce vasodilatation and increase cardiac output, which may alter the maternal hemodynamic response to epidural or spinal anesthesia.
   a. The well-hydrated, vasodilated condition of these women may blunt regional anesthesia-induced hypotension.
   b. Maternal tachycardia may limit the efficacy of ephedrine. Instead, use phenylephrine 50 to 100 µg to treat significant maternal hypotension.
2. Aggressive intravenous hydration may predispose to fluid overload. Incorrectly interpreting tachycardia as a sign of hypovolemia also may result in excessive intravenous fluid infusion.
3. β-Agonists may interfere with pulmonary hypoxic vasoconstriction; this effect may increase the risk of maternal hypoxemia, particularly under general anesthesia.

4. The magnitude of the interaction between β-agonist and anesthetic drugs depends on the time between the cessation of tocolytic therapy and the induction of anesthesia. If time allows, a delay of 2 or more hours may be prudent.

MAGNESIUM SULFATE

1. An effective intravenous tocolytic in doses similar to, or slightly higher than, those used for seizure prophylaxis in women with preeclampsia/eclampsia.
2. Maternal side effects
   a. Vasodilation, flushing, headache, drowsiness, blurred vision, nausea, constipation, chest pain, and postural hypotension.
   b. Magnesium acts at the myoneural junction to cause generalized skeletal muscle weakness and loss of deep-tendon reflexes. Overdose can cause respiratory depression and arrest and even cardiac arrest.
   c. Pulmonary edema, usually related to excessive intravenous fluids, also may occur.
3. Magnesium is excreted primarily through the kidneys; use with caution in patients with compromised renal function.
4. Deep-tendon reflexes are monitored during magnesium therapy. Loss of the patellar reflex occurs with a serum magnesium concentration of about 10 mg per deciliter. Respiratory depression occurs at concentrations of 12 to 15 mg per deciliter.
5. Advantages versus β-agonist therapy
   a. No hyperglycemia and metabolic lactic acidosis
   b. No inotropic and chronotropic effects
   c. No hypokalemia or metabolic stimulation

ANESTHETIC IMPLICATIONS

1. Magnesium and muscle relaxants
   a. Magnesium causes muscle weakness by itself and potentiates the nondepolarizing muscle relaxants, including rocuronium and mivacurium.
   b. Reversal of a nonpolarizing muscle relaxant with an anticholinesterase may be incomplete, as magnesium decreases the sensitivity of the motor end-plate to applied acetylcholine, reducing the efficacy of the reversal process.
   c. Magnesium attenuates succinylcholine fasciculations.
   d. Magnesium does not change the onset or duration of a single dose of succinylcholine.
   e. Magnesium does increase the duration of paralysis after repeated doses or continuous infusion of succinylcholine.
   f. Use a peripheral nerve stimulator.
2. Hemodynamic interactions
   a. Magnesium produces vasodilation, but without increasing cardiac output. Postural hypotension is more likely with magnesium than with β-agonist drugs.
   b. Sympathetic block during regional anesthesia should be unlikely to produce hypotension.
   c. Marked preblock hydration usually is not necessary and may predispose to pulmonary edema.

FETAL EFFECTS

1. Fetal blood concentration of magnesium parallels that in maternal blood.
2. Fetal heart rate variability may decrease.
3. At birth, infants exposed to magnesium may exhibit decreased muscle tone, ileus, and poor feeding.
4. Neonatal weakness and respiratory or cardiac depression are unlikely in the absence of maternal toxicity. If severe neonatal depression is seen in the absence of maternal magnesium toxicity, look for other causes.

Prostaglandin Synthesis Inhibitors

1. Indomethacin is an effective tocolytic.
2. Maternal side effects essentially are those of aspirin: nausea, vomiting, gastritis, peptic ulcer formation, and masking of fever.
3. Like aspirin, it can be associated with thrombocytopenia, and it interferes with platelet function. A large body of data suggests that neuraxial block is safe for patients receiving aspirin or other prostaglandin synthetase inhibitors.
4. Fetal effects
   a. To limit the risk of premature closure of the ductus arteriosus, indomethacin usually is not used after 34 weeks' gestation.
   b. Indomethacin also may be associated with reversible oligohydramnios.
5. With its lack of maternal cardiovascular and other side effects and its ease of administration, indomethacin often is used for initial tocolysis in early pregnancy. It also is a useful adjunct for the temporary control of PML in the mother being transported to a tertiary care center for delivery.

Calcium Channel Blockers

1. Calcium channel blockers, particularly nifedipine, are potent relaxants of uterine muscle and are effective tocolytics.
2. They are potent vasodilators and often incite flushing and hypotension. Other bothersome side effects include nausea and headache.
3. Hemodynamic effects
   a. Magnitude is less than with ritodrine.
   b. Maternal heart rate increases, whereas diastolic blood pressure and mean arterial pressure decrease.
4. Changes in glucose homeostasis accompany nifedipine.
5. Nifedipine does not significantly affect serum electrolytes.

DRUG INTERACTIONS

1. Preterm labor is a syndrome of disorders resulting from a variety of causes associated with different cellular mechanisms. Therefore, it is not unreasonable to use different tocolytic agents concurrently in the hope that their synergistic interactions may halt more resistant cases of preterm labor.
2. The simultaneous use of various tocolytics increases the risk of adverse drug interaction and potentiates some side effects.
   a. Magnesium potentiates the hypotensive effect of nifedipine.

    b. This combination depresses left ventricular contractility more than does either drug alone.
    c. Nifedipine potentiates the effects of magnesium on neuromuscular function.

ANESTHETIC IMPLICATIONS
1. Both inhalation and local anesthetics have calcium channel–blocking properties.
2. In animals, calcium channel blockers potentiate the hemodynamic effects of inhalational anesthetics. If uterine relaxation is indicated, this drug interaction could have significant consequence.
3. Calcium channel blockers also may potentiate the direct myocardial effects of local anesthetics.

Atosiban
1. Atosiban (1-deamino 2D-tyr-(OE+)-4-thr-8-orn-vasotocin/oxytocin Mpa, D-Tyr(E+)^2, Thr^4, Orn^8-oxytocin) is a competitive inhibitor of oxytocin.
2. Preliminary studies in animals and humans report a reduction in preterm uterine activity versus placebo.
3. Atosiban has relatively few side effects.

ANESTHETIC MANAGEMENT
OF THE PRETERM DELIVERY
1. Try to ensure the most atraumatic delivery possible. A sudden, uncontrolled delivery will markedly increase the likelihood of intracerebral hemorrhage, the leading cause of morbidity and mortality in preterm birth. For vaginal delivery, the obstetrician will strive for an atraumatic delivery over a wide episiotomy.
2. The premature infant tolerates asphyxia poorly. The asphyxiated preterm infant has an increased incidence of RDS, IVH, and necrotizing enterocolitis. Before vaginal or cesarean delivery, position the mother carefully to prevent aortocaval compression. Give supplemental oxygen. Avoid or aggressively treat maternal hypotension.
3. Morbidities
    a. Maternal hemorrhage from placenta previa, placenta abruption, or uterine atony from attempted tocolysis can complicate preterm birth.
    b. The incidence of breech presentation in the preterm birth is 25% compared with 3% at term.
    c. Maternal, fetal, and neonatal infection are more common.
    d. Fetal heart rate changes and prolapsed cord are more common.
    e. Expeditious cesarean section is indicated if the fetus shows any evidence of compromise.
    f. Delivery in a tertiary care center, instead of transfer after birth, lowers neonatal mortality.
4. Finally, the anesthetist involved in a preterm birth must be acquainted with the side effects of the various tocolytics and their interactions with anesthetic techniques and drugs.

Vaginal Delivery

1. Lumbar epidural analgesia, initiated early and maintained throughout labor and delivery, is the most desirable option for labor analgesia. Keep the following principles in mind:

   a. The preterm infant may require urgent or emergent cesarean delivery. Make certain that the epidural catheter is functioning properly. Local anesthetics should produce bilateral sensory change that ascends with additional drug.

   b. Minimize the effects of epidural block on the duration of labor. Try not to hinder maternal expulsive efforts during the second stage of labor.

   c. Avoid precipitous delivery. Most obstetricians like to control delivery of the fetal head by gradually stretching the perineum, cutting a generous episiotomy, or using forceps. These maneuvers require good perineal anesthesia.

   d. Avoid drugs that can cause fetal compromise.

Patient Positioning

1. If the fetal head is low in the vagina or labor is progressing rapidly, identify the epidural or subarachnoid space with the mother on her side to prevent fetal head compression.

2. To reduce the risk of cord prolapse, apply this same precaution if the membranes have ruptured but the fetal head remains out of the pelvis or the fetal breech is presenting.

Anesthetic Technique

1. Either epidural or combined spinal–epidural analgesia may be appropriate.

2. Prehydration usually is not needed in these well-hydrated vasodilated women.

3. Induction

   a. Epidural analgesia

      i. Inject drug in small increments via the epidural catheter. (Although drug injection through the epidural needle may provide good initial analgesia, a poorly functioning epidural catheter will be useless for subsequent cesarean section.)

      ii. Fifteen to 20 mL 0.125% bupivacaine with 1 to 2 µg per milliliter fentanyl or 0.5 µg per milliliter sufentanil provides effective analgesia for most women.

      iii. Look for sensory change 15 to 20 minutes after drug injection. The goal is complete perineal analgesia and a sensory level to at least T8.

   b. Combined spinal–epidural anesthesia

      i. May be the preferred technique if labor is progressing rapidly and delivery is imminent.

      ii. Bupivacaine 0.25 mg plus fentanyl 6 µg or sufentanil 1.2 µg will rapidly provide labor analgesia and perineal anesthesia.

4. Maintenance

   a. Use an infusion of bupivacaine (0.083% to 0.125%) with fentanyl 2 mg per milliliter or sufentanil 0.4 µg per milliliter at 10 to 12 mL per hour to maintain the block.

      b. Monitor the block closely to ensure adequate perineal analgesia without excessive maternal motor blockade.
   5. The amount of opioids used in these recommended techniques is very small and appears to be well tolerated by the fetus. The addition of opioid allows a reduction in the concentration of local anesthetic, allowing preservation of some motor power.
   6. Give the mother supplemental oxygen throughout labor.

Alternatives to Neuraxial Analgesia
   1. Analgesia for delivery can be provided by inhalation of 50% nitrous oxide in oxygen.
   2. Intravenous ketamine 0.25 mg per kilogram (15 to 25 mg) can provide additional analgesia and often will allow the use of forceps or vacuum. Should prolonged analgesia be required, additional 0.125- to 0.25-mg per kilogram doses may be used. Avoid loss of consciousness and limit the total dose of ketamine to 1 mg per kilogram before delivery.
   3. Pudendal block or at least local infiltration of the perineum helps decrease the need for systemic analgesics for episiotomy and application of forceps or vacuum.
   4. General anesthesia rarely is required for vaginal delivery. Should it be, take precautions to prevent pulmonary aspiration. Avoid inducing anesthesia when the patient is in the lithotomy position. Use a rapid-sequence induction with cricoid pressure.

Cesarean Section
   1. Cesarean section accounts for a large proportion of preterm deliveries.
   2. Although it offers little or no long-term benefit, the use of cesarean section for very low birth weight infants (500 to 1,499 g) has been rising steadily over the past 15 years.

Choice of Anesthetic
   1. Although the choice of anesthetic can influence neonatal condition at birth, there is little evidence of any long-lasting effects.
   2. Infants delivered using epidural anesthesia usually have higher 1- and 5-minute Apgar scores than those delivered using general anesthesia.
   3. Other factors related to low 1-minute Apgar scores include malpresentation, primiparity, low gestational age, and the presence of RDS and IVH.

Regional Anesthesia
   1. In a breech or nonvertex presentation, doing the block with the patient sitting may predispose to prolapse of the umbilical cord.
   2. A mother who has just received a β-agonist tocolytic should have cautious and minimal intravenous prehydration.
   3. An F_iO_2 of 0.5 from the time of block until delivery may significantly improve neonatal oxygenation at birth.
   4. Preterm patients may develop less extensive sensory blockade after spinal anesthesia than will term patients.[1]

Uterine Relaxation

1. Some have avoided regional anesthesia for cesarean delivery of the preterm infant because general anesthesia provides uterine relaxation if needed for delivery of the head.
2. Intravenous nitroglycerin 50 to 200 µg also is a potent uterine relaxant and is useful in obstetric emergencies such as cesarean delivery of the breech fetus.
3. When preparing for the delivery of a preterm (breech) fetus, consider giving nitroglycerin 100 µg to induce acute uterine relaxation (approximately 30-second onset) to assist in the delivery of the fetal head.

General Anesthesia

1. Occasionally, general anesthesia may be indicated.
2. Do not reduce the dose of the induction agents with proper technique, fetal drug exposure is minimal and not associated with perinatal asphyxia.
3. Use appropriate maneuvers to prevent aspiration.
4. Maintain left uterine displacement until delivery.
5. Use a high F_iO_2 (0.5 to 1.0) until delivery.
6. Maintain anesthesia and help assure maternal amnesia with 0.75 minimum alveolar concentration of a potent inhaled agent.
7. Nitrous oxide can be used if desired.
8. Monitor end-tidal carbon dioxide and avoid maternal hyperventilation.
9. Remember the potential interactions among tocolytics (particularly the β-agonists, magnesium, and the calcium channel blockers), anesthetics, and muscle relaxants.

Management of the Cocaine-addicted or Intoxicated Patient in Preterm Labor

1. Cocaine use during pregnancy is associated with an increased incidence of preterm labor.
2. In addition to causing preterm labor, cocaine use in pregnancy is associated with an increased incidence of intrauterine growth retardation, abruptio placenta, and pregnancy-induced hypertension.

Anesthetic Considerations

1. Long-term intravenous drug users can present problems of venous access. Peripheral veins may be thrombosed. Some addicts even self-inject via their internal jugular veins.
2. These patients are at high risk for infection with human immunodeficiency virus and hepatitis.
3. Acute cocaine intoxication can precipitate a placental abruption and, at the same time, produce sympathetic stimulation that masks the degree of blood loss and volume depletion.
   a. As the drug effect wanes, catecholamine concentrations decrease and blood pressure may fall.
   b. Vasopressors may be needed to restore maternal blood pressure and placental perfusion.
      i. Ephedrine may prove ineffective in cocaine users with depleted catecholamine reserves.

ii.   Phenylephrine, a direct-acting agent, is a good alternative.

4.   Consider the cardiovascular effects of cocaine when choosing anesthetics. Use caution with agents with arrhythmogenic potential in the face of elevated catecholamines (halothane), those that may further stimulate the cardiovascular system (ketamine), or myocardial depressants (high-dose thiopental or volatile agents).

5.   The neonate
   a.   In addition to the usual problems of prematurity, these neonates may be at a higher risk for periventricular hemorrhage, IVH, and necrotizing enterocolitis.
   b.   The fetus acutely intoxicated with cocaine has arterial hypoxemia and increases in blood pressure, heart rate, and cerebral blood flow.
   c.   Neonates of cocaine-addicted mothers have a higher incidence of genitourinary tract and central nervous system defects.

CARE OF THE PREMATURE NEWBORN

1.   Ideally, care of the premature newborn begins well before delivery. When time permits, mother and fetus should be transferred intact to a center that can appropriately care for these infants.

2.   Maternal antenatal corticosteroids can hasten fetal lung maturity and decrease the incidence of RDS.
   a.   They can significantly reduce the risks of RDS, IVH, and death before 28 days of life in very low birth weight infants.
   b.   The most significant risk appears to be a slight increase in the incidence of neonatal sepsis.
   c.   Maternal risks
      i.   Demargination of neutrophils increases the white blood cell count.
      ii.   Corticosteroids interfere with glucose homeostasis and increase blood glucose concentration.
      iii.   Immunosuppression may increase the risk of maternal infection.

3.   Other therapies that appear to improve neonatal outcome include surfactant for the prevention and treatment of RDS and inhaled nitric oxide in the treatment of persistent pulmonary hypertension of the newborn, congenital diaphragmatic hernia, and some forms of congenital heart disease.

4.   At birth, initial care focuses primarily on the prevention or treatment of asphyxia and maintenance of body temperature.
   a.   Although hyperoxia is a concern because of the fear of retrolental fibroplasia and pulmonary oxygen toxicity, one should not hesitate to give a high F_iO_2 (greater than 0.9) if there are signs of hypoxemia.
   b.   If intubation is required, either continuous positive airway pressure or positive end-expiratory pressure will be necessary to maintain alveolar expansion.
   c.   The premature infant has a large surface area for a small mass and rapidly loses heat. Hypothermia can

lead to acidosis and increased oxygen consumption. It should be prevented by immediately drying the neonate at birth and placing the child under radiant heat in an area protected from drafts.

REFERENCE

1. James KS, McGrady E, Patrick A. Combined spinal-extradural anaesthesia for preterm and term caesarean section: is there a difference in local anaesthetic requirements? *Br J Anaesth* 1997;78:498.

Fetal Malpresentation and Multiple Birth

FETAL MALPRESENTATION

Definitions

1. Fetal lie
   a. The relative position of the long axis of the fetus to that of the uterus
   b. It can be longitudinal, transverse, or oblique.
   c. Vertex and breech presentations are longitudinal lies.
   d. A spontaneous vaginal delivery can be achieved only from a longitudinal lie.
2. Presentation: the body part that overlies the pelvic inlet
3. The attitude of the fetal head is either flexion, with the chin approaching the chest, or extension, with the occiput approaching the back.
4. Vertex presentation with flexion is associated with the greatest chance of a safe vaginal delivery, because the fetal skull first enters the pelvis with the smallest presenting diameter.
5. Any variation in presentation or attitude is referred to as a malpresentation, and the prognosis for a safe vaginal delivery is decreased.

Breech Presentation

1. The prevalence of breech presentation decreases with increasing gestational age.
   a. At the end of the second trimester: 25%
   b. At 30 weeks: 17%
   c. At term: 3.5%
2. There are four types of breech presentation, defined by the presenting part and whether the hips and knees are flexed or extended.
   a. Complete: The buttocks present with both hips and knees flexed.
   b. Frank: The buttocks present with the hips flexed and the knees extended. This is the most common breech presentation.
   c. Footling: One or both feet present, and both hip(s) and knee(s) are in extension.
   d. Kneeling: One or both knees present. The hips are extended and the knees are flexed.

Fetal Risks

1. Neonatal mortality with breech presentation is about five times greater than that of term cephalic presentations.
2. Hazards
   a. Umbilical cord accidents, including cord compression and prolapse
      i. Complete breech: 5%
      ii. Footling breech: 10%

iii. Frank breech: 0.5%, the same as with a vertex presentation
   b. Nuchal arm
   c. Difficulty with the aftercoming head
3. These problems can cause either fetal mechanical injury, such as skull fracture or brachial plexus damage, or anoxic brain injury and death.

Maternal Risks
1. Increased morbidity is related to the use of cesarean section for delivery.
2. Vaginal breech delivery also increases maternal risk compared with vertex delivery.
   a. Intrauterine manipulation increases the risk of infection.
   b. Uterine relaxation increases the risk of uterine atony and hemorrhage.

External Cephalic Version
1. The fetus is turned from a breech to a cephalic presentation by using manipulations through the abdominal wall.
2. Successful version will reduce the cesarean section rate for breech presentation.
3. Potential complications of version, although rare, include placental abruption, fetal–maternal hemorrhage, isoimmunization, preterm labor, uterine rupture, fetal distress and death, and maternal mortality.
4. Contraindications to external cephalic version include uterine anomalies, placenta previa, abruptio placenta, and non-reassuring signs of fetal well-being.

ANESTHETIC CONSIDERATIONS
1. The role of neuraxial anesthesia in external version is controversial.
2. Both epidural analgesia and intrathecal opioids improve maternal comfort.
3. Maternal analgesia also may improve chances of successful version.

Obstetric Management
1. Methods of vaginal breech delivery
   a. Spontaneous: The infant delivers without any obstetric manipulations.
   b. Partial extraction: The baby delivers without assistance up to the umbilicus, at which point the obstetrician assists with the delivery of the thorax and aftercoming head.
   c. Total extraction: The obstetrician assists in the delivery of the entire fetus, usually by applying traction to the legs or ankles. Except for the delivery of a second twin, total breech extraction is almost never performed.
2. Currently, the cesarean section rate for breech presentations is 80% to 100%. Although neonatal outcomes may be better after cesarean delivery for breech presentation, maternal morbidity is several times higher.

Anesthetic Considerations

Vaginal Delivery

NEURAXIAL ANALGESIA

1. Because of concerns about prolonged labor and impaired maternal expulsive efforts, breech presentation was once a relative contraindication to epidural analgesia.
2. Today, epidural block is the preferred method of labor analgesia in breech presentation.
3. Effect of epidural analgesia on outcome
   a. Slightly longer second stage of labor
   b. Studies often report fewer breech extractions and better neonatal condition associated with epidural analgesia.

UTERINE RELAXATION

1. During vaginal delivery, immediate uterine relaxation may become necessary to assist in delivery of the aftercoming head.
2. General endotracheal anesthesia with a potent inhalation agent will provide uterine relaxation.
3. Intravenous (IV) nitroglycerin 50 to 100 μg, or sublingual aerosol spray of nitroglycerin 0.8 mg, also will reliably produce uterine relaxation and may preclude the need for general anesthesia.

Cesarean Section

1. Anesthetic considerations for cesarean section of a breech baby are similar to those with vertex presentations.
2. Entrapment of the aftercoming head also may occur during cesarean section because of uterine muscle contraction. Relaxation of the uterus can be accomplished with an inhalational agent or nitroglycerin, as described for vaginal deliveries.

Malpresentation of the Vertex

1. During labor, the smallest anteroposterior (AP) diameter of the fetal skull normally presents into the pelvis.
   a. Before labor, the fetal head is partially flexed, with the occipitofrontal diameter presenting.
   b. As contractions intensify, and the fetus begins to descend into the pelvis, resistance to descent normally forces further flexion of the fetal head, and the chin approaches the chest.
   c. Malpresentation of the vertex occurs when the fetal head is not flexed (i.e., military attitude [no flexion or extension], or brow [partial extension], or face [complete extension] present).
   d. In these situations, a larger AP diameter of the fetal head presents to the maternal pelvis than in the flexed attitude.
2. The most common factor associated with malpresentation of the vertex is cephalopelvic disproportion, due to large fetal size or a contracted maternal pelvis.
   a. Cephalopelvic disproportion may inhibit flexion and rotation of the fetal head.

  b. Other associated risk factors include multiparity, neoplasms, uterine anomalies, abnormal placental size and location, and polyhydramnios.
3. Face presentation
  a. The prognosis for vaginal delivery of a face presentation depends on the direction of the mentum (chin).
  b. Seventy percent to 80% may deliver vaginally in a mentum anterior (chin-up) position.
  c. In the mentum posterior position, the prognosis for vaginal delivery is poor, unless the fetus is very small: The fetal brow is compressed against the maternal symphysis, preventing flexion of the fetal head.
4. Brow presentation
  a. Vaginal delivery is unlikely.
  b. The largest fetal AP diameter presents into the pelvis.
  c. Only with a small, preterm infant will vaginal delivery possibly occur.
  d. Fortunately, most brow presentations spontaneously convert to either a face or occiput presentation.
5. Persistent occiput posterior presentation (OPP)
  a. Occurs in about 5% of births.
  b. Because a larger cephalic diameter presents into the pelvis, the frequency of cephalopelvic disproportion is greater, the length of the first and second stages of labor is longer, and the frequency of operative deliveries higher.
  c. Babies who present as OPP also have an increased incidence of abnormal fetal heart rate tracings.
6. Epidural labor analgesia is associated with malpresentation.
  a. Techniques that use more concentrated local anesthetics are associated with more frequent persistent OPP.
  b. Abnormal labor, associated with malpresentation may be more painful and increase the likelihood that the patient will request epidural analgesia.

Shoulder Presentation

1. Uncommon; about 1 in 350 pregnancies
2. Etiologic factors include placenta previa, prematurity, multiparity, and cephalopelvic disproportion.
3. The risk of cord prolapse is increased.
4. Shoulder presentation requires cesarean section for safe delivery of the fetus.
  a. Difficulty with delivery of the fetus may occur, leading to prolonged uterine incision-to-delivery time.
  b. Uterine contraction may interfere with delivery, and uterine relaxation may be needed.

Compound Presentation

1. Both an extremity and the vertex or breech enter the pelvis.
2. Complicates about 1 in 1,000 deliveries
3. Most commonly associated with prematurity
4. Women with a baby who has a compound presentation may be allowed to labor, as the presenting extremity will usually withdraw as labor progresses.

MULTIPLE BIRTH

Incidence

1. Twin gestation occurs in approximately 1 in 90 pregnancies.
   a. Monozygotic (MZ): occurring from a single ovum
      i. Frequency is fairly constant throughout the world: approximately 4 per 1,000 deliveries.
   b. Dizygotic (DZ): occurring from two ova
      i. Account for two-thirds of twins
      ii. Are as genetically distinct as any other siblings born to the same parents
2. Triplets in 1 in 9,800 pregnancies
3. Quadruplets in 1 in 70,000 pregnancies
4. Risk factors
   a. Older maternal age
   b. Higher parity
   c. Ovulation-inducing drugs

Placentation

1. All DZ twins develop a dichorionic diamniotic placenta.
2. The timing of cell division in MZ twins affects the subsequent placental-membrane relation and has a significant impact on morbidity and mortality (Table 29.1).
3. Monoamniotic placentation occurs in fewer than 2% of all twin pregnancies but also carries a high perinatal mortality rate because of the potential for cord entanglement.

Fetal Risks

1. Twin delivery increases perinatal mortality six-to eightfold.
2. Morbidity and mortality are primarily related to prematurity. Twins deliver prematurely because the uterus does not remain quiescent until term or because of insufficient uterine blood flow.
3. Even when a twin pregnancy reaches term, the infants are still at increased risk. Twins weighing more than 2,500 g are at greater risk of death than are singleton controls.

Table 29.1. Monozygotic twins

Chorion	Amnion	Time to Division (d)	Rate (%)	Perinatal Mortality (%)	Comments
Dichorionic	Diamniotic	0–3	30	9	Two single placentas or one fused placenta
Monochorionic	Diamniotic	4–8	68	25	Cord anomalies, placental vascular nomalies
Monochorionic	Monoamniotic	>8	5	>50	High mortality from cord intertwining

4. Triplet gestation also has a higher perinatal mortality rate than that of singletons, but not greater than that of twins.
5. Second twin
   a. Greater risk of morbidity and mortality than for the first
   b. After delivery of the first twin, partial separation of the placenta, reduced uterine size, and clamping of the first umbilical cord can reduce intervillous blood flow and oxygenation to the second twin.
   c. Continuous fetal heart rate monitoring and improved neonatal resuscitation may improve outcome for the second twin.
6. Specific risks
   a. Malpresentation due to growth retardation and poly-hydramnios
   b. The risk of umbilical cord prolapse increases with the greater incidence of malpresentations, malpositions, and premature rupture of membranes.
   c. Interlocking of twins occurs when the vertex of a breech-presenting first twin interlocks with the chin of a vertex-presenting second twin.
      i. If not recognized before labor, the traction normally applied during delivery of the breech can result in fetal death.
      ii. The incidence of interlocking twins is about 1 in 1,000 twin deliveries and carries a high mortality rate.
7. Conjoined twins
   a. Incidence: one in 50,000 deliveries
   b. Etiology is unknown; it is probably due to incomplete division of an MZ embryo at approximately 13 to 15 days after ovulation.

Maternal Risks

Physiologic Risks
1. The physiologic changes that occur during a singleton gestation are exaggerated in mothers with multiple gestations.
   a. Twinning is associated with an additional 15% increase in cardiac output.
   b. Increased incidence of supine hypotensive syndrome: a 32-week uterus of a twin gestation is as big as a term uterus containing a single fetus and gets progressively larger.
   c. Anemia occurs 2.4 times more often.
2. Hypoxemia, especially in the supine position, also is more likely to occur in the woman with a twin gestation. This risk is related to:
   a. A decrease in the functional residual capacity from displacement of the diaphragm by the enlarged uterus.
   b. An increase in the closing volume.
   c. An increase in oxygen consumption.

Obstetric Risks
1. Pregnancy-induced hypertension and preeclampsia are five times more common during a twin gestation.

2. Uterine atony, because of the overdistended uterus, increases the risk of postpartum hemorrhage by two- to threefold.
3. There also is an increased incidence of antepartum hemorrhage from abruptio placentae and placenta previa.
4. Premature rupture of membranes occurs more frequently in multiple gestations, leading to preterm labor.
   a. Tocolytic agents, especially the β-adrenergic agonists and magnesium sulfate, are associated with maternal pulmonary edema.
   b. Premature rupture of membranes coupled with fetal malpresentation and malposition leads to an increased incidence of umbilical cord prolapse.
   c. Malpresentation also leads to a greater frequency of cesarean section and postoperative infection.
5. Polyhydramnios occurs in approximately 12% of multiple gestations and may herald congenital abnormalities (gastrointestinal and central nervous system).

Obstetric Management
1. Early diagnosis reduces perinatal morbidity and mortality.
2. Prophylactic bed rest, cervical cerclage, prophylactic tocolysis, and early elective hospitalization have been suggested to prevent premature labor and its sequelae. It is difficult, however, to document any benefit from these measures.

Intrapartum Management
1. Obstetricians often elect to deliver twins by cesarean section. However, outside of a few widely accepted indications (Table 29.2), few data support this choice.
2. The intrapartum management of a twin gestation is determined by the intrauterine position of the twins.
   a. Twin A vertex, twin B vertex (42.5%): Most experts agree that vaginal delivery should be attempted.
   b. Twin A vertex, twin B nonvertex (38.4%)
      i. Management is controversial.
      ii. After delivery of the first baby, a decision must be made as how to deliver the second.

Table 29.2.   Factors favoring cesarean delivery with multiple gestation

Malpresentation of twin A
Discordancy, with twin B larger than twin A
Intrauterine death of one fetus
Twin–twin transfusion
Congenital deformities
Decreased uteroplacental reserve (positive oxytocin challenge test or nonreactive nonstress test)
Fetal cardiac decelerations of either twin
Prematurity
Three or more fetuses

(1) Options include external cephalic version, internal podalic version and total breech extraction, or cesarean section.

(2) Internal podalic version and breech delivery yields the same neonatal outcome as vertex delivery.

c. Twin A nonvertex (19.1%): Cesarean delivery is usually chosen.

3. The time between delivery of the first and second twin is not critical as long as fetal heart rate tracing of twin B remains reactive.

4. Although triplets can be safely delivered vaginally, most recommend cesarean section for women with three (or more) fetuses.

Anesthetic Management

Labor and Delivery

1. All women with multiple gestations should have a large-bore IV placed on admission to the labor floor and early consultation with an anesthesiologist.

2. Discuss the delivery plan with the obstetricians early in labor.

3. Because of the increased risk of emergency cesarean section, encourage early placement of an epidural catheter.

a. Epidural analgesia is associated with good neonatal outcome after vaginal delivery of twins.

b. Effective epidural analgesia reduces the need for maternal general anesthesia for intrauterine manipulation or cesarean section of the second twin.

Suggested Technique

1. Epidural or combined spinal-epidural analgesia with a dilute opioid-local anesthetic solution will provide excellent analgesia for labor.

2. At delivery, there are several goals:

a. The patient should be able to push effectively, especially before delivery of twin A.

b. The patient should be have adequate analgesia for possible intrauterine manipulation of twin B.

c. The patient may require an emergency cesarean section for twin B.

d. Suggested technique

   i. Continue dilute opioid-local anesthetic infusion throughout the second stage of labor.

   ii. When delivery of twin A is imminent, inject increments of 0.5% bupivacaine to a total of 10 mL. This additional local anesthetic should provide analgesia for intrauterine manipulation of twin B and establish the beginnings of surgical anesthesia if cesarean section is needed.

   iii. If cesarean section is indicated, inject additional 0.5% bupivacaine or 2% lidocaine with 1:200,000 epinephrine and $NaHCO_3$.

e. If uterine relaxation is needed for intrauterine manipulation of twin B, use either nitroglycerin 50 to 100 μg IV, or general anesthesia with a high concentration of a volatile anesthetic agent.

  f. After delivery, be prepared for uterine atony and postpartum hemorrhage. Uterine atony may require the use of oxytocin, methylergonovine, or 15-methyl prostaglandin $F_{2\alpha}$.

Cesarean Section

1. Twin gestation does not appear to increase the risk of hypotension or the spread of sensory block associated with spinal anesthesia.
2. Elective cesarean section: Any anesthetic is appropriate.
3. Cesarean section in labor
    a. If an epidural catheter was placed for labor and a cesarean section is necessary, use the catheter and extend the level of anesthesia with an appropriate local anesthetic.
    b. Use spinal anesthesia if the patient does not have a functioning epidural catheter.
    c. General anesthesia may be needed for some emergencies.
4. The anesthetic management of triplet and higher order pregnancies is similar to that previously described, except that all the concerns are magnified.
    a. These women may be at greater risk of hypotension associated with the rapid onset of spinal anesthesia.
    b. Combined spinal-epidural anesthesia, with a reduced dose of intrathecal local anesthetic, is a reasonable option.

Neonatal Resuscitation

At birth, numerous physiologic changes must occur as a fetus makes the transition to a neonate. Despite the complexity of this process, only 6% of newborns require life support in the delivery room. This percentage increases quickly among newborns who weigh less than 1,500 g. Hospital policies designating who answers calls for neonatal resuscitation may have important medicolegal consequences for the anesthesiologist.

NEONATAL ADAPTATIONS TO EXTRAUTERINE LIFE

1. Fetal physiology
   a. Pulmonary vascular resistance (PVR) is high, with 90% of right ventricular output shunting across the ductus arteriosus.
   b. Systemic vascular resistance (SVR) is low: 40% of cardiac output flows to the low-resistance placenta.
2. Vaginal delivery
   a. Compression of the infant's thorax expels fluid from the mouth and upper airways.
   b. With crying, the lungs fill with air, surfactant is released, and oxygenation is increased. These changes greatly decrease PVR.
   c. Simultaneously, clamping the umbilical cord removes the low-resistance placental bed from the circulation, increasing SVR.
   d. Within minutes, the right-to-left shunt across the foramen ovale and ductus arteriosus is substantially reduced.
3. Transient hypoxemia or acidosis is well tolerated by a normal newborn, and prompt intervention usually prevents any permanent sequelae.
4. Prolonged hypoxemia or acidosis impedes the transition from fetal to neonatal physiology.
   a. The fetus/neonate initially responds by redistributing blood flow to the heart, brain, and adrenal glands.
   b. Tissue oxygen extraction increases.
   c. Eventually, myocardial contractility and cardiac output decrease.
   d. Hypoxemia and acidosis promote patency of the ductus arteriosus, counteracting the normal neonatal increase in pulmonary artery blood flow.
   e. Ventilatory drive is reduced by both indirect central nervous system and direct diaphragmatic depression.
   f. The net result is a neonate with persistent pulmonary hypertension and little or no ventilatory drive. These babies require prompt intervention.

PREPARATION

1. Equipment and medications should be conveniently located, checked frequently for proper functioning and expiration date, and replenished immediately after use (Table 30.1).
2. At least one person skilled in newborn resuscitation should attend every delivery (i.e., certified to provide neonatal

Table 30.1.   Equipment and medications for neonatal resuscitation

Suction equipment	**Bag and mask equipment**
Bulb syringe	Neonatal resuscitation bag with
Mechanical suction	pressure-relief valve
Suction catheters, 5F–10F	Face masks: newborn and
Meconium aspirator	premature sizes
	Oral airways
Intubation equipment	Oxygen with flowmeter and tubing
Laryngoscope	
Straight blades, 0 and 1	**Medications**
Extra bulbs and batteries	Epinephrine 1:10,000
Endotracheal tubes,	Naloxone hydrochloride, 0.4 mg/mL
2.5–4.0 mm	or 1.0 mg/mL
Stylet	Volume expander
Scissors and gloves	Sodium bicarbonate 4.2%
	(5 mEq/10 mL)
Miscellaneous	Dextrose 10%
Radiant warmer	Sterile water and normal saline
Stethoscope	
ECG	
Adhesive tape	
Syringes and needles	
Alcohol sponges	
Umbilical artery catheterization tray	
Umbilical tape	
Umbilical catheters, 3.5F, 5F	
Three-way stopcocks	
Feeding tube, 5F	

advanced life support [NALS]). Additional personnel should be available if a high-risk delivery is anticipated.

3. Remember Guideline VII of the American Society of Anesthesiologists, *Guidelines for Regional Anesthesia in Obstetrics,* which states:

> Qualified personnel, other than the anesthesiologist attending the mother, should be immediately available to assume responsibility for resuscitation of the newborn. The primary responsibility of the anesthesiologist is to provide care to the mother. If the anesthesiologist is also requested to provide brief assistance in the care of the newborn, the benefit to the child must be compared to the risk to the mother.

ASSESSMENT OF RISK

1. With careful ante- and intrapartum fetal assessment, the need for neonatal resuscitation can be predicted in about 80% of cases.
2. Antepartum assessment includes evaluation for major fetal anomalies and identification of maternal factors that may influence fetal well-being (Table 30.2).

Table 30.2. Maternal and fetal factors associated with need for resuscitation

Maternal diabetes
Pregnancy-induced hypertension
Chronic hypertension
Previous Rh sensitization
Previous stillbirth
Bleeding in the second or third trimester
Maternal infection
Lack of prenatal care
Maternal substance abuse
Known fetal anomalies
Postterm gestation
Preterm gestation
Multiple gestation
Size–dates discrepancy
Polyhydramnios
Oligohydramnios
Maternal drug therapy: reserpine, lithium carbonate; magnesium, adrenergic blocking drugs

3. Intrapartum events often predict the need for neonatal resuscitation (Table 30.3). Intrapartum evaluation includes fetal heart rate (FHR) monitoring with, when indicated, fetal scalp or vibroacoustic stimulation, or fetal scalp-blood sampling for pH determination.

RESPONSE

Intrapartum

1. Identify and correct maternal factors that may impair oxygen delivery to the fetus.
   a. Maternal hypotension or decreased cardiac output from aortocaval compression, sympathectomy, hemorrhage, or cardiac disease
   b. Consider and, if appropriate, treat disease states that may interfere with maternal oxygenation, such as asthma, pneumonia, or pulmonary edema.
2. Uterine hyperstimulation, tetany, abruption, or rupture may interfere with blood flow to the fetus. If needed, stop oxytocin infusion or give a tocolytic agent to reduce uterine tone.
3. Consider umbilical cord prolapse if FHR changes are sudden, severe, and prolonged.

At Birth

1. The first step in neonatal resuscitation is to minimize heat loss (Fig. 30.1).
   a. Cold stress leads to hypoxemia, hypercarbia, and metabolic acidosis.
   b. These promote persistence of the fetal circulation and hinder resuscitation.

Table 30.3.   Intrapartum events associated with need for resuscitation

Cesarean delivery
Abnormal fetal presentation
Premature labor
Rupture of membranes >24 h
Chorioamnionitis
Precipitous labor
Prolonged labor >24 h
Prolonged second state >3–4 h
Nonreassuring fetal heart rate patterns
General anesthesia
Uterine tetany
Meconium-stained amniotic fluid
Prolapsed cord
Abruptio placentae
Uterine rupture
Difficult instrumental delivery
Maternal systemic narcotics within 4 h of delivery

   c. Within the first 20 seconds of life, the newborn should be dried, placed under a radiant warmer, and undergo suctioning of mouth and nose (tracheal suctioning if meconium is present).
2. Next (within 30 seconds of birth) assess neonatal respiration.
   a. If the infant is gasping or apneic, begin positive-pressure ventilation (PPV) at a rate of 40 to 60 breaths per minute with 100% oxygen.
   b. Peak inspiratory pressures of 30 to 40 cm water or higher are necessary for initial lung expansion.
3. The majority of infants requiring any resuscitation will respond to these first two steps.
4. Indications for endotracheal intubation include ineffective bag-and-mask ventilation, anticipated need for prolonged mechanical ventilation, or as a route for administration of medicine.
5. The third step is assessment of neonatal heart rate.
   a. Chest compressions are required in only 0.03% of deliveries.
   b. Neonatal cardiac arrest is generally the result of respiratory failure, producing hypoxemia and tissue acidosis.
   c. Chest compressions should be instituted at a rate of 120 per minute when, after 15 to 30 seconds of PPV, the

Fig. 30.1.   Overview of resuscitation in the delivery room. (Source: Reprinted from American Heart Association and American Academy of Pediatrics. *Textbook of neonatal resuscitation.* Dallas: American Heart Association, 1994, with permission.)

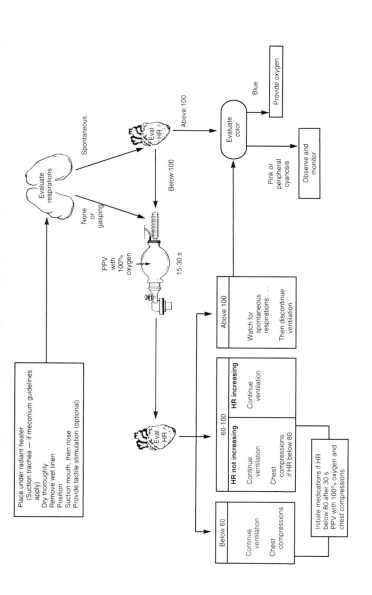

Place under radiant heater
(Suction trachea — if meconium guidelines
apply)
Dry thoroughly
Remove wet linen
Position
Suction mouth, then nose
Provide tactile stimulation (optional)

Evaluate respirations

Spontaneous

None or gasping

PPV with 100% oxygen

15-30 s

Eval HR

Above 100

Below 100

Evaluate color

Blue

Provide oxygen

Pink or peripheral cyanosis

Observe and monitor

Eval HR

Above 100

Watch for spontaneous respirations . . .
Then discontinue ventilation

60-100

HR not increasing

Continue ventilation

Chest compressions
if HR below 80

HR increasing

Continue ventilation

Below 60

Continue ventilation

Chest compressions

Initiate medications if HR below 80 after 30 s
PPV with 100% oxygen and chest compressions

Table 30-4. Medications, dosages, and routes of administration

Medication	Concentration to Administer	Preparation	Dosage/Route	Total Dose/Infant		Rate/Precautions
Epinephrine	1:10,000	1 mL	0.1–0.3 mL/kg IV or ET	**Weight**	**Total mL**	Give rapidly; may dilute with normal saline to 1–2 mL if giving ET
				1 kg	0.1–0.3 mL	
				2 kg	0.2–0.6 mL	
				3 kg	0.3–0.9 mL	
				4 kg	0.4–1.2 mL	
Volume expanders	Whole blood 5% Albumin-saline Normal saline Ringer's lactate	40 mL	10 mL/kg IV	**Weight**	**Total mL**	Give over 5–10 min
				1 kg	10 mL	
				2 kg	20 mL	
				3 kg	30 mL	
				4 kg	40 mL	

Medication	Concentration to Administer	Preparation	Dosage/Route	Weight	Total Dose	Total mL	Rate/Precautions
Sodium bicarbonate	0.5 mEq/mL (4.2% solution) IV	20 mL or two 10-mL prefilled syringes	2 mEq/kg	1 kg	2 mEq	4 mL	Give *slowly*, over at least 2 min Give only if infant is being effectively ventilated
				2 kg	4 mEq	8 mL	
				3 kg	6 mEq	12 mL	
				4 kg	8 mEq	16 mL	

				Weight	Total Dose	Total mL	
Naloxone hydrochloride	0.4 mg/mL	1 mL	0.1 mg/kg (0.25 mL/kg) IV, ET IM, SQ	1 kg	0.1 mg	0.25 mL	Give rapidly
				2 kg	0.2 mg	0.50 mL	IV, ET preferred
				3 kg	0.3 mg	0.75 mL	IM, SQ acceptable
				4 kg	0.4 mg	1.00 mL	
	1.0 mg/mL	1 mL	0.1 mL/kg (0.1 mL/kg) IV, ET IM, SQ	1 kg	0.1 mg	0.1 mL	
				2 kg	0.2 mg	0.2 mL	
				3 kg	0.3 mg	0.3 mL	
				4 kg	0.4 mg	0.4 mL	
				Weight	**Total μg/min**		
Dopamine	$6 \times$ Weight (kg) $\times$ Desired dose (μg/kg/min)		Begin at 5 μg/kg/min (may increase to 20 μg/kg/min if necessary) IV	1 kg	5–20 μg/min		Give as a continuous infusion using an infusion pump
	$\dfrac{}{\text{Desired fluid (mL/h)}}$			2 kg	10–40 μg/min		
	= mg of dopamine per 100 mL of solution			3 kg	15–60 μg/min		Monitor heart rate and blood pressure closely
				4 kg	20–80 μg/min		
							Seek consultation

IM, intramuscular; ET, endotracheal; IV, intravenous; SQ, subcutaneous.
Source: From American Heart Association and American Academy of Pediatrics. *Textbook of neonatal resuscitation.* Dallas: American Heart Association, 1994.

heart rate is below 60 or between 60 and 80 and not increasing. In most neonates with adequate ventilation, cardiac function normalizes quickly. Chest compressions should be stopped when heart rate is greater than 80.

6. These three steps should occur within the first minute of life. Survival is unlikely if the Apgar score is 0 at 10 minutes of age.
7. Medications
    a. Indicated if, after adequate ventilation with 100% oxygen and chest compressions for 30 seconds, heart rate remains below 80 beats per minute
    b. Medications, doses, and routes of administration are given in Table 30.4.
    c. Naloxone hydrochloride is indicated specifically for neonatal respiratory depression due to maternal opioid administration. It should not be given to a neonate exposed to long-term maternal opiates, as it can precipitate acute withdrawal.
    d. Sodium bicarbonate should be used only when ventilation is adequate (or respiratory acidosis will replace metabolic acidosis) and metabolic acidosis is documented or presumed, or all other measures have been unsuccessful.
    e. Routes of administration: umbilical vein, peripheral veins, or endotracheal instillation. While establishing intravenous access, both epinephrine and naloxone can be instilled into the trachea.

ANCILLARY ISSUES
Neonatal Hypoglycemia
1. Approximately 10% of healthy term neonates have transient hypoglycemia.
2. Other neonates at risk include those born of diabetic mothers or mothers who received a large amount of intravenous dextrose during labor.
3. Macrosomic, pre- or postmature neonates also are prone to hypoglycemia.
4. If the glucose concentration is fewer than 40 to 45 mg per deciliter, the neonate should be treated either with oral feedings (2 to 3 mL per kilogram D_{10} in water) or by intravenous infusion (8 mg per kilogram per minute).

Laryngeal Mask Airway
1. The size 1 laryngeal mask airway (LMA) can be used to resuscitate term newborns requiring PPV at birth. The LMA may be especially useful in the management of newborns with airway abnormalities (i.e., Pierre Robin syndrome).
2. Further studies are needed to assess the reliability of this technique of airway management in the neonate requiring resuscitation.

Pulse Oximeter Placement
1. The right-to-left shunt at the ductus arteriosus persists for some time after birth and may affect oxygen saturation readings obtained by pulse oximetry.

2. An oxygen saturation measurement obtained from the right hand is a better index of neonatal cerebral oxygenation than one from the lower extremities.

MEDICOLEGAL ASPECTS FOR THE OBSTETRIC ANESTHESIOLOGIST

1. Hospital policy should define who is responsible for the actual resuscitation and what procedures will be followed if additional personnel are needed.
2. Good Samaritan statutes prevent a person from being liable for negligent acts or omissions committed while voluntarily providing emergency care. The anesthesiologist lacks Good Samaritan immunity when having an employment duty to resuscitate the infant. However, if a duty to the infant does not exist before delivery, it is not suddenly created because the anesthesiologist is present and has a relationship with the mother.[1]
3. A compilation of obstetric anesthesia malpractice suits since 1985 found that 12 of 69 (17.4%) included neonatal resuscitation claims against anesthesia personnel. There was a payout to the plaintiff in ten of the 12 cases.[2]
4. An anesthesiologist expected to perform neonatal resuscitation must maintain a high level of skill in that area. Any obstetric anesthesiologist, even if not a designated resuscitator, should be capable of basic neonatal resuscitation steps that could be initiated in an unanticipated emergency while awaiting designated personnel.

ETHICAL ASPECTS FOR THE OBSTETRIC ANESTHESIOLOGIST

1. When faced with the need to resuscitate a very low birth weight infant (fewer than 750 g), a stillborn infant, or an infant with severe congenital anomalies that may preclude long-term survival, the obstetric health care team may have conflicting feelings about how to proceed.
2. Ideally, parents, neonatology and obstetric staff, and the hospital ethics committee (when necessary) discuss these issues before delivery. In the complete absence of such discussions, it is usually best to attempt resuscitation and then withdraw treatment later if so decided.[3]

REFERENCES

1. Knapp RM. Medicolegal aspects of obstetric anesthesia. In: Ostheimer GW, ed. *Manual of obstetric anesthesia.* New York: Churchill Livingstone, 1992:412.
2. Heyman HJ. Neonatal resuscitation and anesthesiologist liability [Letter]. *Anesthesiology* 1994;81:783.
3. Goldsmith JP, Ginsberg HG, McGettigan MC. Ethical decisions in the delivery room. *Clin Perinatol* 1996;23:529.

Anesthesia for Postpartum Sterilization

OBSTETRIC AND GYNECOLOGIC ISSUES

Advantages

1. After delivery, the fallopian tubes are easily accessible by minilaparotomy. Interval tubal sterilization requires laparoscopy, which has a higher risk of bowel and vascular injury.
2. If post-partum tubal ligation (PPTL) is done within 4 to 12 hours of delivery, additional hospitalization can be avoided.
3. The epidural catheter placed for labor analgesia may be reused.
4. Certain conditions, however, are incompatible with postpartum tubal sterilization. The American College of Obstetricians and Gynecologists (ACOG) recommends that tubal ligation be deferred in patients who have had medical or obstetric complications.[1] Postpartum tubal ligations performed in the labor and delivery ward may be canceled if staffing is insufficient.

Morbidity and Mortality

1. Tubal ligations have a good safety record. The Committee on Obstetrics of ACOG supports the practice of postpartum tubal ligation, barring any maternal or neonatal contraindication.[1] The World Federation of Health Agencies for the Advancement of Voluntary Surgical Contraception endorses tubal ligations performed within 48 hours of delivery.[2]
2. The mortality rate for all tubal sterilizations, interval and postpartum, has been reported as 4 in 100,000 (0.004%).
3. Mask general anesthesia has been a causative factor in many perioperative tubal ligation deaths.
4. Regional block has replaced mask general anesthesia as the most popular anesthetic technique for postpartum surgery. It remains to be seen how this trend will affect anesthesia-related mortality.

POSTPARTUM PHYSIOLOGY

Cardiovascular

1. Cardiac output reaches its peak level immediately after delivery, increasing up to 240% to 270% of nonpregnant values in patients with normal intrapartum blood loss.
   a. The return of blood to the circulation from the involuting uterus causes this increased cardiac output.
   b. Excessive blood loss from lacerations, uterine atony, placenta accreta, or coagulopathy can lead to hypovolemia and decreased cardiac output.
2. Cardiac output gradually returns to nonpregnant values, with most of the decrease occurring within the first 2 weeks after delivery.

Respiratory

1. One to 2 weeks after delivery, minute ventilation is still 28% higher than nonpregnant values.
2. Functional residual capacity returns to within 5% of the nonpregnant value by 1 to 2 weeks after delivery.
3. The anatomic abnormalities associated with difficult intubation in term pregnant patients (obesity, short neck, receding mandible, protruding maxillary incisors, and Mallampati classification of 3 or 4) persist postpartum. In addition, postpartum patients, especially those with preeclampsia, may have developed laryngeal edema during intense, prolonged second-stage Valsalva maneuvers.

Central Nervous System

1. The sensitivity of the parturient to spinal or epidural local anesthetics decreases soon after delivery.
2. Both hormonal and mechanical postpartum changes may contribute to this effect.
   a. Progesterone decreases rapidly after delivery and the spread of intrathecal lidocaine decreases as cerebrospinal fluid progesterone decreases.
   b. Relief of aortocaval compression and decreased intraabdominal pressure also may contribute.

Risk of Aspiration

1. Some of the gastrointestinal changes associated with pregnancy persist after delivery.
2. Decreased esophageal sphincter pressure, delayed gastric emptying, and increased gastric volume increase the risk of aspiration of gastric contents.

Reflux

The incidence of esophageal reflux decreases after delivery.

Gastric Emptying

1. Gastric emptying of liquids is not delayed during pregnancy, in laboring women who do not receive opioids, or in the postpartum period.
2. Gastric emptying of solid food is delayed after delivery.
   a. Most postpartum women will still have gastric food particles 4 hours after eating.
   b. Half of women presenting for postpartum tubal ligation may have residual gastric food.[3]
3. Opioids are the most important cause of delayed gastric emptying in parturients.
   a. Epidural fentanyl 50 or 100 µg or epidural diamorphine 5 mg delay gastric emptying.
   b. Parenteral meperidine 150 mg, diamorphine 10 mg, or pentazocine 60 mg markedly delay gastric emptying; the effects of smaller doses of opioids have not been studied.

Gastric Volume and pH

1. Gastric volume and pH do not differ between nonpregnant and postpartum patients.

2. Drinking 150 mL of water 2 to 3 hours before surgery does not increase gastric volume in postpartum patients compared with NPO postpartum patients or nonpregnant patients.[4]

ANESTHESIA
Regional Anesthesia
1. Advantages
   a. Excellent surgical anesthesia
   b. Avoidance of airway manipulation
   c. When labor epidural catheters are successfully reused, avoidance of an additional anesthetic
2. Patient refusal is a contraindication to regional anesthesia.
   a. The most common reasons for refusal are fear of backache, fear of the needle, fear of seeing or hearing during the procedure, and fear of paralysis. On further discussion, many of these patients will consent to regional anesthesia.

Spinal Anesthesia
1. Spinal anesthesia rapidly provides reliable surgical anesthesia.
2. Lidocaine, meperidine, and bupivacaine are the most frequently used spinal anesthetics.

LIDOCAINE
1. Has quick onset and short duration
2. Has a long history of safe use in spinal anesthesia
3. Recent reports of transient neurologic symptoms, which consist of radicular back and lower extremity pain after isobaric 2% or hyperbaric 5% lidocaine, have led some anesthesiologists (including me) to avoid lidocaine spinal anesthesia.

MEPERIDINE
1. An opioid that produces local anesthetic effects after intrathecal injection
2. Roughly equipotent with lidocaine
3. Versus lidocaine
   a. Shorter duration motor block
   b. Longer time to first analgesic request
   c. More pruritus
4. Respiratory depression is possible. Risk may be greater with concurrent benzodiazepine.

BUPIVACAINE
1. Excellent operating conditions
2. Larger doses produce prolonged blockade.
3. Recommended doses
   a. Patient sitting for induction: 10 mg
   b. Patient in lateral decubitus position for induction: 7.5 mg

Epidural Anesthesia
1. An epidural catheter placed for labor analgesia may be used for postpartum tubal ligation. If reactivation of the catheter is unsuccessful, however, valuable operating room time is lost.

   a. A short delivery-to-surgery time may improve the success of labor epidural reactivation.
   b. Deeper catheter insertion (5 to 8 cm into the epidural space) may improve success rates.
2. Any concentrated local anesthetic, 15 to 20 mL, is appropriate.

Local Anesthesia

1. Patients can undergo postpartum tubal ligations comfortably with only local anesthesia. This option is frequently used in emerging nations underserved by anesthesia providers.
2. Inject dilute local anesthetic (i.e., 20 mL lidocaine, 0.5%) subcutaneously to allow skin incision and entry into the intraperitoneal space and then instill intraperitoneal dilute local anesthetic.
3. Pay attention to the dose of drug used.
4. Supplement with maternal sedation and systemic opioids.

General Anesthesia

   Maternal physiologic changes after delivery affect the response of postpartum patients to some commonly used general anesthetic drugs.

Succinylcholine

1. Diminished activity of plasma cholinesterase prolongs the duration of succinylcholine after delivery but not during gestation.
   a. Postpartum subjects require a lower dose to attain 80% twitch depression.
   b. The time to twitch recovery is longer in postpartum than in nonpregnant patients (685 seconds versus 470 seconds).[5]
2. Metoclopramide also may prolong the duration of succinylcholine. Metoclopramide may directly inhibit acetylcholinesterases, leading to cholinergic effects and inhibiting the degradation of succinylcholine.

Nondepolarizing Muscle Relaxants

1. The postpartum decrease in plasma cholinesterase activity also prolongs the duration of mivacurium (by 3.1 minutes).[6]
2. Vecuronium blockade lasts significantly longer in postpartum patients (63 minutes versus 35 minutes).[7]
3. The duration of atracurium does not differ between postpartum and nonpregnant subjects.

Volatile Anesthetics

1. The minimum alveolar concentration (MAC) of isoflurane is decreased for a short period immediately after delivery.
   a. Less than 12 hours after delivery, isoflurane MAC is 0.75%, which is 28% less than MAC at 6 weeks postpartum.
   b. Isoflurane MAC does not differ between women 12 to 24 hours after delivery (0.95%) and at 6 weeks (1.04%).[8]
2. High concentrations of volatile anesthetics interfere with both spontaneous uterine contraction and the contractile response to oxytocin.

a. Both spontaneous contraction and the response to oxytocin are not inhibited with up to 0.5% of either halothane or enflurane.
b. At higher inhaled concentrations, halothane 2% or enflurane 1.5%, uterine contraction is depressed, an effect that reverses quickly when the volatile anesthetic is discontinued.

ADMINISTERING ANESTHESIA FOR POSTPARTUM TUBAL LIGATIONS

1. Identify the patient early in her labor; obtain early anesthetic consultation.
    a. Carefully examine the airway.
    b. Evaluate any medical and obstetric conditions that might interfere with the planned surgery.
    c. Urge the patient and obstetrician to use epidural rather than systemic opiate analgesia.
2. Postpone or cancel surgery in patients with medical or obstetric conditions that would interact negatively with the anesthesia or surgery.
    a. Immediate postpartum tubal ligation (particularly with a general anesthetic with volatile agent) is not appropriate in patients in whom there is difficulty maintaining uterine tone.
    b. Patients with moderate-to-severe preeclampsia should wait until magnesium therapy is stopped.
    c. Patients with valvular heart disease may not tolerate the stress of a general anesthetic on top of a postpartum increase in cardiac output.
3. Assess the blood loss and intravascular volume status before initiating anesthesia.
    a. Patients should not be hypotensive or tachycardic before tubal ligation.
    b. In patients with adequate predelivery hemoglobins and minimal blood loss, little information is gained by an immediate postpartum hemoglobin.
4. Perform regional anesthesia if possible.
    a. Reactivate an epidural catheter with 15 to 20 mL 2% lidocaine with 1:200,000 epinephrine, or 3% 2-chloroprocaine, which should raise the sensory level to at least the sixth thoracic dermatome.
    b. In patients without an epidural block, spinal anesthesia may be induced by using hyperbaric bupivacaine 7.5 to 10.0 mg.
5. Provide general anesthesia if safe and needed.
    a. Avoid rapid-sequence induction of general anesthesia in patients with identified difficult airways.
    b. Remember, the duration of succinylcholine is moderately prolonged in the postpartum patient.
    c. If volatile anesthetics are given to patients within hours of delivery, MAC is decreased by approximately 30%. High concentrations of these agents may interfere with the effects of oxytocin and cause excessive uterine relaxation.

REFERENCES

1. American College of Obstetrics and Gynecology Committee Opinion. Committee on obstetrics: maternal and fetal sterilization: postpartum tubal sterilization. *Int J Gynecol Obstet* 1992;39:244.
2. World Federation of Health Agencies for the Advancement of Voluntary Surgical Contraception. Safety and voluntary surgical contraception: guidelines for service programs. 1988.
3. Jayaram A, Bowen MP, Deshpande S, Carp HM. Ultrasound examination of the stomach contents of women in the postpartum period. *Anesth Analg* 1997;84:522.
4. Lam KK, So HY, Gin T. Gastric pH and volume after oral fluids in the postpartum patient. *Can J Anaesth* 1993;40:218.
5. Leighton BL, Cheek TG, Gross JB, et al. Succinylcholine pharmacodynamics in peripartum patients. *Anesthesiology* 1986;64: 202.
6. Gin T, Derrick JL, Chan MTV, Chui PT, Mak TWL. Postpartum patients have slightly prolonged neuromuscular block after mivacurium. *Anesth Analg* 1998;86:82.
7. Camp C, Tessem J, Adenwala J, Joyce TH III. Vecuronium and prolonged neuromuscular blockade in postpartum patients. *Anesthesiology* 1997;67:1006.
8. Zhou HH, Norman P, DeLima LGR, Mehta M, Bass D. The minimum alveolar concentration of isoflurane in patients undergoing bilateral tubal ligation in the postpartum period. *Anesthesiology* 1995;82:1364.

32

Postoperative Analgesia

Intramuscular and intravenous (IV) narcotics have long been the mainstay of pain therapy after cesarean delivery. In some hospitals, they are still the most widely practiced analgesic technique. The past two decades have seen a major shift in the methods used for postoperative analgesia in obstetric patients. The discovery, beginning in the 1970s, of widely distributed receptor systems (both opioid and non-opioid) within the central nervous system, combined with the escalating use of regional anesthesia, produced a radically different approach to postoperative pain control.

EPIDURAL ANALGESIA
Morphine

1. A single epidural injection of morphine provides more profound and prolonged analgesia than the same dose of intramuscular morphine.
    a. Most patients who receive epidural morphine after cesarean section report good to excellent analgesia. About half need no other analgesics in the first 24 hours after surgery.
    b. Dose–response studies suggest that pain relief provide by epidural morphine plateaus at doses above 3.75 mg.[1]
    c. Volume of diluent is not a factor in the production of analgesia with epidural morphine.
2. Today morphine remains the most widely used epidural opioid for analgesia after cesarean section.

Side Effects of Epidural Morphine

Some of the initial enthusiasm for epidural morphine was dampened by the high incidence of accompanying side effects.

PRURITUS

1. Nearly all investigators studying epidural morphine have reported itching as a side effect; reports differ only in its frequency and severity.
    a. The pruritus associated with epidural morphine is characteristically mild.
    b. It occurs most commonly on the face or trunk, although it also may be generalized.
    c. In the clinically used range, itching is not significantly related to dose.
2. The exact mechanism by which epidural morphine causes pruritus is unknown. Although pruritus resulting from epidural opioids is often dismissed as a simple μ-receptor–related phenomenon, a careful review of the available data indicates this to be a much more complex issue that awaits further investigation.

NAUSEA AND VOMITING

1. Nausea or vomiting occurs less frequently than pruritus.

2. Not all nausea and vomiting after cesarean delivery is due to epidural opioid, and some find no difference in the incidence of nausea and vomiting between epidural and intravenous morphine.[1]
3. Epidural morphine can cause nausea and vomiting by stimulating the chemoreceptor trigger zone, located in the base of the fourth ventricle of the brain.
   a. Morphine, a highly hydrophilic compound, remains free in the cerebrospinal fluid (CSF) for a long time.
   b. Morphine concentration in the cervical CSF increases slowly.
      i. It is undetectable for the first hour after lumbar epidural injection.
      ii. Cervical CSF concentration peaks 3 to 4 hours after injection.

RESPIRATORY DEPRESSION

1. Recognized as a serious complication of epidural morphine shortly after its introduction to clinical use
2. The incidence of this potentially disastrous complication has been the subject of some debate.
   a. The risk is low enough that it can only be characterized by a large series of patients.
   b. Available data suggest that the frequency of clinically significant respiratory depression after epidural morphine 5 mg or less in the obstetric population is at most 0.2% to 0.3%.
3. Respiratory depression after epidural morphine is often described as "late," with an onset between 6 and 12 hours after administration.
   a. This usually manifests as a decline in respiratory rate that, if untreated, will lead to progressive respiratory acidosis.
   b. The cause is the cephalad migration of morphine within the CSF, which leads to direct central depression of respiration.

HERPES SIMPLEX LABIALIS

1. Morphine reaching the trigeminal nucleus may somehow decrease cell-mediated immunity, leading to recrudescence of latent herpes simplex virus-1 (HSV-1) lesions.
2. Clinical studies report conflicting data about the risk of recurrent HSV lesions associated with neuraxial morphine.
3. The disparity in the findings of these different series may represent differences in the study populations that have not yet been characterized, or other unrecognized factors.
4. Most clinicians do not consider a history of oral herpes infection as a contraindication to epidural morphine.

Treatment of Side Effects

1. Most cases of pruritus are mild and do not require treatment.
   a. Diphenhydramine 25 to 50 mg usually provides adequate symptomatic relief. The sedation associated with diphenhydramine may be as instrumental in providing relief as its antihistaminergic effect.

   b. Naloxone 0.04 to 0.2 mg IV also can relieve the itching, but must be titrated carefully to eliminate pruritus without reversing analgesia. Because of its short duration, a continuous infusion of naloxone may be needed to prevent recurrent itching. Start at 0.4 to 0.6 mg per hour and titrate as needed.
   c. Nalbuphine 5 to 10 mg IV will effectively relieve itching without decreasing analgesia.
   d. Droperidol, ondansetron, and propofol also have been reported to effectively relieve epidural morphine–induced pruritus.
   e. This array of treatments by widely differing classes of agents underscores our lack of knowledge about opioid-related pruritus.
2. Treatment options for nausea and vomiting include antiemetics and opioid antagonists.
   a. Intravenous ondansetron 4 mg and droperidol 0.625 mg are effective.
   b. Intravenous nalbuphine 5 to 10 mg or naloxone 0.1 to 0.2 mg can relieve opioid-induced nausea and vomiting.
3. Early or late, the treatment of choice for respiratory depression is IV naloxone. In severe cases, support ventilation immediately while waiting for naloxone to have effect.

Prevention of Side Effects
1. Naloxone infusion can prevent side effects but must be carefully titrated to avoid reversing analgesia.
2. IV nalbuphine, although an effective treatment, does not prevent side effects after epidural morphine.
3. Naltrexone 5.0 to 12.5 mg is a long-acting, orally administered opioid antagonist that may limit the side effects of epidural morphine, but it also may hinder analgesia.
4. Prophylactic transdermal scopolamine decreases the incidence of nausea and vomiting during the first 24 hours after cesarean delivery. The scopolamine patch must be applied several hours in advance. Some patients then complain of dry mouth.

Other Epidural Opioids
1. Side effects and a long latency complicate the use of epidural morphine for postoperative analgesia.
2. Various other opioids have been used in a quest for a more "perfect" epidural analgesic.

Fentanyl
1. Dose: 50 to 100 μg
2. Comparison with morphine
   a. Faster onset
   b. Shorter duration (2 to 4 hours)
   c. A single dose does not appear to decrease 24-hour morphine consumption.
3. Epidural fentanyl plus epidural morphine may be an effective combination: Fentanyl improves intraoperative and immediate postoperative analgesia.

4. While a single dose of epidural fentanyl has a direct spinal action, systemic absorption during continuous infusion also may play a role.
5. Opioid-related side effects also are common with epidural fentanyl.
    a. Pruritus occurs in up to 100% of patients.
    b. Nausea and vomiting occur less frequently.
    c. Sedation also has been reported.
    d. Respiratory depression occurred in one woman who received epidural fentanyl 100 µg at cesarean delivery.
        i. Unlike epidural morphine, epidural fentanyl produces early-onset respiratory depression.
        ii. This property may lessen the risks of epidural fentanyl, as respiratory depression is likely to occur when the patient is still under the anesthesiologist's direct care and supervision, rather than hours later.

Sufentanil
1. Like fentanyl, the major advantage of epidural sufentanil over epidural morphine is its rapid onset.
2. Epidural sufentanil 30 to 60 µg produces prompt, short-lasting analgesia.
3. Side effects are common.
4. When given intravenously at these doses, sufentanil can produce profound respiratory depression.

Meperidine
1. Epidural meperidine 50 mg provides analgesia for a range of 150 to 200 minutes.
2. Dose–response studies suggest that 25 mg is the minimally effective dose.
3. Side effects are infrequent except at the higher doses (100 mg).

Hydromorphone
1. Commonly known as Dilaudid
2. Its analgesic potency, administered systemically, is roughly twice that of morphine.
3. Doses of 0.6 to 1.0 mg provide good analgesia for about 12 hours.
4. Side effects after epidural hydromorphone are at least as common as those after epidural morphine.

Other Opioids
1. Epidural methadone 4 to 5 mg provides rapid, limited-duration analgesia.
2. Diamorphine (heroin) 2.5 to 5.0 mg reportedly provides over 12 hours of effective analgesia.

Agonist/Antagonists
Butorphanol
1. A mixed opioid agonist/antagonist
    a. It has both agonist and antagonist actions at the µ-receptor.
    b. It is a pure agonist at the ∂- and κ-receptors.

2. Epidural butorphanol 2 mg produces rapid, short-lasting analgesia after cesarean section.
3. The most significant reported side effect is somnolence, lasting approximately 6 hours.
4. Combining epidural morphine and butorphanol for post-cesarean section analgesia may modestly decrease pruritus compared with morphine alone.

Nalbuphine
1. Another mixed opioid agonist/antagonist
   a. Antagonist at the μ-receptor
   b. Agonist at the σ-receptor
   c. Partial agonist at the κ-receptor
   d. Its antagonist properties may limit the potential for respiratory depression and other side effects after epidural administration, but also may limit its analgesic potency.
2. In one study, epidural nalbuphine 10 mg afforded just over an hour of analgesia. Doses of 20 to 30 mg increased the duration to more than 3 hours. The only significant side effect was somnolence, which was seen in up to 50% of patients after 30 mg.[2]

α_2-Agonists
Clonidine
1. An α-adrenergic type 2–receptor agonist
   a. After oral administration, it has significant antihypertensive actions.
   b. After epidural or spinal injection, it produces significant analgesia.
2. A single bolus of clonidine 800 to 900 μg provides about 4 hours of analgesia
3. Bolus plus infusion regimens (400- to 800-μg bolus, 20- to 40-μg per hour infusion) produce adequate analgesia but significant sedation.
4. Smaller doses of clonidine potentiate the effects of epidural opioids.
5. Side effects: sedation, decreases in blood pressure and heart rate

Epinephrine
1. A naturally occurring catecholamine with both α- and β-adrenergic agonist actions.
2. α_2-Adrenergic agonism may be responsible for epinephrine's analgesic properties.
3. Epinephrine has an inconsistent effect on the duration of epidural opioids and may increase the severity of side effects.

Controversies: 2-Chloroprocaine
1. The use of 2-chloroprocaine for epidural anesthesia may impair the analgesic efficacy of epidural morphine.
2. Using even small (7-mL) doses of 2-chloroprocaine to "test" epidural catheters significantly impairs subsequent epidural morphine analgesia.
3. The inhibitory effect of 2-chloroprocaine is not limited to epidural morphine. Epidural fentanyl 50 μg provides signif-

icantly shorter analgesia after lidocaine or 2-chloroprocaine than after bupivacaine or lidocaine with epinephrine.

4. The mechanism of 2-chloroprocaine's inhibitory effect has remained elusive.

5. When using 2-chloroprocaine, be aware that epidural opioid analgesia may not be ideal, and be prepared to offer an alternative form of pain relief.

Summary

1. Clinical recommendations
   a. Adding fentanyl 50 to 100 μg to epidural local anesthetic enhances intraoperative comfort and provides early postoperative analgesia.
   b. Immediately after delivery, give epidural morphine 2 to 4 mg.
   c. Side effects:
      i. Treat pruritus and inadequate analgesia with nalbuphine 5 to 10 mg IV.
      ii. Treat nausea and vomiting with traditional antiemetics (i.e., metoclopramide, ondansetron).

2. These recommendations are applicable to most parturients.
   a. While it is convenient to think of this patient population in terms of means and averages, individual responses are distributed along a bell-shaped curve. It is impossible to predict how any individual will respond.
   b. Despite the fact that most patients will have sufficient analgesia with this regimen, others will require significant additional medications. If a parturient requires significant amounts of additional analgesics in the early postoperative period, do not hesitate to add patient-controlled IV analgesia (see later).

3. Because of the theoretical risk of respiratory depression and the occurrence of side effects, we find standard postoperative orders very useful (Table 32.1).
   a. Nurses check and record respiratory rates hourly for 24 hours after epidural morphine.
   b. If respiratory rate decreases below 8 breaths per minute, the nurse should immediately inject naloxone and notify the anesthesiologist.
   c. In the absence of other sedatives or narcotics, respiratory depression of this degree is extremely uncommon.

SUBARACHNOID ANALGESIA

Morphine

1. Small doses of intrathecal morphine provide prolonged analgesia in patients with acute and chronic pain.

2. In parturients, subarachnoid morphine produces excellent pain relief after cesarean section.

3. Analgesia lasting as long as 44 hours has been reported after as much as 0. 6 mg subarachnoid morphine.

4. Even very small doses of morphine significantly decrease the amount of patient-controlled analgesia (PCA) morphine used after cesarean section.
   a. There is no difference in PCA morphine use after 0.1 to 0.5 mg intrathecal morphine.[3]

Table 32.1.   Postoperative neuraxial opioid orders

1. This patient received epidural/spinal morphine_____ mg at ____ hours on _____ (date).
2. Label chart and cardex: "Spinal/Epidural Morphine—Special Orders"
3. No analgesics, sedatives or antiemetics for 12 hours unless ordered by anesthesiologist.
4. Monitor respiratory rate and level of consciousness/sedation q1h × 24 hours.
5. Call anesthesiologist (Beeper # _____) for:
   a. Respiratory rate <10/min
   b. Moderate-to-severe itching
   c. Marked somnolence (patient should be easily aroused by verbal address or light touch)
   d. Persistent pain
6. Naloxone, one ampule at bedside at all times.
7. Give naloxone, one ampule IV STAT for respiratory arrest and call anesthesiologist STAT.
8. Maintain IV access or heparin lock at all times.
9. Nalbuphine 5 mg IV q4–6h prn pain or itching.
10. Ibuprofen 600 mg PO q6h × 3; give first dose at (Date/time)[a] _____

[a]Give ketorolac 30 mg IV shortly after delivery. Ketorolac 15 mg IV can be substituted for the ibuprofen.

---

    b. Only the incidence of pruritus and the need for treatment interventions increase significantly as the dose of intrathecal morphine increases.

    c. The optimal dose of intrathecal morphine after cesarean section appears to lie between 0.1 and 0.2 mg.

5. Side effects reported after intrathecal morphine are comparable to those seen after epidural morphine.
   a. Pruritus occurs in 40% to 80% of patients and appears to be dose-dependent.
   b. Vomiting occurs rarely after low doses (0.1 mg) of morphine, but in up to one-third of patients receiving larger doses (0.25 mg).
   c. Clinically significant respiratory depression is rare.
6. Intrathecal, like epidural, morphine cannot completely eliminate the need for supplemental analgesics, however, and the best way to ensure excellent analgesia may be through a combination of intrathecal morphine and PCA supplementation.

Fentanyl

1. Subarachnoid fentanyl also has been used at cesarean delivery.
2. Doses greater than 6.25 µg will prolong the time until the patient first requests pain relief but will not decrease 24-hour morphine consumption.

3. Pruritus occurs frequently.
4. Respiratory depression has been reported.

Other Opioids

1. Subarachnoid sufentanil 10 μg
   a. Provides immediate postoperative analgesia but does not decrease 24-hour morphine use.
   b. Pruritus, usually of short duration, occurs in more than half of the patients.
2. Methadone produces analgesia of shorter duration and less consistent quality than does morphine, even at doses as high as 20 mg.
3. Oxymorphone provides approximately 16 hours of analgesia when administered intrathecally, with predictable side effects of pruritus, nausea, and vomiting.

Nonopioids

1. Epinephrine does not appear to augment intrathecal morphine postoperative analgesia.
2. Clonidine
   a. Dose: 150 μg provides up to 6 hours of postoperative analgesia.
   b. Side effects include decreased systolic, diastolic, and mean arterial pressures, and sedation.[4]
3. Neostigmine
   a. Painful stimuli release norepinephrine (NE) from descending inhibitory pathways.
   b. NE stimulates α_2-adrenoreceptors, which activate spinal cholinergic neurons.
   c. Painful stimuli increase NE and acetylcholine (ACh) concentrations in CSF, and spinal neostigmine prevents the breakdown of synaptically released ACh, enhancing analgesia.
   d. In parturients, a single injection of intrathecal neostigmine produces a dose-related decrease in morphine consumption after cesarean section for about 10 hours.
   e. Unfortunately, neostigmine also incites dose-related postoperative nausea and vomiting.[5]

Summary

1. Morphine remains the best choice for postoperative subarachnoid analgesia.
2. Current data suggest that morphine 0.1 mg will provide 24 hours of good to excellent postoperative analgesia for most parturients.
3. If a patient is having significant discomfort, do not hesitate to provide supplemental analgesia, usually PCA morphine.
4. Because of the very small volumes of opioids used with this technique, measure these drugs in tuberculin syringes to minimize the risk of accidental overdose.
5. As with epidural opioid analgesia, close postoperative monitoring of patients is essential. Postoperative orders are identical to those used after epidural opioids (see Table 32.1).

PATIENT-CONTROLLED ANALGESIA

1. In recent years, PCA has become a popular and effective method of providing postoperative analgesia after a wide range of surgical procedures.
2. In most studies, pain relief associated with PCA morphine is not quite that provided by neuraxial morphine, but patient satisfaction is at least as good.
3. Technical issues
    a. Choice of drug
        i.   Only minor differences exist among the commonly used opioids.
        ii. Oxymorphone may produce more nausea.
        iii. Patients receiving fentanyl are more likely to require supplemental doses.
        iv. Meperidine can be detected in breast milk and may decrease neonatal neurobehavioral scores.
    b. Basal infusion
        i.   Provides little or no benefit
        ii. Does not change 24-hour opioid use
        iii. Increases nausea
    c. Settings
        i.   Drug: morphine
        ii. Bolus: 1 to 2 mg
        iii. Lockout: 10 minutes
        iv. Basal infusion: None

Patient-Controlled Epidural Analgesia

1. Epidural PCA (PCEA) allows the use of local anesthetics, opioids, and nonopioid adjuncts for postoperative analgesia.
2. As might be imagined, this approach allows a large and sometimes bewildering array of options.
3. PCEA opioid-only techniques provide better analgesia with less sedation than comparable IV PCA techniques.
4. Fentanyl and sufentanil are the opioids most often used for PCEA administration because of their rapid onset and efficacy.
5. As with patients who receive IV PCA, a basal infusion does not significantly improve the quality of pain relief with PCEA. Background infusion does increase sedation.
6. Local anesthetics, particularly bupivacaine, can be added to PCEA for analgesia after cesarean section.
    a. The concentration of local anesthetic must be carefully chosen to enhance analgesia without producing sensory or motor blockade, as many of these patients are ambulatory within hours of surgery.
    b. Adding local anesthetic to PCEA also may increase the risk of significant complications, such as pressure sores.
7. Clearly, PCEA is an effective technique for analgesia after cesarean section. Whether it offers distinct advantages over epidural or intrathecal morphine is a matter of dispute. PCEA requires maintaining a functioning epidural catheter in the postoperative period, not always a simple task. Further, in many practices, cesarean delivery is more likely to be accomplished with spinal than with epidural anesthesia, which precludes use of the technique or subjects the

parturient to a second procedure. Still, PCEA may be a useful technique for selected patients and populations.

ALTERNATIVE APPROACHES
Ilioinguinal Nerve Block
1. Ilioinguinal nerve block, using bupivacaine 0.5%, may provide some postoperative analgesia after cesarean delivery (via Pfannenstiel incision).
2. Wound infiltration with bupivacaine 0.5% seems comparable to the nerve block.

Nonsteroidal Antiinflammatory Drugs
1. In recent years, several parenteral nonsteroidal antiinflammatory agents (NSAIDs) have been developed.
2. As a sole agent, intramuscular ketorolac 30 mg provides analgesia comparable to meperidine 75 mg.
3. NSAID therapy may decrease postoperative opioid requirements.
   a. Diclofenac, ketoprofen, and tenoxicam decrease systemic opioid use.
   b. NSAIDs also enhance the analgesia provided by intrathecal morphine. With this combination therapy, smaller doses of intrathecal morphine (0.025 to 0.05 mg) plus regularly administered NSAIDs provide similar pain relief as higher doses of morphine, but with fewer side effects.[6]

REFERENCES
1. Palmer CM, Petty JV, Nogarmi WM, Marquez RC, Van Maren G, Alves DM. What is the optimal dose of epidural morphine for post-cesarean analgesia? A dose response study. *Anesthesiology* 1996; 85:A909.
2. Camann WR, Hurley RH, Gilbertson LI, Long ML, Datta S. Epidural nalbuphine for analgesia following caesarean delivery: dose-response and effect of local anaesthetic choice. *Can J Anaesth* 1991;38:728.
3. Palmer CM, Emerson SS, Voulgaropoulos D, Alves D. Dose-response relationship of intrathecal morphine for postcesarean analagesia. *Anesthesiology* 1999;90:437.
4. Filos KS, Goudas LC, Patroni O, Polyzon V. Intrathecal clonidine as a sole analgesic for pain relief after cesarean section. *Anesthesiology* 1992;77:267.
5. Krukowski JA, Hood DD, Eisenach JC, Mallak KA, Parker RL. Intrathecal neostigmine for post-cesarean section analgesia: dose response. *Anesth Analg* 1997;84:1269.
6. Cardoso MMSC, Carvalhlo JCS, Amaro AR, Prado AA, Cappelli EL. Small doses of intrathecal morphine combined with systemic diclofenac for postoperative pain control after cesarean delivery. *Anesth Analg* 1998;86:538.

Postoperative Complications Associated with Regional Anesthesia in the Parturient

HEADACHE

1. Headache is very common postpartum.
   a. Almost 40% of women experience headaches in the first week after delivery.
   b. Many headaches are unrelated to anesthesia.
2. Postdural puncture headache (PDPH) is the most common postoperative complication of regional anesthesia in obstetric patients.
3. A careful history, including symptoms past and present, physical examination, and laboratory tests, if indicated, is essential in guiding proper diagnosis and management.
4. Differential diagnosis of headache
   a. Nonspecific headache: Risk factors include history of migraine, depression, stress, or caffeine withdrawal.
   b. Stress headaches: typically pounding, temporal, or circumferential
   c. Tension headache
      i. Lasts 30 minutes to 7 days.
      ii. Has at least two of the following: pressing/tightening (nonpulsating) character, mild or moderate intensity, bilateral location, and not aggravated by physical activity.
      iii. Nausea and photophobia are absent.
      iv. Treat with acetaminophen or nonsteroidal anti-inflammatory drugs (NSAIDs).
   d. Migraine headache
      i. More common in women, with a prevalence of 15% to 20%
      ii. The hormonal changes of pregnancy improve symptoms in more than 66% of women, but headaches frequently recur postpartum.
      iii. They typically last 4 to 72 hours.
      iv. They have two of the following: unilateral location, pulsating quality, moderate or severe intensity, and aggravation with physical activity.
      v. Nausea, vomiting, or photophobia also are present.
      vi. Prodromes occur in 15% of patients, with visual changes being the most common.
      vii. Treatment: Egotamine tartarate 2 mg is one of the classic treatments for migraine headaches. However, higher dose aspirin, acetaminophen, or NSAIDs also may work. Sumatriptan, a 5-hy-droxytryptamine (5-HT1)-receptor agonist, ad-ministered as 6 mg subcutaneously (SC) or 25 to 100 mg PO, is very effective.

e. Hypertension/preeclampsia/eclampsia
    i. Severe hypertension may cause headaches.
    ii. Preeclampsia is associated with headache, possible visual changes, nausea, and vomiting.
    iii. Postpartum preeclampsia or eclampsia may first manifest as a complaint of headache.
f. Brain tumor
    i. Associated headache is typically generalized.
    ii. It has a dull, deep, aching quality.
    iii. It is usually intermittent and relieved by simple analgesics.
    iv. Symptoms may overlap with migraine and tension-type headache.
    v. In pain clinics specializing in headaches, the incidence of brain tumors is less than 1%.
g. Cortical vein thrombosis
    i. Pregnancy is a hypercoaguable state that may rarely lead to cortical vein thrombosis (CVT), with an incidence of 1 in 6,000.
    ii. The superior longitudinal sinus or the cortical veins may thrombose, impeding venous drainage.
    iii. The increased venous pressure reduces cerebrospinal fluid (CSF) absorption from the arachnoid villi and increases intracranial pressure (ICP).
    iv. Venous stasis may produce arterial stasis and focal cerebral infarction.
    v. Symptoms
        (1) Occur before delivery or within 48 hours after delivery.
        (2) Include severe headache, nausea, focal neurologic signs, seizures, and altered mental status.
    vi. Diagnosis is made by contrast computed tomography (CT) scan, magnetic resonance imaging (MRI), or cerebral angiogram.
    vii. Treatment aims at seizure prophylaxis, and reducing ICP and cerebral edema by mechanical ventilation and steroids.
h. Subdural hematoma
    i. Dural puncture can rarely result in a subdural hematoma.
    ii. Headache should be nonpositional and persistent.
    iii. There also may be symptoms of nausea and/or vomiting, confusion, or altered mental status.
    iv. Focal neurologic signs may be present.
    v. A noncontrast CT scan or MRI will reveal the hematoma.
    vi. Surgical drainage usually is required.
i. Subarachnoid hemorrhage
    i. Symptoms include severe headache, nausea and vomiting, neck stiffness, and decreased mental status.
    ii. Focal neurologic deficits may be present.
    iii. A noncontrast CT scan or MRI will reveal the hematoma.
    iv. Surgery may be required.

    j. Meningitis: septic or aseptic

        i. Infectious meningitis is rare after regional anesthesia.

        ii. Symptoms include severe headache, fever, stiff neck, Kernig and Brudzinski signs (pain when extending the knee with the hip flexed, and flexion of the lower extremities with neck flexion).

        iii. Decreased mental status, vomiting, and seizures also may occur.

        iv. Aseptic meningitis appears like bacterial meningitis, but no organisms are found in the CSF.

    k. Pneumocephalus

        i. Intracranial air may cause sudden severe headache, possibly with neck or back pain.

        ii. Reabsorption of air over a period of several hours to days will eliminate the headache.

    l. Caffeine withdrawal

        i. Patients with a moderate daily dose of caffeine (235 mg; 2.5 cups coffee) may develop caffeine-withdrawal headaches.

        ii. Even people who consume low or moderate amounts of caffeine may have withdrawal syndrome: 52% develop moderate-to-severe headache, 10% depression or anxiety, and even decreased fine-motor performance.

        iii. Caffeine sodium benzoate may be administered intravenously for replacement therapy while the patient has nothing by mouth (NPO).

    m. The hormonal changes of lactation have been reported to cause headaches.

    n. Iatrogenic/medications

        i. Patients receiving $MgSO_4$ may develop flushing, nausea, and headaches.

        ii. The headache may be due to the underlying preeclampsia or to cerebral vasodilatation.

        iii. Allergies to food or flowers also may cause nasal stuffiness, sinusitis, and headaches.

        iv. Hypoglycemia may cause headache and tachycardia.

        v. Electrolyte disturbances also may cause headaches.

    o. Psychogenic

        i. Patients should be told of the risk of headache with any neuraxial anesthetic.

        ii. There is no evidence for widespread psychogenic headaches.

Postdural Puncture Headache

1. PDPH may follow intentional or unintentional puncture of the dura mater.

2. It always has a positional component.

3. Symptoms include a rapid onset of a severe headache, neck pain, and cranial nerve symptoms (vision or hearing changes).

a. Pain originating above the tentorium is transmitted via the trigeminal nerve to the frontal region.
b. Pain from below the tentorium is transmitted via the vagus and upper cervical nerves to the occipital region and neck.
c. Pain may be frontal or circumferential.
d. Nausea and, less frequently, vomiting may occur, but are not typical.
e. Tinnitus, deafness, photophobia, and diplopia also are rare.
f. The sixth cranial nerve has a tortuous intracranial course and is more susceptible to traction; paresis occurs in 1 in 5,000 to 8,000 PDPHs.

Incidence
1. The risk of dural puncture during epidural catheter placement ranges from 0.6% to 2.6%.
2. Risk factors for PDPH include age younger than 40, female, pregnant, increasing needle size, cutting beveled needle, orientation of needle, and history of PDPH.
   a. Bearing down during delivery does not affect the incidence of PDPH.
   b. The rate of CSF leak and the incidence of PDPH are related to the size of the dural hole.
      i. Dural puncture with a 17-gauge epidural needle may cause headache in 50% to 86% of parturients.
      ii. Small gauge blunt or pencil-point spinal needles only carry a 1% to 2% incidence of headache.
      iii. If a cutting-edged needle is used, orienting the needle bevel parallel to the longitudinal axis of the back (caudad–cephalad) decreases the size of the dural hole and the incidence of headache compared with perpendicular orientation.

Pathophysiology
1. The normal adult has 150 mL of CSF and produces about 450 mL per day. The acute loss of as little as 20 mL CSF causes symptoms of PDPH.
2. Loss of CSF may cause sagging of intracranial contents in the upright position, putting traction on pain-sensitive structures like the meninges, cranial nerves, bridging veins, and tentorium.
3. Cerebral vasodilatation resulting from low ICP may produce PDPH.
   a. The symptomatic relief offered by some cerebral vasoconstrictors (e.g., caffeine) supports this theory.
   b. Transcranial Doppler studies show significant changes in cerebral blood flow velocity that correlate with symptoms of PDPH.

HEARING LOSS
1. Auditory side effects of dural puncture may include a transient decrease in low-frequency hearing.
2. Hearing loss may be unilateral and is related to size of dural puncture.
3. Hearing loss resolves after epidural blood patch (EBP).

Course/Treatment

1. Onset
   a. Can be immediate or delayed.
   b. Begins within 2 days of dural puncture in 66% of obstetric patients.
2. Duration
   a. PDPH usually resolves in 1 week (75%).
   b. If untreated, 9% may persist after 6 months.
   c. Prolonged headache for months or even years has rarely been reported.
   d. Average duration of headache after use of 20-, 22-, and 23-gauge (cutting) needles, 5.4, 4.9, and 2.7 days, respectively.[1]
3. Treatment
   a. Symptomatic therapy is usually adequate. Any medication that ameliorates the pain will allow the headache to spontaneously resolve.
   b. Although an EBP is the definitive treatment for PDPH, it is usually elective in nature. If a patient shows signs of cranial nerve traction (diplopia, tinnitus), then EBP becomes an urgent necessity.
   c. Bed rest
      i. Patients do not have a headache while supine.
      ii. The incidence of PDPH is *not* affected by bed rest.
   d. Hydration
      i. Does not increase CSF production.
      ii. Does not reduce the incidence of PDPH.
   e. Abdominal binders
      i. Increase intraabdominal pressure, increasing epidural and vertebral venous pressure, resulting in increased intracranial pressure.
      ii. Use is uncommon but may significantly reduce the incidence of headache.
   f. NSAIDs are effective initial analgesics for PDPH.

CEREBRAL VASOCONSTRICTORS

1. Caffeine has been used to treat PDPH for more than 50 years.
   a. It may work by counteracting the cerebral vasodilatation caused by low ICP.
   b. Intravenous or oral caffeine will provide at least temporary relief of headache in many patients.
   c. Side effects include dizziness and flushing and, rarely, seizures. Toxicity occurs in doses of more than 15 mg per kilogram, when serum caffeine concentrations are greater than 30 mg per milliliter.
2. Theophylline, another methylxanthine, also has been useful to reduce PDPH.
3. Sumatriptan, a serotonin (5-HT1) agonist, has proven inconsistent as a treatment of PDPH.

EPIDURAL SALINE

1. Lumbar epidural saline (10 to 20 mL) will transiently increase lumbar epidural and CSF pressure.
2. It provides temporary relief of PDPH.

3. Excessive epidural volume may produce side effects of back, neck, and orbital pain. Retinal hemorrhages were reported after an epidural bolus of 120 mL saline.

EPIDURAL BLOOD PATCH

1. Considered the definitive treatment for PDPH
   a. Successful treatment rates for EBP are commonly described as greater than 95%.
   b. These high reported success rates may reflect the short duration of follow-up. With longer follow-up, headache may return in 30% of patients.
2. Fifteen to 20 mL blood will extend over three to nine spinal segments. Clot appears to adhere to the dura mater.
3. Mechanism(s) of action
   a. Tamponade effect at site of puncture
   b. Mass effect, producing cephalad displacement of CSF.

Side Effects

1. Transient side effects, including back pain, neck ache, paresthesia, radiculitis, and cranial nerve dysfunction, are seen with up to 35% of EBPs.
2. Occasionally, backache persists for up to 1 month.
3. Rarely, mental status may change after an EBP. In two case reports, patients had other intracranial pathology. These exceedingly rare cases reinforce the need for a proper history and physical examination before performing EBP.
4. EBP does *not* impair the efficacy of subsequent epidural analgesia.[2]

Prophylactic Epidural Blood Patch

1. May decrease the frequency and severity of subsequent PDPH
2. Does not completely prevent PDPH
3. Role in clinical practice
   a. Thirty percent to 50% of women will *not* develop PDPH after dural puncture with a large-gauge needle.
   b. Prophylactic EBP provides no benefit to these patients.
   c. Prophylactic EBP is not part of my routine clinical practice.

Other Treatments

1. Epidural injection of 20 to 30 mL low-molecular-weight dextran (Dextran 40) has been used successfully to treat PDPH.
   a. Side effects include dysesthesia (7%) and burning sensation (3.5%) at time of injection, but no long-term sequelae.
   b. Dextran 40 may be effective because it is slowly absorbed from the epidural space, allowing more time for the dural puncture to heal.
2. Epidural gelatin also has been described in the treatment of PDPH.
   a. Gelatin powder (Gelfoam; Upjohn Co, Kalamazoo, MI) 600 to 700 mg can be dissolved in 10 mL of autologous plasma.
   b. Gelfoam adheres to the area and causes a tissue reaction similar to a blood clot.[3]

Technique for Epidural Blood Patch

1. Unless you expect technical difficulties, position the patient on her side. (It seems cruel to me to place a patient with a severe positional headache in the upright position.)
2. With strict aseptic technique, identify the epidural space at or close to the presumed site of dural puncture.
   a. The lower space may be preferred to a higher interspace because epidural blood spreads more cephalad than caudad.
   b. However, EBP performed slightly above the original puncture site will be effective.
3. After locating the epidural space, have an assistant draw 20 mL of the patient's blood under aseptic conditions.
4. Inject blood slowly.
   a. Stop briefly after each 5 mL.
   b. Inquire about symptoms of back or leg pressure or pain.
   c. Stop injecting with the onset of symptoms. If symptoms resolve promptly, slowly start injecting again.
   d. Stop completely when symptoms return immediately with renewed injection.
   e. Attempt to inject at least 15 mL, but probably no more than 20 mL of blood.
5. Have the patient remain supine for 2 hours to maximize the efficacy of blood patch.
6. Patients may then be discharged with instructions to return to the hospital if the headache returns, gets worse, or if visual or hearing disturbances develop.

Recurrent Headache

1. A single blood patch will provide permanent relief of PDPH in 70% of patients.
2. A second blood patch will cure most of the remaining headaches.
3. If symptoms persist after a second EBP, reconsider your diagnosis. Radiologic imaging may be warranted. A CT scan of the head may reveal other causes of headache (see earlier). I usually do not perform more than two EBPs, and never more than three.

Timing of Epidural Blood Patch

1. Most PDPH will resolve with conservative therapy.
2. There are no strict rules governing the timing of EBP.
   a. I usually offer patients 24 hours of conservative therapy (caffeine, analgesics) and then consider EBP.
   b. Case reports describe effective EBPs months and even years after dural puncture.

BACKACHE

Background

1. Low back pain is nearly ubiquitous in the general population.
2. Chronic back pain is present in 3% to 7% of the adult population.
3. Sciatica accompanies up to 25% of cases of back pain.
4. Herniated lumbar disc has a prevalence of 13% in both those with back pain and the general population.

5. Pain may originate from a herniated intervertebral disc, a nerve root that is compressed or stretched, lumbar facet joints, paraspinous muscle, posterior longitudinal ligament, or from the local blood vessels and nerves.
6. The high prevalence and multiple causes of low back pain must be kept in mind when treating backache during or after delivery.

Pregnancy

1. The physiologic changes of pregnancy predispose to back pain, with an incidence approaching 50%.
    a. Relaxing loosens ligaments.
    b. The increasing size of the gestation exaggerates the lumbar lordosis.
2. Pain also may be caused by compression of the lumbosacral nerves.
    a. Radicular symptoms often accompany low back pain.
    b. True sciatica with a dermatomal distribution is uncommon (1%).
3. After delivery, back pain is very common, occurring in about 40% of new mothers.

Regional Anesthesia

1. Retrospective studies often report an increased incidence of back pain after labor epidural analgesia.
2. Prospective studies, on the other hand, find no increased risk.
3. When discussing back pain and epidural analgesia, remember:
    a. Back pain is common with or without regional anesthesia.
    b. Back pain is a chronic disease: A history of back pain predicts future pain.
    c. Epidural analgesia does not affect the incidence of back pain after delivery in prospective studies.
    d. Epidural injections are used in the treatment of acute back pain.
4. Discussing these points with a parturient anxious about the effects of epidural analgesia on postpartum back pain usually allays her fears.

2-Chloroprocaine

1. The use of 2-chloroprocaine with sodium ethylenediaminetetraacetic acid (EDTA) has been associated with severe back pain lasting up to 36 hours.
    a. Although gross muscle spasm has not been noted, this pain is possibly due to paraspinous muscle spasm caused by localized EDTA-related hypocalcemia.
    b. Intravenous calcium chloride has been used to treat the back pain.[4]
2. The most recent preparation of 2-chloroprocaine (Nesicaine-MPF) lacks EDTA.

Treatment

1. Treatment of back pain is symptomatic with analgesics.
2. Heat and physical therapy may help.
3. Exercise and proper posture are important in the long-term prevention of backache.

INFECTIONS

1. Serious infections related to neuraxial anesthesia are very rare.
2. Rapid diagnosis and treatment are essential.
3. Erythema at the site of epidural insertion is not uncommon because of irritation of the catheter or a minor localized infection.

Prevention

1. Infection can start by introduction of bacteria during a procedure, or when bacteremia causes "seeding" of an indwelling foreign body (e.g., epidural catheter).
2. Strict aseptic technique is essential, not only during insertion of the epidural catheter, but also during subsequent injections.
   a. Wear a face mask when identifying the epidural space and inserting a catheter.
   b. Keep the hub and cap of the epidural catheter sterile.
   c. Inject only sterile solutions.

Epidural Abscess

1. A rare but potentially devastating complication that requires prompt recognition and treatment
2. The estimated incidence is 0.2 to 1.2 per 10,000 tertiary hospital admissions.
3. It usually occurs as a complication of infection elsewhere in the body, with bacteria seeding the epidural space.
4. Epidural analgesia is an uncommon cause of epidural abscess. The reported incidence varies from 1 in 26,000 to 1 in 500,000 epidural anesthetics.
5. Epidural abscess usually becomes symptomatic a few days to weeks after delivery.
   a. Typical symptoms include fever, malaise, headache, and back pain at the level of the infection.
   b. On physical examination, there is tenderness to deep palpation over the site of infection and pain with movement (flexion greater than extension).
   c. On routine laboratory examination, the white blood cell count will be increased with a polymorphonuclear leukocytosis, and blood cultures may be positive for bacteria.
   d. Nerve root pain develops 1 to 3 days after onset.
   e. Neurologic deficits will develop as the abscess progresses and impinges on the spinal cord and its blood supply.
   f. Lower extremity pain, weakness, bowel and bladder dysfunction, and paraplegia may occur.
6. Diagnostic imaging
   a. The preferred technique for spinal infections is MRI with gadolinium enhancement.
   b. If MRI is unavailable, a CT scan also may be used.
   c. A myelogram is less informative and more invasive.
7. Especially if neurologic symptoms are present, spinal decompression by laminectomy must be performed immediately. Treatment with antibiotics but not surgical drainage is not sufficient. Neurologic compromise is usually reversible if the spinal cord is decompressed within 6 to 12 hours of symptoms.

Meningitis

1. Bacterial meningitis is very rare after epidural or spinal anesthesia.
2. Cases of meningitis in parturients are assumed to be related to a breach in sterile technique.
3. Meningitis also has been reported after combined spinal–epidural and continuous spinal anesthesia.
4. Bacterial meningitis
   a. Usually seen 24 to 48 hours after regional anesthesia
   b. Fever, headache, and stiff neck
   c. The CSF will show increased white blood cells (polymorphonuclear), decreased glucose, increased protein, and organisms on Gram stain.
   d. Infectious organism can sometimes be traced to the oropharyngeal flora of the anesthetist.
5. Aseptic meningitis
   a. Appears like bacterial meningitis, except that no organisms are found in the CSF.
   b. Is more common when reusable equipment is improperly cleaned and sterilized.
   c. Is probably due to chemical irritation of the spinal cord and meninges.
   d. Symptoms usually occur 6 to 24 hours after spinal anesthesia, are similar to those of bacterial meningitis, and include headache, fever, stiff neck (nuchal rigidity), and photophobia.
   e. CSF analysis shows increased white blood cells (usually lymphocytosis), normal glucose, increased protein, and no bacteria on Gram stain.

NEUROLOGIC DEFICITS

1. The most feared complication of regional anesthesia is a neurologic deficit.
2. Fortunately, such problems are very rare in obstetric patients.
3. After delivery, most neurologic injuries have obstetric, not anesthetic, causes.

Neurologic Examination and Testing

1. Symptoms of back or extremity pain, weakness, paresthesia, or numbness must be evaluated promptly. Although most of these complaints are minor in origin (e.g., nonspecific low-back discomfort or tenderness at the epidural insertion site), some are potentially catastrophic (i.e., epidural hematoma).
2. The best approach to possible postpartum neurologic deficits is to:
   a. Take a good history.
   b. Perform a full neurologic examination.
   c. Request additional diagnostic testing, if needed.
   d. Decide on management and the need for consultations.

History

1. Elicit the precise onset, location, and radiation of symptoms.
2. Did they start during needle insertion or drug injection?
3. Is the anesthetic block prolonged, or was there a period of full recovery?

4. Is the pain/deficit in a dermatomal pattern, part of a peripheral nerve distribution, or perhaps nonanatomic?
5. Note any history of back pain, numbness, or weakness.
6. Investigate positioning and management of the second stage of labor. Use of forceps and excessive or prolonged hyperflexion of the hips may result in injury to the muscles or nerves.

Physical Examination
1. Perform and document a detailed neurologic examination.
   a. Careful mapping of symptoms may reveal a pattern consistent with a peripheral nerve injury or a single root lesion.
   b. Detailed documentation in the chart is very important to good patient care and may serve in your future defense.
2. Some areas to check on physical examination:
   a. Sensory and motor tone of the paraspinous muscles (soft versus knotted, innervated by the posterior rami of the nerve root)
   b. Tenderness to deep palpation of the processes (transmits pressure to epidural space, pain elicited with an intraspinal mass)
   c. Localized area of erythema or purulence
   d. Sacroiliac joint tenderness

Diagnosis
Routine Tests
1. If the problem is a peripheral nerve injury (e.g., common peroneal nerve), further testing may not be needed.
2. If fever accompanies back pain or headache, a white blood cell count and differential should be performed.
3. An examination of the CSF may rarely be indicated to rule out septic or aseptic meningitis.

Advanced Testing
1. If a patient has symptoms isolated to a particular nerve root, then obtain CT or MRI of the affected area.
   a. History of a recent regional anesthetic does not prove causation.
   b. An occult herniated disc may become symptomatic after the stress of labor and delivery.
2. Neurophysiologic testing can help document the location and severity of an injury.
   a. Electrodiagnostic testing will localize a problem to the central nervous system (CNS) or to the periphery at the individual nerve, root, or plexus.
   b. Electrodiagnostic testing also may help differentiate a neurapraxia, which will resolve in 1 to 5 months, from an axonotmesis with axonal interruption, which may last longer.
      i. Electromyography (EMG) will help to document the time and location of injury.
         (1) After denervation, the muscle fibers begin to discharge spontaneously, but muscle fibrillation potentials do not change for 2 to 3 weeks after nerve injury.

(2) Thus, an EMG with abnormalities within the first week after delivery will document pre-existing disease (i.e., before regional anesthesia).

(3) If an interval change occurs 4 to 6 weeks after delivery, then the injury occurred around the time of delivery.

(4) If the nerve root is injured, both the anterior and posterior rami should be involved.

(5) Thus, the paraspinous area should be affected.

(6) If not, then the level of nerve injury is distal to the nerve root and not caused as a direct result of central regional anesthesia.

ii. Conduction velocity studies can provide immediate information about both motor and sensory nerves.

(1) The conduction velocity represents the fastest-conducting fibers, and surface recordings may miss disease in small-diameter nerve fibers.

(2) Lesions proximal to the dorsal root ganglia do not affect the sensory potential and thus help to distinguish radicular from peripheral nerve disease.

iii. Proximal nerve segments can be indirectly evaluated by using the late-response studies (F responses, H reflex).

(1) The F response is a measure of proximal nerve conduction from the point of peripheral nerve stimulus to the anterior horn cells and back along the nerve.

(2) The H reflex is found in the tibial nerve–soleus system, occurs during submaximal stimulation, and is thought to be a monosynaptic reflex with an afferent and efferent limb.

(3) A prolonged H reflex with a normal F response in the same nerve identifies dorsal root pathology.

iv. Somatosensory evoked potentials (SSEPs) will monitor the dorsal columns of the spinal cord. SSEPs are sensitive to spinal cord damage produced by compression, mechanical distraction, and ischemia.

v. Motor evoked potentials (MEPs) measure the integrity of the descending motor pathways in the anterior part of the spinal cord.

Management

1. Management of a neurologic deficit is specific to the particular injury.
2. A neurologist should be consulted if a deficit is identified.
3. Steroids are frequently used to reduced swelling and inflammation.

4. Physical therapy may be appropriate for intermediate and long-term neurologic deficits.

OBSTETRIC INJURIES
1. Injuries to the nervous system occur during vaginal delivery in patients who do not receive regional or general anesthesia (Table 33.1).
   a. Parturients may experience compression nerve injury, or rarely, an ischemic spinal cord injury.
   b. Incidence: 0.85% of parturients report at least transient postpartum nerve injuries.[5]
   c. Most resolve within 6 months.
2. Specific injuries
   a. The fetal head may compress and injure the lumbosacral plexus as it crosses the ala of the sacrum or the posterior brim of the pelvis.

Table 33.1.   Peripheral nerve injuries in obstetric patients

Nerve	Root Value	Mechanism of Injury	Clinical Picture
Lumbosacral trunk	L4, L5, S1	Forceps Fetal head	Foot drop Quadriceps and hip adductors affected
Femoral nerve	L2, L3, L4	Fetal head Retractor	Quadriceps weakness
			Weak hip flexion
			Absent patellar reflex
			Hypalgesia in thigh and calf
Lateral cutaneous nerve	L2, L3	Stirrups	Hypalgesia in the front thigh
Common peroneal nerve	L4–S2	Stirrups	Foot drop Hypesthesia in the lateral calf
Obturator nerve	L2–L4	Fetal head	Weakness of thigh adduction
			Hypesthesia in the medial aspect of thigh

Nerve may be compressed by the fetal head or by the stirrups because of improper positioning.
Source: From Ramanathan S. *Obstetric anesthesia.* Philadelphia: Lea & Febiger, 1988:102, with permission.

      i. More common in nulliparae with platypelloid pelves, large babies, cephalopelvic disproportion, vertex presentation, and forceps delivery

      ii. Can be unilateral (75%) or bilateral (25%)

      iii. May involve multiple root levels and appear as injuries to the femoral nerve or obturator nerve with sensory impairment in the fourth and fifth lumbar (L4 to L5) dermatomes. The superior gluteal nerve also may be affected.

b. Femoral nerve

      i. Injury decreases sensation over the anterior thigh and medial calf and impairs quadriceps strength, hip flexion, and patellar reflex (see Table 33.1).

      ii. Proximal lesions at the level of the lumbosacral plexus also may impair hip flexion because of iliopsoas weakness.

c. Obturator nerve

      i. It can be compressed against the lateral pelvic wall or in the obturator canal.

      ii. Injury produces decreased sensation over the medial thigh and weakness in hip adduction and internal rotation.

      iii. Electrophysiologic evaluation will differentiate obturator nerve injury from L3 toL4 radiculopathy and lumbar plexopathy.

d. Compression injuries: more common at sites peripheral to the sacrum. Most peripheral nerve injuries are due to positioning problems.

      i. Common peroneal nerve

        (1) Is among the most frequently injured.

        (2) Exits the popliteal fossa by winding around the fibular head before dividing into the deep and superficial branches.

        (3) May be compressed at the level of the neck of the fibula during the lithotomy position in stirrups or with the legs leaning against the bed rail.

        (4) Symptoms

          (a) Paresthesia over the lateral calf and dorsum of the foot

          (b) Foot drop and inversion (i.e., difficulty with dorsiflexion and eversion of the foot)

          (c) Sensory loss on the dorsal surface of the foot just proximal to the first and second toes

      ii. Femoral nerve

        (1) Also may be compressed at the level of the inguinal ligament during flexion of the hip during the second stage of labor

        (2) The use of a squatting bar to keep the hips hyperflexed during the second stage of labor has resulted in femoral nerve injury.

      iii. Lateral femoral cutaneous nerve
        (1) Arises from the lumbar plexus (L2 to L3) and provides sensation to the anterolateral thigh
        (2) The nerve enters the thigh by passing under the lateral inguinal ligament, where it may become compressed.
        (3) Injury produces paresthesia in the anterolateral thigh, also called meralgia paresthetica.
  e. Ischemic injury: also may produce neurologic deficits
      i. The spinal cord may become ischemic during periods of severe hypotension or by compression of its blood supply.
      ii. The lower spinal cord
        (1) About 85% of people have the majority of arterial blood supplied by the artery of Adamkiewicz, which arises from the lower thoracic or upper lumbar segment of the aorta (T9 to L2).
        (2) The other 15% have spinal cord blood supplied by a branch of the iliac arteries when the artery of Adamkiewicz originates high off the aorta (T5). These feeder vessels from the iliac artery may be compressed as they cross the lumbosacral trunk.
      iii. Neurologic deficit also may occur because of anterior spinal artery syndrome.
        (1) Loss of the anterior two-thirds of the spinal cord results in loss of motor function, pain, and temperature below the level of the lesion.
        (2) The dorsal column is supplied by vertebral arteries and carries vibration and joint sensation, which are spared.
        (3) Rarely, vasoconstriction of the anterior spinal artery may result in neurologic injury.
  f. Arteriovenous malformation (AVM) within the spinal cord can cause paraplegia.
      i. The spinal venous pressure may be increased, predisposing the spinal cord to decreased flow and stasis during periods of moderate hypotension or compression.
      ii. Dural AVMs most commonly are seen as pain (of the back, root, or remote) in 39%, leg weakness in 29%, or sensory symptoms in 24%. Progression of symptoms is usually slow, and spontaneous hemorrhage is less common than in spinal cord AVMs.

ANESTHESIA-RELATED NEUROLOGIC DEFICITS
Nerve Trauma
1. A very uncommon cause of neurologic damage
  a. Two-thirds of these neurologic complications are associated with either paresthesia (nerve trauma) or pain during injection (intraneuronal injection).

b. If the patient reports localized pain with insertion of an epidural or spinal needle or catheter, stop immediately!
   i. Differentiate benign pressure from a true paresthesia.
   ii. Transient paresthesia with threading of an epidural catheter is common and is probably related to the catheter-tip design and stiffness.
   iii. The combined spinal–epidural needle-through-needle technique also is associated with frequent transient paresthesae.
   iv. Stop advancing and withdraw immediately in the face of severe radicular pain with involuntary leg movement.
c. Direct trauma to nervous tissue may occur at the level of the spinal cord, nerve root, or peripheral nerve.
   i. Epidural needle insertion is most likely to stimulate a nerve root.
   ii. Spinal needles may touch nerve roots inside or outside of the thecal sac or directly injure the spinal cord.
   iii. Use caution at any level of insertion.

Equipment Problems

1. Epidural catheters usually slide out easily when pulled.
   a. If resistance is encountered on withdrawal, reposition the patient into the exact position used during insertion.
   b. If the catheter starts to stretch, be very cautious. Most catheters are fairly strong and will not break, even when mildly stretched.
   c. Leave recalcitrant catheters in place and wait a few hours. Spontaneous movement of the patient may loosen the catheter.
   d. If pain is encountered during epidural catheter withdrawal, stop immediately!
      i. The catheter may entrap a nerve root.
      ii. An imaging procedure may be necessary (MRI or CT after injecting a little contrast media into the epidural catheter).
      iii. If a knot in the catheter is found or if it is encircling a root, a radiologist may be able to untangle it under fluoroscopy.
2. If a catheter breaks or becomes sheared off (usually during placement), the patient must be informed.
   a. Epidural catheters meet the ANSI Z-29 implantation standards and are nonirritating.
   b. Attempting surgical removal of a catheter fragment will cause more trauma than leaving it in place.
   c. However, if neurologic symptoms are attributable to the catheter fragment (e.g., radicular pain), then surgical removal may become necessary.

Adverse Drug Effect

1. After reports of cauda equina syndrome, the Food and Drug Administration removed microspinal catheters (28- and 30-gauge) from commercial use in 1992.

   a. The small-diameter/high-resistance catheters required slow injection, allowing pooling of local anesthetic in the sacral area.
   b. When doses of 5% lidocaine exceeded 100 mg, localized high concentrations of lidocaine resulted in neurotoxicity and cauda equina syndrome.

Transient Neurologic Symptoms (TNS)
1. A syndrome of pain and dysesthesia in the buttocks, thighs, or calves that can follow spinal anesthesia and resolves within 72 hours
2. Mostly associated with 5% hyperbaric lidocaine
3. Factors associated with TNS include atraumatic small-bore needles with side hole directed caudad, lithotomy position, and high dose and concentration of lidocaine.
4. Hyperbaricity is not a causative factor.
5. Even 2% lidocaine can cause transient radicular pain.

Chemical Contamination
1. The epidural space is remarkably tolerant to chemical contamination.
   a. The epidural space is vascular and has a high degree of systemic absorption.
   b. The dura also serves as a protective barrier to the spinal cord.
2. Subarachnoid injection of chemical contaminants may produce neurotoxicity.

Accidental Intrathecal or Intravascular Injection
1. A drug administered by the wrong route may produce neurotoxicity.
2. Unrecognized intrathecal injection of most local anesthetics may produce excessive sensory and motor block, but prompt diagnosis and treatment should prevent adverse outcomes.
3. Neurologic deficit after accidental intrathecal injection of 2-chloroprocaine has been reported.
   a. The original formulation of epidural 2-chloroprocaine contained sodium bisulfite as an antioxidant. There were several reported cases of cauda equina syndrome when large doses of this formulation were injected into the subarachnoid space.
   b. The manufacturer (Astra Pharmaceuticals) reformulated the drug, decreasing the concentration of bisulfite, and eventually adding EDTA as a preservative. 2-Chloroprocaine containing sodium EDTA was associated with back pain.
   c. Formulations of 2-chloroprocaine without any preservative are now available (Nescaine-MPF).
4. Intravenous injection of local anesthetics can produce convulsions and possibly cardiac arrest.

EPIDURAL HEMATOMA
1. Epidural hematoma is a rare complication of central regional anesthesia, with an estimated frequency of 1 in 150,000 to 1 in 250,000.

2. Most epidural hematomas associated with regional anesthesia occur in patients with a hemostatic abnormality.
3. Epidural hematomas have been noted after both insertion and removal of the catheter in anticoagulated patients. Thus, epidural catheters should be inserted and removed only when the coagulation status is normal.
4. After reports of epidural and spinal hematomas after regional anesthesia in patients receiving low-molecular-weight heparin, the FDA released a public health advisory warning of this risk.[6]

Signs and Symptoms

1. Epidural hematoma is characterized by bilateral leg weakness, urinary incontinence, absent rectal sphincter tone, and decreased lower-extremity reflexes.
2. It may be preceded by sharp pain in the back and legs.
3. Symptoms progress over a few hours.
4. If a hematoma occurs during surgical anesthesia, the sensory level of anesthesia may decrease slightly or not at all. Continued motor paralysis should raise suspicions.
5. If suspected, immediate CT or MRI is indicated.
6. Surgical decompression should occur within 6 hours for the best chance of full neurologic recovery.

REFERENCES

1. Kovanen J, Sulkava R. Duration of postural headache after lumbar puncture: effect of needle size. *Headache* 1986;26:224.
2. Blanche R, Eisenach JC, Tuttle R, Dewan DM. Previous wet tap does not reduce success rate of labor epidural analgesia. *Anesth Analg* 1994;79:291.
3. Ambesh SP, Kumar A, Bajaj A. Epidural gelatin (Gelfoam) patch treatment for post dural puncture headache. *Anaesth Intensive Care* 1991;19:444.
4. Dirkes WE Jr. Treatment of nesacaine-MPF-induced back pain with calcium chloride [Letter; comment]. *Anesth Analg* 1990;70: 461.
5. Wong CA, Scavone BM, Dugan S, et al. The incidence of postpartum nerve injuries. *Anesthesiology* 1999;A8.
6. Lumpkin MM. Reports of epidural or spinal hematomas with the concurrent use of low molecular weight heparin and spinal/epidural anesthesia or spinal puncture. FDA Public Health Advisory 12. U.S. Department of Health and Human Resources.

Subject Index